Royal Liverpool University Hospital – Staff Library

Please return or renew, on or before the last date below.
Items may be renewed **twice**, if not reserved for another
user. Renewals may be made in person, by telephone:
0151 706 2248 or email: library.service@rlbuht.nhs.uk.
There is a charge of 10p per day for late items.

Grayson's

DISEASES
OF THE
CORNEA

Grayson's
DISEASES OF THE CORNEA

ROBERT C. ARFFA, M.D.

Adjunct Associate Professor of Ophthalmology
Medical College of Pennsylvania;
Clinical Assistant Professor of Ophthalmology
University of Pittsburgh School of Medicine and
The Eye and Ear Institute of Pittsburgh
Pittsburgh, Pennsylvania

THIRD EDITION

with 584 illustrations
including 210 in color

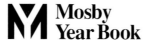

Mosby
Year Book

St. Louis   Baltimore   Boston   Chicago   London   Philadelphia   Sydney   Toronto

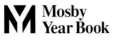

Mosby
Year Book
Dedicated to Publishing Excellence

Editor   Kimberly Kist
Assistant Editor   Penny Rudolph
Project Manager   Patricia Tannian
Production Editor   John Casey
Designer   David Zielinski

Third Edition

Mosby–Year Book, Inc.
11830 Westline Industrial Drive
St. Louis, Missouri 63146

Library of Congress Cataloging in Publication Data
Arffa, Robert C.
    Grayson's diseases of the cornea.—3rd ed. / Robert C. Arffa
       p.   cm.
    Rev. ed. of: Diseases of the cornea / Merrill Grayson. 2nd ed.
  1983.
    Includes bibliographical references and index.
    ISBN 0-8016-0262-9
    1. Cornea—Diseases. I. Grayson, Merrill. 1919- Diseases of
  the cornea. II. Title. III. Title: Diseases of the cornea.
       [DNLM: 1. Corneal Diseases   WW 220 A685g]
  RE336.G76   1991
  617.7'19—dc20
  DNLM/DLC   91-8794
  for Library of Congress   CIP

CL/WA/WA   9 8 7 6 5 4 3 2 1

To Sharon, Rachel, Lauren, and Matthew, without whose understanding and support this would not have been possible.

FOREWORD

Dr. Arffa has written a clear, concise, and readable text that residents and practitioners will find extremely helpful in their studies and practice. Dr. Arffa is an astute clinician, scholar, and stimulating teacher. In this third edition of *Diseases of the Cornea* he has updated therapy and expanded on the clinically relevant material. More photographs have been added, and more comprehensive tables are included, which will be appreciated by the readers.

All who found the original text helpful will be indebted to Dr. Arffa for this new, clearly written text. I certainly am very grateful to him for taking on this extensive task from which we all shall profit.

Merrill Grayson, M.D.
Distinguished Professor Emeritus
of Ophthalmology

PREFACE TO THE
THIRD EDITION

In preparing the third edition of *Diseases of the Cornea* I have tried to maintain the features that I believe have made Dr. Grayson's book so valuable and so popular: its readability, single authorship, clinical orientation, the quantity and quality of illustrations, and the use of tables. As before, it is oriented toward the resident and general practitioner; the most clinically relevant material on each subject is presented. Corneal diseases and corneal manifestations of systemic diseases remain emphasized, but the section on conjunctivitis has been expanded. Coverage of laboratory testing, parasitic keratitis, scleritis, and epithelial healing diseases has been increased. More specific information is given about the treatment of corneal diseases, including indications and results of surgery, but not surgical technique.

I would like to acknowledge some who have assisted me in the preparation of this book. The photography department at the Eye and Ear Institute of Pittsburgh provided most of the photographs added to this edition. Many ophthalmologists obtained the photographs and generously agreed to their use in this text. Diane Curtin took many of the photographs and helped in ferreting them out from the department archives and in selecting and producing them. Jon Coulter has prepared several new illustrations for this edition. Dr. Bruce Johnson supplied many new pathology micrographs.

Dr. Fred M. Wilson II, Dr. Grayson's colleague at Indiana University for many years, has contributed a chapter on the toxicity of topically applied medications.

I would like to thank several colleagues who reviewed chapters for me and made many helpful suggestions: Stuart Fourman, Jerold Gordon, Bruce Johnson, and Lee Wiley.

I also would like to acknowledge and thank the people who taught me cornea (in chronologic order): David Miller, Merrill Grayson, Fred Wilson II, Herbert Kaufman, Richard Thoft, Jerold Gordon, Mel Roat, and the fellows and residents at the Eye and Ear Institute of Pittsburgh.

Robert C. Arffa

Preface to the
First Edition

Resident teaching has always been one of the major aims of my academic career. My desire has been to contribute to this dream by preparing and organizing the material of my major interest in ophthalmology so that it can more easily be assimilated by the student. I hope I have done this with *Diseases of the Cornea*.

Because of the close relationship between the conjunctiva and cornea, some diseases affecting both are discussed in the text. Primary corneal diseases and corneal manifestations of systemic diseases are stressed. Throughout the text, tables provide convenient and rapid association for study. *Diseases of the Cornea* is not to be considered an encyclopedia of corneal disease but a thorough aid to help one correlate and organize the large amount of material concerned. Discussion of therapy is included where it is considered necessary and helpful.

Many colleagues in the field have generously given permission to use their illustrations. Dr. Fred M. Wilson II and I took the color photographs of patients who attended the Cornea Service of the Department of Ophthalmology at Indiana University Medical Center. Kenneth Julian and Gene Louden are to be thanked for their generous aid in preparing many of the illustrations.

I greatly appreciate the work of my associate, Dr. Fred M. Wilson II, whose time, help, suggestions regarding the text, and close association in clinical consultation with numerous problems noted in this book were invaluable.

Merrill Grayson

CONTENTS

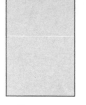

ANATOMY

CONJUNCTIVA

GROSS ANATOMY

The conjunctiva is a mucous membrane that covers the inner surface of the lids and the outer surface of the globe. It allows independent movement of the lids and the globe, provides mucus for lubrication, and contains lymphoid tissue for immunologic protection. The conjunctival epithelium is derived from surface ectoderm.

The conjunctiva begins at the mucocutaneous junction on the lid margin, posterior to the orifices of the meibomian glands. It is firmly adherent to the lids over the tarsi and loosely attached in the fornices and over the globe, except at the limbus. Approximately 2 mm from the tarsal margin is a shallow groove, the subtarsal groove, which marks the transition from the nonkeratinized, stratified squamous epithelium of the lid margin to cuboidal epithelium.

In the primary position the distance between the limbus and fornix is approximately 10 mm, both superiorly and inferiorly (Figs. 1-1 and 1-2). The fornices are maintained by muscular fibers from the

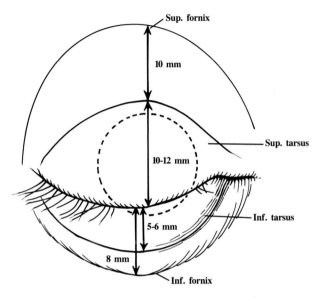

Fig. 1-1. Frontal view of lids and conjunctiva.

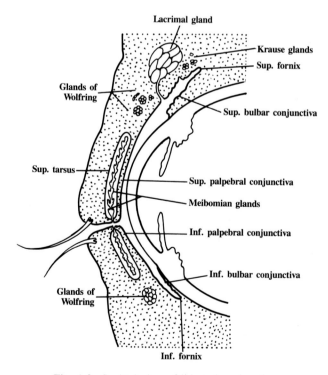

Fig. 1-2. Sagittal view of lids and conjunctiva.

levator palpebra superioris and inferior rectus, respectively. The total surface area of the conjunctiva averages 16 cm^2/eye.

Two specialized conjunctival structures are present medially, the plica semilunaris and the caruncle. The plica semilunaris is a fold of conjunctiva that extends from the superior to inferior fornices. It serves as a source of additional conjunctiva to permit lateral rotation of the globe. The caruncle, which lies medial to the plica, measures approximately 4 × 5 mm. It is essentially modified skin tissue, and like skin contains hairs, sebaceous glands, and sweat glands. Unlike skin, it also contains lacrimal tissue (Krause glands), and the surface epithelium is not keratinized.

MICROSCOPIC ANATOMY

Like all mucous membranes, the conjunctiva has an epithelial layer and a submucosal lamina propria. The structure of the epithelial layer varies greatly in different regions. Stratified squamous epithelium is present on the lid margin, over the most peripheral 2 to 3 mm of the tarsi, and for 2 to 3 mm surrounding the limbus. The remainder of the tarsal conjunctiva and the forniceal conjunctiva has from two to five epithelial cell layers, with cuboidal basal cells, cylindric superficial cells, and up to three layers of polyhedral cells between them (Fig. 1-3). The number of cell layers gradually increases over the bulbar conjunctiva, with the superficial cells becoming flatter and the basal cells taller, and increasing the number of polyhedral layers.

Goblet cells, mucus-secreting apocrine cells, occur in all regions of the conjunctiva. They are most numerous over the tarsi and on the plica and least numerous in the interpalpebral bulbar conjunctiva. Goblet cells are oval or round, with a flattened nucleus near the base of the cell and a large intracellular collection of mucin (Fig. 1-3). The number of goblet cells can increase in some conjunctival inflammations and decrease in destructive conjunctival processes, such as Stevens-Johnson syndrome or cicatricial pemphigoid.[1]

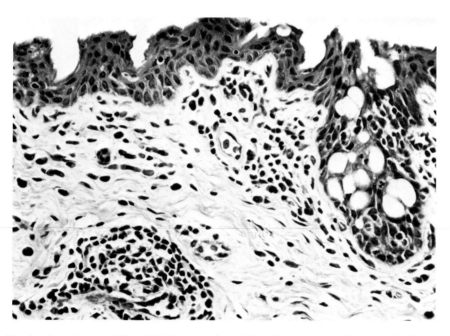

Fig. 1-3. Forniceal conjunctiva. The epithelium contains goblet cells, and nests of lymphoid cells are present in the substantia propria. (Hematoxylin-eosin stain; ×500.) (Courtesy Bruce L. Johnson, Pittsburgh.)

The surfaces of the conjunctival epithelial cells are covered with microvilli and microplicae, as well as a thin glycocalyx and mucin coating.[2] This coating increases the surface area and aids in attachment of the tear film. The basal epithelial cells are attached to a typical basement membrane by hemidesmosomes. Melanocytes may be found among the basal epithelium.

The conjunctival stroma consists of two layers, a superficial lymphoid layer and a deeper fibrous layer. The lymphoid layer is made up of a connective tissue matrix containing a homogeneous-appearing population of lymphocytes (Fig. 1-3). Normally no germinal follicles are present. The lymphoid layer is not present at birth, but begins to form at 6 to 12 weeks of age. Deep to this layer is a fibrous tissue layer, through which runs the conjunctival vessels and nerves. Of variable thickness, this layer is very limited over the tarsus.

Over the globe, a layer of loose areolar tissue separates the conjunctiva from Tenon's layer, also called the episclera. Tenon's layer contains branches of the anterior ciliary arteries, which have passed forward from the insertions of the extraocular muscles. Approximately 3 to 4 mm from the limbus, Tenon's layer and conjunctiva merge. The conjunctiva and its vessels can normally be moved freely over Tenon's layer and its vessels.

Two types of accessory lacrimal glands are present in the conjunctiva: Krause glands, and the glands of Wolfring. Their structures are similar to that of the lacrimal gland. The glands of Krause are located in the upper fornix and in the caruncle, in the submucosal connective tissue. The glands of Wolfring are located in the tarsi, at the upper border of the upper tarsus and the lower border of the lower tarsus (Fig. 1-4).

Vascular Supply and Lymphatic Drainage

The conjunctiva receives its blood supply from the muscular, medial palpebral and lacrimal branches of the ophthalmic artery. The medial palpebral and lacrimal branches form the peripheral, or marginal, arcades of the lids, located between the tarsus and the orbicularis (Fig. 1-5). Branches from these arcades pass through the tarsi to the conjunctiva, at about the level of the subtarsal groove.

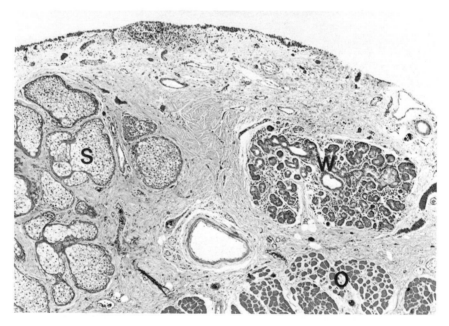

Fig. 1-4. Accessory lacrimal gland of Wolfring *(W)*. Tarsus and sebaceous glands *(S)* and orbicularis muscle *(O)* are also seen. (Hematoxylin-eosin stain; ×80.) (Courtesy Bruce L. Johnson, Pittsburgh.)

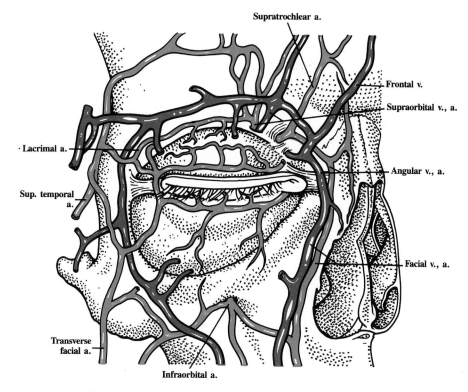

Fig. 1-5. Vascular supply of lids and conjunctiva, frontal view.

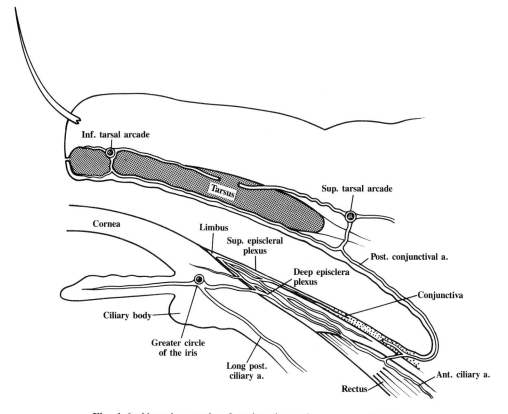

Fig. 1-6. Vascular supply of conjunctiva and cornea, sagittal view.

They supply the entire conjunctiva except for the area lying within 3 to 4 mm of the limbus. In this area there is anastomosis of the conjunctival vessels with the branches of the anterior ciliary arteries in Tenon's layer (Fig. 1-6). The branches from the anterior ciliary artery appear darker than the superficial vessels and do not move with the conjunctiva.

The conjunctival capillaries are fenestrated, similar in structure to those found in the choroid. Under conditions of inflammation, the leakage through these fenestrations can exceed the rate by which the fluid can pass through the conjunctiva to the surface, resulting in chemosis.

Normally, no lymphatics are present in the cornea; however, the conjunctiva has a rich lymphatic network. The lymphatics arise approximately 1 mm from the limbus. Lymphatics in the lateral portions of the conjunctiva drain to the preauricular and intraparotid nodes, and in the medial portions they drain to the submandibular nodes.

INNERVATION

Sensory innervation of the conjunctiva is supplied by the ophthalmic division of the fifth cranial nerve. In general, the nerve supply of the conjunctiva is from the same source as that of the lid, except that the long ciliary nerves innervate the limbal conjunctiva. The only sensory modality perceived is pain, except for some pressure sensation in the marginal tarsal conjunctiva and the caruncle. Autonomic fibers are also present and are associated with blood vessels.

TABLE 1-1. Precorneal Tear Film

LAYER AND SOURCE	LOCATION	FUNCTION
INNERMOST: MUCIN (0.2-0.5 μm)		
Conjunctival goblet cells	Most numerous over tarsi and on plica	Reduces surface tension between the epithelial surface and the tear film to enhance spreading of tear film
		Lubricates the ocular surface; coats and traps debris
MIDDLE: AQUEOUS (6.5 μm)		Source of water, glucose, immunoglobulins, and antimicrobial enzymes
Lacrimal gland	Lacrimal fossa, superior temporal orbit; orbital and palpebral lobes; ducts enter cul-de-sac in superior temporal area	Lacrimal gland is source of reflex section
Accessory lacrimal glands of Krause	Upper conjunctival fornix and caruncle	Accessory glands are primary basal secretors
Accessory lacrimal glands of Wolfring	Adjacent to upper margin of upper tarsus and lower margin of lower tarsus	
SUPERFICIAL LAYER: LIPID (0.5 μm)		
Meibomian glands	About 25 in upper tarsus, 20 in lower tarsus; empty onto lid margin	Retards evaporation of aqueous layer
Gland of Zeis	Palpebral margin of each eyelid; empty directly onto lid margin	
Glands of Moll	Roots of eyelashes; empty into hair follicles	

Modified from Grayson M and Keates RH: Manual of diseases of the cornea, Boston, 1969, Little, Brown & Co, Inc.

TEAR FILM

The integrity of the cornea depends on the presence of a precorneal tear film. This layer lubricates and wets the surface of the cornea, is necessary for the health of the epithelial cells, and provides a smooth optical surface for good visual acuity.

The tear film, approximately 7 μm thick, is thickest immediately after a blink and thins progressively until the next blink, or until the tear film breaks up. It consists of three layers (Table 1-1). The outermost layer, the lipid layer, is approximately 0.5 μm thick and contains low polarity lipids such as waxy and cholesterol esters.[3] Derived from the secretions of the meibomian glands, the lipid layer's primary function is to retard evaporation.

The middle layer, approximately 6.5 μm thick, consists of aqueous tear fluid and contains ions of inorganic salt, glucose, urea, and various proteins, including enzymes, immunoglobulins, complement, and albumin.[4] It is secreted by the main and accessory lacrimal glands. Numerous cells are present in the aqueous tears, derived from the corneal and conjunctival epithelium, the conjunctival lymphoid tissue, and the conjunctival vessels. Lymphocytes are most numerous, followed by desquamated epithelial cells and polymorphonuclear leukocytes.[5]

The third layer of the tear film is a mucin layer, which is 0.2 to 0.5 μm thick, and coats the epithelial cell surfaces. It is derived from the conjunctival goblet cells. The mucin reduces the surface tension between the epithelial surface and the tear film, enhancing spread of the tear film. Mucus in the tear film also lubricates the ocular surface, reducing friction during lid or eye movement, and coating and trapping debris.

CORNEA

GROSS ANATOMY

The cornea is the transparent, anterior portion of the outer shell of the eye, corresponding to a watch crystal. It is spheric but appears slightly elliptic anteriorly because the limbus is more prominent vertically. The cornea anteriorly measures about 12.5 × 11.5 mm (Fig. 1-7). The cornea is thin-

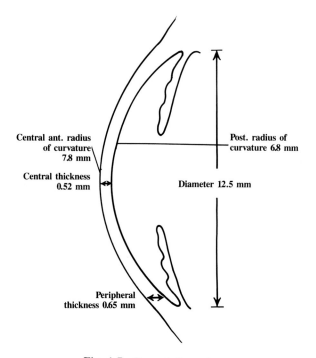

Fig. 1-7. Corneal dimensions.

nest centrally, averaging about 0.52 mm, whereas the periphery is approximately 0.65 mm thick. The central one third of the cornea, called the optical zone, is almost spheric, with an average radius of curvature of 7.8 mm. The peripheral cornea is less curved, but variably so. The posterior corneal surface is nearly spheric, and its radius of curvature has been estimated to be approximately 6.8 mm.[6] Using these numbers, the refractive power of the anterior surface of the cornea is +48.8 diopters (D) and the posterior surface is −5.8 D. The net refractive power of the cornea, therefore, is 43 D, or 70% of the total refractive power of the eye.

In the newborn the cornea is relatively large, averaging 10 mm vertically. Its curvature is also steeper, approximately 51 D at term birth.[7] In premature infants the cornea is smaller in diameter and steeper in curvature: At 34 weeks the corneal diameter averages 8.2 mm,[8] and corneal curvature averages 52 to 53 D. The cornea continues to grows in diameter and flatten with age, reaching close to adult measurements after the first year.[8,9]

MICROSCOPIC ANATOMY

The cornea consists of five layers: epithelium, Bowman's layer, stroma, Descemet's membrane, and endothelium (Fig. 1-8). In the normal state it does not contain blood or lymphatic vessels.

Epithelium. The corneal epithelium is a stratified squamous, nonkeratinizing epithelium. Approximately five cells deep, it is composed of three types of cells: columnar basal, polygonal wing, and flat superficial cells. The superficial cells lie in two layers. On scanning electron microscopy, flat and mostly hexagonal epithelial cells are seen, attached to each other by straight cell boundaries.[10-12] They exhibit numerous microprojections (microvilli and microplicae) and have an extensive fibrillar glycocalyx, or buffy coat, on their surface membrane (Figs. 1-9 and 1-10). The microprojections enhance the adherence of the tear film to the glycocalyx. Tight junctions are present around the entire lateral borders of each cell, serving as an anatomic barrier to passage of substances into the intercellular space.

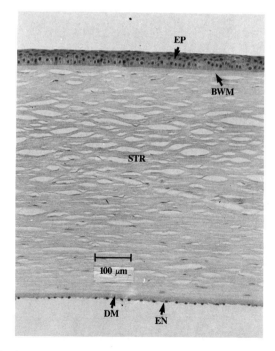

Fig. 1-8. Photomicrograph of a cross section of human cornea showing stratified squamous epithelium *(EP)*, Bowman's layer *(BWM)*, stroma *(STR)*, Descemet's membrane *(DM)*, and endothelium *(EN)*. (Courtesy Nirmala Sundar-Raj, Pittsburgh.)

The wing cell layer is three cells deep; the more superficial the cell, the flatter its appearance. The nuclei of the wing cells lie parallel to the surface. There is extensive interdigitation of the wing cells, with numerous desmosomal attachments. Mats of tonofilaments are present, which maintain cell shape.

The deeply situated basal cells compose the single layer of columnar cells that rest on the basement membrane. These cells are rounded on their anterior surface with oval nuclei arranged perpendicularly to the surface (Fig. 1-11). These cells are mitotically active, and the daughter cells produced move anteriorly to become wing cells. The basal cells also contain arrays of tonofilaments to maintain cell shape. Actin filaments are present and may play a role in cell migration, such as occurs during wound healing.[13] Unlike basal conjunctival cells, the basal surface of the cells is flat, which is

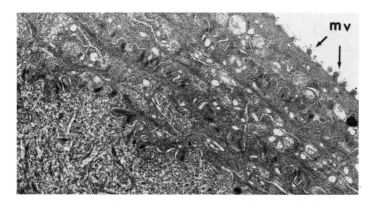

Fig. 1-9. Superficial cells are flat, with microvilli *(mv)* on their surface. (From McTigue JW et al: Clinical application of electron microscopy of the cornea: a course, Chicago, 1968, American Academy of Ophthalmology and Otolaryngology.)

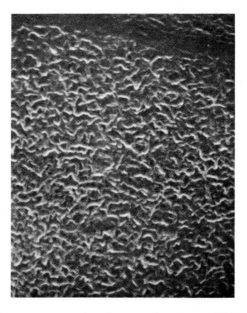

Fig. 1-10. Superficial cell of cornea on scanning electron microscopy exhibits reticulated appearance. (From Kuwabara T: Fine structure of the eye, ed 2, Howe Laboratory of Ophthalmology, Boston, 1970, Harvard Medical School.)

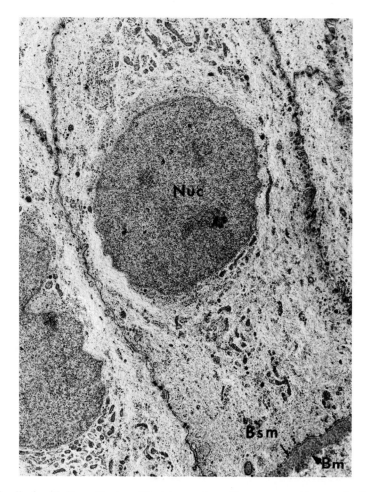

Fig. 1-11. Basal cell of epithelium. Nucleus *(Nuc)* is round, and basement membrane of cell *(Bsm)* borders on Bowman's layer *(Bm)*. (From McTigue JW et al: Clinical application of electron microscopy of the cornea: a course, Chicago, 1968, American Academy of Ophthalmology and Otolaryngology.)

thought to facilitate their adherence. Hemidesmosomes along the basal surface of these cells attach them to the basal lamina.

Other types of cells may be found among the basal epithelial cells. Slender cells with electron-dense cytoplasm and rich rough endoplasmic reticulum are occasionally seen and may be recently divided cells. Lymphocytes and small cells with dark nuclei and multiple dendritic processes are also found. Peripherally, Langerhans cells, antigen-presenting immune cells, are present.

The epithelial cells of the cornea are interdigitated and firmly attached to each other by many desmosomes. These junctions provide mechanical stability to the epithelial layer. Gap junctions are present between all adjacent cells in the epithelium. These serve as conduits through which small molecules may pass from one cell to another.

The cytoplasm of the epithelial cell exhibits a dense matrix containing many fine keratofibrils. The microorganelles generally are sparse but are more evident in basal cells than in wing or superficial cells. Mitochondria are small and not very abundant. The Golgi apparatus and rough endoplasmic reticulum (Fig. 1-12) are relatively small.

Glycogen particles are seen in the epithelial cells, particularly in basal cells (Fig. 1-12, *B*). The

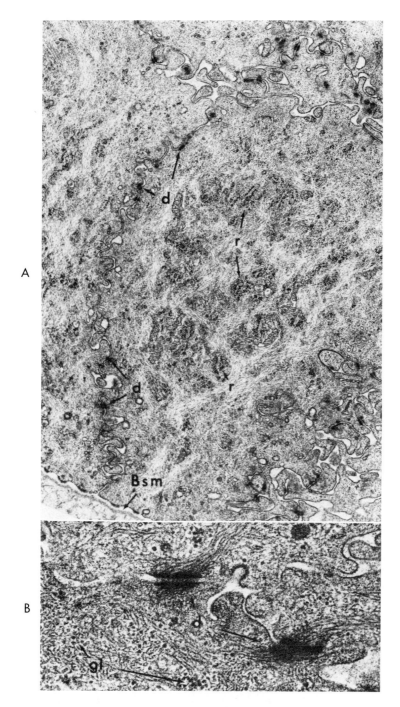

Fig. 1-12. A, Cytoplasm of corneal epithelium contains endoplasmic reticulum *(r),* glycogen, and keratofibrils. Few mitochondria are seen. Cell membranes are joined by conspicuous desmosomes *(d).* Basal lamina of epithelial cell is noted *(Bsm).* **B,** Higher magnification of desmosomal attachments *(d),* glycogen *(gl),* and keratofibrils. (From McTigue JW et al: Clinical application of electron microscopy of the cornea: a course, Chicago, 1968, American Academy of Ophthalmology and Otolaryngology.)

amount present varies in different pathologic conditions; in disease, epithelial glycogen stores may be markedly depleted, and the glycogen particles may disappear from epithelial cells during acute wound healing.[14,15]

Unmyelinated nerve fibers are frequently present in the epithelium. The fibers are usually found among the basal cells, but are rare among the wing cells. The nerve ends without forming a specific end organ, as these would reduce corneal transparency.

Beneath the basal layer of epithelial cells, and produced by these cells, is a basal lamina, or basement membrane. It is approximately 500 Å thick, and by electron microscopy is composed of an anterior clear zone, the lamina lucida, and a posterior dark zone, the lamina densa (Fig. 1-13). Biochemically, it appears to be similar to skin basal lamina, containing type IV collagen,[16] laminin,[16,17] fibronectin, fibrin, and bullous pemphigoid antigen.[18,19] Basement membrane, together with its hemidesmosomes and anchoring fibrils, participates in the adherence of the epithelial cells to the

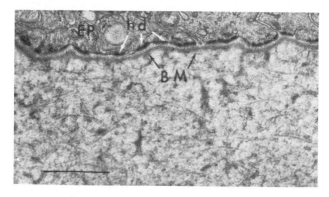

Fig. 1-13. Basement membrane *(BM)* is made up of fine granular material and is composed of two layers: lamina lucida and lamina densa. Hemidesmosomes *(hd)* are noted. Basal epithelial cell is also seen *(EP)*. (From Kuwabara T: Fine structure of the eye, ed 2, Howe Laboratory of Ophthalmology, Boston, 1970, Harvard Medical School.)

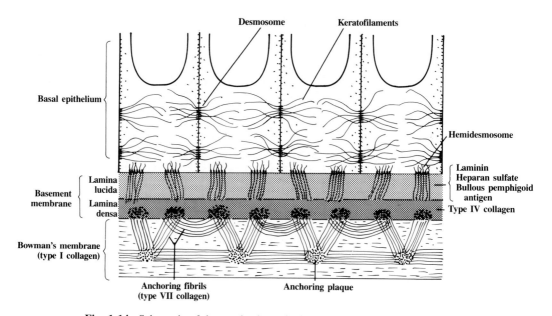

Fig. 1-14. Schematic of the mechanism of adherence of the corneal epithelium.

stroma (Fig. 1-14). Hemidesmosomes attach the basal epithelial cells to the basal lamina and to anchoring fibrils. Anchoring fibrils, composed of collagen type VII, extend from the basal lamina into the superficial stroma, and end in localized plaques, composed of type IV and type VII collagen.[20]

Bowman's layer. Bowman's layer is an acellular zone, 8 to 10 μm thick, beneath the epithelium. The anterior margin is limited anteriorly by the basement membrane of the epithelium, and the posterior border merges into the anterior stromal collagen fibers. Under the light microscope, Bowman's layer appears homogeneous, but by electron microscopy Bowman's layer is seen to consist of randomly arranged, short collagen fibrils (Fig. 1-15). The collagen fibrils are smaller in diameter, approximately two thirds that of stromal fibrils. In the deeper portions, these fibrils increase in diameter and length and gradually transform into the regular stroma.

Bowman's layer is often said to be resistant to trauma, offering a barrier to corneal invasion by microorganisms and tumor cells, but it is not known whether this is true. On the other hand, Bowman's layer is considered to have no regenerative capacity when damaged. A thin layer, with a fine structure identical to that of Bowman's layer, is formed during wound healing; however, this secondary type of layer does not regain its original thickness.

Stroma. The stroma, which constitutes about 90% of the cornea, consists primarily of collagen fibers, stromal cells, and ground substance. It is approximately 78% water. The collagen fibrils account for about 80% of the dry weight of the cornea, the ground substance for about 15%, and cellular elements for only about 5%. It is well known that the collagen fibrils are arranged into 200 to 300 lamellae parallel to the tear surface (Fig. 1-16, *A*). Interlacing lamellae cross each other in a highly regular fashion, at less than 90 degrees in the anterior stroma, and at nearly right angles in the posterior stroma. The lamellae run parallel to each other and to the surface of the cornea, each running the full length of the cornea. Therefore a cross section of the stroma will show some fibrils running nearly parallel to the section, and some running nearly perpendicular (Fig. 1-16, *A*). The layered arrangement of the fibrils facilitates lamellar dissection of the cornea.

The collagen fibrils of the corneal stroma are uniform and small, about 250 to 300 Å in diameter. The fibrils show bandings very similar to those of other collagen fibrils. Cross section reveals that the

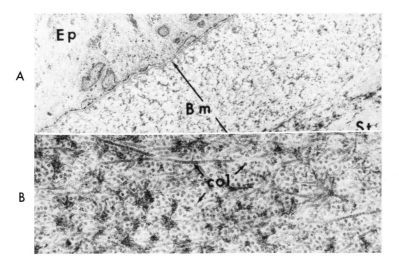

Fig. 1-15. A, Bowman's layer *(Bm)* is noncellular layer seen beneath the epithelium *(Ep)*. **B,** Short and fine collagen fibril material *(col)* intermingling in Bowman's layer. (From McTigue JW et al: Clinical application of electron microscopy of the cornea: a course, Chicago, 1968, American Academy of Ophthalmology and Otolaryngology.)

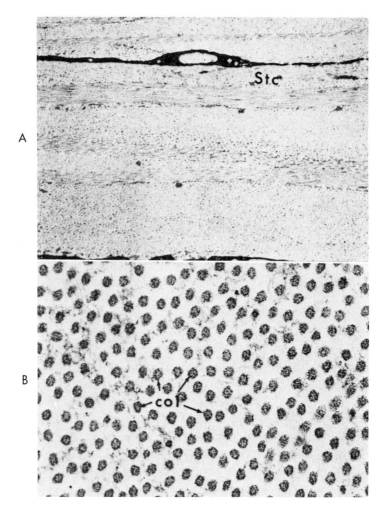

Fig. 1-16. A, Corneal stroma consists of regular arrangement of collagen fibrils parallel to cell surface. **B,** Regularity of 300 Å diameter collagen fiber *(col)* is noted. *Stc,* Stromal cells. (From McTigue JW et al: Clinical application of electron microscopy of the cornea: a course, Chicago, 1968, American Academy of Ophthalmology and Otolaryngology.)

individual fibril is made up of several subunits of extremely fine fibrils (Fig. 1-16, *B*). Type I collagen is the predominant collagen found in the cornea, although types III and V may also be present.[21]

The ground substance surrounding the collagen fibrils is rich in glycosaminoglycans (GAGs). Keratan sulfate and chondroitin sulfate are the primary GAGs of the stroma, in approximately a 3:1 ratio.[22] The ground substance may play a role in maintaining the regular array of collagen fibrils. With stromal edema the individual collagen fibril size does not change, the volume of the ground substance increases, and the space between collagen fibrils increases.

The keratocyte is the predominant cell of the stroma. It is a large flat cell with a number of large processes that extend out from the cell body in a stellate fashion. The cell bodies are seen between packed collagen lamellae, and their processes usually extend within or between the same lamellar plane. Occasionally the tips of the processes touch neighboring cells. Their cytoplasm contains microorganelles, microtubules, some lysosomes, glycogen particles, lipid particles, and various inclusion bodies (Fig. 1-17). The keratocyte is probably derived from neural crest and maintains the col-

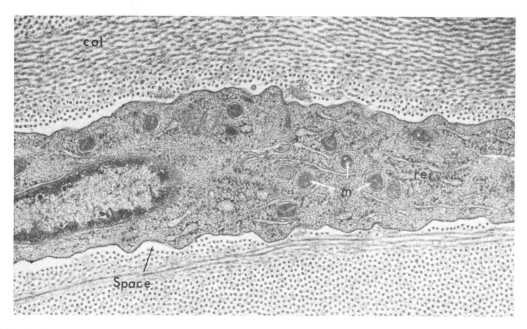

Fig. 1-17. Keratocyte is rich in rough endoplasmic reticulum *(rer)* and mitochondria *(m)*. Small space is seen around keratocyte as it borders stromal collagen *(col)*. (From Kuwabara T: Fine structure of the eye, ed 2, Howe Laboratory of Ophthalmology, Boston, 1970, Harvard Medical School.)

lagen and extracellular matrix of the stroma. Small fibrillar bundles of recently synthesized collagen can be observed adjacent to keratocytes.[23]

In response to stromal injury the keratocytes migrate into the wound area and undergo transformation into fibroblasts. These transformed cells have increased rough endoplasmic reticula and Golgi complexes and reduced cytoplasmic processes. They contribute to the scar formation by proliferation and collagen production.[15] The keratocyte can produce abundant basal lamina in endothelial dystrophy,[23] and in other pathologic conditions, inclusions, such as lipid droplets, can be present. The keratocytes accumulate metabolic products in many conditions, such as cystinosis, multiple myeloma, and lysosomal storage diseases, such as the mucopolysaccharidoses and sphingolipidoses.

In addition to keratocytes, small numbers of polymorphonuclear leukocytes, plasma cells, and macrophages are seen in the normal stroma, located between the lamellae of the collagen fibers.

Descemet's membrane. Descemet's membrane is approximately 10 μm thick in adults, and is a thick basal lamina produced by the endothelium (Fig. 1-18). *Schwalbe's ring* marks the termination of Descemet's membrane peripherally. On electron microscopy Descemet's membrane is seen to be composed of anterior banded and posterior homogeneous zones. The anterior zone is produced in utero, beginning at approximately 4 months of gestation. The posterior portion is produced after birth, and progressively thickens with age. It contains type IV collagen and fibronectin.[24] Peripherally, localized thickenings of Descemet's membrane, called *Hassall-Henle* bodies, are present in the normal eye.

In contrast to Bowman's layer, Descemet's membrane is easily detached from the stroma and after injury regenerates readily. In some pathologic conditions, metallic substances are deposited in Descemet's membrane, for example, copper in Wilson's disease and silver in argyrosis (see Fig. 27-5). The endothelial cell, when stimulated by inflammation, trauma, or genetic disturbances, can produce excess abnormal basal lamina[25] (which also contains type I collagen[26,27]), causing a thickening of Descemet's membrane and Descemet's wart formation. Thus the multiple layers of Descemet's membrane can provide a morphologic record of previous episodes of disease.

Endothelium. A single layer of flat hexagonal cells lies posteriorly on Descemet's membrane. On scanning electron microscopy, one may see the normal flat surface cells with sharply demarcated borders (Fig. 1-19). The endothelial cells, more cuboidal in shape and about 10 μm in height at birth, flatten with age to about 4 μm in adults. The endothelium is probably derived from neural crest. The cell density decreases from approximately 3500 to 4000 cells/mm^2 at birth to 2500 to 3000 cells/mm^2 in the adult cornea, for a total of about 400,000 cells.

Generally there is no mitotic activity in the endothelium after birth. Some endothelial cells die throughout life, resulting in a gradual decrease of the endothelial cell population with age. As cell loss occurs, with aging or trauma, the neighboring cells spread out to cover the vacant area. This results in an increase in cell area and a decrease in cell density. The endothelial cells are capable of preserving function in spite of tremendous enlargement, and generally can maintain corneal function down to cell densities as low as 300 to 600 cells/mm^2.

These cells exhibit great metabolic activity, as indicated by the presence of numerous large mitochondria, smooth and rough endoplasmic reticula, a well-developed Golgi apparatus, and free ribosomes (Fig. 1-20). One may occasionally see a microvillus (Fig. 1-21), but usually the presence of

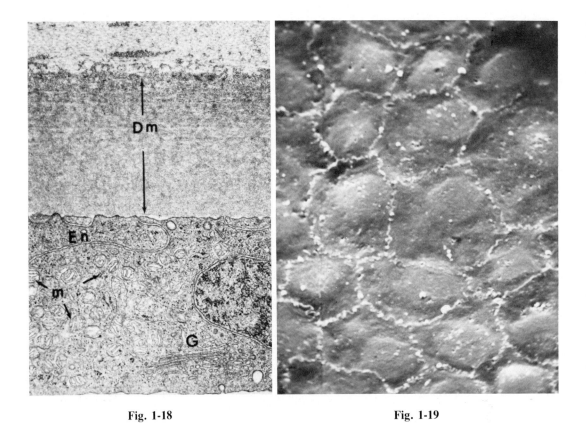

Fig. 1-18   **Fig. 1-19**

Fig. 1-18. Descemet's membrane *(Dm)* is basement membrane of endothelial cells *(En)*. It is rich in Golgi apparatus *(G)* and mitochondria *(m)*. (From McTigue JW et al: Clinical application of electron microscopy of the cornea: a course, Chicago, 1968, American Academy of Ophthalmology and Otolaryngology.)

Fig. 1-19. Normal orderly arrangement of endothelium with clear-cut cell borders. (From Grayson M: Trans Am Ophthalmol Soc 72:517, 1974.)

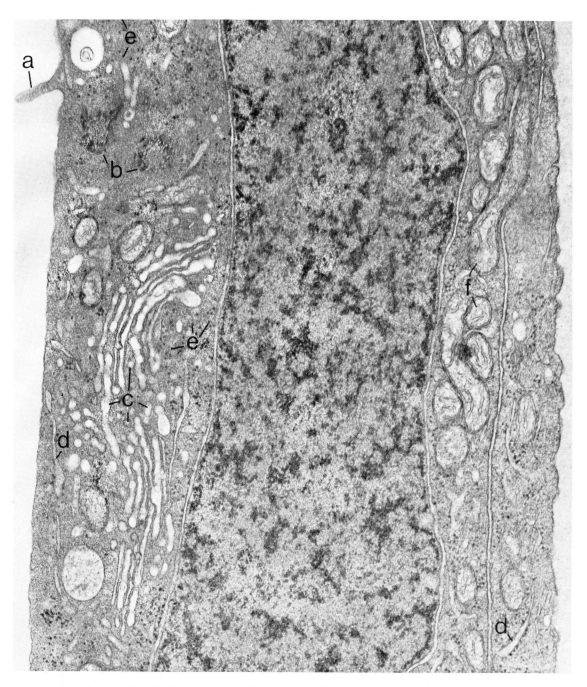

Fig. 1-20. Well-developed Golgi system, abundant mitochondria, and smooth and rough endoplasmic reticulum. *a,* Microvillus; *b,* cisternae; *c,* Golgi system; *d,* endoplasmic reticulum; *e,* ribosomes; *f,* mitochondria. (From Hogan MJ, Alvarado JA, and Weddell JE: Histology of the human eye, Philadelphia, 1971, WB Saunders Co.)

Fig. 1-21. Microvilli *(large arrow)* are sparse in normal endothelium. Endothelial cells are joined by zonular occludens *(small arrow)*.

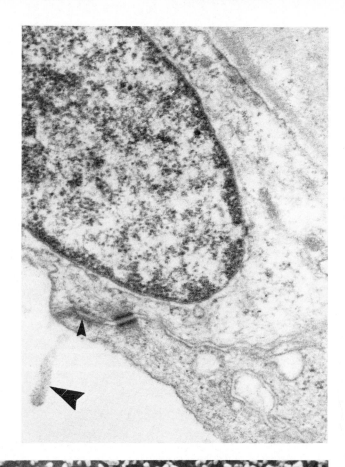

Fig. 1-22. Microvilli noted on endothelial cells in pathologic states. (From Grayson M: Trans Am Ophthalmol Soc 72:517,1974.)

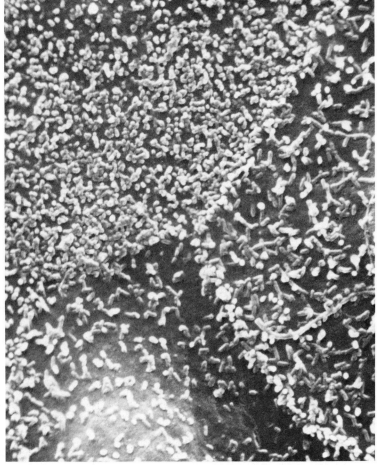

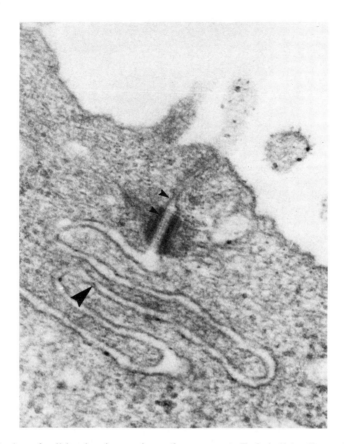

Fig. 1-23. Interdigitation of cell borders is prominent *(large arrow)*. Endothelial cells are joined by zonula occludens *(small arrows)*.

microvilli denotes some pathologic state (Fig. 1-22). A central cilium is present in many endothelial cells; its function is unclear. There is elaborate interdigitation of the lateral walls of adjacent cells (Fig 1-23), and multiple junctional complexes, including zonulae occludentes (Fig. 1-21), maculae occludentes, and desmosomes, are present. There is some resistance to intercellular passage of substances, created by both the elaborate interdigitation of the cell borders, increasing the distance substances must travel, and localized occlusive cell junctions, but even large molecules may penetrate.[28]

The endothelial cell can show great change in response to pathologic stimulation. Even minor corneal injury can elicit a response: The endothelial cells posterior to a corneal epithelial wound may become swollen and develop numerous protrusions immediately after injury. After endothelial trauma damaged endothelial cells slide over the injured area, acting as a reparative element, elaborating new Descemet's membrane where it is absent. In Fuchs' dystrophy the cell appears to have "collapsed," the border is irregular, and the nucleus stands out as a white, raised fluffy structure (Fig. 1-24). Where there is extreme stress, the endothelial cells may undergo transformation into fibroblast-like cells, and elaborate an abnormal posterior collagenous layer (Fig. 1-25).[25]

INNERVATION

Sensory innervation of the cornea is supplied by the first division of the trigeminal nerve by way of the long ciliary and possibly short ciliary branches of the nasociliary nerve (Fig. 1-26). The long

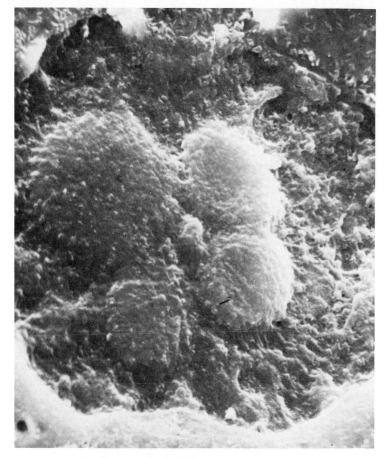

Fig. 1-24. Disorderly arrangement of endothelial cells in Fuchs' dystrophy with irregular cell borders. Note "collapse" of cell and irregular fluffy cell nucleus. (From Grayson M: Trans Am Ophthalmol Soc 72:517, 1974.)

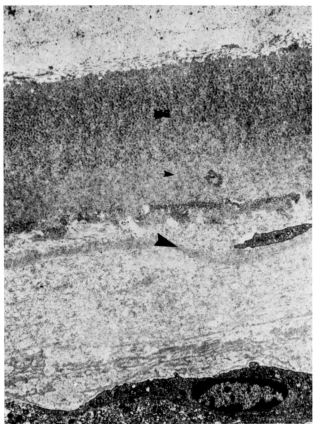

Fig. 1-25. Descemet's membrane consists of anterior banded layer *(medium arrow)* and nonbanded area *(small arrow)*. Multilaminar basement membrane is laid down by altered endothelial cells *(large arrow)*.

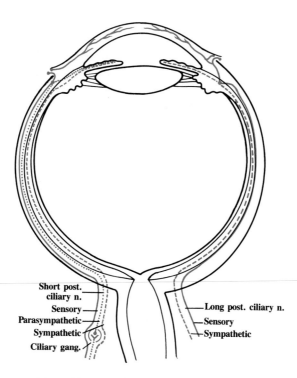

Short post. ciliary n.
Sensory
Parasympathetic
Sympathetic
Ciliary gang.

Long post. ciliary n.
Sensory
Sympathetic

Fig. 1-26. Corneal and conjunctival innervation.

ciliary nerves enter the eye near the optic nerve and pass anteriorly in the suprachoroidal space. They branch several times before reaching the limbus and may anastomose with branches from the short ciliary nerves, which enter the sclera a few millimeters posterior to the limbus. Recurrent branches pass out through the sclera to innervate the limbal conjunctiva and limbal corneal epithelium. About 70 nerve trunks pierce the cornea at the middle one third of its thickness. The nerves lose their myelin sheath after traversing 0.5 to 2.0 mm into the cornea and then continue as transparent axon cylinders. The nerves find their way to beneath Bowman's layer where they form a dense subepithelial plexus. They then pierce Bowman's layer to terminate among the epithelial cells, as simple axon terminals without specialized sensory organs. Some nerve trunks proceed into the deep stroma, dividing in a manner similar to that of the superficial fibers, and ending among the stromal cells.

Sympathetic fibers also innervate the cornea, although their role is unclear. Their cell bodies lie in the superior cervical ganglion, and their axons are carried in the trigeminal nerve, passing with the sensory fibers to the corneal epithelium.[29] In addition to acetylcholine containing sensory fibers and norepinephrine containing sympathetic fibers, substance P-containing fibers have been identified in the subepithelial plexus.[30] There is a relatively high concentration of extraaxonal acetylcholine in the epithelium, as well as acetylcholinesterase and choline acetyl transferase. The role of the acetylcholine is not known.

After sectioning of the nerve trunks at the limbus, there is a migration of neighboring intact nerves into the denervated area; regeneration of damaged fibers usually takes about 9 months. However, reinnervation after penetrating keratoplasty is limited, with central sensation severely reduced or absent even decades later.[31]

Corneal sensitivity is much greater centrally than peripherally, and much greater peripherally than on the conjunctiva. Pain appears to be the only sensation perceived by the corneal nerves.

LIMBUS

The limbus is the semitransparent, vascularized transition zone between the conjunctiva and sclera on one side and the cornea on the other. Clinically the peripheral corneal margin blends inconspicuously with the sclera, and the central extent of the limbus is reasonably defined by a line joining the ends of Bowman's layer and Descemet's membrane.

Several changes occur at the limbus: The stroma of the cornea loses its transparency, and the stromal lamellae lose their orderly arrangement. The individual collagen fibers become larger and varied in diameter and arrangement, acquiring the characteristics of the sclera. Bowman's layer terminates in a rounded end at the central margin of the limbus and gives rise to fibrous connective tissue, in which the subepithelial papillae develop in the zone of the palisade.

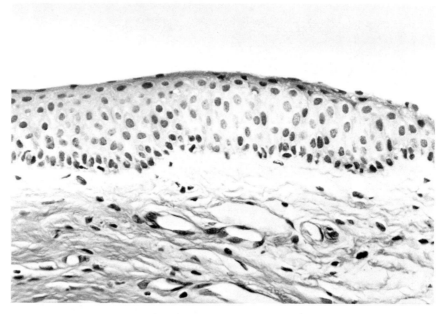

Fig. 1-27. Limbal conjunctiva. The epithelium is approximately 12 layers in thickness. (Hematoxylin-eosin stain; ×500) (Courtesy Bruce L. Johnson, Pittsburgh.)

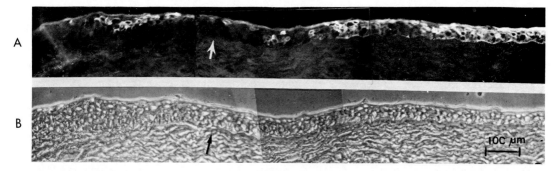

Fig. 1-28. Differential distribution of an epithelial basic keratin *(K3)* in the human cornea and limbus, as determined by immunofluorescence staining with the monoclonal antibody AE5. **A,** Immunofluorescent staining. **B,** Corresponding phase contrast micrograph. Arrows point to the beginning of Bowman's layer. Note in the limbus (to the left of the arrow) K3 is not detectable in the basal and suprabasal cells. In the cornea (to the right of the arrow), K3 is detectable in all the layers in the central regions but is not detectable in the basal cells in the peripheral region. (Courtesy Nirmala Sundar-Raj, Pittsburgh.)

The termination of Bowman's layer is clinically approximately at the apices of the limbal blood vessels. The epithelium of the cornea becomes thicker at the limbus, containing about 12 cell layers (Fig. 1-27). The epithelium projects downward between the subepithelial papillae, which appear as white, radially oriented lines crossing the limbus every 1 to 2 mm. These clinically visible projections are known as the *palisades of Vogt*. Corneal and conjunctival epithelium contain different keratins, allowing for their immunohistochemical differentiation (Fig. 1-28).

The limbus appears to be very important in corneal epithelial regeneration. Limbal epithelium has greater proliferative potential than peripheral or central corneal epithelium[32] and appears to contain a population of stem cells whose daughter cells populate the cornea.[33,34] These cells are probably located at the base of the epithelial pegs. If the limbus is totally destroyed, as in severe alkali burns or Stevens-Johnson syndrome, there is reduced capacity for epithelial regeneration.

REFERENCES

1. Ralph RA: Conjunctival goblet cell density in normal subjects and in dry eye syndromes, Invest Ophthalmol 14:299, 1975.
2. Nichols B, Dawson CR, and Togni B: Surface features of the conjunctiva and cornea, Invest Ophthalmol Vis Sci 24:570, 1983.
3. Brown SI and Dervichian DG: The oils of the meibomian glands: physical and surface characteristics, Arch Ophthalmol 82:537, 1969.
4. Records R: The tear film. In Duane T and Jaeger E, editors: Clinical ophthalmology, vol 4, Philadelphia, 1988, Harper & Row.
5. Norn MS: The conjunctival fluid: its height, volume, density of cells, and flow, Acta Ophthalmol 44:212, 1966.
6. Katz M: The human eye as an optical system. In Tasman W and Jaeger EA, editors: Duane's clinical ophthalmology, vol 1, Philadelphia, 1989, JB Lippincott Co.
7. Donzis PB, Insler MS, and Gordon RA: Corneal curvatures in premature infants, Am J Ophthalmol 99:213, 1988.
8. Isenberg SJ: The eye in infancy, Chicago, 1989, Mosby–Year Book, Inc.
9. Gordon RA and Donzis PB: Refractive development of the human eye, Arch Ophthalmol 103:785, 1985.
10. Harding CV et al: A comparative study of corneal epithelial cell surfaces utilizing the scanning electron microscope, Invest Ophthalmol 13:906, 1974.
11. Hoffman F: The surface of epithelial cells of the cornea under the scanning electron microscope, Ophthalmol Res 3:207, 1972.
12. Pfister RR: The normal surface of corneal epithelium-scanning electron microscopic study, Invest Ophthalmol 12:654, 1973.
13. Gipson IL and Anderson RA: Actin filaments in normal and migrating corneal epithelial cells, Invest Ophthalmol Vis Sci 16:161, 1977.
14. Kuwabara T, Perkins DG, and Cogan DG: Sliding of the epithelium in experimental corneal wounds, Invest Ophthalmol 15:4, 1976.
15. Robb RM and Kuwabara T: Corneal wound healing. I. The movement of polymorphonuclear leukocytes into corneal wounds, Arch Ophthalmol 68:632, 1962.
16. Madri JA et al: The ultrastructural organization and architecture of basement membranes. In Porter R and Whelan J, editors: Basement membranes and cell movement, CIBA Foundation Symposium, vol 108, London, 1984, Pitman Press.
17. Madri JA et al: Ultrastructural localization of fibronectin and laminin in the basement membrane of the murine kidney, J Cell Biol 86:682, 1980.
18. Masutani M et al: Detection of specific collagen types in normal and keratoconus corneas, Invest Ophthalmol Vis Sci 20:738, 1981.
19. Millin JA, Golub BM, and Foster CS: Human basement membrane components of keratoconus and normal corneas, Invest Ophthalmol Vis Sci 27:604, 1986.
20. Gipson IK, Spurr-Michaud SJ, and Tisdale A: Anchoring fibrils form a complex network in human and rabbit cornea, Invest Ophthalmol Vis Sci 28:212, 1987.
21. Freeman IL: Collagen polymorphism in mature rabbit cornea, Invest Ophthalmol Vis Sci 17:171, 1978.
22. Praus R and Brettschneider I: Glycosaminoglycans in embryonic and postnatal human cornea, Ophthalmic Res 7:542, 1975.
23. Kuwabara T: Current concepts in anatomy and histology of the cornea, Contact Intraocular Lens Med J 4:101, 1978.
24. Newsome DA et al: Detection of specific collagen types in normal and keratoconus corneas, Invest Ophthalmol Vis Sci 20:738, 1981.
25. Waring GO, Laibson PR, and Rodrigues M: Clinical and pathologic alterations of Descemet's membrane, with emphasis on endothelial metaplasia, Surv Ophthalmol 18:325, 1974.
26. Kenney C et al: Analyses of collagens from ultrastructurally pure Descemet's membrane and cultured endothelial cells, Invest Ophthalmol Vis Sci 17(suppl):253, 1978.
27. Perlman M, Baum JL, and Kaye GI: Fine structure and collagen synthetic activity of monolayer cultures of rabbit corneal endothelium, J Cell Biol 63:306, 1974.
28. Kreutziger GO: Lateral membrane morphology and gap junction structure in rabbit corneal endothelium, Exp Eye Res 23:285, 1986.
29. Klyce SD et al: Distribution of sympathetic nerves in the rabbit cornea, Invest Ophthalmol Vis Sci 27(suppl):354, 1986.
30. Tervo K et al: Substance P-immunoreactive nerves in the human cornea and iris, Invest Ophthalmol Vis Sci 23:671, 1982.

31. Rao GN et al: Recovery of corneal sensitivity in grafts following penetrating keratoplasty, Ophthalmology 92:1408, 1985.

32. Ebato B, Friend J, and Thoft R: Comparison of limbal and peripheral human corneal epithelium in tissue culture, Invest Ophthalmol Vis Sci 29:1533, 1988.

33. Schermer A, Galvlin S, and Sun T: Differentiation-related expression of a major 64K corneal keratin in vivo and in culture suggests limbal location of corneal epithelial stem cells, J Cell Biol 103:49, 1986.

34. Thoft RA, Wiley LA, and Sundar-Raj N: The multipotential cells of the limbus, Eye 3:109, 1989.

PHYSIOLOGY

METABOLISM

The cells of the cornea—epithelium, keratocytes, and endothelium—are metabolically active and require nutrients for their function. The metabolism of the corneal epithelium is most readily studied and therefore best understood.

EPITHELIUM

The major nutrients required are glucose, oxygen, vitamins, and amino acids. The catabolism of glucose and glycogen is the main energy source for the epithelial cells. Most of the glucose is derived from the aqueous humor; 10% or less comes from the limbal vessels or tears. The epithelium is also able to store large amounts of glycogen, which can be mobilized when the supply of free glucose is insufficient (for example, hypoxia and trauma).

Glucose is catabolized through both aerobic pathways, including the tricarboxylic acid (TCA), or Krebs, cycle and hexose monophosphate shunt, and anaerobic pathways (Fig. 2-1). The relative roles

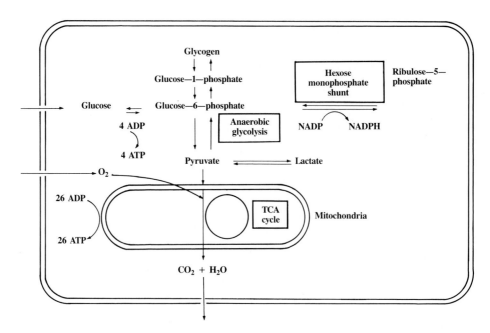

Fig. 2-1. Epithelial glucose metabolism.

of these pathways have not been determined, but it is thought that the TCA cycle is not very active because it takes place in mitochondria, and mitochondria are not very abundant in the epithelium.[1,2] The catabolism of glucose through these pathways produces adenosine triphosphate (ATP) and nicotinamide-adenine dinucleotide phosphate (NADPH), high energy compounds, which are then used in cellular processes.

Anaerobic glycolysis produces pyruvate and lactate, which, under aerobic conditions, can then be converted to CO_2 by the TCA cycle. The CO_2 is readily eliminated, by diffusion across the endothelium and epithelium, and by conversion to bicarbonate by the endothelium. Lactate cannot pass through the epithelium and must diffuse through the stroma and endothelium into the aqueous.[3] During hypoxia or other times of corneal stress, lactate accumulates and can cause localized acidosis and an increased osmotic solute load. This effect can result in epithelial and stromal edema and possibly alter endothelial morphology and function.[3]

Most of the oxygen taken in by the cornea is consumed by the epithelium and the endothelium. Oxygen is supplied mainly by diffusion from the tear film. The oxygen tension in the aqueous is probably 30 to 40 mm Hg,[4] and this is not sufficient to meet epithelial metabolic needs. When the eye is open, atmospheric oxygen enters the tears, and the partial pressure of oxygen is approximately 155 mm Hg. When the lids are closed, oxygen enters the tears only by diffusion from the conjunctival blood vessels, and the partial pressure falls to about 55 mm Hg.[5]

The use of contact lenses and intrastromal lenses for correction of refractive errors has increased our awareness of corneal oxygenation and nutrition. Successful contact lens wear requires adequate supply of oxygen to the epithelium. With wear of oxygen-impermeable (for example, polymethylmethacrylate [PMMA]) lenses tear flow beneath the lens must carry oxygenated tears to the central epithelium (Fig. 2-2, *B*). Hydrophilic soft contact lenses and oxygen-permeable (for example, silicone, fluoropolymer) rigid lenses supply oxygen both by diffusion through the lens and by tear flow (Fig. 2-2, *C,D*). Oxygen supply is most limited beneath the upper lid and during sleep, when tear oxygen tension is reduced. When impermeable lenses, for example, polysulfone, are placed in the

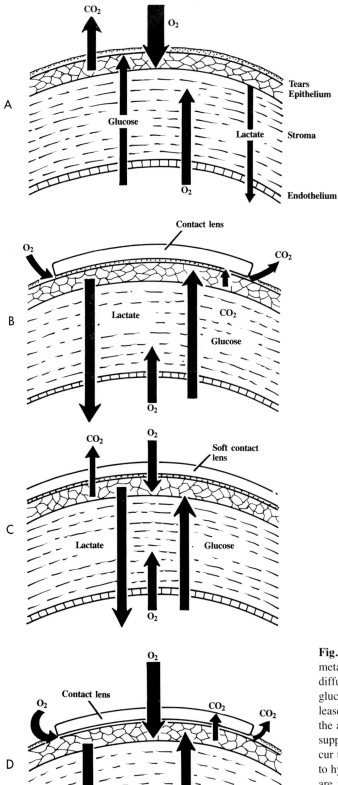

Fig. 2-2. Effect of contact lens wear on epithelial metabolism. **A,** Normal state. Most of the oxygen diffuses through the tears from the atmosphere; glucose is supplied by the aqueous; CO_2 is released into the atmosphere; lactate diffuses into the aqueous. **B,** During PMMA lens wear, oxygen supply and CO_2 release are impaired and must occur through passage of tears beneath the lens. Due to hypoxia, glucose demand and lactate production are increased. **C,** During hydrophilic contact lens wear, oxygen supply is improved because some O_2 can pass through the lens, but glucose demand and lactate production are moderately increased. **D,** With highly oxygen-permeable rigid contact lenses, oxygen supply, glucose demand, and lactate production are near normal.

corneal stroma, glucose and other nutrients must diffuse around the lens to reach the anterior epithelium and keratocytes. If the lenses are too large or too anterior, such that the supply of nutrients is inadequate, the anterior cornea melts.

Amino acids, vitamins, and other nutrients are supplied to the epithelium principally by the aqueous humor.

ENDOTHELIUM

The endothelium appears to contain the same aerobic and anaerobic glycolytic pathways as the epithelium, although their activities are lower. The major energy source is glucose, which is derived from the aqueous humor. The ability of the endothelium to store glycogen is not known. Unlike the epithelium, the endothelial oxygen need is met by the aqueous. Glutathione is also important for normal endothelial function.[6] Most likely it plays a role in the elimination of free radicals and toxic peroxides formed during light exposure.[7,8]

CONTROL OF STROMAL HYDRATION

The control of corneal stromal hydration is essential for transparency. Water accounts for 78% of the weight of the cornea, higher than most connective tissue elsewhere in the body. Hydration can also be described as the ratio of water (by weight) to dry weight of tissue. The normal hydration of the cornea is 3.45. If the hydration is increased to 6.8, or 87% of the weight of the cornea, the thickness doubles.

Several mechanisms play a role in the regulation of corneal hydration (Fig. 2-3):
1. Barrier function of the epithelium and endothelium
2. Swelling pressure of the stroma
3. Ionic transport by the epithelium and endothelium
4. Intraocular pressure
5. Evaporation of water from the corneal surface

BARRIER FUNCTION OF THE EPITHELIUM AND ENDOTHELIUM

Both the epithelium and the endothelium act as barriers to the movement of water and ions into the stroma. The greatest resistance to electrolyte diffusion lies in the epithelium, primarily the surface

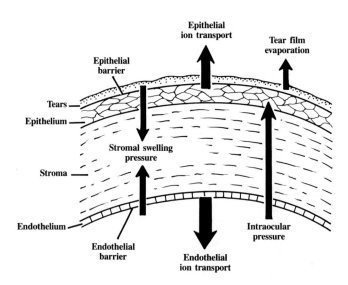

Fig. 2-3. Control of stromal hydration.

layers.[9-11] The epithelial cell outer membranes are relatively impermeable to the passage of ions, and the epithelial cells are connected to surrounding cells by tight junctions, which, although not as effective as the cell membranes, also significantly impede ion flow.[12]

Comparatively the endothelium is 200 times more permeable to electrolytes than the epithelium, but it is still 10 times more resistant than the stroma.[9-11] The resistance to intercellular passage of ions is created by both the elaborate interdigitation of the cell borders, increasing the distance substances must travel, and by localized occlusive cell junctions.[13]

SWELLING PRESSURE OF THE STROMA

If the epithelium and endothelium are removed, the corneal stroma will swell to approximately twice normal thickness as a result of imbibement of water by the stromal ground substance. The glycosaminoglycans (GAGs) of the ground substance are negatively charged and repel each other. Also, they have a tendency to take on cations to preserve ionic charge neutrality (Donnan's equilibrium). The stromal swelling pressure is approximately 50 to 60 mm Hg at normal thickness and decreases exponentially as the stroma swells.[14,15] Therefore at normal thickness the stromal swelling pressure must be counterbalanced by a force that moves water out of the stroma.

IONIC TRANSPORT BY THE EPITHELIUM AND ENDOTHELIUM

It was demonstrated in the 1950s that active metabolic processes are necessary for maintenance of normal stromal hydration.[16,17] Lowering corneal temperature, blocking anaerobic glycolysis, or depriving the cornea of oxygen or glucose will lead to stromal swelling. It was also suspected that the endothelium played the greater role, since its removal had the greater effect.

It is now well established that the endothelium is responsible for active dehydration of the cornea.[18] Although it was originally referred to as an endothelial "fluid pump," the mechanism appears to be one of active transport of ions from the stroma into the aqueous, with passive, secondary movement of water. The exact process remains unclear, but the endothelium actively transports bicarbonate,[19,20] and probably sodium,[21] from the stroma to the aqueous. This ion transport creates an osmotic gradient (2 to 3 mOsm), which balances the swelling pressure of the corneal stroma.[22,23]

There is also evidence for ion transport in the corneal epithelium, which may also play a role, although certainly a much smaller one. The epithelium secretes chloride into the tears by active transport,[24,25] which is regulated by a beta-adrenergic receptor and is mediated intracellularly by adenylate cyclase.[26] The adrenergic receptors probably respond to catecholamines released by the sympathetic nerve fibers present in the epithelium, and possibly also to other neurotransmitters.[27] In the frog[28] and in the rabbit[29] the corneal epithelium is capable of secreting chloride and fluid and thinning the stroma. However, this has not been demonstrated in primates.

INTRAOCULAR PRESSURE

In the normal eye intraocular pressure (IOP) has little effect on the stromal thickness. However, when the IOP exceeds the stromal swelling pressure, epithelial edema occurs. Thus with a normal cornea epithelial edema occurs when the IOP exceeds 55 mm Hg. However, if endothelial function decreases and the stroma thickens to 0.60 mm, epithelial edema will occur at an IOP of approximately 30 mm Hg. After penetrating keratoplasty corneal thickness is much more responsive to IOP; increasing the IOP thins the donor cornea, whereas decreasing it thickens the donor. The mechanism for this process has not been established, but it is thought to be related to the anterior stromal lamellae bearing the stress of IOP.[30]

EVAPORATION OF WATER FROM THE CORNEAL SURFACE

Evaporation of water from the tear film results in hypertonicity of the tears and draws water from the epithelial cells, and subsequently the stroma. Evidence for this effect is that the cornea is 5%

thinner during waking hours than during sleep.[31] Also, in patients with borderline endothelial function, vision is often worse in the morning and improves over the day. However, the ability of tear evaporation to thin the stroma is normally quite limited because blinking and reflex tearing rapidly restore isotonicity. Only in eyes without normal tear flow or surfacing can significant stromal thinning occur (for example, dellen).

CORNEAL TRANSPARENCY

The cornea transmits approximately 90% of light in the visible spectrum. (However, all light with a wavelength of 300 nm or less, and the majority of light with a wavelength greater than 1400 nm, is absorbed.) The need for corneal transparency is obvious, but the mechanism by which this is achieved has long been obscure. The lack of blood and lymph vessels, the absence of myelin sheaths around the corneal nerves, and proper hydration of the stroma are certainly necessary. Why then is the corneal stroma transparent, whereas other tissues with similar mixtures of collagen fibrils and ground substance, for example, sclera, are not? Dry collagen has a refractive index of 1.55, whereas the ground substance has a refractive index of 1.35; normally such disparity produces light scatter, and the tissue is opaque.

Maurice[32] suggested that the tight packing and regular lattice arrangement of the stromal collagen fibrils is responsible. Light scattered by individual fibers is cancelled by destructive interference with scattered light from neighboring fibers. As long as the fibers are regularly arranged and separated by less than a wavelength of light, the cornea will remain transparent. However, if the stroma is edematous, the space between the fibers increases, destructive interference no longer occurs, light is scattered, and corneal transparency is reduced.

More recently, it has been determined that a regular lattice arrangement of the collagen fibers is not necessary for transparency. In Bowman's layer the collagen fibrils are irregularly arranged, and the shark cornea also contains regions of disorganized collagen fibrils.[33] Goldman and Benedek[33,34] and others[35] concluded that appreciable light scattering did not occur unless regional fluctuations in refractive index exceeded 2000 Å. (Visible light is 4000 to 7000 Å.) The corneal stroma does not scatter light because its collagen fibrils are small in diameter (approximately 300 Å) and closely spaced (approximately 550 Å). Corneal clouding occurs when variations in refractive index occur over areas greater than 2000 Å in diameter. Stromal swelling can increase interfibrillar distance to greater than this amount.[36]

DRUG PENETRATION
MIXING IN THE TEARS

When drugs intended to act in the corneal stroma or anterior chamber are administered as a drop, they must overcome several obstacles before they can exert their therapeutic effect. The penetration of any drug is affected by its concentration on the surface and the time of contact, that is, for topical ocular medications, the concentration achieved in tears and the persistence of the medication in the tears.

The volume of a drop from a standard medication bottle is approximately 40 µl. The volume of tears on the surface of the eye is only about 10 µl,[37] and therefore much of the medication is immediately lost onto the eyelashes. Some extra volume can be retained (up to 25 µl), but blinking or squeezing of the lids in response to the drop reduces the excess. In addition, the medication becomes diluted by tears already in the eye to approximately 25% of that in the drop.[38] Therefore both the volume and concentration of the drop are immediately reduced. Smaller, more concentrated drops of medication would be more effective, but they are not marketed because of increased manufacturing costs.

After initial mixing the drug is progressively diluted by new tear secretion. In the normal eye, with a relatively nonirritating drug, the concentration is reduced about 90% by tearing alone in 20 minutes. Tear concentration is also reduced by absorption of the drug into the eye; and for some lipophilic drugs, for example, pilocarpine, the combination of absorption and dilution reduced tear concentration to 10% of its starting value in only 4 minutes.[39] If the drop is irritating, reflex tearing occurs and the dilution is even more rapid. Irritation is primarily caused by a pH or osmolality far from that of the tears.

Ophthalmic ointments are composed of drug particles suspended in an oleaginous base. The purpose of ointment administration is to increase the time that drug is present in the tears. The ointment is retained in the cul-de-sac and gradually melts, releasing the drug into the tears. This theoretic advantage is not always realized, however; aqueous levels of tetracycline and chloramphenicol were found to be higher after administration of ointment preparations than solutions,[40,41] but levels of dexamethasone were much lower.[42]

CORNEAL PENETRATION

Topically applied drugs reach the corneal stroma and aqueous only through the cornea; nearly all drug penetrating the conjunctiva is carried away by blood vessels. To penetrate the cornea, a drug must pass through both the epithelium and the stroma, which are very different types of barriers. Because the epithelium is cellular and composed largely of lipid membranes, nonpolar substances penetrate readily, but polar, or hydrophilic, substances penetrate poorly. The stroma, on the other hand, is composed primarily of water, and polar groups pass through it more easily. Because drugs have to pass through both barriers, those soluble in both lipid and water exhibit the best penetration.

Many ophthalmic medications are weak bases. Weak bases tend to penetrate well because they exist in an equilibrium between a neutral and an ionic form. The neutral form penetrates the epithelium well; once in the stroma the equilibrium shifts to favor the ionic form. The ions are able to pass through the stroma to the endothelium, where the reverse process occurs.

If the epithelium is not intact, such as after a corneal abrasion or during treatment of an infectious ulcer, hydrophilic drugs are much more effective. Inflammation also increases drug penetration, but to a lesser extent. Some preservatives and surfactants present in drug formulations, such as benzalkonium chloride, impair the integrity of the epithelial barrier and increase penetration.

REFERENCES

1. Kinoshita JH: Some aspects of the carbohydrate metabolism of the cornea, Invest Ophthalmol 1:178, 1962.
2. Thoft RA and Friend J: Corneal epithelial glucose metabolism, Arch Ophthalmol 88:58, 1971.
3. Klyce SD: Stromal lactate accumulation can account for corneal edema osmotically following epithelial hypoxia in the rabbit, J Physiol 321:49, 1981.
4. Klyce SD and Beuerman RW: Structure and function of the cornea. In Kaufman HE et al, editors: The cornea, New York, 1988, Churchill Livingstone.
5. Efron N and Carney LG: Oxygen levels beneath the closed eyelid, Invest Ophthalmol Vis Sci 18:93, 1979.
6. Dikstein S and Maurice DM: The metabolic basis of the fluid pump of the cornea, J Physiol (Lond) 221:29, 1955.
7. Riley MV et al: Oxidized glutathione in the corneal endothelium, Exp Eye Res 30:607, 1981.
8. Ng MC and Riley MV: Relation of intracellular levels and redox state of reduced glutathione to endothelium function in the rabbit cornea, Exp Eye Res 30:511, 1980.
9. Maurice DM: The permeability to sodium ions of the living rabbit's cornea, J Physiol (Lond) 112:367, 1951.
10. Maurice DM: Cornea and sclera. In Davson H, editor: The eye, ed 3, New York, 1984, Academic Press.
11. Mishima S and Hedbys BO: The permeability of the corneal epithelium and endothelium, Exp Eye Res 6:10, 1967.
12. Marshall WS and Klyce SD: Cellular and paracellular pathway resistances in the "tight" Cl⁻-secreting epithelium of the rabbit cornea, J Membr Biol 73:275, 1983.
13. Kreutziger GO: Lateral membrane morphology and gap junction structure in rabbit corneal endothelium, Exp Eye Res 23:285, 1986.
14. Dohlman CH, Hedbys BO, and Mishima S: The swelling pressure of the corneal stroma, Invest Ophthalmol Vis Sci 1:158, 1962.
15. Hedbys BO and Dohlman CH: A new method for the determination of the swelling pressure of the corneal stroma in vitro, Exp Eye Res 1:122, 1963.
16. Davson H: The hydration of the cornea, Biochem J 59:24, 1955.
17. Harris JE and Nordquist LT: The hydration of the cornea, Am J Ophthalmol 40:100, 1955.
18. Maurice DM: The location of the fluid pump in the cornea, J Physiol (Lond) 221:43, 1972.

19. Hodson S and Miller F: The bicarbonate ion pump in the endothelium which regulates the hydration of the rabbit cornea, J Physiol 263:563, 1976.

20. Hull DS et al: Corneal endothelium bicarbonate transport and the effect of carbonic anhydrase inhibitors on endothelial permeability and fluxes and corneal thickness, Invest Ophthalmol Vis Sci 16:883, 1977.

21. Lim JJ and Ussing HH: Analysis of presteady-state Na^+ fluxes across the rabbit corneal endothelium, J Membr Biol 65:197, 1982.

22. Fischbarg J et al: The mechanism of fluid and electrolyte transport across corneal endothelium: critical revision and update of a model, Curr Eye Res 4:351, 1985.

23. Wiederholt M, Jentsch TJ, and Keller SK: Electrical sodium-bicarbonate symport in cultured corneal endothelial cells, Pflugers Arch 405:S167, 1985.

24. Klyce SD, Neufeld AH, and Zadunaisky JA: The activation of chloride transport by epinephrine and Db cyclic-AMP in the cornea of the rabbit, Invest Ophthalmol 12:127, 1973.

25. Wiederholt M: Physiology of epithelial transport in the human eye, Klin Wochenschr 58:975, 1980.

26. Klyce SD and Wong RKS: Site and mode of adrenaline action on chloride transport across the rabbit corneal epithelium, J Physiol 266:777, 1977.

27. Klyce SD, Beuerman RW, and Crosson CE: Alteration of corneal epithelial transport by sympathectomy, Invest Ophthalmol Vis Sci 26:434, 1985.

28. Zadynaisky JA and Lande MA: Active chloride transport and control of corneal transparency, Am J Physiol 221:1837, 1981.

29. Klyce SD: Enhancing fluid secretion by the corneal epithelium, Invest Ophthalmol Vis Sci 16:968, 1977.

30. McPhee TJ, Bourne WM, and Brubaker RF: Location of the stress-bearing layers of the cornea, Invest Ophthalmol Vis Sci 26:869, 1985.

31. Mishima S and Maurice DM: The effect of normal evaporation on the eye, Exp Eye Res 1:46, 1961.

32. Maurice DM: The structure and transparency of the cornea, J Physiol 136:263, 1957.

33. Goldman JN and Benedek GB: The relationship between morphology and transparency in the nonswelling corneal stroma of the shark, Invest Ophthalmol 6:574, 1967.

34. Benedek GB: Theory of transparency of the eye, Appl Optics 10:459, 1971.

35. Farrell RA, McCally RL, and Tatham PER: Wavelength dependencies of light scattering in normal and cold swollen rabbit cornea and their structural implications, J Physiol 233:589, 1973.

36. Goldman JN et al: Structural alterations affecting transparency in swollen human corneas, Invest Ophthalmol 7:501, 1968.

37. Mishima S et al: Determination of tear volume and tear flow, Invest Ophthalmol 5:264, 1966.

38. Maurice DM: Kinetics of topically applied ophthalmic drugs. In Saettone MF, Bucci M, Speiser P, editors: Ophthalmic drug delivery: biopharmaceutical, technological and clinical aspects, New York, 1987, Springer-Verlag.

39. Sieg JW and Robinson JR: Mechanistic studies on transcorneal permeation of pilocarpine, J Pharm Sci 65:1816, 1976.

40. Hanna C et al: Ocular penetration of topical chloramphenicol in humans, Arch Ophthalmol 96:1258, 1978.

41. Massey JT et al: Effect of drug vehicle on human ocular retention of topically applied tetracycline, Am J Ophthalmol 81:151, 1976.

42. Cox WV, Kupferman A, and Leibowitz HM: Topically applied steroids in corneal disease. II. The role of drug vehicle in stromal absorption of dexamethasone, Arch Ophthalmol 88:549, 1972.

HISTORY AND EXAMINATION

HISTORY

Because diagnosis can often be made by examination alone, ophthalmologists may neglect taking a thorough history. However, an organized and directed history can be very informative and provide valuable clues to the diagnosis, as well as prevent pitfalls in treatment. Specific forms may be used to facilitate the completion of a comprehensive external disease history and examination and to ensure that necessary portions are not omitted. A form used by Dr. Grayson is shown in Figs. 3-1 and 3-2. As in a general medical examination, the physician should first obtain the patient's chief complaint and record it in the patient's own words. Then the history of the present illness, past ocular history (including medications), general medical history (including systemic medications and allergies), and family history should be obtained.

| WISHARD MEMORIAL HOSPITAL | | Indianapolis, Indiana | INDIANA UNIVERSITY HOSPITALS |

CORNEA - EXTERNAL DISEASE HISTORY

Revised 1-75

M6322600
WMH61-704

DATE_____ REFERRED BY_____

COMPLAINTS: OD ☐   OS ☐   OU ☐

Decr. Vision ☐	Photophobia ☐	Discharge ☐	Other ☐
Dryness ☐	Itching ☐	Lids Sealed ☐	
F.B. Sensation ☐	Redness ☐	Opacity ☐	
Burning ☐	Tearing ☐	Mass ☐	
Pain ☐	Epiphora ☐	Blepharitis ☐	

☐ In-Patient   ☐ Out-Patient

PRESENT ILLNESS:

Trigger: ☐

Worsened By: ☐

Improved By: ☐

Daily Variation: ☐

Seasonal Variation: ☐

Adenopathy: ☐

MEDICATIONS:

EYE: GENERAL:

PAST HISTORY:

ALLERGY:

FAMILY HISTORY:

_____ M.D.
SIGNATURE

MED. REC. COPY

CORNEA-EXTERNAL DISEASE HISTORY   **B-70**

| B-CLIN. NOTES | E-LAB | G-X-RAY | K-DIAGNOSTIC | M-SURGERY | Q-THERAPY | T-ORDERS | W-NURSING | Y-MISC. |

Fig. 3-1. Comprehensive form can aid in obtaining complete background history.

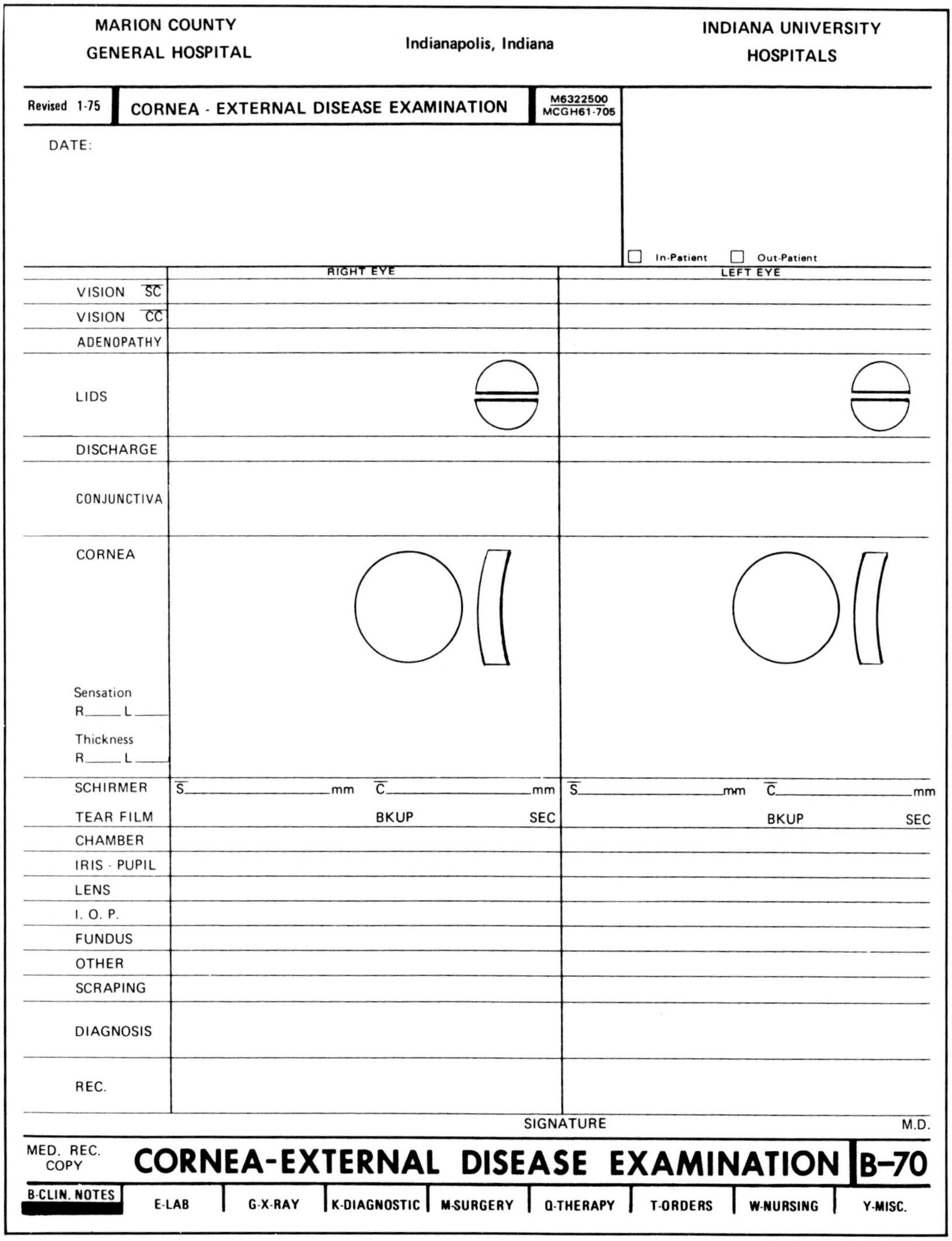

MARION COUNTY GENERAL HOSPITAL	Indianapolis, Indiana	INDIANA UNIVERSITY HOSPITALS

Revised 1-75	CORNEA - EXTERNAL DISEASE EXAMINATION	M6322500 MCGH61-705	

DATE:

☐ In-Patient   ☐ Out-Patient

	RIGHT EYE	LEFT EYE
VISION $\overline{SC}$		
VISION $\overline{CC}$		
ADENOPATHY		
LIDS		
DISCHARGE		
CONJUNCTIVA		
CORNEA		
Sensation R____ L____		
Thickness R____ L____		
SCHIRMER	$\overline{S}$____mm $\overline{C}$____mm	$\overline{S}$____mm $\overline{C}$____mm
TEAR FILM	BKUP SEC	BKUP SEC
CHAMBER		
IRIS - PUPIL		
LENS		
I. O. P.		
FUNDUS		
OTHER		
SCRAPING		
DIAGNOSIS		
REC.		

SIGNATURE   M.D.

MED. REC. COPY	**CORNEA-EXTERNAL DISEASE EXAMINATION**	**B-70**

B-CLIN. NOTES	E-LAB	G-X-RAY	K-DIAGNOSTIC	M-SURGERY	Q-THERAPY	T-ORDERS	W-NURSING	Y-MISC.

Fig. 3-2. Comprehensive form can aid in performance of complete examination.

HISTORY OF PRESENT ILLNESS

Triggering mechanisms, daily or seasonal variations, associated factors, and factors that improve or worsen the symptoms should be elicited. Following are some common symptoms and their associated diseases.

A sensation of dryness in the eyes or burning suggests keratoconjunctivitis sicca. This sensation may be associated with dryness of the mouth or other signs of Sjögren's syndrome. The ocular symptoms are usually worse in the afternoon. They may be aggravated in a dry atmosphere, such as inside a home with dry air heat during the winter. Reading and watching television also tend to worsen the symptoms. The dry eye is in essence a compromised one and is prone to infection, delayed healing, and adverse effects from topical medications. Therefore keratoconjunctivitis sicca must be thought of and tested for in the presence of these problems.

Sharp pain, followed by foreign body sensation, photophobia, and tearing may signal a corneal erosion. The symptoms may last minutes to 2 to 3 days and can occur repeatedly. Spontaneous erosions occur most often upon awakening, but may occur at any time of the day or even during sleep.

Worsening of eye irritation in the morning is typical of blepharitis, nocturnal lagophthalmos, and floppy lid syndrome. The complaint of decreased vision in the morning, improving in the afternoon, usually connotes early corneal decompensation due to edema.

Photophobia is a prominent complaint when there is infiltration of the cornea with inflammatory cells, an epithelial defect, or iritis. It is seen in phlyctenulosis, exposure to ultraviolet light (sunlamp), severe keratoconjunctivitis, corneal erosions or abrasions, and infectious keratitis. It may be observed in some systemic syndromes, such as Sjögren's syndrome and Richner-Hanhart syndrome, and with some intracranial lesions.

Itching, especially of the inner canthi, is an important complaint to note because of its association with allergic states. Seasonal variation is usually a hallmark of external inflammation due to airborne allergens, such as pollen.

The presence and type of discharge are important clues to the nature of the underlying disease. If the eyelids are sealed in the morning, a polymorphonuclear response should be suspected. This response may occur in bacterial and chlamydial infections, but also in viral conjunctivitis if the conjunctival inflammation is severe, such as when membranes are present. Purulent discharge suggests bacterial and chlamydial disease. A mucoid, ropy discharge is highly suggestive of an allergic condition or keratoconjunctivitis sicca.

Watery tearing and epiphora are common complaints. The patient may state that the "tears run down the face." It can be most annoying and require constant wiping, which in itself is irritating to the skin of the lids. Usually, tearing is related to ocular irritation or inflammation, but blockage of the lacrimal drainage system must be considered. Examination of the lacrimal drainage system is also indicated in the presence of repeated episodes of bacterial conjunctivitis or when there are findings suggestive of canalicular or lacrimal sac inflammation.

A patient may report a newly noted pigmentation or mass of the lid, conjunctiva, cornea, or iris. Inquiry should be made as to the duration of its presence and whether it has increased in size, bled, become inflamed, or changed in color. Obtaining old photographs may be helpful.

A full description of the characteristics of ocular pain aids in determining the cause. The type of pain, chronicity, location, onset, frequency, duration, and aggravating and relieving conditions should be investigated.

The patient's nutritional status can play a role in external disease. A nutritional history may be indicated, particularly in patients who are emaciated, severely debilitated, or impoverished. Faddish or other unusual dietary habits can lead to vitamin or protein insufficiency or hypervitaminosis.

Injury, present or past, and its nature must be thoroughly investigated. Inquiry as to whether the injury occurred on the job or in the garden is important. If the cornea was struck with vegetable matter and subsequently develops an infiltrate or ulcer, fungal keratitis must be suspected. If a liquid has been splashed in the eye, it is important to determine the exact chemical contents and concentrations in the liquid. One should also determine the amount of the liquid, the duration of exposure, the amount of time that elapsed before irrigation, and the amount of irrigation. Grant's[1] *Toxicology of the Eye* is very useful in determining the potential adverse effects of the chemicals involved.

If a foreign body is suspected, it is important to determine its composition, whether it is inert or toxic, and whether it may carry infectious agents. Its size and the velocity on impact should also be estimated.

Contact lens wear is often associated with external disease. If a patient wears contacts, the types of lenses, wearing pattern, age of the lenses, cleaning and disinfection regimen, and solution types and ages should be investigated. Use of tap water, homemade saline solutions, and saliva are important to elicit because of their association with *Acanthamoeba* keratitis.

MEDICATIONS

It is most important to note what medications, both topical and systemic, have been used and for how long. It is also vital to determine all components of combined medications, including any preservatives present. Topical therapy may mask underlying disease, interfere with laboratory testing, or be the cause of signs and symptoms. For example, topical antibiotic administration can prevent growth of causative organisms in culture. Steroid use can suppress a disease and make it more difficult to diagnose. Steroids also can promote corneal ulceration, cataract development, and glaucoma. Common preservatives, such as thimerosal or benzalkonium chloride, can cause an allergic conjunctivitis, a toxic follicular reaction, or epithelial keratitis. Other drugs can cause follicular responses, calcific band keratopathy, conjunctival scarring, or pigmentation of the conjunctiva and cornea (see Chapter 28). Topical anesthetic agents are occasionally inappropriately prescribed or self-administered by patients and can result in severe corneal changes.

Systemically administered medications may cause conjunctival scarring (for example, practolol), decrease tear production or blink rate, or cause deposits in the lens and cornea (see Chapter 27). Systemic immunosuppression predisposes to infection and probably to recurrence of herpes simplex or herpes zoster as well.

PAST OCULAR HISTORY

The past history of eye disease should be obtained, including previous episodes of inflammation and infection, surgery, and injury. As an example, the presence of inferior conjunctival scarring may suggest a diagnosis of cicatricial pemphigoid; however, the scarring may be due to years of phospholine iodide use or an old alkali injury.

GENERAL MEDICAL HISTORY

Investigation of a patient's past history of systemic disease should include skin, cardiovascular, neurologic, mucous membrane, collagen, metabolic, and immune diseases. Many external disease problems are associated with these entities, as will be seen in ensuing chapters. Investigation as to whether the patient is an immunocompromised host is important, especially when treating an infection or contemplating surgery. For example, prior exposure of the lids or eyes to radiation treatment can contribute to keratinization, cicatrization, and telangiectasia of the conjunctiva, as well as to drying of the eye and epithelial disease.

OTHER HISTORY

The family history is very important. A number of corneal conditions are hereditary, and in some, such as the corneal dystrophies, manifestations can be limited to the cornea. In addition, a large number of other hereditary conditions, primarily involving other organ systems, can cause external disease. Thus no external ocular problem should be handled without considering the patient's general health, capability of response to infection, family history, previous ocular history, and medication use.

CLINICAL EXAMINATION

The examination of the eyes is begun after establishing the history of the case. In making this examination too much stress can not be laid upon the necessity of proceeding systematically, since otherwise important matters can very readily be overlooked. We first examine the patient with regard to his general physical condition as well as with regard to the expression of his countenance, and then, in observing the eyes themselves, proceed gradually from the superficial parts—lids, conjunctiva, and cornea—to the deeper portions. (Fuchs E: *Textbook of Ophthalmology,* 1892, D. Appleton & Co., New York.)

GENERAL APPEARANCE

As stressed by Fuchs, it is important not to proceed directly to biomicroscopic examination of the eye, but instead to observe first the patient's general condition, then the face and skin, and then to perform a flashlight examination of the lids and conjunctiva. Note whether a patient is debilitated, has poor hygiene, or is obese, as this may suggest a floppy lid syndrome or increased risk of wound dehiscence postoperatively. Assess the patient's ability to provide an accurate history, to comprehend the nature of the disease, and to comply with therapy.

VISUAL ACUITY

Uncorrected and best-corrected vision should be determined. If normal vision cannot be obtained with the patient's correction, a pinhole test or refraction should be performed. Astigmatism, regular or irregular, is often overlooked as a cause of unexplained decreased vision and can be diagnosed with a keratometer or photokeratoscope, as described below, or by temporary hard contact lens fitting. A hard contact lens will correct astigmatism and indicate how much of the decreased vision can be attributed to this mechanism. A number of devices, such as the Potential Acuity Meter* blue-field entoscope, and laser interferometer, can help determine visual impairment due to corneal and lenticular opacities.

SKIN

Observation of the condition of the patient's skin is vital to a complete examination. Skin diseases, particularly those involving the face, commonly cause external disease of the eye. Acne rosacea and eczema are common diseases that can easily be overlooked, particularly when examining a patient in a darkened room. Therefore their responsibility for problems of the conjunctiva and cornea goes unrecognized. Discoid lupus, bullous pemphigoid, epidermolysis bullosa, and seborrheic dermatitis are other skin diseases associated with external eye disease.

LYMPH NODES

Investigation for lymphadenopathy is an important part of the external disease examination. One should look for palpable, as well as grossly visible, preauricular and submandibular nodes. Small palpable preauricular nodes are seen in the following conditions:

1. Trachoma
2. Vaccinia
3. Inclusion conjunctivitis

---

*Mentor, Norwell, MA

4. Primary herpes simplex
5. Adenoviral conjunctivitis
6. Hyperacute conjunctivitis *(Neisseria)*
7. Lid conditions such as hordeola, impetigo, and cellulitis
8. Dacryoadenitis
9. Toxic reaction to drugs such as idoxuridine
10. Newcastle disease

It is rare for a routine bacterial conjunctivitis to produce a preauricular node. The only exception is hyperacute conjunctivitis.

Grossly visible preauricular nodes are usually associated with localized conjunctival nodules or ulcerations (Parinaud's oculoglandular syndrome) or follicular conjunctival response. These conditions are discussed in Chapter 6.

LIDS

The lid margins, bases of the lashes, and meibomian gland orifices should be examined routinely for signs of inflammation. Yellowish collars surrounding a lash (see Fig. 13-1) suggest staphylococcal blepharitis. Staphylococcal infection of the lids is one of the most common causes of a chronic red eye. Collarettes are composed of fibrin, which forms around the base of the lash and is lifted from the lids as the lash grows out. A small ulcerated area around the base of the lash may be seen. In chronic staphylococcal blepharitis, other lid margin problems, such as broken lashes, loss of lashes, and thickening of the lid margins, may be present. The cornea is often affected, most commonly with an inferior epithelial keratitis. Less often an acutely inflamed eye, marginal corneal infiltrates, superficial corneal vascularization, or phlyctenules may develop. These problems are discussed at greater length in other chapters.

Large greasy scales (scurf) attached to the lashes (see Fig. 13-5) indicate seborrheic blepharitis. Seborrheic blepharitis is noninfectious and commonly associated with seborrheic dermatitis. It can also be associated with conjunctival and corneal inflammation. Blepharitis can be associated with ulceration of the skin of the lid margin. Ulcerative blepharitis most commonly occurs at the lateral canthus, when it is called angular blepharitis (see Fig. 6-8). A number of infectious agents can produce this picture, including *Moraxella*. In meibomitis, inflammation is noted around the orifices of the meibomian glands, and the secretions are thickened (see Fig. 13-6). Corneal and conjunctival inflammation can occur. A more thorough discussion of blepharitis and meibomitis can be found in Chapter 13.

Many tumors may arise from the lids, some of which may be associated with corneal disease. *Molluscum contagiosum* lesions (see Fig. 13-11) are easy to overlook and can be associated with a chronic follicular conjunctivitis. Commonly, acute and chronic inflammatory masses arise from inflammation of skin structures at the lid margin. A *hordeolum* is an acute nodular inflammation of the eyelid. It may be infectious, usually caused by *Staphylococcus aureus,* or sterile. External hordeola involve the anterior lamellae of the lid and may arise from the Zeis glands, sweat glands, or hair follicles. Internal hordeola affect the posterior lamellae and arise from the meibomian glands. In contrast to these, a *chalazion* is a relatively quiet, chronic granulomatous reaction to sebaceous material extruded from a Zeis or meibomian gland.

It is important to assess lid function. Incomplete blinking *(lagophthalmos)* or decreased blink rate may not be noted unless specifically tested for. Lagophthalmos may result in corneal drying and subsequent irritation, infection, vascularization, or ulceration. Lagophthalmos may occur only during sleep and often must be inferred from observation of corneal changes. Ectropion (Fig. 3-3) and entropion often cause corneal or conjunctival disease and should be noted.

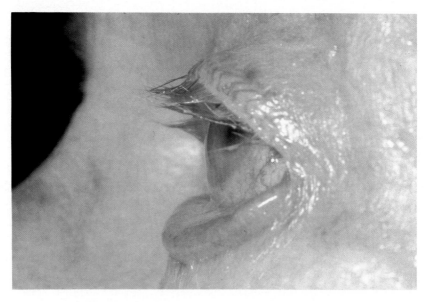

Fig. 3-3. Ectropion. (Courtesy John Stuart, Pittsburgh.)

CONJUNCTIVA

Chemosis. Chemosis is accumulation of fluid within or beneath the conjunctiva (Fig. 3-4). It most commonly is caused by allergic conjunctivitis but can result from orbital inflammation, severe intraocular inflammation (for example, endophthalmitis), or with severe infectious conjunctivitis, such as the hyperacute conjunctivitis of gonorrhea or epidemic keratoconjunctivitis. Systemic diseases, such as Graves' disease or trichinosis, can result in chemosis. Chemosis rarely occurs in the absence of other signs of inflammation. In one such case, subclinical myositis was responsible.

Papillae. Papillae and follicles in the conjunctiva must be identified and differentiated to help solve problems in inflammatory external disease. Characteristics of papillae and follicles include the following:

FOLLICLE	PAPILLA
Discrete, round, elevated lesion of conjunctiva	Elevated polygonal hyperemic areas separated by paler areas
Diameter of 0.5 to 5.0 mm	0.3 to 2.0 mm; "giant" if >1.0 mm
Usually located in inferior palpebral conjunctiva, although they can be seen superiorly	May be seen anywhere on conjunctiva, or at limbus; giant papillae usually over superior tarsus
Vascular network grows around follicle; vessels disappear toward center of follicle	Central fibrovascular core noted in each papilla with central blood vessel, which, when reaching surface, forms arborized vascular figure
Represents new formation of lymphoid tissue	Composed of polymorphonuclear leukocytes and other acute inflammatory cells; epithelial hypertrophy
Histopathologically composed of lymphocytes, macrophages, and plasma cells; may form lymphoid follicles	
No histologic difference between follicles caused by irritants, infections, or in folliculosis	Connective tissue septae are anchored into deeper tissues, resulting in polygonal outline; giant papillae occur when these septae rupture

Papillae can occur only where the conjunctiva is fastened down to the underlying tissue by anchoring septae, such as over the tarsi, and at the bulbar limbus. The anchoring septae normally divide the

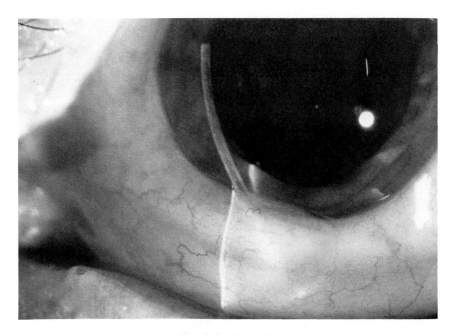

Fig. 3-4. Chemosis.

conjunctiva into a mosaic pattern of polygonal papillae, each less than 1 mm in diameter. A central fibrovascular core is present within each papilla.

A papillary response is a nonspecific sign of conjunctival inflammation and results from edema and polymorphonuclear cell infiltration of the conjunctiva (Fig. 3-5). Giant papillae result from breakdown of the fine fibrous strands that compose the anchoring septae. With the breakdown of the attachments, larger papillae, greater than 1 mm, may develop, most commonly in the upper tarsal conjunctiva. Papillae in the tarsal conjunctiva tend to be flat-topped, whereas those found at the limbus are more dome-shaped. Small white dots *(Trantas' dots)*, composed of eosinophils, may be seen on the surface of limbal papillae in vernal conjunctivitis (see Fig. 19-6). When the everted upper tarsal conjunctiva is examined, the superior edge often appears to contain large papillae. This finding is normal, resulting from the decrease in the density of the anchoring septae. Giant papillae in the remaining tarsal conjunctiva can be seen in vernal conjunctivitis, keratoconjunctivitis of atopic dermatitis, and as a reaction to foreign material, such as contact lenses, prostheses, and suture material (Fig. 3-6).

Follicles. Follicles may be seen in the normal conjunctiva, particularly in younger patients. The follicle is produced by a lymphocytic response, sometimes with a germinal center (Fig. 3-7). The newborn is incapable of developing a follicular response for the first 6 to 12 weeks of life. Follicles appear as smooth, translucent elevations of the conjunctiva, sometimes with vessels over the peripheral surface (see Fig. 8-1). They are most easily appreciated in the upper tarsal conjunctiva and the lower cul-de-sac, the latter usually exhibiting the greater response. However, they can also be seen at the limbus (Fig. 3-8). It is extremely important for the ophthalmologist to determine if a significant follicular response is present because it is a relatively specific inflammatory response and helps define the differential diagnosis. This is discussed further in Chapter 6.

The following are relatively common conditions in which acute follicular conjunctivitis occurs:

1. Adenoviral keratoconjunctivitis
2. Adult inclusion conjunctivitis
3. Herpes simplex (primary)

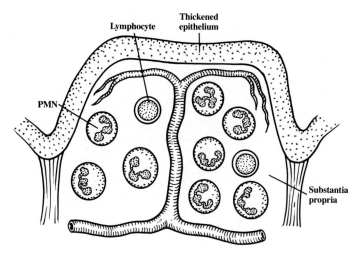

Fig. 3-5. Schematic diagram of a papilla.

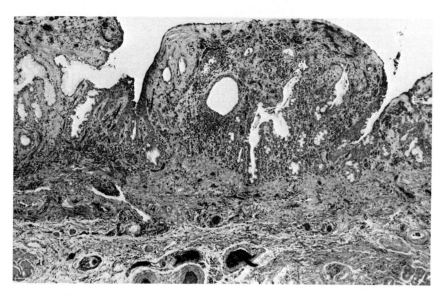

Fig. 3-6. Papilla of superior tarsal conjunctiva in vernal conjunctivitis showing proliferation of fibrovascular connective tissue and chronic inflammatory infiltrate. (Hematoxylin-eosin stain, ×80.) (Courtesy Bruce L. Johnson, Pittsburgh.)

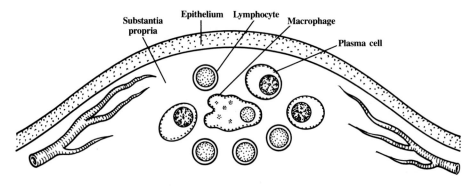

Fig. 3-7. Schematic diagram of a follicle.

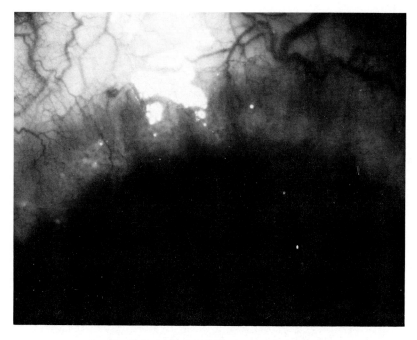

Fig. 3-8. Limbal follicles in vernal catarrh.

4. Enterovirus
5. Acute hemorrhagic conjunctivitis
6. Newcastle disease
7. Acute trachoma

Chronic follicular conjunctivitis commonly occurs in these conditions:

1. Adult inclusion conjunctivitis
2. Trachoma
3. Toxic reaction to drugs
4. Molluscum contagiosum
5. *Moraxella* conjunctivitis
6. Parinaud's oculoglandular syndrome
7. Axenfeld's syndrome
8. Merrill-Thygeson syndrome
9. Benign lymphoid hyperplasia (folliculosis)

It is an error to speak of follicles of sarcoid because the conjunctival masses are actually yellow-white or opaque granulomas.

Membranes. Both membranous and pseudomembranous conjunctivitis are striking clinical signs (Fig. 3-9). Membranes are composed primarily of fibrin that has coagulated on the epithelial surface. Little distinction exists between pseudomembranes and true membranes, except that true membranes might leave a raw surface when peeled off and cause bleeding, thus signifying more intense conjunctival inflammation. A variety of infectious agents can produce pseudomembranous or membranous conjunctivitis. Formerly it was caused principally by the diphtheria organism *(Corynebacterium diphtheriae)* and beta-hemolytic streptococci; but now, in this country, adenoviral conjunctivitis is the most common cause, followed by primary herpetic conjunctivitis. A partial differential diagnosis follows:

1. Beta-hemolytic streptococci
2. Adenoviral keratoconjunctivitis, commonly type 8

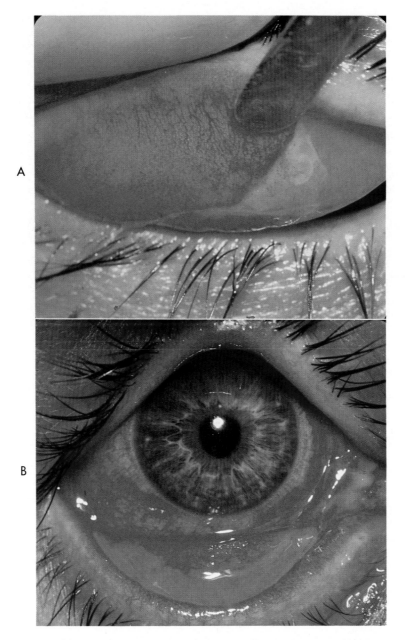

Fig. 3-9. Membrane formation on tarsal conjunctiva in case of epidemic keratoconjunctivitis. **A,** Upper lid. **B,** Lower lid.

3. Primary herpes simplex
4. Vernal conjunctivitis
5. Neonatal inclusion conjunctivitis
6. Diphtheria
7. *Candida*
8. Chemical burns
9. Cicatricial pemphigoid

10. Stevens-Johnson syndrome
11. Lyell's disease (toxic epidermal necrolysis)
12. Ligneous conjunctivitis

Scarring. The ordinary acute or chronic conjunctivitis heals without cicatrization. In fact, the epithelium can be severely damaged without provoking the formation of scar tissue. Scars form only when there is destruction of stromal tissue. There may be severe infiltration and edema of the stroma, as in gonococcal ophthalmia of the adult, without scar formation.

Every possible effort should be made to prevent conjunctival cicatrization because of its long-term complications, such as entropion and trichiasis. A deficiency of mucus may result from loss of conjunctival goblet cells, and closure of lacrimal ducts can lead to keratoconjunctivitis sicca. Nontraumatic conjunctival scarring can result from a variety of conjunctival and systemic inflammatory diseases, including those causes of membranous conjunctivitis listed earlier. Scarring after membranous conjunctivitis tends to be diffuse and nonspecific in appearance, with no predilection for the conjunctiva of either lid, upper or lower.

Special types of scarring, with characteristic morphologic features and location, are seen in trachoma, ocular cicatricial pemphigoid, and atopic keratoconjunctivitis. Severe shrinkage, such as in cicatricial pemphigoid, also occurs occasionally in a few other diseases.

The scar pathognomonic of trachoma is at the limbus. It is the so-called *Herbert's peripheral pit* and consists of the cicatricial remains of a limbal follicle (see Fig. 8-6). Less characteristic, but still diagnostically important, are the stellate scars resulting from cicatrization of necrotic conjunctival follicles. Diffuse scarring may also occur, leading to bowing of the upper tarsus, or ectropion if severe enough. *Arlt's line,* a cicatricial line near the lid border of the upper tarsus, can occur in other diseases, but also suggests trachoma, as does an S curve of the upper lid border caused by cicatrization. In trachoma, scarring is always more prominent on the upper lid than on the lower lid.

In atopic keratoconjunctivitis the scars are focal and tend to occur in the centers of the giant papillae. There also can be diffuse shrinkage of the lower fornix, but even in this instance symblepharon, entropion, and trichiasis tend not to occur. Vernal conjunctivitis does not normally scar the conjunctiva, but radical treatment of the disease frequently does.

Conjunctival scarring may also be seen in dermatitis herpetiformis and epidermolysis bullosa, other mucous membrane diseases, lymphogranuloma venereum, exfoliative dermatitis, sarcoidosis, and with chronic use of some topical medications and systemic administration of practolol.

Keratinization. Keratin may be seen in conditions of drying, superior limbic keratoconjunctivitis, vitamin A deficiency, and squamous neoplasia.

Telangiectasia and sludging. Telangiectasia and sludging of the circulation of the conjunctival vessels can occur in a number of systemic diseases. Telangiectasia of conjunctival vessels is seen in the following:

1. Ataxia-telangiectasia
2. Diabetes mellitus
3. Fabry's disease (see Fig 21-5)
4. Sickle cell anemia
5. Degos syndrome
6. Osler-Weber-Rendu disease
7. Polycythemia vera
8. Radiation (late)
9. Arteriosclerosis
10. Fucosidosis
11. G_{M_1} gangliosidosis

Sludging within conjunctival vessels occurs in multiple myeloma and sickle cell disease. Engorgement of conjunctival veins may be seen in cavernous sinus thrombosis, or with arteriovenous fistulas affecting the orbital circulation.

TEAR FILM AND LACRIMAL SYSTEM

Examination of the tear film is extremely important. Keratoconjunctivitis sicca is a very common disease, one that is often overlooked. It should be considered in cases of unexplained conjunctival injection, corneal thinning, persistent epithelial defect, or poor wound healing. The tear meniscus, tear breakup time, and Schirmer's tests may be used to facilitate diagnosis, as discussed in Chapter 14.

Attention should be focused next on the lacrimal drainage system. Canaliculitis or dacryocystitis should be suspected if there is a complaint of discharge from the eye and pouting of the punctum is present on examination, or if tenderness and swelling is noted in the area of the canaliculi or lacrimal sac (Fig. 3-10). An attempt should be made to express purulent material from the canaliculus and sac. *Canaliculitis* is usually caused by *Actinomyces israelii*, a gram-positive, branching filamentous bacterium, whose unusual structure facilitates its lodging in the canaliculus. An incision along the length of the canaliculus may be necessary to remove concretions formed during infection.

The following organisms are most likely to cause canaliculitis:

1. *Actinomyces israelii*
2. *Candida albicans*
3. *Aspergillus niger*
4. Primary herpes simplex
5. Herpes zoster
6. Vaccinia
7. Syphilis
8. Tuberculosis

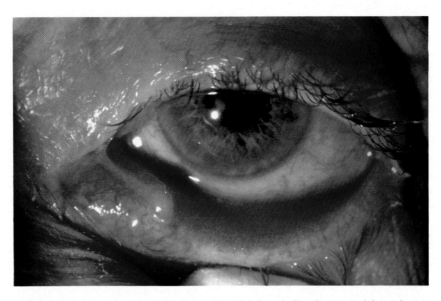

Fig. 3-10. Canniliculitis. Nasal lid margin is thickened and injected. Purulent material can be expressed from punctum.

Swelling, inflammation, and tenderness over the lacrimal sac area (below the medial canthus) are seen in *dacryocystitis*. This condition is usually accompanied by pain, tearing, and purulent discharge; but the only symptom may be occasional epiphora. In any patient with such a complaint or with recurrent conjunctivitis pressure should be applied over the lacrimal sac to look for reflux of mucopurulent material. The following organisms are most likely to cause dacryocystitis:

Acute dacryocystitis

   1. *Staphylococcus aureus*

   2. Beta-hemolytic streptococcus

Chronic dacryocystitis

   1. *Streptococcus pneumoniae*

   2. *Haemophilus influenzae*

CORNEA

Superficial vascularization. Normally superficial limbal vessels do not extend onto the cornea for more than 1 mm. Any growth beyond the normal limbal arcade is called *pannus*. Pannus may be accompanied by subepithelial fibrous tissue or stromal scarring, in which case the clarity of the stroma is reduced. Vascular pannus can be divided into micropannus, where vessels extend only 1 to 2 mm beyond the normal arcade, and gross pannus, where they extend more than 2 mm.

If a gross pannus is seen, the physician should consider the following:

1. Trachoma
2. Phlyctenulosis
3. Acne rosacea
4. Atopic keratoconjunctivitis
5. Contact lens wear
6. Staphylococcal blepharitis
7. Herpes simplex keratitis

If a micropannus is visible, the following disorders are common causes:

1. Inclusion conjunctivitis
2. Childhood trachoma
3. Staphylococcal blepharitis
4. Contact lens wear
5. Superior limbic keratoconjunctivitis
6. Vernal conjunctivitis

Vital stains. Fluorescein and rose bengal dyes should be applied routinely when diagnosing corneal and conjunctival diseases. Fluorescein will travel wherever water can enter the cornea, wherever there is bare stroma, or where the barrier function of the surface epithelium is lost. Rose bengal stain is a red aniline dye chemically related to fluorescein. It stains damaged and devitalized epithelial cells, as well as mucus. Rose bengal is particularly useful in keratoconjunctivitis sicca, superior limbic keratoconjunctivitis, and any eye with milder epithelial injury. It produces irritation, so it is best applied after topical anesthesia. It stains the skin and clothing, so care must be taken in application. To reduce the volume instilled, one may either break a wooden applicator stick and place a drop on the obliquely broken surface, or take some of the dye up into the hollow end of a plastic applicator stick. One should avoid testing of sensation, Schirmer's tests, or applanation tonometry before evaluating the ocular surface with these dyes.

Filaments. Filamentary keratitis is a nonspecific clinical sign, but the specific etiologic factors usually can be determined by examination (Table 3-1). Epithelial filaments appear as small mucoid de-

TABLE 3-1. Filaments

ETIOLOGIC GROUP	SPECIFIC DISEASE	USUAL LOCATION AND NUMBER OF FILAMENTS
Viral	Herpes simplex (transitory)	Usually single filament
Surgical	After cataract extraction	Diffuse if eye is occluded
	Bullous keratopathy (transitory)	
Trauma	After corneal abrasion and erosion (transitory)	Usually single layer of filaments
Mechanical	Occlusion (including ptosis)	Diffuse
Other	Keratoconjunctivitis sicca	Interpalpebral
	Psoriasis (rare)	
	Superior limbic keratoconjunctivitis	Upper one third of cornea
	Neurotrophic keratopathy	Interpalpebral
	Toxicity from topical ophthalmic medications	Lower one third of cornea

posits adherent to the corneal surface (Fig. 3-11). They stain with fluorescein and rose bengal. The mechanism of their formation is controversial. Filaments consist of a coil of epithelial cells attached to the cornea at one end, with adherent mucus and other debris. Following is a list of the conditions that should be considered when filamentary keratitis is observed:

1. Superior limbic keratoconjunctivitis
2. Ptosis or lid occlusion in adults
3. Keratoconjunctivitis sicca
4. Neuroparalytic keratopathy
5. Recurrent erosions
6. Corneal trauma
7. Neurotrophic keratopathy
8. Herpes simplex keratitis
9. Chronic bullous keratopathy
10. Toxicity from topical ophthalmic medications

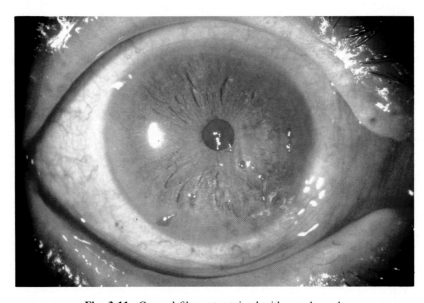

Fig. 3-11. Corneal filaments stained with rose bengal.

Epithelial staining. *Punctate epithelial keratitis* can result from any disease of the corneal epithelium. Some of the more common causes include the following:

GENERAL GROUPING	SPECIFIC DISEASE
Viral	Herpes simplex
	Herpes zoster
	Molluscum contagiosum
	Measles
	Mumps
	Infectious mononucleosis
	Adenoviral disease
	Vaccinia
	Newcastle
Chlamydia	Trachoma
	Inclusion conjunctivitis
Bacterial	Staphylococcal blepharitis
Systemic immune disease	Keratoconjunctivitis sicca
Traumatic and mechanical	Posttraumatic erosion
	Exposure
	Trichiasis
Allergy	Vernal catarrh
Nutritional	Vitamin A deficiency
Toxic	Drug-induced disease
Neurologic	Neurotrophic keratitis
Unknown	Superior limbic keratoconjunctivitis
	Thygeson's superficial punctate keratitis

It may be visible with illumination, or only after instillation of fluorescein or rose bengal. The pattern of the staining, both on the conjunctiva and on the cornea, may be suggestive of an etiology, but often a systematic history and examination are required to determine the cause. Some common staining patterns are illustrated in Fig. 3-12.

Findings Associated with Superficial Epithelial Keratopathy

LID DISEASE	CONJUNCTIVAL LESIONS
Blepharitis	Follicles
Meibomitis	Adenovirus
Lid position abnormalities	Trachoma
Entropion	Molluscum contagiosum
Ectropion	Primary herpes simplex
Lagophthalmos	Herpes zoster
Ichthyosis	Adult chlamydial keratoconjunctivitis
Urbach-Wiethe disease	Drug toxicity
Lid warts	Giant papillae
Molluscum contagiosum	Vernal catarrh
Ulcers or vesicles of lid, as seen in herpes simplex, herpes zoster, vaccinia	Contact lens wear
Psoriasis	Membrane (conjunctival)
	Epidemic keratoconjunctivitis
	Hyperacute conjunctivitis
	Ligneous conjunctivitis
	Stevens-Johnson syndrome
	Scarring of conjunctiva
	Pemphigoid
	Trachoma
	Epidemic keratoconjunctivitis
	Atopic disease
	Lye burns
	Stevens-Johnson syndrome
	Lyell's disease (Ritter) (toxic epidermal necrolysis)

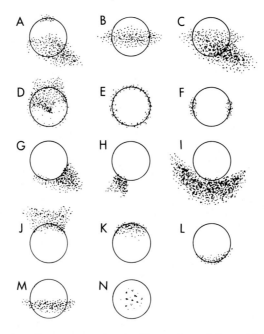

Fig. 3-12. Staining patterns (usually more prominent with rose bengal than with fluorescein) of various conditions. **A,** Drug-induced toxicity or allergy. **B,** Keratoconjunctivitis sicca. **C,** Keratoconjunctivitis sicca with superimposed drug toxicity or allergy. **D,** Contact lens–induced keratoconjunctivitis. **E,** Perilimbal staining in soft contact lens wearer without papillary keratoconjunctival reaction. **F,** Typical hard contact lens–induced staining. **G,** Staining caused by inferonasal gravitation of increased amounts of conjunctival mucus, especially in patients who rub their eyes. **H,** Staining from recent insertion of Schirmer strip. **I,** Factitious (self-induced) conjunctivitis from rubbing or scraping of inferior conjunctiva or from instillation of irritating substance into lower cul-de-sac. **J,** Superior limbic keratoconjunctivitis. **K,** Fine punctate epithelial keratopathy, worse above, of vernal catarrh, "floppy eyelid" syndrome, or early contact lens–induced keratoconjunctivitis. **L,** Staphylococcal blepharokeratoconjunctivitis. **M,** Lagophthalmos. **N,** Focal epithelial keratitis, as caused by adenovirus, molluscum contagiosum, rubeola, inclusion conjunctivitis, or Thygeson's superficial punctate keratitis. (Modified from Wilson FM: Trans Am Ophthalmol Soc 81:854, 1983.)

Characteristic Distributions of Superficial Keratopathy

LOCATION	ETIOLOGIC FACTOR
Lower third	Staphylococcal blepharitis
	Exposure
	Entropion
	Drug toxicity
	Acne rosacea
Interpalpebral	Keratitis sicca
	Neurotrophic keratitis
	Exposure keratitis (lagophthalmos)
	Ultraviolet exposure
	X-ray exposure
Upper third	Trachoma
	Inclusion conjunctivitis
	Superior limbic keratoconjunctivitis
	Vernal catarrh
	Molluscum contagiosum
Central	Epidemic keratoconjunctivitis
	Inclusion conjunctivitis

LOCATION	ETIOLOGIC FACTOR
Diffuse	Verruca vulgaris
	Mumps
	Infectious mononucleosis
	Acute conjunctivitis—bacterial and viral
	Drug toxicity
	Severe vernal
	Keratoconjunctivitis sicca (severe)
	Vitamin A deficiency
	Edema of epithelium
	Contact lens keratopathy
Random	Erosion
	Trichiasis
	Foreign body
	Herpes simplex keratitis

Inferior staining is characteristic of staphylococcal blepharitis, exposure, and rosacea. Interpalpebral staining is characteristic of conditions such as keratoconjunctivitis sicca, medicamentosa, lagophthalmos, neurotrophic keratitis, and ultraviolet exposure. Staining in the superior portion of the cornea usually occurs in vernal catarrh, in superior limbic keratoconjunctivitis, and in the presence of a foreign body in the upper lid. Sectoral staining may occur in conditions such as trichiasis and trauma.

Focal epithelial keratitis is a term that can be used to describe the coarser or grouped epithelial lesions, which may be seen in a number of diseases (Fig. 3-13). These lesions appear like the cytopathologic effect caused by some viruses in culture, and in many cases, represent a similar process occurring in the corneal epithelium. The following diseases cause these lesions:

1. Adenoviral keratoconjunctivitis
2. Thygeson's superficial punctate keratitis
3. Herpes simplex
4. Herpes zoster

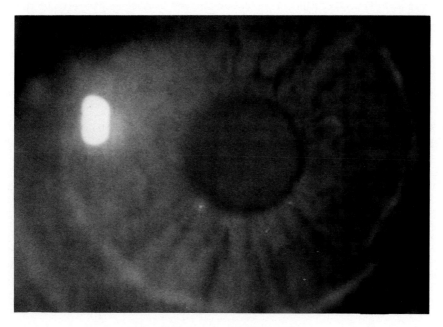

Fig. 3-13. Focal epithelial keratitis.

5. Adult inclusion conjunctivitis
6. Drug toxicity
7. Vaccinia
8. Measles
9. Mumps
10. Varicella

Other characteristic epithelial lesions include the following:

1. Syncitial: Vernal
2. Dendritic: Herpes simplex, herpes zoster, mucoid plaque, healing epithelial defect, tyrosinosis
3. Stellate: Herpes zoster and herpes simplex
4. Linear: Foreign body, trichiasis

Subepithelial nummular opacities. Subepithelial nummular opacities that do not stain can follow active epithelial lesions, or they may occur without clinical epithelial involvement. The following are some of the more common causes:

ETIOLOGIC AGENT	SPECIFIC ENTITY
Viral	Herpes simplex
	Herpes zoster (round irregular)
	Epidemic keratoconjunctivitis
	Acute hemorrhagic conjunctivitis
	Newcastle disease
Unknown	Nummular (Dimmer)
	Padi keratitis
Rare forms	Leprosy (rare)
	Onchocerciasis (more common)
Chlamydia	Trachoma
	Inclusion conjunctivitis (round, as seen in epidemic keratoconjunctivitis)

Sensation. It is important to recognize decreased corneal sensation because it is a pathologic condition of the eye that frequently results in corneal disease and because its presence has etiologic significance. Corneal sensation can be determined qualitatively with a cotton applicator, or quantitatively with an esthesiometer, such as the Cochet-Bonnet[2] (Fig. 3-14). The cornea should be examined with fluorescein before the corneal sensation is tested because this testing may leave punctate staining or even linear staining. One should never touch what appears to be an infected area of the cornea and then touch an uninvolved area of the cornea with the same testing device; always use a separate cotton applicator for each eye when there is infection.

Measurement of corneal sensitivity with the Cochet-Bonnet esthesiometer is performed as follows: With the patient fixating straight ahead, the nylon filament is moved perpendicularly toward the

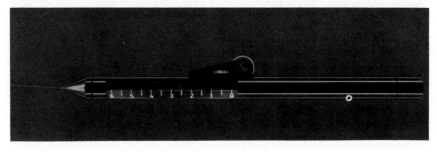

Fig. 3-14. Cochet-Bonnet esthesiometer.

cornea until it hits the cornea and begins to bend. This is repeated with progressively shorter lengths of filament until a response is obtained in 50% of stimulations.

Fifth cranial nerve injury from any cause may decrease corneal sensation, but herpes simplex and herpes zoster infections are probably the most common. A more complete discussion is given in Chapter 15.

Increased visibility of corneal nerves. The corneal nerves may be seen in normal eyes as fine branching white lines that originate at the limbus in the midstroma and become more anterior centrally (Fig. 3-15). The following conditions may be associated with increased visibility of the corneal nerves[3]:

1. Fuchs' dystrophy
2. Keratoconus
3. Neurofibromatosis
4. Refsum's syndrome[4]
5. Ichthyosis
6. Leprosy
7. Congenital glaucoma
8. Failed corneal graft
9. Multiple endocrine neoplasia[5]
10. Use of *Cannabis sativa* (marijuana)[6]
11. Deep filiform dystrophy
12. Aging
13. Ectodermal dysplasia
14. Posterior polymorphous dystrophy
15. Primary amyloidosis
16. Siemen's disease (keratosis follicularis spinulosa decalvans)

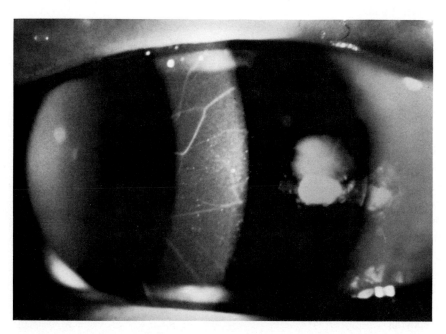

Fig. 3-15. Increased visibility of corneal nerves in multiple endocrine neoplasia type IIb. (Courtesy Richard W. Yee, San Antonio.)

Corneal nerves may become secondarily thickened as a consequence of injury (hyperregeneration). This condition was described by Wolter[7-9] and is seen with trauma, keratoplasty, granulomatous uveitis, congenital glaucoma, retinopathy of prematurity, congenital cataract, intraocular foreign bodies, phthisis bulbi, band keratopathy, and increased age. In these conditions the nerve fibers are irregularly thickened and course irregularly through the stroma into the epithelium.

Inflammation of one or several corneal nerves, with stromal infiltration surrounding them, has been called *radial keratoneuritis* and can be seen in *Acanthamoeba* keratitis (see Fig. 10-15).

Verticillata. Whorllike opacities are occasionally seen in the corneal epithelium and result from accumulation of substances within the corneal epithelium. The vortex pattern (see Fig. 27-11) reflects the growth pattern of the epithelial cells. The oldest cells and those that have undergone the greatest number of divisions are located slightly below the center of the cornea, and the youngest and least divided cells tend to be in highest concentration near the limbus. Therefore materials that progressively accumulate in epithelial cells are seen in highest concentration centrally, and least near the limbus. Many of the drugs associated with this picture exhibit cationic amphiphilia, and it has been hypothesized that: (1) these drugs may penetrate lysosomes and form complexes with polar lipids; and (2) these complexes are unable to pass from the lysosomes or be degraded, resulting in progressive accumulation.[10]

The following have been associated with cornea verticillata[11]:
1. Fabry's disease
2. Amiodarone[12,13]
3. Iron
4. Chloroquine and related drugs (hydroquinone, benoquin)
5. Chlorpromazine
6. Indomethacin[14]
7. Meperidine hydrochloride (Demerol)
8. Quinacrine
9. Tamoxifen
10. Tangier disease
11. Striate melanokeratosis
12. Melkersson-Rosenthal syndrome
13. Tilorone
14. Naproxen[15]
15. Suramin[16]
16. Clofazimine[17]

Crystals. Although uncommon, crystals in the cornea are a striking finding and have great diagnostic significance. Crystals are found in the following conditions:
1. Schnyder's crystalline dystrophy
2. Lecithin cholesterol-acyltransferase deficiency
3. Tangier disease
4. Secondary lipid keratopathy
5. Band keratopathy
6. Cystinosis
7. Tyrosinosis
8. Hyperuricemia (gout)
9. Multiple myeloma and other dysproteinemias (see Fig 19-37)
10. Porphyria
11. Marginal crystalline dystrophy of Bietti
12. Diffenbachia plant (calcium oxalate)[18]

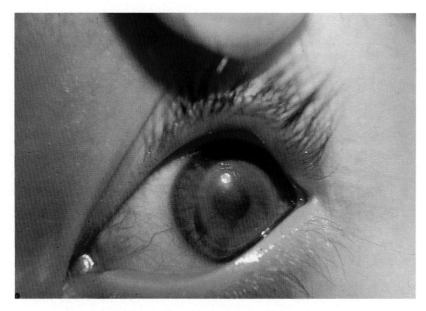

Fig. 3-16. Ring infiltrate. Reaction is similar to Wessely ring.

Ring infiltrates. Partial or complete ring-shaped stromal infiltrates (Fig. 3-16) can be seen in a number of conditions. The classic form of ring infiltration is the Wessely ring reaction, which is seen 10 to 12 days after experimental introduction of antigen into the cornea. The ring, which consists primarily of antigen-antibody complexes, complement, and polymorphonuclear leukocytes, slowly migrates centripetally and diminishes in intensity until the cornea is clear. Occasionally, pannus can result.`

This type of ring infiltrate, presumably also the result of an immunologic response, can be seen in patients with severe corneal burns, corneal foreign bodies, bacterial (especially *Pseudomonas*), herpetic, *Acanthamoeba,* or fungal keratitis, and abuse of topical anesthetic agents.

INTRAOCULAR PRESSURE MEASUREMENT

Applanation tonometry may be inaccurate when there is corneal surface irregularity or astigmatism. Errors in astigmatic corneas are reduced by measuring the pressure with the tonometer mires divided in the axis halfway between the steeper and flatter axes. With marked corneal irregularity a MacKay-Marg tonometer or pneumotonometry (Fig. 3-17) is necessary. I find MacKay-Marg more accurate, but these units are no longer available. Both devices tend to give a higher reading than by applanation, by approximately 4 mm, and can give a minimum reading of 4 to 10 mm, even in the presence of an open eye. Recently a hand-held device, the Tono-Pen* was found to be as accurate as a MacKay-Marg tonometer.[19] These devices can measure intraocular pressure fairly accurately with a soft contact lens in place, as long as it is not an aphakic lens.[20,21]

MEASUREMENT OF CORNEAL THICKNESS

The normal central corneal thickness is 0.52 mm. Any greater thickness indicates endothelial dysfunction. Measurement of corneal thickness is therefore valuable in determining the functional status of the endothelium such as in the following situations: assessing risk of corneal decompensation be-

---

*Bio-Rad, Santa Anna, CA 92705.

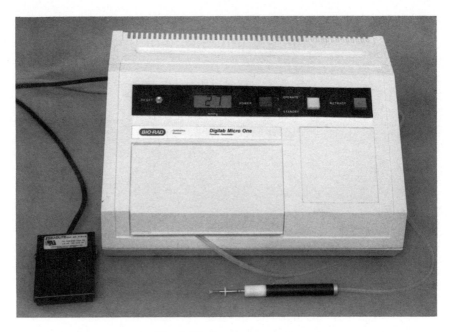

Fig. 3-17. Pneumotonometer.

fore cataract surgery, determining the health of a corneal graft, or guiding treatment of a case of herpetic disciform edema. With practice, fairly accurate corneal thickness measurements can be obtained with an optical pachymeter attached to the slit-lamp microscope (Fig. 3-18). Ultrasonic pachymeters (Fig. 3-19) can give rapid measurements and can more easily yield peripheral thicknesses. When a given cornea is tested with multiple ultrasonic devices, the measurements vary considerably,

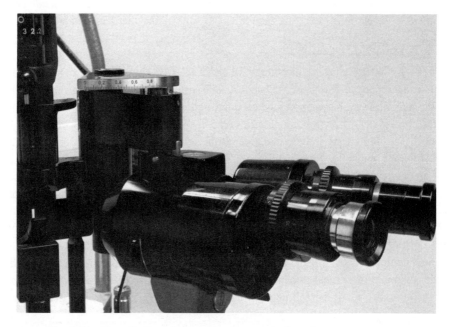

Fig. 3-18. Haag-Streit optical pachymeter attached to slit-lamp microscope.

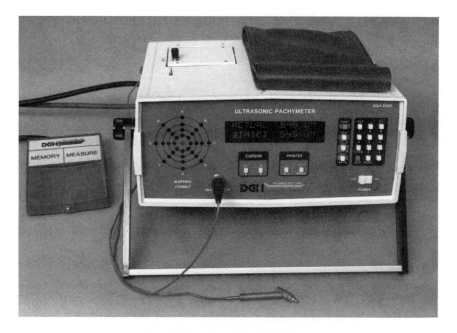

Fig. 3-19. Ultrasonic pachymeter.

but most units are internally consistent.[22] Pachymetry can also be obtained with some specular microscopes.

SPECULAR MICROSCOPY

A specular microscope (Fig. 3-20) permits visualization and photography of the endothelial cell layer. From these photographs endothelial cell density can be estimated. Corneal thickness generally does not begin to increase until there has been considerable loss of endothelial cells; lesser degrees of endothelial cell loss and qualitative changes can be determined by specular microscopy (Fig. 3-21). Repeated endothelial cell counts are useful to assess the effect of different types of injury, such as cataract extraction, vitreous touch, intraocular lens implants, or corneal transplantation. Specular microscopy is used routinely to evaluate donor tissue for suitability for transplantation. It may be useful in assessing the ability of the cornea to withstand intraocular procedures such as cataract surgery or secondary lens implantation.

CORNEAL TOPOGRAPHY

The corneal surface, or more accurately, the air-tear interface, is the most powerful refractive surface of the eye, accounting for approximately two thirds of the eye's total refractive power. The power of the surface is inversely proportional to its radius of curvature. This radius of curvature, which can be determined optically using a keratometer, is used to estimate the refractive power of the cornea. An illuminated ring is placed at a fixed distance from the corneal surface, and the size of the reflected image of the ring is determined by the curvature of the corneal surface. Measurement in different meridians can indicate the axis and amount of corneal astigmatism. Knowledge of the corneal curvature is important in fitting contact lenses, measuring and correcting astigmatism, calculating intraocular lens implant power, and planning and analyzing refractive surgical procedures. The keratometer may also be used to observe corneal surface irregularity.

The keratometer measures the corneal curvature at approximately 1.5 mm from the visual axis. In

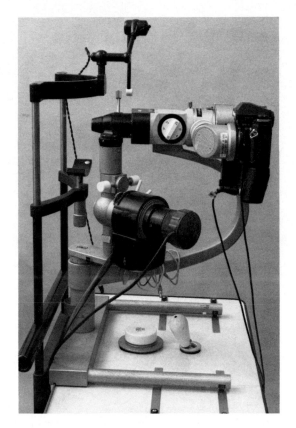

Fig. 3-20. Specular microscope.

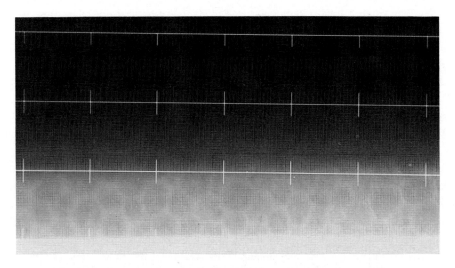

Fig. 3-21. Specular photograph of endothelium showing polymegathism.

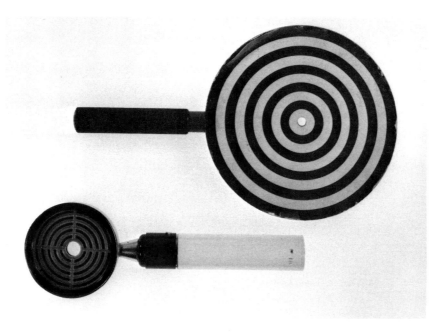

Fig. 3-22. Placido disc devices.

most cases the curvature over the visual axis is fairly uniform, and this single measurement is sufficiently descriptive. However, if the cornea does not have regular astigmatism, with the major axes 90 degrees apart, its accuracy is reduced. Keratometry also provides no information about the shape of the peripheral cornea. Keratoscopy is a means of getting information about the shape of the entire cornea. This method was originally devised by Placido,[23] and the simplest device for obtaining these images is called a Placido disc. A series of concentric illuminated white rings are placed on a disc that is held in front of the cornea (Fig. 3-22). When the examiner looks through the window in the center of the disc, he or she sees the reflections of the rings, and the position, size, and spacing of these rings are determined by the corneal shape. A photokeratoscope permits photography of the reflected images, and several commercial systems are available (Figs. 3-23 and 3-24). From these images quantitative data about the corneal curvature can be obtained by computer analysis,[24] but, to date, these systems have limited distribution.

Photokeratoscopy is useful in diagnosing and staging keratoconus[25-27] and other corneal thinning disorders, guiding suture removal after cataract and corneal transplant surgery,[28] observing and treating corneal astigmatism, and planning and evaluating other refractive procedures.[29-31]

OTHER OCULAR STRUCTURES

It is essential to perform a complete ocular examination even if pathology initially appears to be isolated to the cornea. Of course, other, unrelated diseases can be present. More relevant, however, is the frequent presence of other signs that provide clues to the diagnosis of corneal disorders. For instance, the association of iritis with noninfiltrative stromal and epithelial disease is suggestive of herpes viruses; sectoral iris atrophy suggests herpes zoster; in the presence of corneal decompensation, corectopia, polycoria, and peripheral anterior synechiae suggest the iridocorneal endothelial syndrome; an anterior subcapsular cataract suggests atopic keratoconjunctivitis.

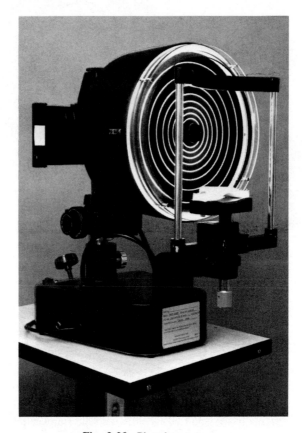

Fig. 3-23. Photokeratoscope.

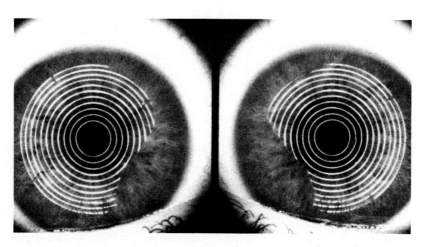

Fig. 3-24. Photokeratoscope picture of normal corneas.

REFERENCES

1. Grant WM: Toxicology of the eye, ed 3, Springfield, Ill, 1986, Charles C Thomas, Publishers.
2. Cochet P and Bonnet R: L'esthesie corneenne, Clin Ophthalmol 4:12, 1960.
3. Mensher JH: Corneal nerves, Surv Ophthalmol 19:1, 1974.
4. Baum JL, Tannenbaum M, and Kolodny EH: Refsum's syndrome with corneal involvement, Am J Ophthalmol 60:699, 1965.
5. Colombo CG and Watson AG: Ophthalmic manifestations of multiple endocrine neoplasia, type three, Can J Ophthalmol 11:290, 1976.
6. Dawson WW: Cannabis and eye function, Invest Ophthalmol 15:243, 1976.
7. Wolter JR: Regeneration and hyper-regeneration of corneal nerves, Ophthalmologica 151:588, 1960.
8. Wolter JR: Hyper-regeneration of corneal nerves in bullous keratopathy, Am J Ophthalmol 58:31, 1964.
9. Wolter JR: Hyper-regeneration of corneal nerves in a scarred transplant, Am J Ophthalmol 61:880, 1966.
10. Lullman H, Lullmann-Rauch R, and Wassermann O: Lipidosis induced by amphiphilic cationic drugs, Biochem Pharmacol 27:1103, 1978.
11. D'Amico DJ and Kenyon KR: Drug-induced lipidoses of the cornea and conjunctiva, Int Ophthalmol 4:67, 1981.
12. Wilson FM, Schmitt TE, and Grayson M: Amiodarone-induced cornea verticillata, Ann Ophthalmol 12:657, 1980.
13. Kaplan LJ and Cappaert WE: Amiodarone keratopathy, Arch Ophthalmol 100:601, 1982.
14. Burns DA: Indomethacin, reduced retinal sensitivity, and corneal deposits, Am J Ophthalmol 66:825, 1968.
15. Szmyd L and Perry HD: Keratopathy associated with the use of naproxen, Am J Ophthalmol 99:598, 1985.
16. Teich SA et al: Toxic keratopathy associated with suramin therapy, N Engl J Med 314:1455, 1986.
17. Walinder PE, Gip L, and Stempa M: Corneal changes in patients treated with clofazimine, Br J Ophthalmol 60:526, 1976.
18. Ellis W, Barfort P, and Mastman GJ: Keratoconjunctivitis with corneal crystals caused by the diffenbachia plant, Am J Ophthalmol 76:143, 1973.
19. Rootman DS et al: Accuracy and precision of the Tono-Pen in measuring intraocular pressure after keratoplasty and epikeratophakia and in scarred corneas, Arch Ophthalmol 106:1697, 1988.
20. Rubenstein JB and Deutsch TA: Pneumotonometry through bandage contact lenses, Arch Ophthalmol 103:1660, 1985.
21. Meyer RF, Stanifer RM, and Bobb KC: MacKay-Marg tonometry over therapeutic soft contact lenses, Am J Ophthalmol 86:19, 1978.
22. Reader A and Salz JJ: Differences among ultrasonic pachymeters in measuring corneal thickness, J Refract Surg 3:7, 1987.
23. Duke-Elder S and Abrahms D: The dioptric imagery of the eye. In Duke-Elder S and Leigh AG: System of Ophthalmology, vol 5, Ophthalmic optics and refraction, St Louis, 1970, Mosby–Year Book, Inc.
24. Klyce SD: Computer-assisted corneal topography: high resolution graphic presentation and analysis of keratoscopy, Invest Ophthalmol Vis Sci 25:1426, 1984.
25. Rowsey JJ, Reynold AE, and Brown R: Corneal topography, Arch Ophthalmol 99:1093, 1981.
26. Maguire LJ and Bourne WD: Corneal topography of early keratoconus, Am J Ophthalmol 108:107, 1989.
27. Rabinowitz YS and McDonnell PJ: Computer-assisted corneal topography in keratoconus, J Refract Corneal Surg 5:400, 1989.
28. Binder PS: Selective suture removal can reduce postkeratoplasty astigmatism, Ophthalmology 92:1412, 1985.
29. Rowsey JJ et al: PERK corneal topography predicts refractive results in radial keratotomy, Ophthalmology 93(suppl):94, 1986.
30. Maguire LJ et al: Corneal topography in myopic patients undergoing epikeratophakia, Am J Ophthalmol 103:404, 1987.
31. Maguire LJ: Corneal topography of patients with excellent Snellen visual acuity after epikeratophakia for aphakia, Am J Ophthalmol 109:162, 1990.

LABORATORY EVALUATION

CYTOLOGY

Cytology is a relatively underused aid in the diagnosis of external ocular disease. In infectious diseases the responsible organisms may frequently be seen, and in many diseases clues may be obtained from the types of inflammatory cells present and from changes in the conjunctival epithelial cells. Cytology is of particular benefit in the diagnosis of allergic diseases, such as hayfever conjunctivitis, atopic keratoconjunctivitis, and vernal conjunctivitis. The presence of eosinophils in a specimen is a fairly specific finding that limits the differential to a few diseases, including those just listed. In conjunctival or corneal infections, isolation and identification of the organism by culture is the primary goal; however, this is not always possible. In some cases, culture of the organism is difficult, such as with chlamydia, syphilis, or mycobacteria, or requires a prolonged period of incubation, as with some fungi. Pretreatment with antibiotics may prevent growth in culture, and cytologic examination of specimens may be the only way to identify the responsible organism. Also, in some cases, such as with *Pseudomonas* keratitis, *N. gonococcus* conjunctivitis, or endophthalmitis, extensive ocular damage may occur before the organism can be identified in culture. Rarely, malignancy may be an unidentified cause of chronic conjunctivitis, and it can be detected with cytology.

TECHNIQUE

Specimens should be taken from the site of most active inflammation. Any portion of the ocular surface can be scraped to yield an adequate specimen. In most cases the conjunctiva will be either uniformly affected, or the inferior fornix will be most involved, so specimens are obtained from the inferior fornix. However, other sites, such as the upper tarsal conjunctiva in trachoma and the limbal conjunctiva in limbal vernal, often yield more information.

Topical anesthesia with proparacaine is usually sufficient, but sometimes greater anesthesia is required for conjunctival specimens. Is those cases a pledget soaked in proparacaine can be applied to the site before scraping. Local application of tetracaine or cocaine also can be used. A platinum spatula, such as a Kimura spatula, is held at 45 degrees to the surface and is passed multiple times in the same direction until sufficient material is obtained. Enough pressure is applied to blanch the conjunctival vessels. If membranes are present, they should be stripped from the area first and placed on a slide, and then the bed should be scraped. For corneal ulcers, all loose material should be removed first, and then the bed scraped. Jeweler's forceps may be helpful in obtaining infected stroma. The sample is smeared on a glass slide that has been cleaned with alcohol. If possible, a 10 mm diameter specimen is obtained. At least two specimens should be obtained, and more if specific stains or tests will be required.

FOLLICULAR EXPRESSION

One may express follicles with the use of ring forceps. This method is valuable in differentiating trachomatous follicles from nontrachomatous ones. Trachoma follicles are soft, probably as a result of the necrotizing effect of the chlamydial organism, and express easily. They contain lymphocytes, plasma cells, monocytes, macrophages, and Leber cells.

EXUDATE SMEAR

An exudate smear is easier to obtain but does not provide as much information as a scraping. It requires only removing the exudate present on the lid margin or within the conjunctival sac with a glass rod or the wooden end of an applicator stick and smearing it onto a microscope slide.

The exudate smear contains only cells that have been sloughed from the conjunctiva, such as

TABLE 4-1. Stains for Corneal and Conjunctival Cytology

STAIN	TIME	USES	COMMENTS
Gram stain	10 min	Bacteria, yeasts	Differentiates gram-positive and gram-negative bacteria
Giemsa (Fig. 10-2)	45-60 min	Cytology, fungi, chlamydial inclusions, bacteria (all stain blue)	Does not reveal intranuclear inclusions
Wright	15 min	Cytology, especially hematologic	Not as good as Giemsa for cytology
PAP	30 min	Tumor cells, inclusions	Relatively complicated
PAS (periodic acid-Schiff) (Fig. 10-8)	25 min	Fungi	
Calcofluor white (Fig. 4-1)	1 min	Fungi,[1,2] *Acanthamoeba*[7]	Requires fluorescence microscope; may be difficult to interpret
Acridine orange (Fig. 4-2)	1 min	Fungi, bacteria, *Acanthamoeba*	Requires fluorescence microscope
Methenamine silver[5] (Fig. 4-3)	1-2 hr	Fungi	Relatively complicated; gelatin-coated slides for modified technique
Potassium hydroxide (KOH)/ Ink-KOH[2,6] (Fig. 4-4)	5 min-12 hr	Fungi	Difficult to read early
Acid fast (Ziehl-Nielsen)	10 min	Mycobacteria, *Nocardia, Actinomyces*	

aged or keratinized epithelial cells, inflammatory cells, and occasionally organisms. This technique is especially good for demonstrating eosinophils; occasionally, one may find eosinophils in an exudate smear when they are not seen in a scraping.

STAINING

A great number of stains are available for examination of specimens, but in most cases Gram and/or Giemsa stains are used. Gram stain is used to identify bacteria, and Giemsa is used for cellular

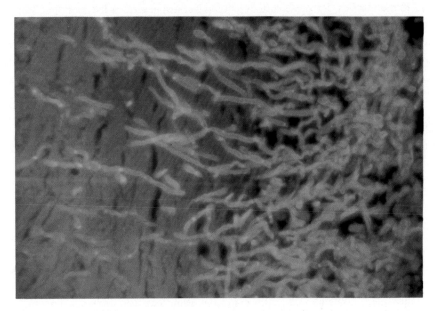

Fig. 4-1. Fungal keratitis stained with calcofluor white.

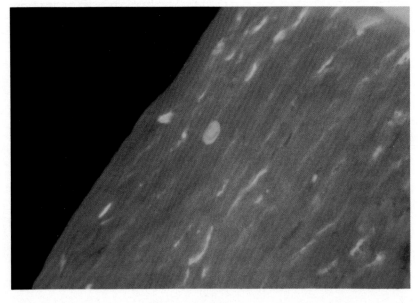

Fig. 4-2. *Acanthamoeba* cyst (orange) stained with acridine orange. (Courtesy Regis P. Kowalski, Pittsburgh.)

identification and morphology, fungi, and chlamydial inclusions. These and other commonly used stains are described in Table 4-1.

Calcofluor white[1,2,7,8] and acridine orange[3,4,9] have been used with increasing frequency, particularly for detection of *Acanthamoeba* and fungi (Figs. 4-1 and 4-2). These organisms can be easily missed with other stains, both in cytology and histologic sections. Both stains require fluorescence microscopy, but are very rapid and easy to perform.

Recently immunologically based methods have been developed for identification of organisms in scrapings. These are described in a separate section.

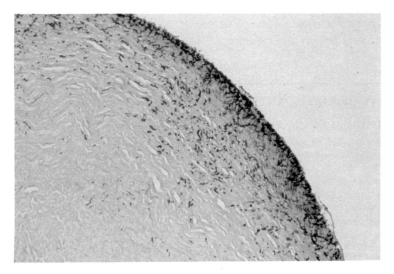

Fig. 4-3. Actinomyces keratitis stained with methenamine silver. (Courtesy Michael W. Belin, Albany, NY.)

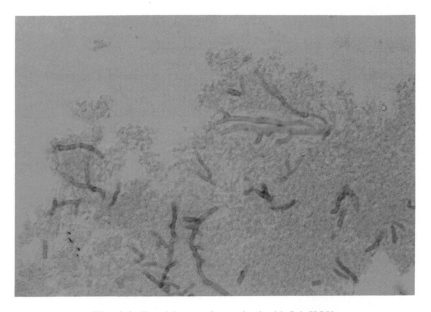

Fig. 4-4. Fungi in scraping stained with Ink-KOH.

CELLS

The important types of cells seen and their significance are described in this section.[10] Unless otherwise indicated, the cells are described as they appear with Giemsa stain. The conditions associated with various cell types are summarized in the box below.

Normal conjunctival epithelium. With scraping of a normal conjunctiva epithelial cells come off in sheets. The cells have large central nuclei, which are oval and uniform in size and may have prominent nucleoli (Fig. 4-5). With Giemsa stain, the nuclei are dark blue to purple, and the cytoplasm is pale blue and slightly granular. The nucleus to cytoplasm ratio is approximately 1:2. Keratin is not normally visible in the cytoplasm.

Keratinization and pyknosis of epithelial cells. Epithelial cells become keratinized with exposure, drying, or mechanical trauma. It also occurs with conjunctival scarring, as in cicatricial pemphigoid, erythema multiforme, trachoma, vitamin A deficiency, superior limbic keratitis, and after irradiation. Keratinization is identified by the presence of faint red granules in the cytoplasm and increasing

---

CYTOLOGY OF CONJUNCTIVAL SCRAPINGS

POLYMORPHONUCLEAR CELLS

Bacterial infection, except *Moraxella*
   and *Branhamella catarrhalis*
Fungal infection
Chlamydial infection
Membranous conjunctivitis (any cause)
Necrosis of conjunctiva (any cause)
Staphylococcal conjunctival phlyctenulosis

**MONONUCLEAR CELLS
(LYMPHOCYTES)**

Viral infection
Thyroid conjunctival hyperemia

**MIXED, POLYMORPHONUCLEAR
PREDOMINATE**

Chlamydial infection, chronic
Most cases of chronic conjunctivitis
Catarrhal ulcers
Superior limbic keratoconjunctivitis
Pemphigoid
Erythema multiforme
Reiter's syndrome
Acne rosacea
Chemical burns
Some drug reactions

MIXED, LYMPHOCYTES PREDOMINATE

Early viral infections
Viral infections with membranes
Most drug reactions
Keratoconjunctivitis sicca
Tuberculous conjunctivitis
Luetic conjunctivitis

BASOPHILS

Trachoma
Vernal catarrh
Chronic conjunctivitis

EOSINOPHILS

Vernal catarrh
Atopic keratoconjunctivitis
Hayfever conjunctivitis
Occasionally in drug allergies
Erythema multiforme
Pemphigoid

PLASMA CELLS

Trachoma

KERATINIZED EPITHELIAL CELLS

Keratoconjunctivitis sicca
Pemphigoid
Chemical burns
Erythema multiforme
Superior limbic keratoconjunctivitis
Squamous metaplasia
Vitamin A deficiency
Trachoma
Radiation
Severe membranous conjunctivitis
Some drug reactions

GOBLET CELLS

Keratoconjunctivitis sicca
Chronic conjunctivitis

MULTINUCLEATED EPITHELIAL CELLS

Herpes simplex infection
Varicella-zoster infection
Chlamydial infection
Measles
Cytomegalovirus infection
Newcastle virus conjunctivitis
Squamous neoplasia
Radiation

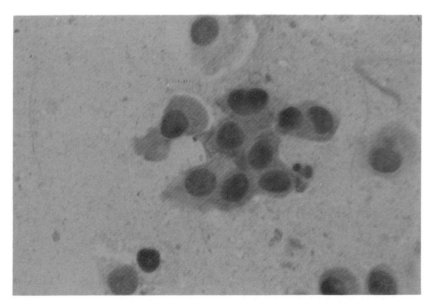

Fig. 4-5. Scraping containing normal conjunctival epithelium (Giemsa). (Courtesy Regis P. Kowalski, Pittsburgh.)

eosinophilia of the cytoplasm. With increasing cellular injury and degeneration the cell becomes pyknotic. The cytoplasm and nucleus shrink and become increasingly basophilic, and eventually the nucleus is lost (Fig. 4-6).

Leukocytes. The polymorphonuclear leukocyte (PMN) is the most common inflammatory cell in ocular specimens. The nucleus is segmented into two to five portions and is basophilic. The cytoplasm may stain pink or blue and may contain bluish granules.

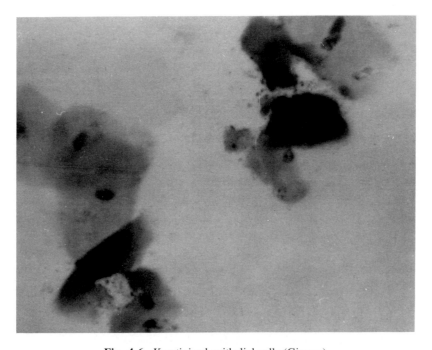

Fig. 4-6. Keratinized epithelial cells (Giemsa).

All bacterial infections except those caused by *Branhamella catarrhalis* and *Moraxella* evoke a polymorphonuclear response. PMNs also are seen in the presence of membranes or necrosis of the conjunctiva, whatever the cause. They are also prominent in trachoma, inclusion conjunctivitis, lymphogranuloma venereum, psittacosis, Reiter's syndrome, psoriasis, erythema multiforme, and drug toxicity. Phlyctenulosis of the conjunctiva characteristically shows little exudate unless it is caused by staphylococci, in which case PMNs will be the predominant cell.

The intensity of the polymorphonuclear response may vary according to the stage of the disease. For example, in acute gonococcal conjunctivitis an intense PMN response occurs, with marked fibrin formation, but in later stages, while the PMNs continue to predominate, there is an increased number of mononuclear cells. In very early viral conjunctivitis PMNs may predominate. In general, in chronic infections PMNs will predominate, with mononuclear cells present in a moderate amount. The exception is staphylococcal conjunctivitis, in which the PMNs are present in marked numbers, even in chronic conjunctivitis.

Lymphocytes are smaller cells, with a nonsegmented, dark staining nucleus and scant bluish cytoplasm (Fig. 4-7). They are the predominant cells in viral conjunctivitis. They also are common in chronic conjunctivitis, chlamydial infections, and hypersensitivity diseases; but PMNs are usually more plentiful. Rarely, they may be the predominant cells in tuberculosis, syphilis, and trachoma.

Monocytes are larger mononuclear cells, with a folded, kidney-bean shaped nucleus, and abundant cytoplasm. Like lymphocytes, they are usually found in viral infections.

Plasma cells are lymphocytes actively producing antibody. They have an eccentric dark nucleus, with a cartwheel chromatin pattern (Fig. 4-7). There is a clear halo adjacent to the nucleus and an eccentric, basophilic cytoplasm. Although these are prominent subepithelially in many types of conjunctivitis and associated with immune-mediated disorders, they rarely are present in scrapings. They are found in trachoma because in this condition the follicles readily rupture with scraping and plasma cells are released.

Eosinophils are never seen in a scraping from a normal eye. They are leukocytes with bilobed nuclei and pink granules in the cytoplasm (Fig. 4-8). The cells are quite fragile, and frequently only

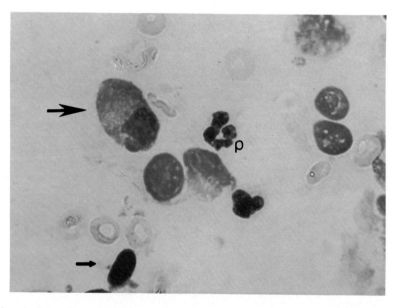

Fig. 4-7. Conjunctival scraping containing mononuclear cell *(small arrow)*, polymorphonuclear cell *(P)*, and plasma cell *(large arrow)* (Giemsa). (Courtesy Regis P. Kowalski, Pittsburgh.)

broken cell remnants and free granules are observed. Eosinophils usually indicate allergic inflammation—hayfever, atopic dermatitis, or vernal conjunctivitis. A few eosinophils are seen in drug and cosmetic allergies, except for phospholine iodide or pilocarpine sensitivity. Eosinophils also may be observed in ocular cicatricial pemphigoid.

Basophils (mast cells) are small bluish cells that contain large, dark blue cytoplasmic granules (Fig. 4-9). They are also seen in allergic disorders, particularly vernal conjunctivitis. Small numbers of basophils may be present in trachoma.

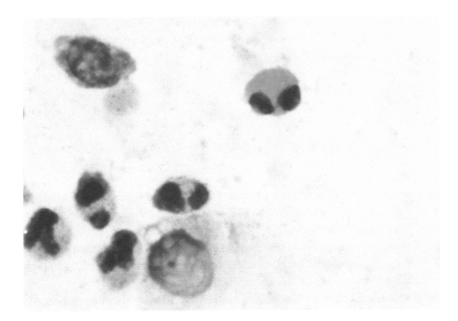

Fig. 4-8. Conjunctival scraping reveals eosinophils in case of cicatricial pemphigoid (Giemsa).

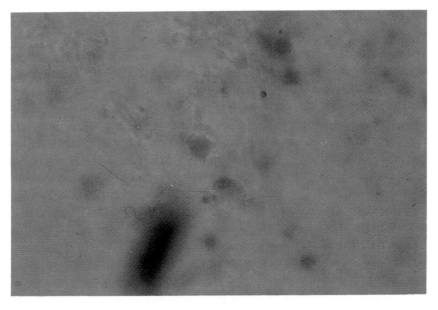

Fig. 4-9. Mast cells (Unna's stain; ×1000).

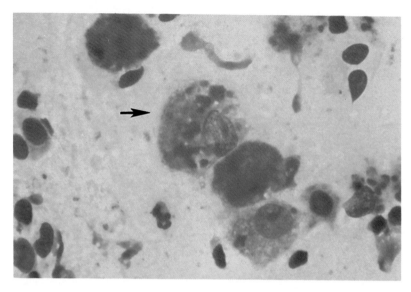

Fig. 4-10. Leber cell *(arrow)* (Giemsa). (Courtesy Regis P. Kowalski, Pittsburgh.)

Leber cells are merely very large macrophages. They are often several times the size of epithelial cells and contain phagocytized cellular debris (Fig. 4-10). They are more numerous in trachoma but may be seen in other types of conjunctivitis.

Goblet cells. Goblet cells contain a large, pink-staining mass of mucoid material. The nucleus is pushed aside to the cell wall and is purple. Goblet cells may be observed in scrapings from normal eyes and are increased in scrapings in keratoconjunctivitis sicca.

Multinucleated epithelial cells. Multinucleated epithelial cells may result from either failure of the nucleus to completely divide during mitosis or fusion of several cells. In the former case, they tend to be close to normal size and are seen in many forms of conjunctival inflammation, including viral and chlamydial infections, allergy, and after irradiation. Fusion of multiple cells produces giant cells, which contain 5 to 20 nuclei. These are seen only in herpetic infections, simplex or zoster (see Fig. 12-20). Tumor cells also may be multinucleated, but these usually exhibit other abnormal characteristics, as described later.

Epithelial cell inclusions. Epithelial cell inclusions occur in viral and chlamydial infections and can be diagnostic. The types of inclusions seen in external ocular infections are listed in Table 4-2. Viral inclusions are best demonstrated with PAP staining, and even then can be difficult to appreciate. Inclusions in molluscum contagiosum are readily appreciated with hematoxylin and eosin staining of specimens from skin lesions. They appear as eosinophilic cytoplasmic masses (Fig. 4-11).

The inclusions of trachoma and inclusion conjunctivitis are readily identifiable with Giemsa staining. The classic chlamydial inclusion, Halberstaedter-Prowazek, is seen as a mass of basophilic granules capping the nucleus (see Fig. 8-3). It is composed of elementary bodies, the infectious form of the organism, containing DNA. Individual elementary bodies may also be seen as uniform, round, reddish-blue or purple granules, 0.3 μm in size, in epithelial cells, PMNs, or extracellularly. These swell to 1 μm, or about the size of a staphylococcus, when they enter an epithelial cell and produce RNA, after which they are called reticulate or initial bodies.

Melanin granules, 0.3 to 1.0 μm, may be seen within epithelial cells. They are deep brown in an unstained slide and greenish-black after Giemsa staining. Mascara may also be seen as pigmented granules within epithelial cells. Nuclear debris may be phagocytosed by epithelial cells, and this stains a uniform dark blue, with a clear circumscribed border.

TABLE 4-2. Viral and Chlamydial Inclusions

DISEASE	LOCATION		STAINING (GIEMSA)		IODINE STAIN
	CYTOPLASMIC	NUCLEAR	EOSINOPHILIC	BASOPHILIC	
Herpes simplex (Cowdry's type A)	−	+	+	−	
Varicella-zoster (Lipschütz)	−	+	+	−	
Variola (Guarnieri)	+	+	+	−	
Vaccinia (Guarnieri)	+	−	+	−	
Newcastle	+	−	+	−	
Molluscum (Henderson-Paterson)	+	−	+	−	
Adenovirus	−	+	+(early)	+(late)	
Trachoma	+	−	−	+	+
Inclusion conjunctivitis (Halberstaedter-Prowazek)	+	−	−	+	+
Lymphogranuloma venereum	+	−	−	+	−
Psittacosis	+	−	−	+	−

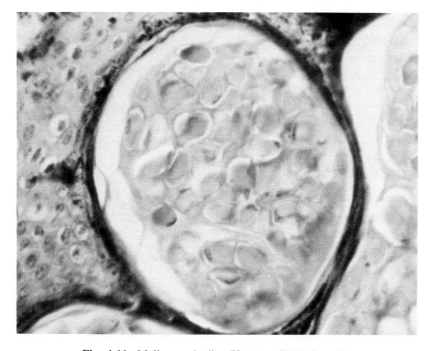

Fig. 4-11. Molluscum bodies (Hematoxylin-eosin stain).

Tumor cells. Several morphologic abnormalities are suggestive of neoplasia (Fig. 4-12):
1. Increased nucleus to cytoplasm ratio
2. Increase in chromatin content, producing hyperchromasia (may also be seen in pyknosis or if the slide is overstained)
3. Aberrant chromatin pattern, with elongation and irregularity in outline
4. Enlarged nucleoli, or an increase in number (usually four or more)
5. Increased mitotic figures and abnormal mitotic figures

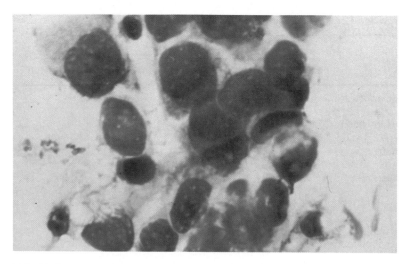

Fig. 4-12. Malignant cells in scraping (Giemsa). (Courtesy Regis P. Kowalski, Pittsburgh.)

6. Multinucleated cells, with associated nuclear changes
7. Bizarre cell shapes
8. Irregularity of cells, variable cell size, and lack of distinct cell boundaries

PAP stain is preferable for evaluation of these characteristics in cytology specimens. However, if tumor is suspected, a biopsy should be performed; cytology alone is not sufficient for diagnosis.

ORGANISMS

The Gram stain characteristics of the most common ocular pathogens are as follows:

BACTERIA	DISTINGUISHING CHARACTERISTICS
GRAM-POSITIVE COCCI	
Staphylococci	Irregular groups or clusters of spheres that may vary in size and staining qualities
Streptococcus pneumoniae	Lancet-shaped diplococci; may see capsule
Other streptococci	Usually oval or elliptic cocci; often in chains
Micrococci	Usually in tetrads
Peptostreptococcus	May occur in pairs or chains
Peptococcus	
GRAM-POSITIVE RODS*	
Corynebacteria	Club-shaped bacillus, often with barred metachromatic granules or terminal masses at the poles
Propionibacterium	Pleomorphic
Clostridia	Slender, motile rod
GRAM-POSITIVE FILAMENTS	
Actinomyces	Intertwining, branching filaments with or without clubs and diphtheroid forms
Nocardia	Intertwining, branching filaments without terminal clubs
GRAM-NEGATIVE RODS	
Pseudomonas aeruginosa	Slender, motile rod with straight parallel sides and curved ends
Klebsiella pneumoniae	Short, fat rod with capsule, often diplobacilli
Bacteroides	Thin, filamentous rods
Haemophilus influenzae	Small coccobacillary rods, may have capsules

*Gram-positive rods and gram-negative cocci are relatively uncommon, and incorrect staining should be suspected.

BACTERIA	DISTINGUISHING CHARACTERISTICS
Moraxella	Diplobacilli, plump rods arranged end-to-end; polar staining, round or rectangular ends; largest of the gram-negative rods
Escherichia coli	Rods without distinguishing characteristics
Proteus	
Serratia	
Citrobacter	
Enterobacter	
Azotobacter	
Acinetobacter	
GRAM-NEGATIVE COCCI*	
Neisseria	Kidney-shaped diplococci; often intracellular; may not decolorize well after antibiotic exposure

*Gram-positive rods and gram-negative cocci are relatively uncommon, and incorrect staining should be suspected.

CULTURE

Diagnosis and appropriate treatment of conjunctival and corneal infections require isolation and identification of the causative organism(s).

MEDIA

Different media must be used because of the varying requirements of ocular pathogens. The commonly used media are described in Table 4-3. Eye cultures should be directly inoculated onto the culture media, rather than into a carrier, because the sample size is small, and many eye pathogens are fastidious organisms.

Mannitol-salt agar plates are helpful to the microbiologist in preliminary identification of staphylococci. Nearly all *S. aureus* isolates will ferment mannitol, whereas many nonaureus species will

TABLE 4-3. Common Media

MEDIA	ORGANISMS	COMMENTS
Blood agar (5% sheep's blood)	Majority of aerobic bacteria; saprophytic fungi	Room temperature for fungi
Chocolate agar	*Haemophilus, Neisseria, Moraxella*	5%-10% CO_2
Sabouraud dextrose agar	Fungi	room temperature
Mannitol-salt agar	Staphylococci, diphtheroids, *Proteus*	37° C air
Thayer-Martin	*Neisseria*	10% CO_2
Lowenstein-Jensen	Mycobacteria, *Nocardia*	
Middlebrook-Cohn	Mycobacteria, *Nocardia*	
E. Coli seeded agar (non-nutrient agar with *E. coli* overlay)	*Acanthamoeba*	
CDC anaerobic blood agar	Bacterial anaerobes	Incubate in anaerobic chamber
Enriched thioglycollate broth	Aerobic and anaerobic bacteria	Better than blood agar for anaerobes and small inoculums
Brain-heart infusion (BHI)	Bacteria, fungi	Fastidious organisms
Chopped meat-glucose	Anaerobes, part. *Clostridia*	
Loeffler's	*C. diptheria*	

not. Therefore only mannitol-positive isolates are tested for coagulase or protein-A, for identification of *S. aureus,* which saves time and expense.

Blood agar, mannitol-salt agar, and chocolate agar are normally used for lid and conjunctival cultures. If a specific organism is suspected, other media may be necessary.

In general, two blood agar plates and one each of chocolate agar, mannitol-salt agar, Sabouraud dextrose agar, and enriched thioglycollate broth are inoculated for corneal ulcers. One blood agar plate and the chocolate agar are incubated in 5% CO_2 at 37° C, and the mannitol-salt plate and enriched thioglycollate broth are incubated in air at 37° C. Another blood agar and the Sabouraud plate are left at room temperature. If another organism is suspected, or if an infection is not responding to therapy, other media are used.

Chlamydial and viral isolation is more difficult, more expensive, and not as widely available as bacterial cultures. However, if available, they can be useful in some patients. For viral and chlamydial cultures, transport media are required. The viral transport media may not be usable for chlamydia because they often contain antibiotics that inhibit their growth. Chlamydial media, however, can be used for both viral and chlamydial transport.

Chlamydiae are normally grown in cultures of cycloheximide-treated McCoy cells. After inoculation with a specimen, the culture is incubated for 48 to 72 hours, and then examined for cytoplasmic inclusions using Giemsa stain. This can be facilitated by use of fluorescein-tagged monoclonal antibodies to the chlamydia.[11]

Viruses also must be grown in cell cultures. A large number of cell lines are available for different viruses. Currently in our laboratory cell line A549, a human lung carcinoma cell line, is used because it supports growth of herpes simplex, herpes zoster, adenoviruses, and cytomegalovirus, as well as other, less common ocular pathogens. The tissue cultures must be examined several times per week for up to 4 weeks for evidence of cellular damage due to viral reproduction (cytopathic effect). Once growth is observed, the causative virus must be identified by other means.

TECHNIQUE

Conjunctiva and lids. Anesthesia with topical proparacaine is sufficient. A cotton-tipped or calcium alginate swab is used. These swabs should be moistened with a broth, such as Mueller-Hinton or trypticase soy, or sterile saline because doing so increases the recovery of organisms. For lid cultures the anterior margins of the upper and lower lids are swabbed several times. The swab is then rolled onto the media. There is no need to culture the upper and lower lids on separate media.

Conjunctival cultures are usually obtained from the tarsal surface of the lower lid. The patient is told to look up, the lower lid is pulled down, and a moistened applicator is used to swab back and forth over the tarsal conjunctiva.

Both eyes are routinely cultured, even if only one is affected. It is convenient and economical to use only one plate for lid and conjunctival cultures from both eyes. A patterned inoculation (Fig. 4-13) facilitates this procedure. For viral cultures a sterile plastic-handled cotton or Dacron swab (calcium alginate should not be used, since it binds and inactivates some viruses[12]) should be moistened with the viral transport medium and rubbed against the superior and inferior tarsal conjunctiva. The tip of the swab is then broken off and placed in the transport medium. Rose bengal should not be applied before obtaining viral cultures because it markedly reduces viral titers.[13]

Cornea. Corneal cultures are best obtained with the aid of a slit-lamp or operating microscope. Proparacaine should be used for anesthesia because cocaine and tetracaine are more bactericidal. A flamed and cooled platinum spatula is used to scrape the leading edge and bed of the ulcer. If loose material is present on the surface, it should be removed first and placed on a slide. A jeweler's forceps or hypodermic needle can sometimes yield a better specimen, particularly for smaller lesions. The specimens are first applied to microscope slides for examination. As discussed earlier, at least

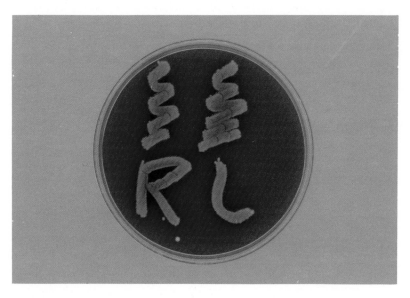

Fig. 4-13. Patterned inoculation of lid and conjunctival specimens (*R* and *L* indicate right and left lid cultures, respectively; conjunctival specimen is placed above ipsilateral lid specimen).

two slides should be prepared, and they should be cleaned and dried before use. Multiple areas of a large ulcer should be scraped. The spatula is flamed and cooled again, and the media are inoculated. Each scraping should be used to inoculate one medium; multiple C streaks are used on the agar plates.

For viral cultures of corneal lesions it is best to scrape the lesion and transfer the material to a cotton swab, which is then placed in the transport medium.

INTERPRETATION

The growth of aerobic bacteria from conjunctiva or cornea usually becomes apparent on standard media within 48 hours and often is evident after only 12 hours. A sample can be taken and examined with Gram stain to give a preliminary identification.

It is often difficult to tell whether an organism in culture is responsible for ocular infection. One aid is that any organism growing outside the C streaks on solid media should be considered a contaminant. Some criteria have been recommended for distinguishing pathogens from nonpathogens. First, clinical signs of infection should be present. Then, according to Liesegang and Forster,[6] one of the following must be present: (1) growth of an organism in two or more media, (2) confluent growth of a known ocular pathogen in one solid medium, or (3) growth in one medium of an organism identified in cytology. Jones[14] recommended that 10 or more colonies of bacterial growth should be present on one solid medium, and that for fungi any detectable growth on any two media or growth on one medium with positive cytology is sufficient.

These recommendations have limitations, however, because often only one medium is suitable for a pathogen and only a few viable organisms of a pathogen may be obtained. Therefore clinical judgment must often be used. One should consider the likelihood of an organism to be a pathogen, the likelihood of it producing the observed clinical picture, and the relative risk of treatment versus not treating a pathogen. Bacterial and fungal organisms present in normal conjunctiva and their approximate incidence are as follows[15-21]:

Bacterial and Fungal Organisms in Normal Conjunctiva

ORGANISM	INCIDENCE (%)
S. epidermidis	75-90
Propionibacteria	80
Diphtheroids	35-55
S. aureus	5-20
Alpha-hemolytic streptococci	2-7
Pseudomonas	0-6
H. influenzae	1.5-3
S. pneumoniae	1-4
Other gram-negative rods	4-7
Total fungi*	10-20
Aspergillus	1-7
Candida	0.5-3

*Higher rate of positive fungal cultures in warmer climates, for example, Phillipines and India.

Many organisms that are commensals under some circumstances or in some individuals can produce serious disease in other individuals or under different conditions.

BIOPSY

INDICATIONS

Conjunctiva. Tissue specimens are often valuable in the diagnosis of ocular and systemic disease. The most obvious indication for biopsy is when there is a question of malignancy. Because conjunctival malignancies may be subtle, a biopsy should be considered in any case of chronic conjunctivitis of undetermined etiology. Sarcoid commonly produces conjunctival granulomas, and a biopsy of suspicious lesions may prove diagnostic and prevent more invasive procedures. Several infectious diseases, including tuberculosis, leprosy, and syphilis, can produce conjunctival granulomas, sometimes in association with visible enlargement of preauricular nodes (that is, Parinaud's oculoglandular syndrome—see Chapter 7). The causative organisms can often be identified in conjunctival biopsy specimens.

The following dermatologic diseases affect the conjunctiva and may be diagnosed from conjunctival biopsies:

Dermatologic Diseases and Immunopathologic Findings

DISEASE	IMMUNOPATHOLOGIC FINDINGS
Cicatricial pemphigoid	Antibody deposited on epithelial BM: IgG, IgA, IgM, complement[22-27] Increased epithelial mitotic rate[28]
Erythema multiforme	C3, IgM, fibrin in vessel walls[29]
Epidermolysis bullosa acquisita*	IgG, IgA, IgM, complement deposits in epithelial BM[30-33]
Pemphigus vulgaris	Epithelial intercellular IgG, IgA, IgM, complement[34]
Adult linear IgA disease	Linear deposits of IgA, IgG along epithelial BM[35]
Toxic epidermal necrolysis	Intercellular IgG, IgM, C3[27]
Molluscum contagiosum	Eosinophilic cytoplasmic inclusions

*Immunopathologic changes demonstrated in skin and conjunctival involvement are common, but immunopathologic examination of conjunctiva has not been reported.

In most cases, diagnosis requires immunopathologic examination for antibodies or complement components.

The following lists some of the many metabolic diseases that exhibit characteristic changes in the conjunctiva[36,37]:

Metabolic Diseases

DISEASE	FINDINGS
Cystinosis	Intracellular crystals[38,39]
Oxalosis	Crystals
Primary familial amyloidosis (rarely secondary systemic)	Amyloid[40]
Fabry's disease	Intracytoplasmic lamellar inclusions[41-43]
Mucolipidoses	Vacuolization of epithelium; intracytoplasmic lamellar or fibrillogranular inclusions[44-49]
Mucopolysaccharidoses	Intracytoplasmic accumulation of acid mucopolysaccharide[50-52]
Tyrosinemia, type II	Intracytoplasmic whorled membranous inclusions[53]
Fucosidosis	Intracytoplasmic multilaminate inclusions in epithelium[54,55]

Conjunctival goblet cell content and mitotic rate may be useful in ocular surface diseases such as cicatricial pemphigoid (CP), vitamin A deficiency, erythema multiforme, and keratoconjunctivitis sicca. In each of these diseases there is loss of goblet cells. In CP, vitamin A deficiency, and atopic dermatitis, an increase in the normal mitotic rate of the conjunctival epithelium has been observed.[28,56] In contrast to the other diseases, increased goblet cell density is found in atopic dermatitis.[57]

Cornea. Corneal stromal biopsies are not often performed because of their destructive effect. However, if an unidentified destructive corneal process is progressing despite current treatment, biopsy is indicated to attempt to make the diagnosis. Obviously, reluctance to remove tissue is much greater when the process involves the visual axis, but biopsy is still indicated in some cases. For example, infections due to fungi,[58] acanthamoeba,[59,60] and atypical mycobacteria[61] have been diagnosed by biopsy when cultures and scrapings did not reveal the organism.

TECHNIQUE

It is often best to check with the pathologist to determine the optimum handling and fixation method before obtaining a specimen. These procedures vary greatly depending on the studies required.

Conjunctiva. Sufficient anesthesia usually can be obtained with a proparacaine-soaked pledget held against the biopsy site. The specimen should be handled as little as possible because crushing the tissue prevents histologic analysis. One edge of the area is picked up with toothed forceps, tenting the tissue, and Wescott scissors are used to snip off a specimen. Multiple pieces may be obtained; if they are from different areas, they should be fixed and labeled individually. If malignancy is suspected, a map of the lesion and location of biopsies should be made.

Cornea. Limited biopsies may be performed at the slit-lamp microscope with a sharp blade and jeweler's forceps. Topical anesthesia is administered, and the lids are held open manually or with a speculum. At the base of the ulcer a piece of infiltrated tissue is grasped and cut free with the blade. Several small pieces can be removed for culture and staining.

If these procedures are insufficient, or if no ulceration is present, lamellar keratectomy is required. Keratectomy must be performed in the operating room and involves removal of a 2 to 5 mm diameter section, one third to one half of stromal depth.[62]

FIXATION

Most specimens will be examined only histologically with light microscopy and can be fixed in 10% formalin. These small specimens tend to curl up in solution, so it is best to lay them flat on a carrier before placing them in the formalin. A wet cellulose sponge or a tongue blade may be used for this purpose. Some have recommended dried cucumber slices, to which the biopsy specimen is attached by albumin fixative.[63,64]

Several diseases are characterized by the presence of crystal in the conjunctiva, and in two of the diseases, cystinosis and oxalosis, the crystals are soluble in formalin. (Also, in advanced gout crystals may be found in the subcutaneous tissue of the lids, and these crystals are also soluble in formalin.) Therefore if a biopsy is performed for diagnosis of one of these diseases the tissue should be fixed in absolute alcohol.

Tissues on which immunopathologic examination is planned should be placed in a Petri dish, with a small amount of saline solution. They must be fresh-frozen in a special mounting medium, such as optimal cutting temperature (OCT), a procedure that should be performed by the laboratory. For electron microscopy, glutaraldehyde solutions are recommended.

IMMUNOPATHOLOGIC TESTS

Many tests have been developed to detect specific antigens in specimens using monoclonal antibodies. These tests are becoming more widely available, more specific, and easier to perform. Commercial tests are now available for detection of a number of ocular pathogens, particularly viruses and chlamydia (described in sections on specific pathogens). A specific antibody is allowed to react with the specimen, and detection of antibody attachment is accomplished by one of several methods. Immunoperoxidase techniques are probably most common today. The monoclonal antibody is labeled with peroxidase, and the presence of the enzyme is detected by its reaction with chromogens, which can be observed with light microscopy. Another common method is by fluorescence; the monoclonal antibody is labeled with fluorescein, and with a fluorescence microscope the amount and location of antibody binding is determined.

Serologic tests are also available for most viruses and for chlamydia. Patient antibodies against an agent can be detected and quantified. Single measurements of titers may be useful, but usually both acute and convalescent titers are required to make the diagnosis of an acute infection. Obviously, this method is not useful in recurrent or long-standing disease.

DERMATOLOGIC DISORDERS

As mentioned previously, immunopathologic techniques help diagnose a number of dermatologic disorders associated with conjunctival scarring (see columnar material on p. 76).

LYMPHOID LESIONS

Immunopathologic techniques have been used to distinguish reactive lymphoid hyperplasia from lymphoma and to classify lymphomas. Light chain monoclonality suggests lymphoma, whereas polyclonality suggests lymphoid hyperplasia.[65] Knowles et al.[66] presents a good review of the characterization of lymphoid tumors.

INFECTIOUS DISEASES

Chlamydia. It is often difficult to establish the diagnosis of chlamydial infection, particularly in adults. Chlamydial cultures are not widely available and are frequently negative despite the presence of infection.[67,68] Typical inclusions in Giemsa-stained specimens, while diagnostic, are rarely seen in adults. Equal difficulty has been encountered in the diagnosis of genital infections, and much of the development in techniques has been performed by researchers in this field.[69]

Two direct tests are commercially available for examining conjunctival specimens: (1) Microtrak,* a fluorescein-tagged monoclonal antibody, and (2) Chlamydiazyme,† an enzyme immunosorbent assay (EIA). In the first test the fluorescein-tagged antibodies are reacted with a smear, and the slide is then examined with a fluorescence microscope for fluorescent chlamydial elementary bodies. The test is relatively easy to perform but requires experience to interpret accurately. In reported series the sensitivity has varied from 60% to 100%, and the specificity from 50% to 100%.[67,68,70-73] In our experience this test is difficult to interpret and should be read only by those with a great deal of experience.

In the EIA, the swab is placed in a solution and reacted with peroxidase-labeled antibodies. The presence of chlamydial antigen is indicated by a change in the color of the solution after addition of a chromogen substrate of the peroxidase. In a report of adult chlamydial conjunctivitis this test had a sensitivity of 71% and a specificity of 97%, which was better than the direct fluorescent test.[73] This test is easy to interpret but relatively difficult to perform. In patients with active trachoma both of these tests have been less sensitive, particularly in cases with mild disease.[74,75]

Serum assays for chlamydial antibodies are also available and may be useful in the diagnosis of ocular disease.[76,77] As mentioned earlier, an acute rise in titer is the most accurate means of serum diagnosis, but single high titers are suggestive. In a recent study[78] a single serum titer $>1:128$‡ had a sensitivity of 90% and a specificity of 76% compared with culture.

Herpes simplex. Several immunologic tests are available for detection of herpes simplex types I and II in ocular specimens. Probably the most accurate of these is the enzyme immunosorbent assay,§ which has been approved by the FDA.[79,80] Unfortunately, this test is both expensive and time consuming (5 hours). An immunofiltration system, designed by Cleveland and Richman,[81] appears to be nearly as accurate and much more practical, and it can also be used for detection of chlamydia and adenovirus. Although this system is not commercially available at the time of this writing, it is expected to become so in the near future.

OTHER TESTS

IMPRESSION CYTOLOGY

If a piece of cellulose acetate filter paper is pressed against the conjunctiva, surface epithelial cells adhere to it when it is removed. The filter paper can be stained and the morphology of the surface epithelium examined. This simple, noninvasive method can be used to assess goblet cell density and epithelial cell differentiation (Fig. 4-14).[82,83] With this technique, squamous metaplasia and goblet cell loss have been demonstrated in cicatricial pemphigoid and keratitis sicca.[84,85] It also can be used in place of conjunctival scraping to diagnose infectious conjunctivitis, allergic conjunctivitis, and mucopolysaccharidosis.[86]

LIMULUS LYSATE TEST

The limulus lysate test is a simple, rapid, and fairly accurate method for detecting endotoxin in corneal specimens.[6,87,88] Endotoxin is lipopolysaccharide in the cell wall of gram-negative enteric organisms, and its detection would therefore indicate that one of these organisms was present in the specimen. The horseshoe crab *Limulus polyphemus* produces cells, coelomic amebocytes, which cause clotting when exposed to endotoxin. The natural response of this organism to gram-negative bacterial infection is disseminated intravascular coagulation. This endotoxin activation of the coagulation pathway has been adapted as a sensitive in vitro assay for the presence of bacterial li-

---

*Syva, Palo Alto, CA.
†Abbott Laboratories, North Chicago, IL 60064.
‡Pharmacia Diagnostics (Electronucleosis), Columbia, MD 21046.
§Herpcheck, Dupont–New England Nuclear Division, Billerica, MA 01862.

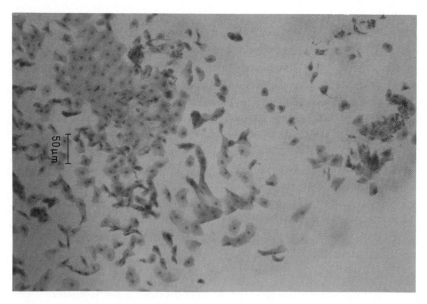

50 µm

Fig. 4-14. Impression cytology. Normal cells on the left with blue cytoplasm and diffusely staining nuclei. Squamous metaplasia on the right with larger cells, smaller, more densely staining (pyknotic) nuclei, and red staining cytoplasm. (Courtesy Melvin I. Roat, Pittsburgh.)

popolysaccharide. It becomes positive earlier than bacterial cultures and is unaffected by the presence of antibiotics; therefore it theoretically allows accurate diagnosis of partially treated patients with gram-negative corneal infections. The test cannot be used to assess the effectiveness of antibacterial therapy because endotoxin persists in the corneal debris for several days despite negative cultures taken from ulcer areas.[88] To perform the test, material from corneal scrapings is emulsified in a test tube with the amebocyte lysate reagent. If endotoxin is present, a visible clot is formed. In our experience at the University of Pittsburgh this test has produced many false-positive results.

REFERENCES

1. Sutphin JE et al: Improved detection of oculomycoses using induced fluorescence with Cellufluor, Ophthalmology 93:416, 1986.
2. Arffa RC et al: Calcofluor white and ink-potassium hydroxide preparations for identifying fungi, Am J Ophthalmol 100:719, 1985.
3. Groden LR et al: Acridine orange and Gram stains in infectious keratitis, Cornea 9:122, 1990.
4. Mattman LH: Cell wall deficient forms, Cleveland, 1974, CRC Press.
5. Forster RK, et al: Methenamine silver–stained corneal scraping in keratomycosis, Am J Ophthalmol 82:261, 1976.
6. Liesegang TJ and Forster RF: Spectrum of microbial keratitis in South Florida, Am J Ophthalmol 90:38, 1980.
7. Wilhelmus KR et al: Rapid diagnosis of *acanthamoeba* keratitis using calcofluor white, Arch Ophthalmol 104:1309, 1986.
8. Marines HM, Osato MS, and Font RL: The value of calcofluor white in the diagnosis of mycotic and *acanthamoeba* infections of the eye and adnexa, Ophthalmology 94:23, 1987.
9. Gomez JT, et al: Comparison of acridine orange and Gram stains in bacterial keratitis, Am J Ophthalmol 106:735, 1988.
10. Stenson S: Cytologic diagnosis. In Karcioglu ZA, editor: Laboratory diagnosis in ophthalmology, New York, 1987, Macmillan.
11. Munday PE, et al: A comparison of the sensitivity of immunofluorescence and Giemsa for staining *Chlamydia trachomatis* inclusions in cycloheximide-treated McCoy cells, J Clin Pathol 33:177, 1980.
12. Bettoli EJ et al: The role of temperature and swab materials in the recovery of herpes simplex virus from lesions, J Infect Dis 145:399, 1982.
13. Roat MI et al: The antiviral effects of rose bengal and fluorescein, Arch Ophthalmol 105:1415, 1987.
14. Jones DB: Polymicrobial keratitis, Trans Am Ophthalmol Soc 79:95, 1975.
15. Reyes AC, Punsaland AP, and Sulit HL: Mycotic flora of the conjunctiva, Philipp J Ophthalmol 2:119, 1970.
16. Pardos GJ and Gallagher MA: Microbial contamination of donor eyes: a retrospective study, Arch Ophthalmol 100:1611, 1982.
17. McCulley JP, Dougherty JM, and Deneau DG: Classification of chronic blepharitis, Ophthalmology 89:1173, 1982.

18. Allansmith MR, Ostler HB, and Butterworth M: Concomitance of bacteria in various areas of the eye, Arch Ophthalmol 82:37, 1969.

19. Locatcher-Khorazo D and Shegal BC: Microbiology of the eye, St Louis, 1972, Mosby–Year Book, Inc.

20. Ainley R and Smith B: Fungal flora of the conjunctival sac in healthy and diseased eyes, Br J Ophthalmol 49:505, 1965.

21. Hammeke JC and Ellis PP: Mycotic flora of the conjunctiva, Am J Ophthalmol 49:1174, 1960.

22. Griffith MR et al: Immunofluorescent studies in mucous membrane pemphigoid, Arch Dermatol 109:195, 1974.

23. Furey N et al: Immunofluorescent studies of ocular cicatricial pemphigoid, Am J Ophthalmol 80:825, 1975.

24. Mondino BJ, Brown SI, and Rabin BS: Autoimmune phenomena of the external eye, Ophthalmology 85:801, 1978.

25. Mondino BJ et al: Autoimmune phenomena in ocular cicatricial pemphigoid, Am J Ophthalmol 83:443, 1977.

26. Rogers RS et al: Immunopathology of cicatricial pemphigoid: studies of complement deposition, J Invest Dermatol 68:39, 1977.

27. Proia A, Foulks GN, and Sanfilippo FP: Ocular cicatricial pemphigoid with granular IgA and complement deposition, Arch Ophthalmol 103:1669, 1985.

28. Thoft RA et al: Ocular cicatricial pemphigoid associated with hyperproliferation of the conjunctival epithelium, Am J Ophthalmol 98:37, 1984.

29. Kasmierowski JA and Wuepper KD: Erythema multiforme: immune complex vasculitis of the superficial cutaneous microvasculature, J Invest Dermatol 71:366, 1978.

30. Richter BJ and McNutt NS: The spectrum of epidermolysis bullosa acquisita, Arch Dermatol 115:1325, 1979.

31. Yaoita H et al: Epidermolysis bullosa acquisita: ultrastructural and immunologic studies, J Invest Dermatol 76:288, 1981.

32. Woodley D et al: Identification of the skin basement autoantigen in epidermolysis acquisita, N Engl J Med 310:1007, 1984.

33. Woodley D: Epidermolysis bullosa acquisita, Prog Dermatol 22:1, 1988.

34. Bean SF, Halubar KK, and Gillett RB: Pemphigus involving the eyes, Arch Dermatol 111:1484, 1975.

35. Leonard JN et al: The relationship between linear IgA disease and benign mucous membrane pemphigoid, Br J Dermatol 110:307, 1984.

36. Libert J: Diagnosis of lysosomal storage diseases by the ultrastructural study of conjunctival biopsies, Pathol Annu 15 (part 1):37, 1980.

37. Van Hoof F et al: The assay of lacrimal tear enzymes and the ultrastructural analysis of conjunctival biopsies: new techniques for the study of in-born lysosomal diseases, Metab Ophthalmol 1:165, 1977.

38. Kenyon KR and Sensenbrenner JA: Electron microscopy of cornea and conjunctiva in childhood cystinosis, Am J Ophthalmol 78:68, 1974.

39. Sanderson PO et al: Cystinosis: a chemical, histopathologic, and ultrastructural study, Arch Ophthalmol 91:270, 1974.

40. Blodi FC and Apple DJ: Localized conjunctival amyloidosis, Am J Ophthalmol 88:346, 1979.

41. Riegel EM et al: Ocular pathology of Fabry's disease in a hemizygous male following renal transplantation, Surv Ophthalmol 26:247, 1982.

42. Weingeist TA and Blodi FC: Fabry's disease: ocular findings in a female carrier: a light and electron microscopic study, Arch Ophthalmol 85:169, 1971.

43. Frost P, Tanaka Y, and Spaeth GL: Fabry's disease-glycolipid lipidosis: histochemical and electronmicroscopic studies of two cases, Am J Med 40:618, 1966.

44. Kenyon KR and Sensenbrenner JA: Mucolipidosis II (I-cell disease): ultrastructural observations of conjunctiva and sclera, Invest Ophthalmol 10:555, 1971.

45. Libert J et al: Ocular findings in I-cell disease (mucolipidosis type II), Am J Ophthalmol 83:17, 1977.

46. Quigley HA and Goldberg MF: Conjunctival ultrastructure in mucolipidosis 3 (pseudo Hurler polydystrophy), Invest Ophthalmol 10:568, 1971.

47. Kenyon KR et al: Mucolipidosis IV: histopathology of conjunctiva, cornea and skin. Arch Ophthalmol 97:1106, 1979.

48. Zwann J and Kenyon KR: Two brothers with presumed mucolipidosis IV, Birth Defects 18:381, 1982.

49. Riedel KG et al: Ocular abnormalities in mucolipidosis IV, Am J Ophthalmol 99:125, 1985.

50. Kenyon KR et al: Ocular pathology of the Maroteaux-Lamy syndrome (systemic mucopolysaccharidosis type VI): histologic and ultrastructural report of two cases, Am J Ophthalmol 73:718, 1972.

51. Quigley HA and Goldberg MF: Scheie syndrome and macular corneal dystrophy: an ultrastructural comparison of conjunctiva and skin, Arch Ophthalmol 85:553, 1971.

52. Kenyon KR et al: The systemic mucopolysaccharidoses: ultrastructural and histological studies of conjunctiva and skin, Am J Ophthalmol 73:811, 1972.

53. Charlton KH et al: Pseudodendritic keratitis and systemic tyrosinemia, Ophthalmology 88:355, 1981.

54. Libert J, Van Hoof F, and Tonduer M: Fucosidosis: ultrastructural study of conjunctiva and skin and enzyme analysis of tears, Invest Ophthalmol 15:626, 1976.

55. Hoshino M et al: Fucosidosis: ultrastructural study of the eye in an adult, Graefe's Arch Clin Exp Ophthalmol 227:162, 1989.

56. Rao V et al: Conjunctival goblet cells and mitotic rate in children with measles and vitamin A deficiency, Arch Ophthalmol 105:378, 1987.

57. Roat MI, Sossi G, and Thoft RA: Increased conjunctival epithelial mitosis and goblet cell frequency in atopic keratoconjunctivitis, Invest Ophthalmol Vis Sci 30(suppl):83, 1989.

58. Ishibashi Y, Hommura S, and Matsumoto Y: Direct examination vs culture of biopsy specimens for the diagnosis of keratomycosis, Am J Ophthalmol 103:636, 1987.

59. Moore BM et al: *Acanthamoeba* keratitis associated with soft contact lenses, Am J Ophthalmol 100:396, 1985.

60. Moore MB et al: Radial keratoneuritis as a presenting sign in *Acanthamoeba* keratitis, Ophthalmology 93:1310, 1986.

61. Moore MB, Newton C, and Kaufman HE: Chronic keratitis caused by *Mycobacterium gordonae,* Am J Ophthalmol 102:516, 1986.

62. Newton C, Moore MB, and Kaufman HE: Corneal biopsy in chronic keratitis, Arch Ophthalmol 105:577, 1987.

63. Erie JC, Collyer SK, and Campbell RJ: Dehydrated cucumber slices as a mount for conjunctival biopsy specimens, Am J Ophthalmol 99:539, 1985.

64. Campbell RJ: Tissue diagnosis: eyelid and conjunctiva. In Karcioglu ZA, editor: Laboratory diagnosis in ophthalmology, New York, 1987, Macmillan.

65. Levy N et al: Reactive lymphoid hyperplasia with single class (monoclonal) surface immunoglobulin, Am J Clin Pathol 80:300, 1983.

66. Knowles DM et al: The application of monoclonal antibodies to the characterization and diagnosis of lymphoid neoplasms: a review of recent studies, Diagn Immunol 1:142, 1983.

67. Schachter J et al: Evaluation of laboratory methods for detecting acute tric agent infection, Am J Ophthalmol 70:377, 1970.

68. Taylor HR, Agarwala N, and Johnson SL: Detection of experimental *Chlamydia trachomatis* eye infection on conjunctival smears and in tissue culture by use of fluorescein-conjugated monoclonal antibody, J Clin Microbiol 20:391, 1984.

69. Stamm WE and Holmes KK: Chlamydial infections: what should we do while waiting for a diagnostic test? West J Med 135:226, 1981.

70. Potts MJ et al: Rapid diagnosis of *Chlamydia trachomatis* infection in patients attending an ophthalmic casualty department, Br J Ophthalmol 70:677, 1986.

71. Hawkins DA et al: Rapid, reliable diagnosis of chlamydial ophthalmia by means of monoclonal antibodies, Br J Ophthalmol 69:640, 1985.

72. Bialasiewicz AA and Jahn GJ: Evaluation of diagnostic tools for adult chlamydial keratoconjunctivitis, Ophthalmology 94:532, 1987.

73. Sheppard JD et al: Immunodiagnosis of adult chlamydial conjunctivitis, Ophthalmology 95:434, 1988.

74. Tabbara KF and Rahi A: Enzyme immunoassay in the detection of chlamydial antigens in patients with trachoma, Ophthalmology 94(suppl):123, 1987.

75. Taylor PB, Burd EM, and Tabbara KF: Comparison of diagnostic laboratory techniques in the various stages of trachoma, Ophthalmology 94(suppl):123, 1987.

76. Darougar S et al: Rapid serological test for diagnosis of chlamydial ocular infections, Br J Ophthalmol 62:503, 1978.

77. Wang S and Grayston J: Immunologic relationship between genital TRIC, lymphogranuloma venereum, and related organisms in a new microtiter indirect immunofluorescence test, Am J Ophthalmol 70:367, 1970.

78. Arffa RC, Kowalski RP, and Springer DS: The value of serology in the diagnosis of adult chlamydial keratoconjunctivitis, Ophthalmology 95(suppl):145, 1988.

79. Kowalski RP and Gordon YJ: Evaluation of immunologic tests for the detection of ocular herpes simplex virus, Ophthalmology 96:1583, 1989.

80. Lee AF et al: Comparative laboratory diagnosis of experimental herpes simplex keratitis, Am J Ophthalmol 109:8, 1990.

81. Cleveland PH and Richman DD: Enzyme immunofiltration staining assay for the immediate diagnosis of herpes simplex virus and varicella-zoster virus directly from clinical specimens, J Clin Microbiol 25:416, 1987.

82. Egbert PR, Lauber S, and Maurice DM: A simple conjunctival biopsy, Am J Ophthalmol 84:793, 1977.

83. Tseng SCG: Staging of conjunctival squamous metaplasia by impression cytology, Ophthalmology 92:728, 1985.

84. Nelson JD, Havener VR, and Cameron JD: Cellulose acetate impressions of the ocular surface: dry eye states, Arch Ophthalmol 101:1869, 1983.

85. Nelson JD and Wright JC: Conjunctival goblet cell densities in ocular surface disease, Arch Ophthalmol 102:1049, 1984.

86. Maskin SL et al: Diagnostic impression cytology for external eye disease, Cornea 8:270, 1989.

87. McBeath J, Forster RK, and Rebell G: Diagnostic limulus lysate assay for endophthalmitis and keratitis, Arch Ophthalmol 96:1265, 1978.

88. Walters RW et al: Limulus lysate assay for early detection of certain gram-negative corneal infections, Arch Ophthalmol 97:875, 1979.

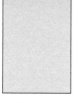

CHAPTER

5

CONGENITAL ANOMALIES

Dysgenesis of the lids
- Cryptophthalmos
- Ankyloblepharon

Abnormalities of corneal size
- Megalocornea
- Microcornea

Abnormalities of corneal shape and curvature
- Cornea plana
- Oval cornea
- Keratectasia
- Generalized posterior keratoconus
- Corneal astigmatism

Anterior segment dysgenesis
- Posterior embryotoxon
- Axenfeld's anomaly and syndrome
- Rieger's anomaly and syndrome
- Circumscribed posterior keratoconus

- Peters' anomaly
- Sclerocornea
- Congenital cornea guttata
- Congenital hereditary endothelial dystrophy
- Congenital hereditary stromal dystrophy
- Posterior polymorphous dystrophy
- Aniridia

Congenital mass lesions of the cornea
- Dermoids
- Other choristomas
- Keloids

Other causes of corneal opacification at birth

Penetrating keratoplasty for congenital corneal opacities

Chromosomal aberrations

This chapter describes the more common congenital anomalies of the anterior segment. These are characterized by alterations in structure caused by abnormalities in development. The abnormalities are present at birth, differentiating them from most corneal dystrophies and systemic disorders of metabolism. The etiology can be genetic, infectious, traumatic, toxic, or a combination of these influences. Most often these etiologic factors affect development between the sixth and sixteenth weeks of gestation, when differentiation of the anterior segment occurs. Developmental anomalies generally fall into three categories: developmental arrest, abnormal differentiation, or a combination of the two.

DYSGENESIS OF THE LIDS
CRYPTOPHTHALMOS

Cryptophthalmos is a condition is which the lids fail to form and the exposed corneal and conjunctival epithelium undergo metaplasia into skin (dermoid transformation). There are no lashes or brows, and in many cases the lacrimal gland and canaliculi also are absent.[1,2] Incomplete forms oc-

83

cur, with nasal or superior involvement only. There is no treatment; incision into the skin enters the globe.

This condition is usually inherited as an autosomal recessive trait and may be unilateral or bilateral. It can be associated with systemic abnormalities, including craniofacial anomalies, syndactyly, cardiac anomalies, genitourinary anomalies, and mental retardation.[1-4] Renal agenesis has been reported in siblings of patients with this condition.[2]

ANKYLOBLEPHARON

In some cases the upper and lower lids are formed but fused in front of a normal cornea. Brows and lashes are present, in contrast to cryptophthalmos. The lids can be incised, although they may fuse again.[5,6]

ABNORMALITIES OF CORNEAL SIZE

MEGALOCORNEA

Megalocornea is defined as a cornea that measures 13 mm or more in horizontal diameter. It is not associated with glaucoma and is nonprogressive. The condition is usually bilateral and transmitted as a sex-linked recessive trait; 90% of patients are male (Fig. 5-1). Occasionally it is transmitted as an autosomal dominant trait, and rarely as an autosomal recessive trait.

The cornea is clear and is histologically normal. Often the anterior chamber is deep, and the ciliary body and lens are enlarged.[7] High myopia, due to increased corneal curvature, and with-the-rule astigmatism can be present. Megalocornea can be associated with other ocular abnormalities, including anterior embryotoxon, Krukenberg's spindle,[8] hypoplasia of the iris stroma, mosaic corneal dystrophy,[9,10] miosis, and heavy pigmentation of the trabecular meshwork. Ectopia lentis, glaucoma, and cataract can develop later in life. Megalocornea also can be associated with systemic syndromes, including Marfan's syndrome, Apert's syndrome,[11] and mucolipidosis type II.[12]

Megalocornea may result from failure of the anterior tips of the optic cup to grow far enough toward each other, allowing the large remaining space to be occupied by the cornea. It may also reflect an exaggeration of the normal tendency for the cornea to be relatively large, compared with the rest of the eye, from embryonic life to age 7. Finally, megalocornea may result from a spontaneously arrested congenital glaucoma. It is interesting to note that megalocornea and congenital glaucoma can occur in different members of the same family, and, rarely, megalocornea can occur in one eye of a patient and congenital glaucoma in the other.

MICROCORNEA

The term "microcornea" is used when the corneal diameter in an otherwise normal-sized eye is 10 mm or less. If the entire eye is small but otherwise normal the condition is called *nanophthalmos;* if the entire eye is small and malformed, *microphthalmos* is said to exist.

Fig. 5-1. Infant with bilateral megalocornea. (Courtesy David A. Hiles, Pittsburgh.)

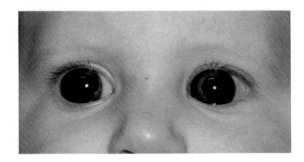

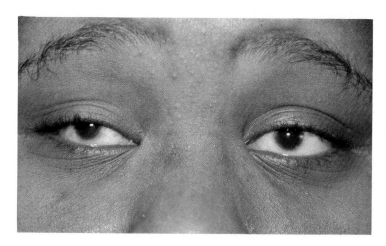

Fig. 5-2. Bilateral microcornea.

Microcornea occurs unilaterally and bilaterally at the same rate (Fig. 5-2). It can be transmitted as an autosomal dominant or recessive trait. If the globe is otherwise normal, visual acuity can be good. The corneal curvature can be flat or steep, and because the axial length also varies greatly, any refractive error can exist. Glaucoma can occur congenitally or in adulthood, secondary to angle closure, with the crowded anterior segment. Microcornea has been associated with a wide variety of ocular and systemic conditions; the more common ones include the following:

Ocular	*Systemic syndromes*[13]
Microblepharon	Ehlers-Danlos[14]
Corneal leukoma	Weill-Marchesani[15]
Cornea plana	Rieger's[16]
Iris coloboma	Waardenburg's[17]
Corectopia	Norrie's
Persistent pupillary membrane	Turner's[18]
Microphakia	Trisomy 13-15[19]
Congenital cataract	Progeria
Congenital glaucoma	Rubella[20]
Angle-closure glaucoma	
Open-angle glaucoma	

The etiology is unknown, but may be an overgrowth of the anterior tips of the optic cup, leaving less than the normal space for the cornea.

ABNORMALITIES OF CORNEAL SHAPE AND CURVATURE
CORNEA PLANA

In cornea plana corneal curvature is 43 diopters (D) or less, most commonly 30 to 35 D. The curvature is the same or less than that of the sclera. In fact, cornea plana may be a form of sclerocornea: Some peripheral scleralization of the cornea occurs in all cases, making the limbus indistinct.[21-24] Diffuse opacification of the central cornea can also be seen.

The condition is commonly associated with microcornea and the following ocular abnormalities:

Ocular		*Systemic*
High refractive errors (particularly hyperopia)	Anterior synechiae	Osteogenesis imperfecta
	Aniridia	Hurler's syndrome
Pseudoptosis	Congenital cataract	Trisomy 13
Microphthalmos	Ectopia lentis	
Blue sclera	Glaucoma	
Iris coloboma	Retinal aplasia	
	Choroidal coloboma	

The anterior chamber is usually shallow. In spite of the flattened cornea the refractive error is not consistently hyperopic, since the axial length varies. The refractive error can be corrected with spectacles or contact lenses.[25]

Cornea plana can be inherited as an autosomal dominant or recessive trait; the recessive form is more severe. It is thought to result from a developmental arrest in the fourth month, at which time the cornea begins to increase its curvature relative to the sclera.

OVAL CORNEA

A vertically oval cornea may be seen in Turner's syndrome,[18] Rieger's anomaly, and in microphthalmos with coloboma.[13] It can also develop after intrauterine interstitial keratitis (usually luetic).

The cornea normally appears to be slightly oval horizontally as a result of the extension of the limbus onto the cornea vertically. This condition is exaggerated in sclerocornea.

KERATECTASIA

Keratectasia is a bulging, opaque cornea that protrudes through the palpebral aperture. The stroma is variably thinned and scarred. Usually unilateral, most cases probably result from an intrauterine keratitis with perforation. The corneal tissue subsequently undergoes metaplasia to skinlike tissue (dermoid transformation). Keratectasia also may be caused by a failure of mesenchyme to migrate into the developing cornea, with subsequent thinning, bulging, and metaplasia.

Congenital anterior staphyloma is similar to keratectasia, but uveal tissue lines the ectatic cornea.

GENERALIZED POSTERIOR KERATOCONUS

Generalized posterior keratoconus is a rare congenital condition in which the entire posterior surface of the cornea is more curved than normal.[5,26,27] Central corneal thinning can result, but the anterior surface is normal. The cornea usually is clear and vision is normal, but stromal haze can be present. The condition is usually unilateral and nonprogressive, and there is no evidence of hereditary transmission. All reported cases have occurred in women.

The condition is probably a developmental arrest, since the posterior corneal curvature usually is more marked in the embryonic cornea. This should not be confused with circumscribed posterior keratoconus, in which there is a localized craterlike defect in the posterior corneal surface and frequent stromal opacity.

CORNEAL ASTIGMATISM

Most cases of primary corneal astigmatism are minor and accompany myopia. However, high degrees of idiopathic astigmatism can occur in a hereditary pattern, usually autosomal dominant.[28] The correlation in the amount of astigmatism between monozygotic twins is not higher than that between dizygotic twins, suggesting that genetic factors are not the major determinant.[29]

ANTERIOR SEGMENT DYSGENESIS

Anterior segment dysgenesis (ASD) is a spectrum of corneal, iris, angle, and lens abnormalities that appear to be related to abnormal development of the mesenchyme forming the anterior segment of the eye.[30,31] These abnormalities were previously referred to as mesodermal dysgenesis or anterior chamber cleavage syndrome, but Wilson[32] has suggested the term ASD because the embryonic mesenchyme is probably derived from neural crest, not mesoderm, and anterior chamber cleavage probably does not occur during development. Most likely, ASD represents abnormal migration or differentiation of the secondary mesenchyme.[33]

During early development of the embryo, primary mesenchyme separates the surface ectoderm and the lens vesicle. The paraxial (secondary) mesenchyme then migrates centrally across the opening of the optic cup in three successive waves. The first wave gives rise to the corneal endothelium, the second to the corneal stroma, and the third to the iris stroma. The anterior chamber is absent, the space being filled with primary or secondary mesenchyme. This tissue gradually recedes, forming the anterior chamber, pupillary aperture, and last, the angle recess. Throughout most of corneal development the vascular pupillary membrane is closely associated with the developing endothelium.[34]

Incomplete migration of the secondary mesenchyme across the front of the eye or incomplete recession of the mesenchyme could be responsible for the following disorders: posterior embryotoxon, Axenfeld's anomaly, Rieger's anomaly, Peters' anomaly, congenital peripheral anterior synechiae, and posterior keratoconus. Abnormal differentiation of the mesenchyme could lead to congenital hereditary endothelial dystrophy, congenital hereditary stromal dystrophy, posterior polymorphous dystrophy, sclerocornea, and congenital cornea guttata.

The conditions described in the next sections are separated relatively arbitrarily, based on common combinations of findings and historical appellations. Because these diseases occur as a spectrum of anterior segment changes, many cases will not fit into a specific category. Nevertheless, it is useful for instruction and recognition to review the traditional descriptions.

POSTERIOR EMBRYOTOXON

Posterior embryotoxon is a thickened and centrally displaced anterior border ring of Schwalbe (Figs. 5-3 and 5-4). *Schwalbe's ring* is a circumferential collagenous band, located peripherally on the posterior surface of the cornea, at the juncture of Descemet's membrane and the trabecular meshwork. In most people it is visible only on gonioscopy, but in approximately 15% of otherwise normal eyes it is sufficiently anteriorly displaced to become visible.[35] It is seen as a reluent irregular line or ridge up to 2 mm central to the limbus, and the posterior corneal surface between the line and the limbus is translucent. It is most often seen temporally and nasally. Occasionally it is dislocated from the cornea and hangs in the angle area.

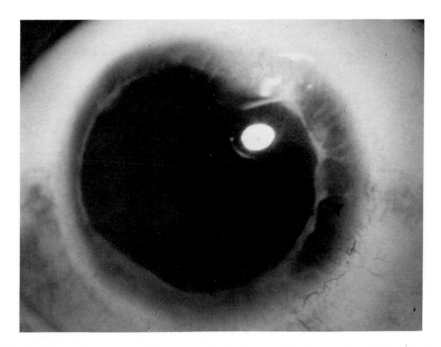

Fig. 5-3. Posterior embryotoxon is thick, centrally displaced anterior border ring of Schwalbe *(arrow).*

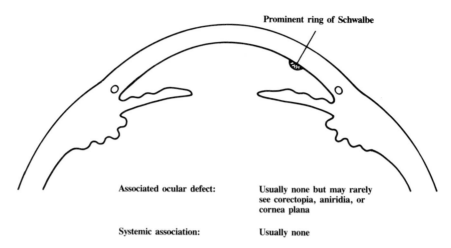

Fig. 5-4. Posterior embryotoxon in otherwise normal eye.

Posterior embryotoxon is often inherited as an autosomal dominant trait. Usually the eye is otherwise normal, but other signs of ASD, including Axenfeld's anomaly, cornea plana, corectopia, and aniridia may be present.

Axenfeld's Anomaly and Syndrome

In Axenfeld's anomaly, iris strands extend across the angle to insert into a prominent Schwalbe's ring (Figs. 5-5 and 5-6). About 50% of these patients develop glaucoma, in which case it is called Axenfeld's syndrome.[36] The glaucoma most often appears during childhood or young adulthood, but may develop during infancy. Both Axenfeld's anomaly and syndrome are dominantly inherited. Skeletal anomalies, such as hypertelorism, facial asymmetry, and hypoplastic shoulder, are occasionally present.[21] Axenfeld's anomaly can rarely be associated with systemic disease.[37]

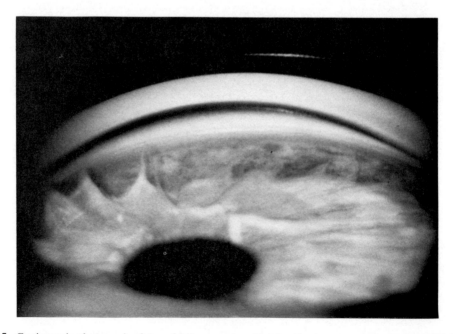

Fig. 5-5. Gonioscopic photograph of Axenfeld's anomaly with iris adhesions to prominent ring of Schwalbe.

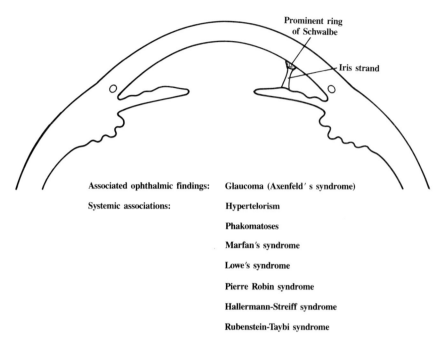

Prominent ring
of Schwalbe

Iris strand

Associated ophthalmic findings: Glaucoma (Axenfeld's syndrome)

Systemic associations: Hypertelorism

                                   Phakomatoses

                                   Marfan's syndrome

                                   Lowe's syndrome

                                   Pierre Robin syndrome

                                   Hallermann-Streiff syndrome

                                   Rubenstein-Taybi syndrome

Fig. 5-6. Axenfeld's anomaly.

RIEGER'S ANOMALY AND SYNDROME

In Rieger's anomaly one sees a prominent Schwalbe's ring, iris strands extending to Schwalbe's ring, and hypoplasia of the iris stroma (Figs. 5-7 and 5-8).[30,38,39] The iris abnormalities range from mild stromal thinning to marked hypoplasia and hole formation. In some cases the sphincter is easily seen, and there are no crypts, furrows, or collarette. The deep iris stroma may appear to be made up of delicate radial fibrils, which give the iris a gray-brown, stringy appearance. An abnormality of the

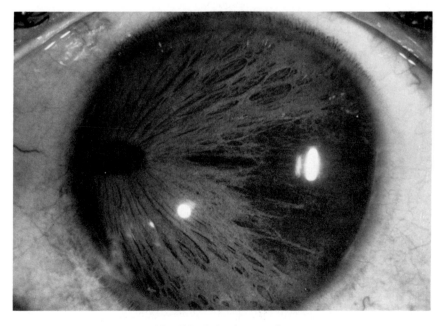

Fig. 5-7. Reiger's anomaly.

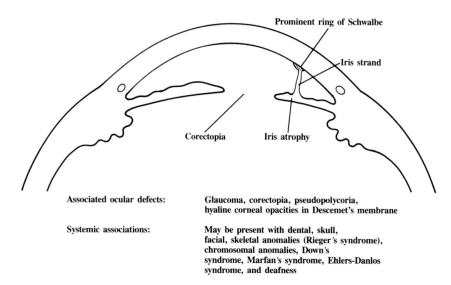

Fig. 5-8. Reiger's anomaly.

shape of the pupil is present in approximately 70% of cases.[40] The iris abnormalities are usually stable, but in a small percentage of patients they will progress.[41-44] Glaucoma occurs in 50% to 60% of these patients and usually develops between 5 and 30 years of age.

Iridodysgenesis with cataract is a variation of Rieger's anomaly in which posterior embryotoxon is absent, juvenile cataract is present, and the inheritance is autosomal recessive.[30,38] *Goniodysgenesis with glaucoma* is Rieger's anomaly without posterior embryotoxon.[30,38]

Rieger's syndrome is the combination of Rieger's anomaly and nonocular developmental anomalies, particularly skeletal anomalies. Maxillary hypoplasia, a broad, flat nasal root, and microdontia or anodontia can be associated with Rieger's syndrome. Other associated systemic abnormalities include malformations of the limbs and spine, deafness, mental retardation, osteogenesis imperfecta, and Marfan's, Down's, and Ehlers-Danlos syndromes.[37,40,45]

Rieger's anomaly and syndrome are inherited as an autosomal dominant trait in about 75% of cases,[40] with 95% penetrance and extreme variation in expressivity.[38,39] In one case there was presumptive isochromosome of the long arm of chromosome 6,[46] and another had a pericentric inversion of chromosome 6.[47] Both Axenfeld's and Rieger's anomalies have been described in the same pedigree.[48,49]

In view of the similarity of the two conditions, a single term: "Axenfeld-Rieger syndrome" has been proposed to encompass the spectrum of changes seen in both.[41,50] However, other disorders, for example, Peters' anomaly, posterior embryotoxon, and posterior keratoconus, are probably part of the same spectrum, which is better described by the term ASD.

CIRCUMSCRIBED POSTERIOR KERATOCONUS

Circumscribed posterior keratoconus is a rare disorder, characterized by one or more localized crater defects on the posterior corneal surface, with a concavity facing toward the anterior chamber[30,51-54] (Fig. 5-9). The lesion is usually unilateral, single, and central, but bilateral, eccentric, and multiple lesions can be present.[51] A nebular stromal haze can overlie the involved area. The anterior surface is normal, visual acuity is usually not affected, and progression does not occur.

Descemet's membrane and endothelium are present in the involved area; however, Descemet's membrane may show abnormal anterior banding, a multilayered configuration, and posterior excres-

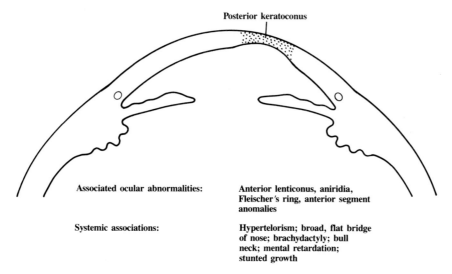

Fig. 5-9. Posterior keratoconus.

cences.[53] These findings suggest an early onset, probably before the sixth month of gestation.[55] Most likely it is the result of abnormal migration or differentiation of the secondary mesenchyme that forms the corneal stroma.[32]

Circumscribed posterior keratoconus may accompany other anterior segment anomalies, including aniridia, anterior lenticonus, Fleischer ring, and other signs of ASD. Associated systemic findings can include hypertelorism, poorly developed nasal bridge, brachydactyly, bull neck, mental retardation, and growth retardation.

Most cases are sporadic, but familial cases have been reported.[56] Similar findings can be seen after trauma. In the past, some have used the term "von Hippel's internal ulcer" synonymously with posterior keratoconus. However, in the former, Descemet's membrane and endothelium are absent in the crater, and vascularization and anterior synechiae may be present. These cases may be a form of Peters' anomaly, caused by intrauterine infection or more extensive anterior segment dysgenesis.

PETERS' ANOMALY

Peters' anomaly refers to a central corneal opacity (corneal leukoma) associated with a posterior corneal defect.[57-59] It encompasses a variety of abnormalities and probably can result from multiple etiologies. In some cases the central leukoma and adherent iris strands are the only signs, and the lens is clear (Figs. 5-10, *A* and 5-11); this has been called the mesodermal form of Peters' anomaly. The iris adhesions usually arise from the iris collarette and extend to the margin of the leukoma. This form is rarely associated with the types of peripheral anomalies seen in Axenfeld's and Rieger's syndromes (Fig. 5-10, *C*). Microcornea, sclerocornea, and infantile glaucoma can be present. It can be bilateral or unilateral and is sporadic, although recessive and dominant pedigrees have been reported.[60]

In other cases the lens is cataractous or is apposed to the leukoma (Figs. 5-10, *B* and 5-12). The corneal opacity tends to be denser than in the previously mentioned cases, and associated ocular and systemic abnormalities are more frequent. These abnormalities include aniridia, sclerocornea, microphthalmos with choroidal coloboma, trisomy 13-15, congenital heart defects, genitourinary disorders, mental retardation, cleft lip and palate,[61] and skeletal anomalies.[40,62]

In all cases Descemet's membrane and endothelium are absent in the area of the opacity.[58-60,63] Bowman's layer may also be absent centrally. In cases where the lens is adherent to the corneal

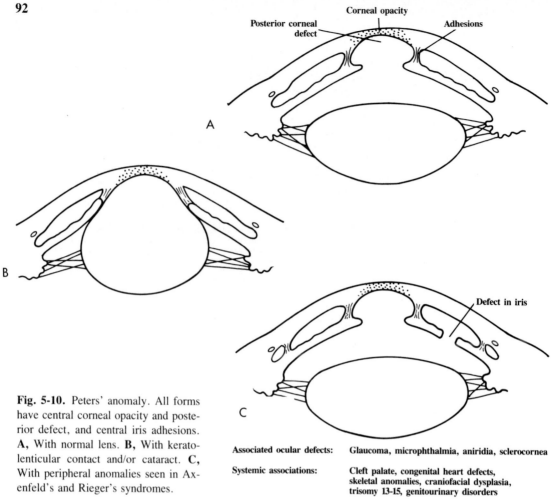

Posterior corneal defect

Corneal opacity

Adhesions

Defect in iris

Fig. 5-10. Peters' anomaly. All forms have central corneal opacity and posterior defect, and central iris adhesions. **A,** With normal lens. **B,** With keratolenticular contact and/or cataract. **C,** With peripheral anomalies seen in Axenfeld's and Rieger's syndromes.

Associated ocular defects:	Glaucoma, microphthalmia, aniridia, sclerocornea
Systemic associations:	Cleft palate, congenital heart defects, skeletal anomalies, craniofacial dysplasia, trisomy 13-15, genitourinary disorders

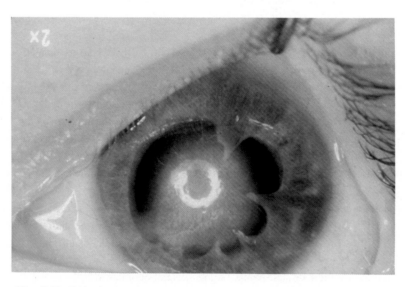

Fig. 5-11. Peters' anomaly. Central corneal opacity with adherent iris strands.

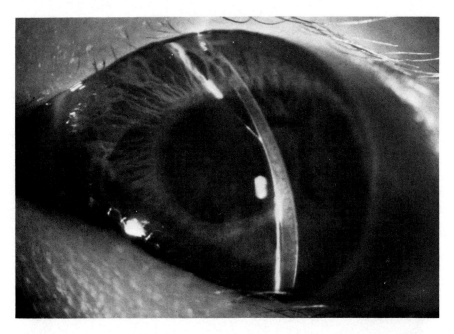

Fig. 5-12. Peters' anomaly with lens-cornea touch. (Courtesy Milton C. Pettapiece, Pittsburgh.)

stroma, the lens capsule can be present or absent. Histochemically, corneas with Peters' anomaly contain much more fibronectin than normal.[64]

A number of pathogenetic mechanisms have been proposed. Dysgenesis of the mesenchymal tissue forming the central iris endothelium and corneal stroma may cause the form of Peters' anomaly limited to the cornea and iris. Intrauterine inflammation could interfere with development of the regional surface ectoderm and neuroectoderm or even cause perforation. Evidence of inflammation is present in some cases, as was described for posterior keratoconus, and the term "von Hippel's internal corneal ulcer" also can be applied to these cases. Faulty separation of the lens vesicle from the surface ectoderm can be responsible for some cases of lens-cornea adhesion (surface ectodermal Peters's anomaly). However, histologic studies suggest that in most cases the lens developed normally and later advanced forward.[59,63,65] This movement may result from dislocation of an abnormal lens, as in aniridia and microphthalmos with coloboma, or from displacement by a retrolenticular mass, as in microphthalmos with persistent hyperplastic primary vitreous.

SCLEROCORNEA

Sclerocornea is a congenital anomaly characterized by nonprogressive, noninflammatory opacification of the peripheral or entire cornea with vascularization[66] (Fig. 5-13). The sclera appears to extend onto the cornea, with opacification and deep or superficial vascularization. It can involve only the peripheral cornea or the entire cornea (total sclerocornea) (Fig. 5-14). When the condition is total the central cornea is slightly less opaque than the periphery. Involved areas have fine, superficial, uninflamed vessels that are extensions of the normal episcleral and conjunctival vessels. In most cases the corneal curvature is flattened (cornea plana). Visual acuity can be severely reduced when the central cornea is involved.

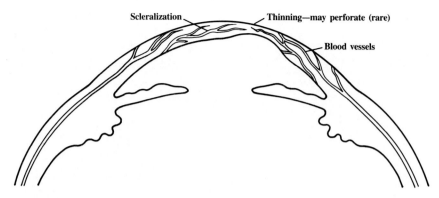

Fig. 5-13. Sclerocornea.

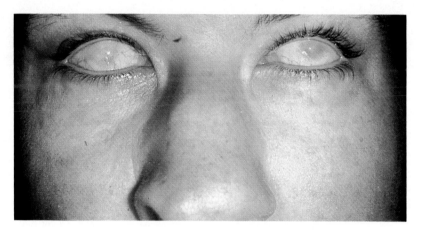

Fig. 5-14. Sclerocornea involving entire corneal area.

Sclerocornea is usually bilateral and affects males and females equally. Most cases are sporadic, but it can be inherited as an autosomal dominant or recessive trait; the dominant forms are less severe.[67,68] It can be associated with the following ocular and systemic abnormalities:

Ocular	*Systemic*[69]
Microphthalmos	Cerebellar anomalies
Blue sclera	Cranial anomalies
Cornea plana	Decreased hearing (Lobstein's syndrome)[21]
Angle anomalies (ASD)	Deformities of the hands and feet
Aniridia	Cryptorchidism
Iris coloboma	Occult spina bifida
Cataract	Hereditary osteoonychodysplasia[70]
Glaucoma (open and closed angle)	Hallermann-Streiff syndrome
Choroidal coloboma	Mieten's syndrome[71]
	Osteogenesis imperfecta
	Others

Histologic examination demonstrates collagen fibers of increased diameter in the superficial stroma, greater than in the posterior stroma, which is typical of sclera but not normal cornea.[72] Bowman's layer is usually absent, and Descemet's membrane and the endothelium can be normal, abnormal, or absent.[68,69,71] Anterior chamber angle abnormalities, such as anterior synechiae, are frequently present.[69,73]

Most likely, the wave of mesenchymal tissue that normally forms the corneal stroma forms tissue resembling sclera instead. The tissue destined to become sclera and cornea is a homogeneous sheet until the limbal anlage develops during the seventh to tenth weeks. The limbal anlage appears to be necessary for development of the increased curvature of the corneal surface. Lack of formation of the limbal anlage or its central displacement may be responsible for sclerocornea.[72]

Penetrating keratoplasty can be performed, particularly if the condition is total bilaterally. Glaucoma is a relatively frequent postoperative complication and bodes a poor prognosis.

CONGENITAL CORNEA GUTTATA

Corneal guttae are rarely seen as a congenital anomaly. The condition is stationary but can be associated with deep stromal opacification. Sometimes it occurs as a familial condition. Two different dominant pedigrees have been described in which congenital cornea guttata was associated with other congenital malformations: in one with anterior polar cataract[74] and in another with mandibulofacial dysostosis, a condition thought to result from a defect in neural crest cell migration during the fourth week of gestation.[75] Both associations suggest that congenital cornea guttata is related to abnormal cellular migration in the anterior chamber during early development.

CONGENITAL HEREDITARY ENDOTHELIAL DYSTROPHY

Congenital hereditary endothelial dystrophy (CHED) is characterized by bilateral diffuse corneal edema that is present at birth or develops within a few years of life. It can be inherited either as an autosomal dominant or autosomal recessive trait. CHED is discussed further in Chapter 18.

CONGENITAL HEREDITARY STROMAL DYSTROPHY

Congenital hereditary stromal dystrophy (CHSD) is a rare condition that is inherited as an autosomal dominant trait.[76] It is present at birth and is nonprogressive. The corneal stroma exhibits a flaky, feathery cloudiness, which is more prominent centrally and fades peripherally. The stromal collagen fibrils are abnormal in form, size, and arrangement.[76]

POSTERIOR POLYMORPHOUS DYSTROPHY

Posterior polymorphous dystrophy (PPD) is often seen as a congenital anomaly. Most often present are localized endothelial abnormalities, which are stable or slowly progressive. Occasionally, patients have cloudy corneas at birth. PPD can be associated with the types of iris and angle anomalies seen in ASD.[77] It is discussed further in Chapter 18.

ANIRIDIA

Aniridia is a congenital hypoplasia of the iris that can be hereditary (autosomal dominant) or sporadic. It is associated with glaucoma, cataracts, foveal hypoplasia, ectopia lentis, and Wilms tumor (in the sporadic cases). It is also often associated with corneal opacification.[78,79] Beginning after 2 years of age, bilateral superficial vascularization and opacification can be seen at the limbus in one or more locations, usually in the vertical meridians. This phenomenon progresses slowly, extending centrally and circumferentially, and can involve the visual axis, reducing vision (Fig. 5-15). The cause of the corneal changes is not known. Schirmer's tests are abnormal in many of the patients,[78] but this is not sufficient to explain the corneal disease.

There is no known treatment for the corneal opacification. Lamellar or penetrating keratoplasty can be performed, but they can be complicated by management of glaucoma, difficulties with epithelial healing, and recurrent scarring.

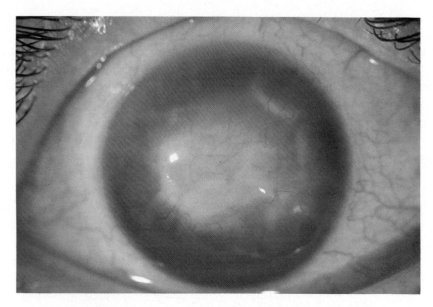

Fig. 5-15. Corneal scarring and cataract formation in aniridia.

CONGENITAL MASS LESIONS OF THE CORNEA

DERMOIDS

Dermoids are choristomas, congenital masses of tissue not normally present in the location in which they are found.[80,81] (This is in contrast to hamartomas, which are abnormal growths of tissue normally present at the site.) Most likely, tissue destined to become skin is displaced to the surface of the eye during fetal development. Dermoids can occur over the cornea, limbus, or conjunctiva.[80,82] They most commonly are seen at the limbus, particularly inferotemporally. They are round or ovoid, yellowish-white, solid, vascularized, and domelike (Fig. 5-16). They can involve the central or entire cornea or form a ring around the circumference of the limbus.[83,84] Hairs can protrude from the mass.

These lesions are present at birth, and they occasionally enlarge, especially at puberty. They can decrease vision by covering the visual axis or by inducing astigmatism. Often a line of lipid material develops along the central edge of the tumor, which also can impair vision.

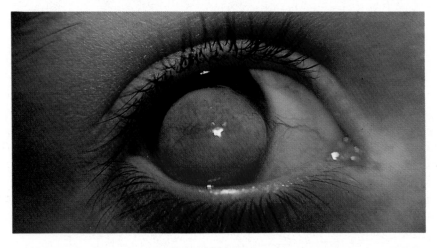

Fig. 5-16. Dermoid of cornea.

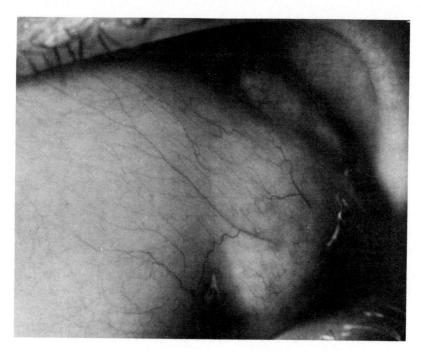

Fig. 5-17. Dermolipoma.

The walls are of dermal origin, composed of dermislike collagen, and can contain cutaneous adnexal structures, such as sebaceous glands, sweat glands, hairs, and fat. A dermolipoma is a dermoid in which fat is prominent, and the cutaneous adnexal structures are usually absent (Fig. 5-17). Limbal and corneal dermoids always extend into the corneal stroma and can extend into the anterior chamber.

Approximately 30% of individuals with *Goldenhar's syndrome* (oculoauricolovertebral dysplasia) have epibulbar dermoids.[85] They most commonly occur unilaterally and at the inferotemporal limbus. Other ocular findings of Goldenhar's syndrome include lid colobomas, microphthalmos, iris coloboma, aniridia, Duane's syndrome, and miliary aneurysms of the retina.[80,85,86] Abnormalities of the structures derived from the first and second branchial arch are common: preauricular appendages (Fig. 5-18), pretragal fistulas, vertebral anomalies, mandibular and malar hypoplasia, and hemifacial microsomia can be seen. Other systemic abnormalities also can be present.[80,85]

Due to the posterior extension of corneal dermoids, they cannot be totally excised without deep lamellar or penetrating keratoplasty. Shaving of the elevated portion can reduce astigmatism and improve cosmesis but not remove the opacity.

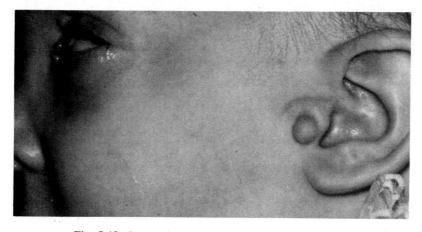

Fig. 5-18. Pretragal appendage in Goldenhar's syndrome.

OTHER CHORISTOMAS

Lacrimal tissue also can be displaced to the ocular surface during fetal development *(ectopic lacrimal gland)*.[87] Sweat glands, hairs, smooth muscle, and sebaceous gland tissue can be present in the mass. Ectopic lacrimal gland tends to be fleshy, with raised translucent nodules and abundant vascularization. Like dermoids, they can extend into the corneal stroma and can exhibit slow growth, particularly during puberty. Surgical removal can be complicated by the presence of soft lacrimal tissue in the corneal stroma.

Osseous and neuroglial choristomas also can be found on the bulbar surface.[88] Osseous choristomas are usually located in the upper temporal quadrant, tend to have sharp edges, and often times spare the cornea.

KELOIDS

A keloid is an exuberant growth of fibrous tissue that occurs in response to injury or as a congenital cornea mass.[89] They are chalky white, glistening solid tumors that show variable posterior extension.[90]

OTHER CAUSES OF CORNEAL OPACIFICATION AT BIRTH

Many of the conditions discussed previously cause corneal opacification at birth. The following conditions also can cause diffuse corneal opacification at birth or during infancy and must be included in the differential diagnosis:

CONDITION	CHARACTERISTICS
PRESENT AT BIRTH	
Congenital glaucoma	Elevated IOP, increased corneal diameter, epithelial and stromal edema, Descemet's ruptures, bilateral 75%
Birth trauma	History of forceps use, unilateral, stromal edema, Descemet's ruptures
Congenital rubella	Bilateral, cataract, miosis, microphthalmos, iritis, glaucoma, retinopathy
Congenital syphilis	Bilateral, inflammatory signs, retinopathy, systemic signs (rare at birth)
PROGRESSIVE OPACIFICATION, CAN BE EVIDENT BEFORE 6 MONTHS	
Cystinosis	Bilateral, stromal crystals, renal disease, autosomal recessive
Mucopolysaccharidosis: Hurler's (MPS1-H) and Scheie's (MPS1-S)	Bilateral, diffuse corneal clouding, abnormal facies, skeletal dysplasia, ± optic atrophy, ± retinopathy, autosomal recessive
Fabry's disease	Bilateral, superficial whorllike opacities, renal failure, skin lesions, X-linked recessive
Mucolipidosis, especially types II and IV	Bilateral, may have abnormal facies, macular cherry-red spot, autosomal recessive

In addition to rubella and syphilis, many other infectious agents can cause intrauterine keratitis, including *Neisseria gonorrhoeae,* staphylococci, herpes simplex, and influenza virus. The process can still be active at birth, or resolved, leaving a leukoma, keratectasia, or congenital anterior staphyloma. Zellweger syndrome (see Chapter 24) and G_{M1} gangliosidosis also can present with early corneal clouding.

PENETRATING KERATOPLASTY FOR CONGENITAL CORNEAL OPACITIES

Penetrating keratoplasty can be successful in infants (Fig. 5-19), but the surgery and the postoperative care can be more demanding.[91-96] Often other ocular abnormalities, such as glaucoma, strabismus, and aphakia, complicate management and interfere with vision. Frequent examinations with

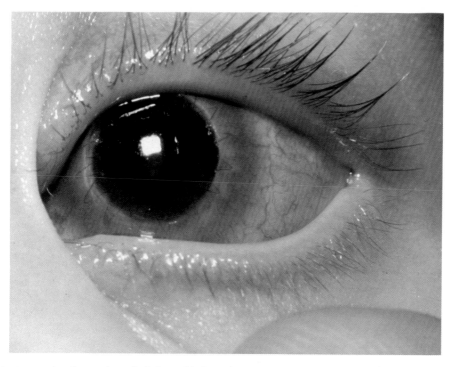

Fig. 5-19. Penetrating keratoplasty in infant with Peters' anomaly. (Courtesy Stuart I. Brown, La Jolla, Calif.)

the infant under anesthesia are required, and the sutures must be removed 4 to 6 weeks after surgery. If a clear graft is obtained, refractive correction and amblyopia therapy are essential for visual rehabilitation. In the most recent report the Emory group[95] reported that 60% of grafts were clear at 1 year. However, the visual results were more disappointing. Preoperative vascularization and necessity for lensectomy and vitrectomy correlated with poor graft survival.

The decision to perform surgery should take into consideration whether retinal, lens, or angle abnormalities are present, whether the disease is unilateral or bilateral, and whether the family can cooperate with the taxing regimens required. In bilateral cases surgery is indicated in an attempt to obtain some useful vision. Surgery can be performed for unilateral disease, particularly if conditions are favorable, but in most cases it is not worthwhile.

CHROMOSOMAL ABERRATIONS

Corneal diseases are rarely associated with a chromosomal aberration, and most chromosomal aberrations are not associated with corneal disease.[97] Most associations have been noted in only a few cases; however, a few associations occur often enough to be worth mentioning.

Trisomy 21 (Down's syndrome) is the most common of all chromosomal disorders, and is frequently associated with keratoconus.

Trisomy 17-18 (Edwards syndrome) is associated with anterior corneal opacities, cataracts, and pupillary abnormalities.[98,99] Three different types of chromosome 18 deletion defects can be associated with corneal abnormalities: short arm deletion with posterior keratoconus; long arm deletion with microcornea, corneal opacities, Peters' anomaly, oval cornea, and ASD; and ring chromosome with corneal leukomas.[100]

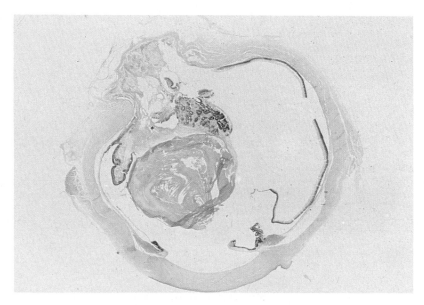

Fig. 5-20. Retinal dysplasia in trisomy 13.

In trisomy 13 (Bartholin-Patau syndrome) dysgenesis of the cornea, iris, and anterior chamber angle and retinal dysplasia are seen (Fig. 5-20). The cornea can be poorly defined, with opacification or scleralization. Nonspecific, spotty corneal opacities may be present.[101,102]

Turner's syndrome (XO) can be associated with blue sclera, oval cornea, corneal opacities, or cataracts.[18]

REFERENCES

1. Goldhammer Y and Smith JL: Cryptophthalmos syndrome with basal encephaloceles, Am J Ophthalmol 80:146, 1975.
2. Codère F, Brownstein S, and Chen MF: Cryptophthalmos syndrome with bilateral renal agenesis, Am J Ophthalmol 91:737, 1981.
3. Ide CH and Wollschlaeger PB: Multiple congenital abnormalities associated with cryptophthalmos, Arch Ophthalmol 81:638, 1969.
4. Bergsma D, editor: Birth defects: atlas and compendium, Baltimore, 1973, Williams & Wilkins Co.
5. Duke-Elder S: System of Ophthalmology, vol 3, part 2, Normal and abnormal development: congenital deformities, St Louis, 1964, Mosby–Year Book, Inc.
6. Reinecke RD: Cryptophthalmos, Arch Ophthalmol 85:376, 1971.
7. Vail DT: Adult hereditary anterior megalophthalmos sine glaucoma: a definite disease entity, Arch Ophthalmol 6:39, 1931.
8. Friede R: Megalocornea congenita, a phylogenetic anomaly, Graefes Arch Clin Ophthalmol 148:716, 1948.
9. Malbran E: Megalocornea with mosaic-like dystrophy, Arch Ophthalmol 74:130, 1965.
10. Young AI: Megalocornea and mosaic dystrophy in identical twins, Am J Ophthalmol 66:734, 1968.
11. Calamandrei D: Megalocornea in due pazienti con syndrome craniosinotoscia, Q Ital Ophthalmol 3:278, 1950.
12. Libert J et al: Ocular findings in I cell disease (mucolipidosis type II), Am J Ophthalmol 83:617, 1977.
13. Warburg M: The heterogeneity of microphthalmia in the mentally retarded. In Bergsma D, editor: The eye, vol 7, Baltimore, 1971, Williams & Wilkins Co.
14. Durham DG: Cutis hyperelastica (Ehlers-Danlos syndrome) with blue scleras, microcornea, and glaucoma, Arch Ophthalmol 49:220, 1953.
15. Feiler-Ofry V, Stein R, and Godel V: Marchesani's syndrome and chamber angle anomalies, Am J Ophthalmol 65:862, 1968.
16. Henkind P, Siegel IM, and Carr RE: Mesodermal dysgenesis of the anterior segment: Rieger's anomaly, Arch Ophthalmol 73:810, 1965.
17. Goldberg G: Waardenburg's syndrome with fundus and other anomalies, Arch Ophthalmol 76:797, 1966.
18. Lessel S and Forbes AP: Eye signs in Turner's syndrome, Arch Ophthalmol 76:211, 1966.
19. Ginsberg J and Boue KE: Ocular pathology of trisomy 13, Ann Ophthalmol 6:113, 1974.
20. Boniuk V and Boniuk M: Congenital rubella syndrome, Int Ophthalmol Clin 8:487, 1968.

21. Desvignes P et al: Aspect iconographique d'une cornea plana dans une maladie de Lobstein, Arch Ophtalmol (Paris) 27:585, 1967.
22. Erikkson AW, Lehmann E, and Forsius H: Congenital cornea plana in Finland, Clin Genet 4:301, 1973.
23. Forsius H: Studien über cornea plana congenita. Bei 19 kranken in 9 familien, Acta Ophthalmol (Copenh) 39:203, 1961.
24. Felix CH: Kongenitale familiäre cornea plana, Klin Monatsbl Augenheilkd 74:710, 1925.
25. Dada VK, Verma LK, and Sachdev MS: Comprehensive visual and cosmetic rehabilitation of cornea plana, Cornea 7:102, 1988.
26. Ross JVM: Keratoconus posticus generalis, Am J Ophthalmol 33:801, 1950.
27. Jacobs HB: Posterior conical cornea, Br J Ophthalmol 41:31, 1957.
28. Francois J: Heredity in ophthalmology, St Louis, 1971, Mosby–Year Book, Inc.
29. Teikari JM and O'Donnell JJ: Astigmatism in 72 twin pairs, Cornea 8:263, 1989.
30. Waring GO, Rodrigues MM, and Laibson PR: Anterior chamber cleavage syndrome: a stepladder classification, Surv Ophthalmol 20:3, 1975.
31. Reese AB and Ellsworth RM: The anterior chamber cleavage syndrome, Arch Ophthalmol 75:307, 1966.
32. Wilson FM: Congenital anomalies. In Smolin G and Thoft RA, editors: The cornea: scientific foundations and clinical practice, Boston, 1983, Little, Brown & Co.
33. Bahn CF et al: Classification of corneal endothelial disorders based on neural crest origin, Ophthalmology 91:558, 1984.
34. Cintron C, Covington HI, and Kublin CL: Morphogenesis of rabbit corneal endothelium, Curr Eye Res 7:913, 1988.
35. Forsius H, Erikksson A, and Fellman J: Embryotoxon corneae posterius in an isolated population, Acta Ophthalmol 42:42, 1964.
36. Sugar HS: Juvenile glaucoma with Axenfeld syndrome, Am J Ophthalmol 59:1012, 1969.
37. Brear DR and Insler MS: Axenfeld's syndrome associated with systemic abnormalities, Ann Ophthalmol 17:291, 1985.
38. Henkind P and Friedman AH: Iridogoniodysgenesis with cataract, Am J Ophthalmol 72:949, 1971.
39. Henkind P, Siegel IM, and Carr RE: Mesodermal dysgenesis of the anterior segment: Rieger's anomaly, Arch Ophthalmol 73:810, 1965.
40. Alkemade PPH: Dysgenesis mesodermalis of the iris and the cornea, Springfield, Ill, 1969, Charles C Thomas, Publishers.
41. Shields MB: Axenfeld-Rieger syndrome: a theory of mechanism and distinctions from the iridocorneal endothelial syndrome, Trans Am Ophthalmol Soc 81:736, 1983.
42. Cross HE and Maumenee AE: Progressive spontaneous dissolution of the iris, Surv Ophthalmol 18:186, 1973.
43. Judisch GF, Phelps CD, and Hanson J: Rieger's syndrome: a case report with a 15-year follow-up, Arch Ophthalmol 97:2120, 1979.
44. Gregor S and Hitchings RA: Rieger's anomaly: a 42-year follow-up, Br J Ophthalmol 64:56, 1980.
45. Dark AJ and Kirkham TH: Congenital opacities: patient with Rieger's anomaly and Down's syndrome, Br J Ophthalmol 52:631, 1968.
46. Tabbara KF, Khouri FP, and der Kaloustian VM: Rieger's syndrome with chromosomal anomaly: report of a case, Can J Ophthalmol 8:488, 1973.
47. Heinemann M, Breg R, and Cotlier E: Rieger's syndrome with pericentric inversion of chromosome 6, Br J Ophthalmol 63:40, 1979.
48. Falls JF: A gene producing various defects of the anterior segment of the eye, Am J Ophthalmol 32:41, 1949.
49. Pearce EH and Kerr CB: Inherited variations in Rieger's malformation, Br J Ophthalmol 49:530, 1969.
50. Shields MB et al: Axenfeld-Rieger syndrome: a spectrum of developmental disorders, Surv Ophthalmol 29:387, 1985.
51. Collier J: Le kératocône posterieur, Arch Ophtalmol (Paris) 22:376, 1972.
52. Townsend WM, Font RL, and Zimmerman LE: Congenital corneal leukomas. III. Histopathologic findings in 13 eyes with paracentral defect in Descemet's membrane, Am J Ophthalmol 77:400, 1974.
53. Wolter FR and Haney WP: Histopathology of keratoconus posticus circumscriptus, Arch Ophthalmol 69:357, 1963.
54. Butler TM: Keratoconus posticus, Trans Ophthalmol Soc UK 50:551, 1930.
55. Krachmer F and Rodrigues MM: Posterior keratoconus, Arch Ophthalmol 96:1867, 1978.
56. Haney WP and Falls HF: The occurrence of congenital keratoconus posticus circumscriptus in two siblings presenting a previously unrecognized syndrome, Am J Ophthalmol 52:53, 1961.
57. Peters A: Über Angeborene Defektbildung der Descemetschen Membran, Klin Monatsbl Augenheilkd 44:27, 1906.
58. Townsend WM: Congenital corneal leukomas. I. Central defect in Descemet's membrane, Am J Ophthalmol 77:80, 1974.
59. Townsend WM, Font RL, and Zimmerman LE: Congenital corneal leukomas. II. Histopathologic findings in 19 eyes with central defect in Descemet's membrane, Am J Ophthalmol 77:192, 1974.
60. Stone DL et al: Congenital central corneal leukoma (Peters' anomaly), Am J Ophthalmol 81:173, 1976.
61. Ide CH et al: Dysgenesis mesodermalis of the cornea (Peters anomaly): associated cleft lip and palate, Ann Ophthalmol 98:1059, 1980.
62. Kivlin JD et al: Peters anomaly as a consequence of genetic and nongenetic syndromes, Arch Ophthalmol 104:61, 1986.
63. Nakaniski I and Brown SI: The histopathology and ultrastructure of congenital central corneal opacity (Peters' anomaly), Am J Ophthalmol 72:801, 1971.
64. Lee CF et al: Immunohistochemical studies of Peters' anomaly, Ophthalmology 96:958, 1989.
65. Heckenlively J and Kielar RP: Congenital perforated cornea in Peters' anomaly, Am J Ophthalmol 88:63, 1979.
66. Howard RO and Abrahams IW: Sclerocornea, Am J Ophthalmol 71:1254, 1971.

67. Block N: Les differents types de sclerocornée, leurs modes d'heredité et les malformations congénitales concomitantes, J Genet Hum 15:133, 1965.

68. Rodrigues MM, Calhoun J, and Weinreb S: Sclerocornea with an unbalanced translocation (17p, 10q), Am J Ophthalmol 78:49, 1974.

69. Friedman AH et al: Sclerocornea and defective mesodermal migration, Br J Ophthalmol 59:683, 1975.

70. Fenske HD and Spitalny LA: Hereditary osteo-onychodysplasia, Am J Ophthalmol 70:604, 1970.

71. Waring GO and Rodrigues MM: Ultrastructure and successful keratoplasty of sclerocornea in Mieten's syndrome, Am J Ophthalmol 90:469, 1980.

72. Kanai A et al: The fine structure of sclerocornea, Invest Ophthalmol 9:687, 1971.

73. Goldstein JE and Cogan DG: Sclerocornea and associated congenital anomalies, Arch Ophthalmol 67:761, 1962.

74. Dohlman CH: Familial congenital cornea guttata in association with anterior polar cataract, Acta Ophthalmol (Copenh) 29:445, 1951.

75. Nucci P et al: Mandibulofacial dysostosis and cornea guttata, Am J Ophthalmol 108:204, 1989.

76. Witschel H et al: Congenital hereditary stromal dystrophy, Arch Ophthalmol 96:1043, 1978.

77. Grayson M: The nature of hereditary deep polymorphous dystrophy of the cornea: its association with iris and anterior chamber dysgenesis, Trans Am Ophthalmol Soc 72:516, 1974.

78. Mackman G, Brightbill FS, and Optiz JM: Corneal changes in aniridia, Am J Ophthalmol 87:497, 1979.

79. Grove JH, Shaw MW, and Bourque G: A family study of aniridia, Arch Ophthalmol 65:81, 1961.

80. Benjamin SN and Allen F: Classification of limbal dermoid choristomas and branch arch anomalies, Arch Ophthalmol 87:305, 1927.

81. Mansour AM et al: Ocular choristomas, Surv Ophthalmol 33:339, 1989.

82. Daily EG and Lubowitz RM: Dermoids of the limbus and cornea, Am J Ophthalmol 53:661, 1962.

83. Mattos J, Contreras F, and O'Donnell FE: Ring dermoid syndrome: a new syndrome of autosomal dominantly inherited bilateral, annular limbal dermoids with corneal and conjunctival extension, Arch Ophthalmol 98:1059, 1980.

84. Henkind P et al: Bilateral corneal dermoids, Am J Ophthalmol 76:972, 1973.

85. Baum JL and Feingold M: Ocular aspects of Goldenhar's syndrome, Am J Ophthalmol 75:250, 1973.

86. Mansour AM et al: Ocular findings in the facioauriculovertebral sequence (Goldenhar-Gorlin syndrome), Am J Ophthalmol 100:555, 1985.

87. Pokorny KS et al: Epibulbar choristomas containing lacrimal tissue: clinical distinction from dermoids and histologic evidence of an origin from the palpebral lobe, Ophthalmology 94:1249, 1987.

88. Boniuk M and Zimmerman LE: Epibulbar osteoma (episcleral osseous choristoma), Am J Ophthalmol 53:290, 1962.

89. O'Grady RB and Kirk HQ: Corneal keloids, Am J Ophthalmol 73:206, 1972.

90. Weizenblatt S: Congenital malformations of cornea associated with embryonic arrest of ectodermal and mesodermal structures, Arch Ophthalmol 52:415, 1954.

91. Picetti B and Fine M: Keratoplasty in children, Am J Ophthalmol 61:782, 1966.

92. Brown SI: Corneal transplantation of the infant cornea, Trans Am Acad Ophthalmol Otolaryngol 78:OP461, 1974.

93. Waring GO and Laibson PR: Keratoplasty in infants and children, Trans Am Acad Ophthalmol Otolaryngol 83:OP283, 1977.

94. Schanzlin DJ, Goldberg DB, and Brown SI: Transplantation of congenitally opaque corneas, Ophthalmology 87:1253, 1980.

95. Stulting RD et al: Penetrating keratoplasty in children, Ophthalmology 91:1222, 1984.

96. Cowden JW: Penetrating keratoplasty in infants and children, Ophthalmology 97:324, 1990.

97. Jay M: The eye in chromosome duplications and deficiencies, New York, 1977, Marcell Dekker.

98. Ginsberg J, Perin EV, and Sueoka ET: Ocular manifestations of trisomy 18, Am J Ophthalmol 66:59, 1968.

99. Mullaney J: Ocular pathology in trisomy 18 (Edward's syndrome), Am J Ophthalmol 76:246, 1973.

100. Yanoff M, Rorke LB, and Niederer BS: Ocular and cerebral abnormalities in chromosome 18 deletion defect, Am J Ophthalmol 70:391, 1970.

101. Apple DJ, Holden JD, and Stallworth B: Ocular pathology of Patau's syndrome with unbalanced O-D translocation, Am J Ophthalmol 70:383, 1970.

102. Roch LM, Petrucci JV, and Varaber AB: Studies on the development of the eye in 13-15 trisomy syndrome, Am J Ophthalmol 60:1067, 1965.

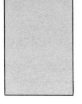

CONJUNCTIVITIS I: FOLLICULAR, NEONATAL, AND BACTERIAL

ACUTE AND CHRONIC FOLLICULAR CONJUNCTIVITIS

The presence of follicles is a relatively specific finding that limits the differential diagnosis to a small number of disorders. It is useful to further categorize these disorders as acute (less than 2 weeks in duration) and chronic (having a longer duration of symptoms). The classifications overlap somewhat because some diseases can manifest themselves as either acute or chronic follicular conjunctivitis.

Follicles must be differentiated from papillae, as was discussed in Chapter 3. Granulomatous lesions must also be differentiated. Fig. 6-1 shows the solitary, solid, raised, rounded, opaque lesion characteristic of sarcoid granuloma.

ACUTE FOLLICULAR CONJUNCTIVITIS

Acute follicular conjunctivitis usually has a rapid onset and often is unilateral early in the infection. The second eye usually becomes involved within a week. The disorder frequently is accompanied by preauricular lymphadenopathy. Following are some of the diseases considered in this category:

1. Epidemic keratoconjunctivitis (EKC) (most commonly adenovirus type 8)

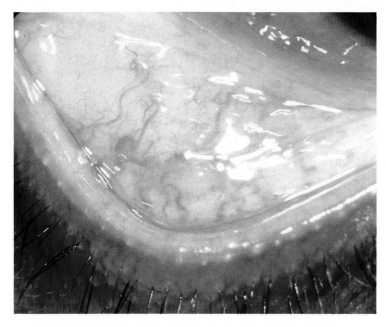

Fig. 6-1. Sarcoid granuloma of the conjunctiva.

2. Pharyngoconjunctival fever (PCF) (most commonly adenovirus types 3 and 7)
3. Primary herpes simplex keratoconjunctivitis (HSV type I, in rare cases type II)
4. Adult inclusion conjunctivitis *(Chlamydia trachomatis)*
5. Epidemic hemorrhagic keratoconjunctivitis (picornavirus)
6. Newcastle disease conjunctivitis (Newcastle disease virus)
7. Acute trachoma *(C. trachomatis)*
8. Neonatal inclusion conjunctivitis *(C. trachomatis)*

These diseases are considered in further detail in subsequent chapters, but the chief characteristics are given in Table 6-1.

CHRONIC FOLLICULAR CONJUNCTIVITIS

Subacute and chronic follicular conjunctivitis can be diagnosed in cases that continue for longer than 2 weeks. These patients may report an acute onset, with persistent disease, or insidious disease development. The conjunctivitis can continue for months or years. The following diseases and related conditions should be considered:

1. Trachoma
2. Inclusion conjunctivitis
3. Molluscum contagiosum
4. Drug-induced conjunctivitis (eserine, idoxuridine, and eye cosmetics)
5. Bacterial conjunctivitis (*Moraxella* organisms and in rare cases other bacteria in adolescents only)
6. Axenfeld's chronic follicular conjunctivitis (orphan conjunctivitis)
7. Chronic follicular conjunctivitis of Merrill-Thygeson type
8. Parinaud's oculoglandular syndrome (cat-scratch fever and others)
9. Folliculosis of childhood

Table 6-2 offers the pertinent details of the diseases just listed. The conditions are outlined thus to give an overall view of these diseases.

Laboratory procedures useful in the diagnosis of follicular conjunctivitis include the following:

1. Bacterial cultures to rule out a primary or secondary bacterial infection
2. Scrapings of the conjunctiva, to reveal cytologic characteristics, including cell types and viral and chlamydial inclusions
3. Immunologic studies for herpes simplex, adenovirus, and chlamydia

OPHTHALMIA NEONATORUM

Conjunctivitis in the neonate should be considered separately because the causes and presentations differ from those in older patients. The infections usually are acquired from the birth canal, and this is reflected in the types of agents seen. The relative frequency of different causes varies, depending on the prevalence of the organisms in the birth canal (of different venereal diseases) and the type of prophylaxis used.

Most commonly, however, no infectious cause is identified. Some of these cases are chemical; some may be undiagnosed chlamydial infection. The neonatal conjunctiva rapidly acquires an indigenous flora, and most bacterial species are equally likely to be present in inflamed and quiet eyes.[1-4] Therefore it is difficult to determine even whether a cultured organism is the cause of clinical disease. Most cases of ophthalmia neonatorum are self-limited and leave no permanent sequelae even if untreated. However, it is probably wise to treat any potential pathogen with appropriate antibiotics.

The most important bacterial agents to recognize are *Neisseria gonorrhoeae* and *Pseudomonas* organisms, because they can rapidly cause extensive ocular injury and, in the case of *Pseudomonas* infections, even death. Herpes simplex conjunctivitis also is important to recognize because it often is associated with disseminated disease, which has a high rate of morbidity and mortality. Early treatment with systemic antiviral therapy can greatly improve the outcome.

The most common agents, typical presentations, and current recommendations for treatment are given in Table 6-3. Clinical criteria are helpful in differentiating between the various agents and in determining initial therapy, but laboratory diagnosis is essential. Clinical signs often are nonspecific, and follicles and adenopathy cannot develop in the newborn for 6 to 12 weeks. The time of onset of disease is approximate and is determined by the time and duration of exposure, the size of the inoculum, the incubation period of the organism, and the effectiveness of the prophylaxis. If membranes are broken before delivery, ocular exposure can occur earlier, and the time before onset of signs is shorter. These infections also can occur in babies delivered by cesarean section, either by previous rupture of membranes or by postnatal inoculation.

The most common prophylaxis today is probably Credé's method, using silver nitrate 1%.[5] This treatment was intended primarily to prevent infection with *Neisseria gonorrhoeae* and is not thought to be effective against *Chlamydia trachomatis,* which currently is the most common cause of infectious neonatal conjunctivitis. The silver nitrate treatment also frequently causes a chemical conjunctivitis (discussed later in this chapter), and if accidentally administered in a stronger solution, it can cause corneal injury. Therefore many have suggested the use of other agents, particularly tetracycline and erythromycin ointments.[6,7] In a recent large prospective trial in Kenya, tetracycline and silver nitrate were found equally effective in preventing gonococcal infection, and, surprisingly, both were similarly effective against chlamydia.[8] Either tetracycline or erythromycin is probably preferable to silver nitrate because these drugs appear to be at least as effective and are nontoxic.

Scrapings and cultures are necessary (see Chapter 4). Giemsa-stained scrapings and direct fluorescent monoclonal antibody testing are used for diagnosis of chlamydial infection. Gram-stained scrapings and culture, including blood agar and chocolate or Thayer-Martin media, are necessary for

Text continued on p. 114.

TABLE 6-1. Diagnostic Features of Acute Follicular Conjunctivitis*

DISEASE	DISCHARGE AND CONJUNCTIVAL APPEARANCE	CORNEA
Epidemic keratocon-junctivitis (EKC)	Watery discharge Hyperemia and chemosis Pseudomembranes in one third of cases, which may result in scars Course of 7 to 14 days Often subconjunctival hemorrhages Follicular response in upper and lower fornices, mostly lower Rare chronic papillary conjunctivitis	Fine, diffuse, slightly elevated epithelial punctate keratitis early; persists 3 weeks in types 8 and 19; affects entire cornea Focal epithelial keratitis on 7th to 13th day Subepithelial opacities (14th to 20th day) at sites of epithelial lesions in 50% of cases; may last months (usually) or years May have stromal infiltration and edema, severe keratitis No pannus (no vascularization)
Pharyngoconjunc-tival fever	Scant watery discharge Hyperemia, chemosis Follicular; may have papillary reaction in upper and lower fornices No scars	Fine epithelial keratitis affecting entire cornea Occasionally subepithelial infiltrates (especially types 3, 4, and 7) but milder and smaller than in EKC No pannus
Acute trachoma* (usually occurs in children)	Diffuse follicular response typically most prominent on upper tarsal plate, often seen at limbus; trachoma follicles soft, can be necrotic Papillary hypertrophy Conjunctival scarring, especially of upper lid Arlt's line; horizontally linear scar at junction of posterior two thirds and anterior one third of tarsal conjunctiva Pain, mucopurulent discharge, photophobia	Fine epithelial keratitis; fine punctate, subepithelial infiltrates; fine keratitis may last until disease subsides Superior pannus (2 to 3 mm early) Marginal corneal infiltrates Occasionally dense focus of cellular infiltrates (trachoma pustule) Cicatrized limbal follicles (Herbert's pits) May result in markedly scarred and vascularized cornea
Adult chlamydial keratoconjunc-tivitis (inclusion conjunctivitis)*	Mild to moderate mucopurulent discharge Never membranous in adults Worse below No conjunctival cicatrization Redness, chemosis Follicular reaction	Superficial punctate to slightly course epithelial keratitis Sometimes subepithelial infiltrates (smaller than in EKC), which may leave scars Superior micropannus

*These entities also can be classified with chronic follicular conjunctivitis.

LABORATORY FINDINGS	ETIOLOGIC FACTORS	EPIDEMIOLOGIC AND OTHER CHARACTERISTICS
Mononuclear response except for polymorphonuclear leukocytes with pseudomembranes Immunoperoxidase test specific and sensitive first week Fourfold increase of antibody titer between acute and convalescent sera Adenovirus can be recovered in cell culture up to 2 weeks after onset, rarely longer	Adenovirus, most commonly types 8 and 19 Transmission from respiratory tract to eye, eye to eye, hand or instrument to eye; frequently acquired from eye care personnel Incubation period is 2 to 14 days Other eye usually involved in 2 to 7 days	Age group: 20 to 40 years Incidence in men greater than in women Eye is infectious up to 14 days Acute systemic symptoms only in children; hyperacute eye involvement Lymph nodes; prominent palpable, tender, and occasionally visible (90% of cases) Vision may be decreased from subepithelial corneal infiltrates
Mononuclear response FA studies of conjunctival smears detect adenovirus The virus can be recovered in cell culture A rising serum antibody titer is useful	Adenovirus, most commonly types 3 and 7 Adenovirus 7 may be more frequent in summer Transmission mainly via respiratory secretions, but also by contaminated swimming pools Incubation period is 3 to 14 days	Pharyngitis and fever Lymph nodes small and palpable but not visible or tender (90% of cases) Occurs in schools and swimming pools Lasts 7 to 14 days No sequelae

Basophilic, cytoplasmic epithelial inclusions (infrequent)
Mainly polymorphonuclear response; may have equal numbers of polymorphonuclear and mononuclear cells in chronic phase
Cytologic findings of expressed follicle:
  1. Leber's cell (macrophages)
  2. Plasma cells
  3. Lymphoblasts
Antibody in tears and serum to *C. trachomatis*
	C. trachomatis types A-C
	Incubation period 1 to 3 weeks
	Secondary bacterial infection common in endemic areas
		Well described since 1500 B.C.
		Other complications are trichiasis, distichiasis, keratitis sicca
		Preauricular nodes: palpable, rarely tender or visible
		Most commonly eye-to-eye transmission
		Multiple reinfections and bacterial superinfections important in pathogenesis of severe disease

Polymorphonuclear response May have 50% polymorphonuclear and 50% mononuclear cells in chronic phase Basophilic, intracytoplasmic, epithelial inclusions FA-stained conjunctival scrapings and serum titers may be helpful	*C. trachomatis* (types D-K)	Venereal, hand-to-eye transstransmission Persists for 3 to 12 months in untreated cases Lymph nodes: palpable, sometimes tender or visible Otitis media in 15% of cases Rarely swimming pool transmission (chlorine inhibits agent)

Continued.

TABLE 6-1. Diagnostic Features of Acute Follicular Conjunctivitis—cont'd

DISEASE	DISCHARGE AND CONJUNCTIVAL APPEARANCE	CORNEA
Neonatal inclusion conjunctivitis	Purulent discharge Papillary hypertrophy and pseudomembranes are main features in infants (nonfollicular) May become follicular if duration is longer than 6 weeks May cause mild conjunctival scarring Usually 4 to 12 days postpartum	May have fine superficial epithelial keratitis Superior micropannus
Herpes simplex virus primary (nonneonatal)	Usually unilateral Scant watery discharge unless pseudomembranous (50% of cases) Follicles often masked by membrane May have conjunctival scars after membrane formation Pain, photophobia	Fine epithelial keratitis (punctate, stellate) Dendrites after 7 days Decreased corneal sensitivity Stromal disease can develop Pannus extremely uncommon
Newcastle disease	Scant watery discharge Primarily affects inferior conjunctiva May have papillary or follicular conjunctivitis If present, follicles are prominent on lower lid Usually unilateral Pain, redness, tearing	Cornea rarely affected, but fine punctate epithelial keratitis and occasionally small subepithelial infiltrates can be seen No pannus
Acute hemorrhagic conjunctivitis	Serous to mucoid discharge Chemosis early, in first 24 hours Bilateral subconjunctival pinpoint hemorrhages in upper palpebral or bulbar conjunctiva; becomes more profuse temporally on bulbar conjunctiva; takes 1 to 2 weeks to absorb Follicles, but not prominent No pseudomembranes Pain, photophobia, redness	May have fine keratitis
Infectious mononucleosis (Epstein-Barr virus)	Acute conjunctivitis Membranous or follicular Subconjunctival hemorrhage	Fine epithelial keratitis; microdendrites Nummular keratitis: lesions are in the peripheral cornea, at all levels; may become confluent or vascularized

LABORATORY FINDINGS	ETIOLOGIC FACTORS	EPIDEMIOLOGIC AND OTHER CHARACTERISTICS
Early (first 2 days) one may see mononuclear cells, later, polymorphonuclear cells Can have equal number of polymorphonuclear and mononuclear cells in chronic phase Large number of basophilic, intracytoplasmic, epithelial inclusions on Giemsa stain FA-stained conjunctival scrapings positive in most cases	*C. trachomatis* (types D-K)	Untreated cases last 3 to 12 months Neonate contracts disease from mother's birth canal May have node late in disease Pneumonitis may be a complication Systemic erythromycin treatment indicated
Mononuclear cells; polymorphonuclear leukocytes when pseudomembranes are present Multinucleated giant cells Virus can be isolated in cell culture Direct immunologic or serologic tests may be helpful	Herpes simplex virus, usually type I	Usually occurs in children but can occur in adults Type I: direct transfer from relatives and friends, blister to eye Vesicles on lid Ulcerative blepharitis Lymph nodes: small, palpable, occasionally tender or visible Duration: 2 weeks
Mononuclear response	Newcastle disease virus (a paramyxovirus)	Droplet (finger to eye) transmission from poultry to human Occurs only with occupational exposure (poultry workers, veterinarians, laboratory workers) Lymph nodes: palpable, small sometimes tender No sequelae Duration: 7 to 10 days
Mononuclear response in early stages, polymorphonuclear in later stage Virus can be isolated during first 2 days	Enterovirus: most commonly enterovirus type 70, coxsackie type A24	Massive epidemics in Asia, Africa, and Americas Hand-to-eye transmission Incubation period less than 24 hours Small preauricular node (sometimes absent) No ocular sequelae, rarely neurologic complications (radiculomyelitis) Anterior uveitis Lasts 10 days or less
Serum antibody titers	Epstein-Barr virus	Uveitis, episcleritis, retinal hemorrhages, papillitis, and retinal edema

TABLE 6-2. Diagnostic Features of Chronic Follicular Conjunctivitis and Related Conditions

DISEASE	CONJUNCTIVA	CORNEA
Molluscum contagiosum	Pseudotrachomatous reaction Conjunctival scarring Follicular conjunctivitis Occlusion of punctum May have molluscum on conjunctiva	Fine epithelial keratitis superiorly Superior pannus
Drug-induced follicular conjunctivitis	Pseudotrachomatous picture Keratinization Drying	Fine or blotchy epithelial keratitis Pseudodendrite Keratinization Pannus Limbal follicles can occur with IDU No Herbert's pits, as in trachoma
Axenfeld's chronic follicular conjunctivitis	No bulbar conjunctival follicles Follicles mainly on lower fornix and tarsus, but also on upper tarsus Heals in 1 to 2 years without scars	No keratitis No pannus
Merrill-Thygeson chronic follicular conjunctivitis	Follicles mainly on lower fornix and tarsus, but also on upper tarsus Heals in 4 to 5 months without scars	Epithelial keratitis, mainly above Micropannus in some cases
Oculoglandular (Parinaud's) syndrome	Focal granulomatous conjunctivitis Granulomas may be surrounded by follicles May have conjunctival ulcers	Usually no involvement; however, it depends on etiology
Moraxella	Tarsal follicles Subacute conjunctivitis with moderate discharge Angular blepharoconjunctivitis	Occasionally marginal (catarrhal) infiltrate

CYTOLOGIC FINDINGS	ETIOLOGIC FACTORS	REMARKS
Molluscum bodies (eosinophilic, cytoplasmic inclusions) in biopsy of lid margin nodule Mononuclear response	Molluscum contagiosum virus (a poxvirus) White painless lid lesions with umbilicated center Incubation period 14 to 50 days	Molluscum of lid should be eradicated by curretting of lesion Often in adolescents and young adults with molluscum on other parts of body as well as lids; may spread venereally Self-limited unless cellular immunity is depressed, but ocular disease may persist for months and can result in visual loss No lymph node enlargement
Polymorphonuclear leukocytes and lymphocytes	"Toxic" reaction Agents causing epithelial keratitis include IDU, miotics, (for example, eserine and diisopropyl fluorophosphate [DFP]), adenine arabinoside, neomycin, gentamicin, tobramycin, and preservatives	Seen after prolonged use of medicines May see follicles without germinal centers with atropine Palpable preauricular adenopathy occurs rarely (IDU) Epithelial keratitis may last several weeks after stopping medication
Mononuclear	May be a slow virus	Seen in orphanages No symptoms No lymph node enlargement
Mononuclear	Unknown	Cannot transfer to monkeys or rabbits
No inclusions		May be transmitted by sharing of eye makeup No lymph node enlargement
Mixed mononuclear and polymorphonuclear leukocytes	Cat-scratch disease (gram-negative filamentous bacteria) most common Others: tularemia, sporotrichosis, tuberculosis, sarcoid (node rarely enlarged), coccidioidomycosis, lues	May have contact with kitten Lymph node visibly enlarged May have fever, malaise Serum and skin tests, plus anaerobic and aerobic cultures (Gram, Giemsa and acid-fast stains), chest x-ray
Gram-negative diplobacilli on smear Much fibrin and only scant polymorphonuclear leukocytes	*M. lacunata*	Adolescent patient Most common in southwestern United States Other bacteria, especially those in lacrimal system (that is, *Streptococcus* and *Haemophilus*), occasionally cause follicular conjunctivitis No lymph node enlargement

Continued.

TABLE 6-2. Diagnostic Features of Chronic Follicular Conjunctivitis and Related Conditions—cont'd

DISEASE	CONJUNCTIVA	CORNEA
Eye makeup–induced follicular conjunctivitis	Insidious or asymptomatic Pigment (mascara) in "follicles" on tarsal and forniceal conjunctiva	No keratitis
Folliculosis of childhood	No inflammation Upper lid can be mildly involved Semilunar fold is spared Follicles tend to be prominent in fornix and fade out toward lid margins	No corneal disease

TABLE 6-3. Differential Diagnosis and Treatment of Ophthalmia Neonatorum

AGENTS	DAY OF ONSET AFTER EXPOSURE	LABORATORY FINDINGS	TYPE OF DISCHARGE
Neonatal inclusion disease (*Chlamydia trachomatis*)	5 to 10 days	Polymorphonuclear cells Basophilic cytoplasmic inclusions Positive FA test	Purulent
Silver nitrate irritation (Credé method)	24 hours	Polymorphonuclear cells	Purulent in severe cases
Neisseria gonorrhoeae	3 to 5 days; shorter if very severe After 5 days indicates exposure after birth	Intraepithelial gram-negative diplococci	Mucopurulent
Staphylococcus aureus	5+ days	Gram-positive cocci and polymorphonuclear cells	Catarrhal to mucopurulent

CYTOLOGIC FINDINGS	ETIOLOGIC FACTORS	REMARKS
Pigment granules only	Incorporation of makeup granules in conjunctival cysts: uncertain whether true follicles develop	In user of cosmetics No lymph node enlargement
Mononuclear cells occasionally	Physiologic change of childhood and adolescence	Seen in children and can be associated with generalized lymphoid hyperplasia Newborn cannot have follicles until 6 weeks of age

PRESENCE OF MEMBRANE	PRESENCE OF FOLLICLES	CORNEAL INVOLVEMENT	RECOMMENDED TREATMENT
+/− May result in conjunctival scars	None in newborn; may develop in 6 weeks Response may be papillary early	Superior micropannus in treated cases Fine epithelial keratopathy	Erythromycin ethyl succinate 125 mg/kg every 6 hours for 14 days Topical tetracycline four times a day for 2 weeks
+ In severe cases		If severe, may have keratopathy, corneal scarring	Proper administration of drug (1%) Clear discharge away Do not use stock bottles of silver nitrate; concentration of drug may be 90%
−	−	Marginal or central ulcer or ring abscess Perforation	For conjunctivitis: Aqueous penicillin G 10 million U daily for 5 days, or ceftriaxone 50 mg/kg IM (one dose) Also, topical saline lavage and erythromycin ointment (0.5%) four times daily
−	−	Punctate keratopathy	Erythromycin ointment (0.5%) six times daily for 2 or 3 weeks

Continued.

TABLE 6-3. Differential Diagnosis and Treatment of Ophthalmia Neonatorum

AGENTS	DAY OF ONSET AFTER EXPOSURE	LABORATORY FINDINGS	TYPE OF DISCHARGE
Streptococcus pneumoniae	5+ days	Gram-positive cocci in chains and polymorphonuclear cells	Purulent
Haemophilus	5+ days	*H. aegyptius:* gram-negative with epithelial parasitism *H. influenzae:* no epithelial parasitism; gram-negative coccobacillus	Catarrhal, in severe cases purulent
Coliform species	5+ days	Gram-negative nonencapsulated rods in and among polymorphonuclear cells	Copious Purulent
Primary herpes (type II)	3 to 15 days	Multinucleated giant cells Positive FA test	Nonpurulent Watery
Candida	5+ days	Pseudohyphal budding yeast forms Polymorphonuclear cells	— Sometimes conjunctival necrosis

bacterial identification. It is absolutely imperative to rule out *N. gonorrhoeae* and *N. meningitidis;* the preceding laboratory hints aid in this differentiation.

INCLUSION CONJUNCTIVITIS OF THE NEWBORN

Inclusion conjunctivitis of the newborn (inclusion blennorrhea) is caused by infection with *Chlamydia trachomatis,* serotypes D through K. *C. trachomatis* encompasses a group of different agents that are responsible for trachoma, inclusion conjunctivitis of the newborn and adult, and lymphogranuloma venereum (see Chapter 8). The diseases these agents cause are distinct entities, and the disease entity depends on the serotype of chlamydia involved: types A through C for trachoma types D through K for inclusion conjunctivitis, and types L_1 through L_3 for lymphogranuloma venereum.[9,10]

The reservoir of infection with *C. trachomatis* types D through K is the urethra or cervix; the disease is transmitted venereally. The infant is infected during passage through the birth canal.[11-13] Inclusion conjunctivitis is the result of contamination of the eye by genital secretion. The disease may

PRESENCE OF MEMBRANE	PRESENCE OF FOLLICLES	CORNEAL INVOLVEMENT	RECOMMENDED TREATMENT
–	–	Ulcer may develop or punctate keratopathy, resembling staphylococcal keratitis	Erythromycin ointment (0.5%) or sulfacetamide sodium (Sulamyd) (10%) six times daily
–	–	Rare, but may develop punctate keratopathy, especially with *H. aegyptius* (Koch-Weeks conjunctivitis)	*H. aegyptius* and *H. influenzae:* 10% sulfacetamide or erythromycin ointment (0.5%) six times daily
–	–	Rare	Irrigation of conjunctival sac Neomycin (0.5%) or tetracycline six times daily
±	– In newborn may develop in 6 to 12 weeks	Epithelial or stromal disease	Debridement and patching Topical trifluorothymidine nine times daily Vidarabine 15 mg/kg/ day for 10 days
–	–	Occasional marginal corneal ulcer	5% natamycin or 1% flucytosine drops

be transmitted by fingers or fomites to the eye and often occurs in those who harbor the genital infection. Eye-to-eye transmission is extremely rare.

Inclusion conjunctivitis of the newborn is the most common infectious type of ophthalmia neonatorum, affecting as many as 3% of all newborns, according to some publications.[14,15] This is because approximately 5% to 13% of pregnant women have chlamydial infection of the cervix, and 30% to 40% of their babies will develop conjunctivitis.[13,16-20] An even higher percentage of the babies develop serologic or other systemic evidence of chlamydial infection, indicating that subclinical systemic spread via conjunctiva or other mucous membranes occurs.

Inclusion conjunctivitis appears as a purulent or mucopurulent papillary conjunctivitis (Fig. 6-2).[21-23] The incubation period usually is 5 days but can vary from 4 to 12 days. No follicles appear in the newborn state, but they can develop if the disease persists, usually between 6 weeks and 3 months of age. Preauricular adenopathy also does not appear unless the infection persists. Swelling of the lids and conjunctiva is common. A conjunctival pseudomembrane may be present. Superficial vascularization of the cornea as a micropannus can be seen, as well as a fine epithelial keratitis and,

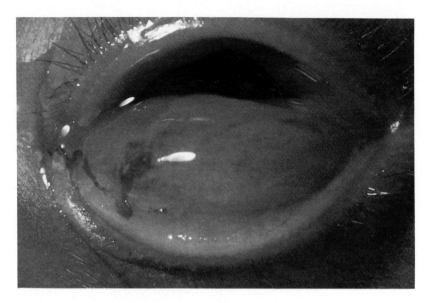

Fig. 6-2. Infantile inclusion conjunctivitis.

on occasion, underlying areas of stromal haze and infiltrate. Although these areas can occur anywhere in the cornea, they usually are more numerous in the periphery. Mild scarring of the conjunctiva is seen if conjunctival disease has been membranous.[15,24] If left untreated the disease may resolve in 3 to 4 weeks or may last for many months; the average duration is 4½ months.[13] The longer the disease goes untreated, the greater the possibility that the patient will be left with a micropannus (Fig. 6-3) or subepithelial corneal scar.[24-26]

Systemic disease can also develop, particularly pneumonitis, which occurs in 10% to 20% of infants.[27-30] Chlamydial pneumonia usually develops at 60 to 90 days of age, and preceding or concurrent conjunctivitis is present in half of these infants.[29] Rhinitis,[25] otitis, vaginitis,[25] and hearing loss[31] have also been reported.

Laboratory diagnosis of chlamydial conjunctivitis is reviewed in Chapter 8. In children Giemsa-stained scrapings and direct fluorescent antibody testing are more helpful because epithelial cell inclusions are present in greater numbers. Oral erythromycin treatment, as recommended by the national Centers for Disease Control (see Table 6-3), usually is sufficient, but persistent cases have been reported.[32] Therefore smears or cultures should be repeated after treatment.

GONOCOCCAL CONJUNCTIVITIS

In every case of ophthalmia neonatorum, gonococcal infection must be ruled out because of the possibility of blinding complications. In the last century neonatal gonococcal conjunctivitis accounted for up to 25% of the inmates in institutions for the blind.[33] The advantage of prophylactic treatment with silver nitrate was first demonstrated by Credé in 1881.[5] This treatment, combined with better treatment and recognition of gonococcal venereal infection, has reduced the incidence to approximately 0.06%.[7] Untreated, approximately 40% of newborns exposed to *N. gonorrhoeae* will develop conjunctivitis.[8] Infection can occur in a number of ways: despite prophylaxis or if it is incorrectly performed or delayed; as a result of prolonged exposure stemming from premature rupture of membranes; or through postnatal inoculation.

The incubation period for this infection usually is 3 to 5 days. However, with premature rupture of the membranes the infant can be infected in utero, and conjunctivitis will become evident earlier.

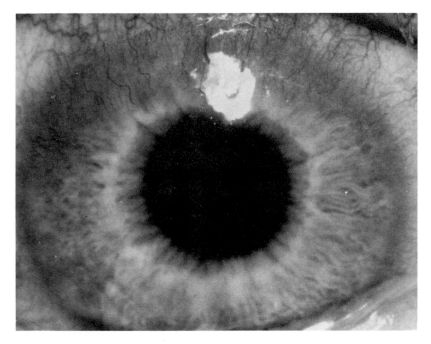

Fig. 6-3. Micropannus in an untreated case of inclusion conjunctivitis in a newborn.

Later infections usually are acquired after birth. Approximately 75% of cases are bilateral. Edema of the lids with severe chemosis and watery or serosanguineous exudate may occur. Membranes or pseudomembranes can develop. If untreated, copious purulent discharge may ensue.

The organism can penetrate intact corneal epithelium. The more severe the conjunctivitis and the longer it is left untreated, the more likely the cornea is to be affected. The cornea may break down, with ulceration either centrally or marginally. Several peripheral ulcers can become confluent and form a ring abscess.

Gram stain is about as sensitive as culture, and often cases are diagnosed by Gram stain but are culture negative.[21] Therefore both tests are required. Systemic treatment is required and probably is sufficient. Topical treatment can be used in addition (see Table 6-3). The incidence of penicillin-resistant strains is increasing, particularly in Africa. In these cases kanamycin, spectinomycin, and cefotaxime are effective. Single-dose administration of cefotaxime (50 mg/kg IM) is curative and simple.[34-36]

Other Bacteria

Certain bacteria are isolated more frequently from eyes with conjunctivitis than from noninflamed eyes, including *Staphylococcus aureus, Streptococcus pneumoniae, Haemophilus, Streptococcus viridans, Escherichia coli,* and *Pseudomonas aeruginosa.*[2,21,26] Any of these, and most likely other bacteria, can cause neonatal conjunctivitis (Fig. 6-4). The clinical characteristics usually are nonspecific, and each can be difficult to differentiate from gonococcal infection. However, some points can be made.

S. aureus conjunctivitis is common and may become serious because of infants' immature immunity. Usually the disease occurs initially as a mild catarrhal conjunctivitis with hyperemia and mucoid or mucopurulent secretion.[22] There may be some edema of the lids. A fine epithelial keratopathy can be present. Scrapings will show gram-positive cocci with polymorphonuclear cells. Unlike with the adult disease, staphylococcal conjunctivitis does not become chronic in the newborn.

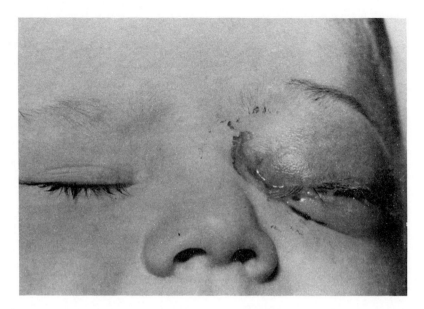

Fig. 6-4. Neonatal bacterial conjunctivitis. (Courtesy of Kenneth Cheng, Pittsburgh.)

The conjunctivitis caused by *H. influenzae* usually is a severe purulent conjunctivitis with edema of the lids, in contrast to the conjunctivitis caused by *H. aegyptius,* which usually is a mild disease with only a small amount of mucoid exudate. On scrapings and Gram stains, *H. influenzae* shows no epithelial parasitism and appears as a tiny, gram-negative coccobacillus, whereas *H. aegyptius* shows epithelial parasitism and appears as a long, fine, gram-negative bacillus.

E. coli is the most common of the coliform bacteria to cause neonatal conjunctivitis. The disease usually is an acute, purulent conjunctivitis with severe chemosis of the conjunctiva, swelling of the lids, and copious purulent secretion. Streptococcal conjunctivitis exhibits a similar picture.

Pseudomonas aeruginosa is an uncommon but important cause of neonatal conjunctivitis. When it occurs in premature infants in a neonatal care unit, it may cause keratitis, endophthalmitis, septicemia, and even death.[21,37] However, it also can cause a mild conjunctivitis or even be isolated from noninflamed eyes.

Herpes Simplex

Herpes simplex virus (HSV) is an uncommon cause of conjunctivitis in the newborn. Usually HSV type II is responsible, but in rare cases it can be type I. The conjunctivitis can be seen in isolation, combined with other ocular lesions, or with disseminated disease. It can be associated with vesicular blepharitis, corneal epithelial lesions, stromal keratitis, cataracts, or necrotizing chorioretinitis.[38,39] Conjunctivitis is occasionally the first sign of disease in a neonate who subsequently develops disseminated herpes simplex, but more commonly it occurs in isolation or several days after manifestations of infection develop at other sites. Overall, conjunctivitis is seen in about 5% to 10% of cases of neonatal herpes.

The conjunctivitis can begin anywhere from 3 days to 2 weeks after birth, with 7 days being the average. The clinical appearance is not distinctive. There is moderate injection, lid edema, and in most cases a nonpurulent exudate with a mononuclear response (see Fig. 12-1). However, if a membrane is present, numerous polymorphonuclear leukocytes are seen. In some cases a serosanguineous discharge is seen. Follicles are not present. Typical skin lesions are present somewhere on the body in one third to one half of patients with eye disease,[39] sometimes as a vesicular blepharitis.

Corneal involvement is also seen in about 10% of cases. Geographic epithelial lesions are most common, but dendrites and diffuse stromal keratitis have also been seen.[40] Necrotizing chorioretinitis and cataracts also can occur. In one case the virus was cultured from the lens 18 months after neonatal infection.[41]

If a herpetic infection is strongly suspected, scrapings may be examined for multinucleated epithelial cells and intranuclear inclusions, and culture and immunopathologic studies may be performed. The finding of typical herpetic skin or corneal involvement also can aid in the diagnosis. The conjunctival inflammation of neonatal herpes simplex resolves spontaneously in 2 to 3 weeks. Systemic and topical antiviral treatment is indicated. Parenteral vidarabine has been shown to reduce morbidity and mortality.[42] The use of acyclovir is currently being examined (see Table 6-3).

CHEMICAL CONJUNCTIVITIS

Chemical conjunctivitis is mild and lasts only a few days. It appears within 24 hours after instillation of the silver nitrate. However, in concentrations higher than 1%, silver nitrate can be most irritating and can cause conjunctival ulceration or corneal opacities.

BACTERIAL CONJUNCTIVITIS

PATHOGENESIS

The ocular surface resists infections through several mechanisms. The mechanical action of the lids and the washing effect of tear flow help by physically removing pathogens. Antimicrobial enzymes, including lysozyme, lactoferrin, and beta-lysin, are present in the tears, as well as secretory IgA antibody. Ceruloplasmin and IgG may also play a role.[43] The intact epithelial surfaces serve as mechanical barriers that inhibit penetration by organisms. The normal, nonpathogenic flora of the ocular surface inhibit growth of foreign bacteria and limit their own population size. This may be accomplished through release of antibiotic-like substances or by means of acidic metabolic end products.[44] The rich blood supply and the lymphoid layer of the conjunctiva provide a rapid and abundant supply of inflammatory cells and mediators.

Conjunctival infection occurs when an organism is able to overcome the host resistance; this depends on the virulence of the organism and the status of host resistance. A less virulent organism may exist as a commensal in one person's eye and cause a conjunctivitis in another person's eye; this has been demonstrated for *S. aureus*.[45]

Each of the mechanisms of resistance can be impaired in disease states. Decreased tear production occurs in keratoconjunctivitis sicca, and tear stagnation occurs with lacrimal duct obstruction. Exposure or poor lid function can lead to localized drying and impairment of the mechanical barrier of the surface. Trauma, including contact lens wear, scarring, or severe nutritional deficiency (particularly vitamin A), also makes the surface less resistant to infection. Antibiotic use can alter the normal flora and allow growth of pathogens that are resistant to the antibiotic. Local and systemic immunosuppression impairs the host's ability to respond to infection. Poor hygiene may lead to frequent inoculation with pathogenic organisms.

The virulence of an organism also determines how often it produces disease and the severity of the disease. Virulence is related to the organism's ability to adhere to the surface, to resist the tear enzymes, to penetrate the epithelium, and to destroy tissue and spread within it. Many bacteria elaborate toxins that impair host response and contribute to the signs and symptoms of disease (see Chapter 9). For example, gonococci are able to invade normal epithelium because of pili that attach to sugar chains on the epithelial cell surface.[46] The epithelial cell phagocytoses the bacteria, and the bacteria multiplies intracellularly, resulting in destruction of the cell and eventual subepithelial invasion.

CLINICAL MANIFESTATIONS

The manifestations of bacterial conjunctivitis depend on the virulence of the organism, as previously described, and the host's response. Fortunately, in most cases bacterial conjunctivitis is self-limiting; the host can overcome the infecting agent, and there are no sequelae. However, some agents can cause more severe disease and result in conjunctival or corneal scarring.

Commonly bacterial conjunctivitis is divided into acute, hyperacute, and chronic forms. A chronic conjunctivitis is one that lasts 4 weeks or longer. Hyperacute infections are distinguished from acute infections by the presence of copious purulent discharge and lid swelling. The bacteria most commonly associated with these forms of conjunctivitis are the following:

Acute conjunctivitis
   Staphylococcus aureus
   Haemophilus aegyptius
   Haemophilus influenzae
   Streptococcus pneumoniae
Hyperacute conjunctivitis
   Neisseria gonorrhoeae
   Neisseria meningitidis
Chronic conjunctivitis
   Staphylococcus aureus
   Moraxella lacunata
   Acinetobacter (Mimeae)
   Escherichia coli, Klebsiella, and other coliforms
   Proteus
   Pseudomonas

TABLE 6-4. Isolates in Bacterial Conjunctivitis at The Campbell Laboratory, Eye and Ear Hospital of Pittsburgh, 1983-1986*

ORGANISM	PATIENT AGE (YRS)			
	0-10	11-60	>60	TOTAL(%)
Staphylococcus aureus	23	86	45	154 (34.1%)
Haemophilus sp.	55	53	12	120 (26.6%)
Streptococcus pneumoniae	21	54	3	78 (17.3%)
Moraxella sp.	3	29	1	33 (7.3%)
Alpha-hemolytic streptococci	8	17	0	25 (5.5%)
Pseudomonas sp.	2	3	5	10 (2.2%)
Proteus sp.	0	3	4	7 (1.6%)
Acinetobacter sp.	3	2	1	6 (1.3%)
Beta-hemolytic streptococci	1	2	2	5 (1.1%)
Neisseria sp.	0	1	0	1 (0.2%)
Others†	2	3	7	12 (2.7%)
Total	118	253	80	451 (100%)

*Includes only cases in which the patient's age was known.

†*Bacillus sp., Enterobacter sp., Escherichia coli, Klebsiella sp., Serratia sp.,* fewer than 5 isolates each.

Acute bacterial conjunctivitis. The patient with acute bacterial conjunctivitis usually develops watering and irritation of the eyes, followed shortly by mucopurulent discharge and sticking of the lids together in the morning (Fig. 6-4). Most often both eyes are involved, although symptoms in one may precede those in the other by 1 to 2 days. On examination, the conjunctiva is diffusely injected, and the mucopurulent exudate may be seen in the fornix or inspissated on the lid margin. Petechial hemorrhages may be present, particularly in *S. pneumoniae* or *Haemophilus* infections. A diffuse, punctate keratopathy can be seen during the first 2 to 3 days. Marginal corneal infiltrates may be present, more commonly in infections caused by *Haemophilus*.[47] Preauricular adenopathy is not present. Giemsa-stained scrapings typically reveal a predominantly polymorphonuclear response (except in infections caused by *Branhamella catarrhalis*). Gram stain may reveal the causative organism. Cultures will isolate the pathogen and guide specific therapy. However, in most cases the cost and inconvenience of obtaining cultures exceed the benefit. If the conjunctivitis is more severe or prolonged or if the eye has been compromised, cultures should be obtained.

Pneumococcal conjunctivitis is more common in children and in colder climates. Without treatment it resolves after 7 to 11 days, leaving no sequelae.[33] *Haemophilus* conjunctivitis is relatively more common in young children (under 5 years of age), but it may be seen at any age (Table 6-4). It also is more common in the warmer regions of the United States. *Haemophilus* conjunctivitis lasts 9 to 15 days and tends to be more severe than that caused by *Pneumococcus*. In young children (under 36 months of age) a severe preseptal cellulitis may develop, with swelling and a bluish discoloration of the lids. Fever, irritability, and upper respiratory tract infection usually are present.[48,49] It is important to recognize this condition, because septicemia, meningitis, septic arthritis, and endogenous endophthalmitis can occur. Systemic treatment is indicated to prevent these complications.

Streptococcus pyogenes and *Corynebacterium diphtheriae* can produce a severe conjunctivitis with membrane formation. Conjunctivitis is the most common ocular complication of Lyme disease and may be an early sign of that disorder.[50,51] There can be a follicular response.

Hyperacute bacterial conjunctivitis. Hyperacute conjunctivitis is typically caused by *Neisseria,* either *N. gonorrhoeae* or *N. meningitidis,* and the former is by far the most common. It usually is acquired by autoinoculation from infected genitalia and therefore is seen most often in adolescents and young adults although it can occur at any age. It appears to be more common in warmer months.[52]

As with acute conjunctivitis, hyperacute conjunctivitis typically begins as redness and irritation but rapidly progresses to copious purulent discharge, swelling of the lids, pain, and tenderness (Figs. 6-5 and 6-6). There is marked hyperemia and chemosis of the conjunctiva, and membranes may form. Tender preauricular adenopathy can be present. Unilateral and bilateral involvement are equally common. Corneal involvement is common, with punctate keratopathy the most frequent finding. Stromal infiltration or ulceration most often develops in the periphery, beneath an overlying fold of edematous conjunctiva. Corneal involvement can occur at any time, even within 24 hours, but is more common the longer the infection is left untreated. Ulceration can progress and perforation occur despite topical antibiotic treatment, and early peripheral corneal infiltration can develop during the first 1 to 3 days of parenteral therapy.[52,53] It is not clear whether the corneal ulceration is caused by invasion by the organism or is noninfectious, resulting from bacterial toxins or products of inflammation.[53]

In conjunctival scrapings the exuberant polymorphonuclear response is evident. Gram-negative diplococci are seen within the inflammatory cells. Culture on chocolate agar or Thayer-Martin media is indicated to isolate the organism and determine antibiotic sensitivity.

With appropriate therapy the discharge abates within 48 hours, and the other signs gradually resolve over 1 to 2 weeks. Corneal and conjunctival scarring can result.

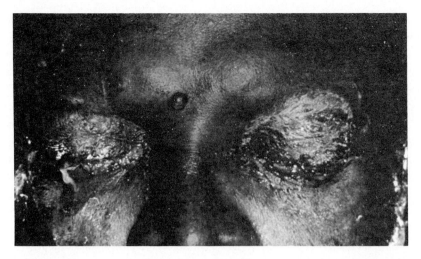

Fig. 6-5. Discharge-coated lids in gonococcal conjunctivitis. (Courtesy of Thomas Roussel, Miami.)

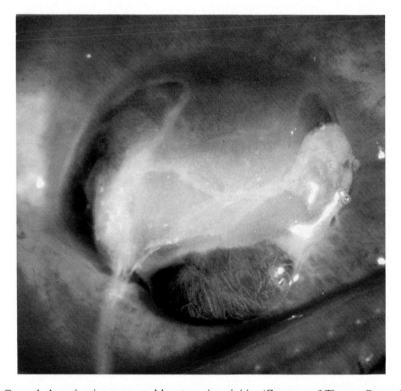

Fig. 6-6. Corneal ulceration in gonococcal keratoconjunctivitis. (Courtesy of Thomas Roussel, Miami.)

Chronic bacterial conjunctivitis. Staphylococcal blepharoconjunctivitis is a common disease with many manifestations. Chronic conjunctival seeding occurs, and conjunctival cultures often yield the organism, but most of the bacteria reside on the lid. Conjunctival and corneal inflammation probably are related to the toxins produced by the staphylococci and the body's immunologic response to the organism and these toxins. These topics are considered in Chapters 13 (blepharitis) and 19 (immunologic diseases).

A number of other bacteria can cause a chronic conjunctivitis.[47,54] *Moraxella* organisms are probably the most common and are seen mainly in young adults. The infection can manifest itself either as a chronic follicular conjunctivitis (Fig. 6-7) or as an angular blepharoconjunctivitis (Fig. 6-8). The latter is characterized by ulceration of the lateral lid margins and conjunctival injection, which is most evident laterally. This is thought to be caused by a proteolytic enzyme produced by the *Moraxella* bacteria. *Proteus* is the only member of the enteric species that produces a marked conjunctival response.[54]

The symptoms of chronic bacterial conjunctivitis are relatively nonspecific. Irritation, redness, and mild mattering of the lids are the most common complaints. The findings include injection, mild

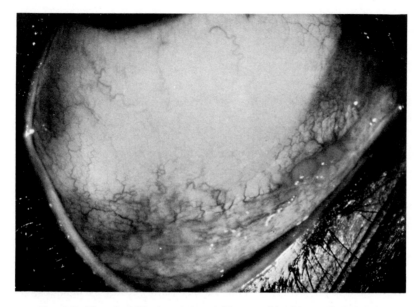

Fig. 6-7. Chronic follicular conjunctivitis caused by *Moraxella* infection.

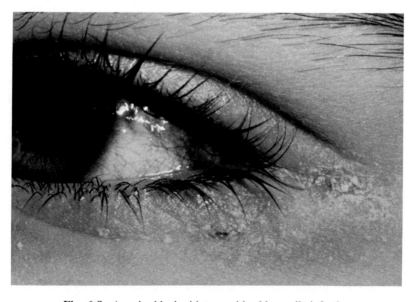

Fig. 6-8. Angular blepharitis caused by *Moraxella* infection.

papillary response, and mucoid or mucopurulent exudate. If staphylococcal blepharitis is present, additional findings may include redness and maceration of the lid margins, crusting, collarettes, inferior punctate keratitis, catarrhal infiltrates, and phlyctenulosis.

TREATMENT

For most cases of bacterial conjunctivitis, topical antibiotic therapy is sufficient. As mentioned previously, ideally antibiotic selection is based on isolation of the causative organism and determination of sensitivity. However, in most cases this is not necessary, and broad-spectrum antibiotic administration is used. Using drops or ointment four times per day usually is sufficient. Sulfacetamide 10% to 15% and neomycin-polymyxin B combination are good broad-spectrum agents, although the latter has a relatively high rate of allergic reactions. The aminoglycosides gentamicin and tobramycin are less appropriate. They are not effective against *S. pneumoniae* and 7% to 8% of *S. aureus* and are associated with significant risk of hypersensitivity and toxicity. Chloramphenicol has broad-spectrum activity, but its use is discouraged because of the very rare risk of aplastic anemia.[55] Treatment should be continued for at least 2 days after symptoms and signs resolve, usually 5 to 7 days.

Hyperacute conjunctivitis caused by *Neisseria* requires systemic therapy. Whenever it is suspected, systemic therapy should be initiated immediately and not delayed until culture confirmation is obtained.

The Centers for Disease Control recommends the following treatment for gonococcal conjunctivitis in adults: aqueous penicillin G 10 million units intravenously (IV) daily for 5 days.[56] For beta-lactamase–producing strains the recommended treatment is cefotaxime 500 mg intravenously four times daily for 5 days or ceftriaxone 1 g intramuscularly (IM) or intravenously daily for 5 days.

However, recent studies have found a single intramuscular dose of ceftriaxone (1 g or 50 mg/kg in patients weighing less than 20 kg)[35] or a single oral dose of norfloxacin (1200 mg in adults)[57] also to be effective.

If keratitis is present an agent effective against penicillinase-producing strains should be administered initially, since delaying treatment can have a devastating result. A multidose regimen is also probably safer. Ullman et al.[36] recommended the following:

1. Ceftriaxone 1 g (25 to 40 mg/kg) intravenously every 12 hours for 3 days (in patients allergic to penicillin, substitute spectinomycin 2 g intramuscularly every 12 hours for 2 days)
2. Topical saline lavage
3. Topical erythromycin, gentamicin, or bacitracin ointment four times daily
4. Treatment for *Chlamydia trachomatis* infection (see Chapter 8)

The value of topical antibiotic administration is unclear, but it certainly is not necessary. Bacitracin, erythromycin, and penicillin are the most effective topical agents. Frequent irrigation helps remove purulent debris and toxic byproducts. Routine treatment for chlamydial infection is recommended by some because of the high incidence of coinfection.

When staphylococcal blepharoconjunctivitis is present, lid scrubs followed by application of bacitracin, erythromycin, or sulfacetamide ointment are performed once or twice times daily for at least 1 month (see Chapter 13).

PARINAUD'S OCULOGLANDULAR SYNDROME

In 1889 Henri Parinaud, a Parisian ophthalmologist, described three butchers who developed a self-limited disease characterized by conjunctival "granulations" and suppurative preauricular adenopathy, which he believed to be caused by an infectious agent transmitted by animals.[58] In 1913 Frederick Verhoeff, an American ophthalmologist, reported that a filamentous organism, *Leptothrix*, was present in the conjunctiva of patients with Parinaud's syndrome,[59] and he later isolated the organism.[60] Since that time it has become evident that the cases described by Parinaud and Verhoeff were

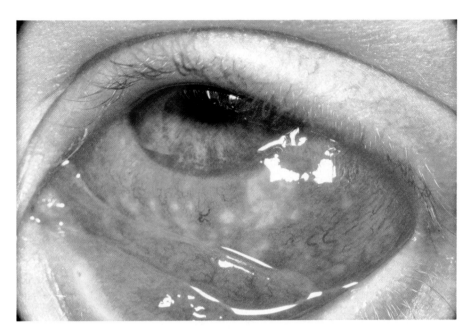

Fig. 6-9. Conjunctival ulcerations in Parinaud's oculoglandular syndrome.

most likely manifestations of cat-scratch disease (CSD), an infectious disease acquired from cats and caused by a filamentous bacterium. However, the term "oculoglandular syndrome" has become more broadly applied, and its definition varies, depending on the source. It is most commonly used to describe any condition in which conjunctival granulomas or ulcerations are associated with preauricular or submandibular adenopathy (Fig. 6-9).

Such a broad definition encompasses a spectrum of diseases, as shown in the box on p. 126, but the most common remains cat-scratch disease. The manifestations vary, depending on the etiologic agent, but usually are not specific enough to permit diagnosis without laboratory identification.

DIAGNOSTIC EVALUATION

Which procedures are performed depends on which of the possible causative agents are suspected, based on history and examination. As a minimum, conjunctival scrapings and culture should be performed. Special media are required for many of the agents, such as blood-dextrose-cysteine agar for *Francisella tularensis,* Lowenstein-Jensen for mycobacteria, and Sabouraud agar for *Sporotrichum schenckii.* Biopsy of the conjunctival lesion for culture and examination is frequently helpful. Skin tests are available for CSD, Lymphogranuloma venereum, coccidioidomycosis, glanders, and tuberculosis. Serologic tests are useful in tularemia, syphilis, infectious mononucleosis, rickettsial infection, and coccidioidomycosis.

CAT-SCRATCH DISEASE

Cat-scratch disease appears to be a relatively common disorder that often goes unrecognized. Eye involvement, manifested as Parinaud's oculoglandular syndrome, occurs in approximately 4% of patients.[61] It is caused by an infectious agent similar to that described by Verhoeff,[60] a pleomorphic gram-negative bacillus.[62-64] This agent has been observed in and cultured from affected lymph nodes and conjunctiva and can produce similar disease in the armadillo.[62] The disease is transmitted by cats, usually immature ones, through a scratch or bite, contact with an open wound, or direct inoculation of mucous membranes. Person-to-person transmission does not appear to occur. Patients with

CAUSES OF PARINAUD'S OCULOGLANDULAR SYNDROME

COMMON	OCCASIONAL	RARE
Cat-scratch disease	Tuberculosis	Chancroid
Tularemia	Syphilis	*Pasteurella multocida*
Sporotrichosis	Coccidioidomycosis	*Yersinia pseudotuberculosis*
		Yersinia enterocolitica
		Leprosy
		Glanders
		Lymphogranuloma venereum
		Listeria
		Actinomycosis
		Blastomycosis
		Mediterranean fever
		Mumps
		Infectious mononucleosis
		Caterpillar hair
		Rickettsia

From Chin GN and Hyndiuk RA: Parinaud's oculoglandular conjunctivitis. In Duane TA and Jaeger EA, editors: Clinical ophthalmology, vol 4, Philadelphia, 1988, Harper & Row, Publishers Inc; and Chin GN and Noble RC: Ocular involvement in *Yersinia enterocolitica* infection presenting as Parinaud's oculoglandular syndrome, Am J Ophthalmol 83:19, 1977.

Parinaud's syndrome probably inoculate the eye with their hand after touching a cat, but a cat may also directly contact the eye.

Three to 5 days after inoculation of the skin, a papule develops. This becomes vesicular, crusts, and resolves, leaving a macule similar to that seen after chickenpox. Seven to 14 days after conjunctival inoculation, a soft, granulomatous nodule develops in the palpebral conjunctiva. It usually is surrounded by follicles and associated with injection, chemosis, and watery discharge. Involvement is unilateral. The patient reports photophobia, irritation, and foreign body sensation.

Regional lymphadenopathy develops within 1 to 2 weeks, usually involving 2 to 3 nodes. The nodes are firm and usually nontender. They typically regress over weeks to months, but 10% to 30% progress to suppuration. In most cases a mild systemic illness occurs, with aching, malaise, anorexia, and mild temperature elevation. In rare cases more severe complications occur, such as encephalopathy, pneumonia, or thyroiditis. The conjunctival granuloma may ulcerate, but it usually disappears over a few weeks, leaving no scar. No treatment is necessary, and antibiotics do not appear to shorten the course or lessen the risk of complications.

The CSD skin test is very helpful in diagnosis, since it is positive in 99% of patients with the disease versus approximately 4% of the general population.[61] Conjunctival or lymph node biopsy specimens should be examined with Warthin-Starry stain to observe the organism.[65] Intravenous gentamicin may be useful in patients with systemic disease.[66]

TULAREMIA

Tularemia is acquired through bites from infected ticks or deer flies, by handling or ingesting infected animal tissue, or by inhaling infected aerosols. All rodents can be sources of infection, but rabbits are the most common source. In most cases a focal ulcer forms at the site of inoculation, with enlargement of local lymph nodes and a systemic reaction that includes fever, myalgia, headache, and malaise. Systemic spread of infection occurs, resulting in granulomatous lesions throughout the reticuloendothelial system and causing pneumonia in a significant percentage of patients. In rare cases pericarditis and meningitis can occur.

Eye involvement is characterized by necrotizing conjunctivitis with tender lympadenopathy.[67] It is unilateral in about 90% of cases. The incubation period averages 3 days, but ranges from 1 to 14 days. The patient reports pain, photophobia, itching, tearing, chemosis, and mucopurulent discharge. Several yellowish conjunctival nodules appear and develop shallow ulceration. They usually are located on the tarsal conjunctiva. The enlarged regional nodes may suppurate and require incision and drainage. Systemic symptoms are more prominent than in CSD. Also, more severe ocular complications can occur, including corneal ulceration, optic neuritis, panophthalmitis, and dacryocystitis.[67]

Diagnosis is made by culture of *Franciscella tularensis* from the skin or conjunctival lesion, affected lymph node, or serum. Blood-glucose-cysteine agar, or other specific media must be used. Serologic diagnosis can be made by demonstrating rising titers.

The recommended treatment is streptomycin 1 g per day intramuscularly for 7 days. Tetracycline (25 mg/kg/day in three to four divided doses) or chloramphenicol (50 mg/kg/day in three to four divided doses) may be used but are less effective.[68]

SPOROTRICHOSIS

Sporotrichosis results from inoculation of the skin or mucous membrane with *Sporotrichum schenckii*. This organism is found in soil and decaying vegetation and on thorns. The most common means of acquiring the infection is through injury by a thorn, cactus, or brier. Nodular reactions are seen at the site of inoculation and along the draining lymphatics. The organism is a rare cause of Parinaud's syndrome.[69,70] The incubation period for conjunctival disease is 11 to 17 days. Small yellow nodules are seen that progress to ulceration. Large subcutaneous nodules may occur in the eyelid skin; these break down and form deep ulcers. Painful adenopathy also is present.[33] Generalized symptoms are rare. Diagnosis is based on culture of the fungus from the conjunctiva or lymphatic lesions. Treatment is with oral iodide. Potassium iodide (up to 4.5 to 9 ml of a saturated solution per day in divided doses) is given until 1 to 2 months after resolution of signs and symptoms.[71]

TUBERCULOSIS

The conjunctiva may be the primary site of tuberculosis infection or may become secondarily involved from the spread of extraocular disease. Most cases occur in individuals under 20 years of age. A wide range of manifestations can be seen, and these have been well described by Duke-Elder.[33,72-74] An acute conjunctivitis may occur with purulent discharge, and membranes can develop. The conjunctiva can instead be quiet and may contain yellow or gray nodules surrounded by follicles, pedunculated growths, or small miliary ulcers. Regional adenopathy may be present, particularly in primary cases, and the nodes can suppurate. The diagnosis is made by biopsy of the conjunctiva or node. Once the diagnosis is made, systemic treatment is administered. Excision of larger conjunctival masses can also be helpful.

SYPHILIS

Direct inoculation of the organism into the conjunctiva can result in primary conjunctival syphilis. The lesion appears similar to chancres occurring elsewhere: after an incubation period of 2 to 4 weeks, an indurated papule develops, ulcerates, and gradually enlarges with surrounding induration. There is little pain or discharge, but the lids become swollen, and the preauricular nodes enlarge and harden.[33,75] Simple conjunctivitis or scleritis can be seen in secondary syphilis, and in tertiary syphilis a gumma can involve the conjunctiva.

SEXUALLY TRANSMITTED DISEASES THAT CAN AFFECT THE EXTERNAL EYE

In addition to syphilis and gonorrhea, which have already been discussed, a number of sexually transmitted diseases can affect the external eye. Adult inclusion conjunctivitis is a relatively common

TABLE 6-5. Sexually Transmitted Diseases

DISEASE	LABORATORY FINDINGS	TYPES OF DISCHARGE	PRESENCE OF FOLLICLES
Inclusion conjunctivitis	Polymorphonuclear leukocytes Rare inclusions (basophilic and cytoplasmic) Direct and serum immunologic tests	Mucopurulent No membrane	Positive Lower lid
Neisseria conjunctivitis	Polymorphonuclear leukocytes Gram-negative diplococci (intracellular)	Purulent or mucopurulent	Pseudomembrane on occasion
Pthirus pubis	Nits and adult organisms in lashes	Watery	Positive Severe, resulting from toxicity of parasites' feces
Reiter's syndrome	HLA B-27 76% ANA negative	Mucopurulent	Papillary response
Verrucae (viral wart)	Mononuclear reaction	None	Negative Papillary response
Molluscum contagiosum	Mononuclear response	None	Positive

*Adult dose of trisulfapyrimidines (triple sulfa), 2 to 4 g immediate loading dose followed by maintenance dose of 2 to 4 g (about 70 mg/kg) four times a day for at least 3 weeks. Do not use in pregnancy or for nursing mothers. Trisulfapyrimidine tablets (Terfonyl) contain equal amounts of sulfadiazine, sulfamerazine, and sulfamethazine.

CORNEAL INVOLVEMENT	OTHER SIGNS	TREATMENT
Superior micropannus Fine or focal epithelial keratitis Sometimes subepithelial infiltrates	Preauricular node on occasion	Tetracycline 250 mg orally four times a day for 3 weeks Do not prescribe for pregnant women or children under 8 years Or give three trisulfapyrimidine tablets* (70 mg/kg) daily, not to exceed 40 g/day for 3 to 4 weeks, Or, erythromycin 250 mg four times a day for 3 weeks
May be severe with peripheral and marginal ulcers Perforation may result	Iridocyclitis Urethritis Preauricular adenopathy	For conjunctivitis: Aqueous penicillin G 100,000 U/kg/day IV in four doses for 7 days; or ceftriaxone 50 mg/kg in one dose; or norfloxacin 1200 mg orally For penicillin-allergic: gentamicin 2 to 2.5 mg/kg IV every 8 hours for 3 days Also topical saline lavage and erythromycin ointment four times daily
Mild epithelial keratitis	Parasite found in axillary, body, chest and perianal hair	Remove nits manually Physostigmine ointment twice a day for 10 days, or 20% fluorescein solution Shampoo with Kwell
Epithelial keratitis Subepithelial infiltrates Loss of central epithelium	Nongranulomatous iritis Urethritis Arthritis Keratoderma blennorrhagica Other mucocutaneous lesions Some cases associated with chlamydial disease or dysentery	Treat chlamydial infection, if present Topical steroids for keratitis or iritis
Fine epithelial keratitis	Pedunculated or sessile lobulated skin lesion	Lid lesions can be removed; cauterize base Conjunctival lesions are best left alone; will regress in time If removing lesions, use $-80°$ C cryoapplication for 1 minute; repeat
Can develop: fine epithelial keratitis, superior micropannus "Pseudo-trachoma" Macropannus can be seen rarely	Umbilicated, raised, white non-inflamed nodule on lid or conjunctiva	Currettage of central core of molluscum

Continued.

TABLE 6-5. Sexually Transmitted Diseases—cont'd

DISEASE	LABORATORY FINDINGS	TYPES OF DISCHARGE	PRESENCE OF FOLLICLES
Lymphogranuloma venereum	May see chlamydial inclusions in macro-phages	None	Positive Papillary response May have granulomas (Parinaud's oculo-glandular syn-drome)
Syphilis (primary conjunctival)	VDRL, RPR positive in active disease FTA-ABS positive for life	None	Negative Papule, ulcerates

disease that results from ocular inoculation with genital fluids containing *Chlamydia trachomatis* (see Chapter 8). Reiter's syndrome can occur after venereal infection by chlamydia or other organisms (see Chapter 7). *Pthirus pubis,* the crab louse, usually resides in the pubic area but can infect the eyelashes. It causes blepharoconjunctivitis, which can be severe and can elicit a follicular response (see Chapter 13). The virus that causes venereal warts (condylomata acuminatum) can also cause ver-rucal lesions on the lid or conjunctiva. These can result in a mild papillary conjunctivitis and fine epithelial keratitis. Molluscum contagiosum can also be transmitted sexually.[76]

Other diseases that in rare cases may cause an oculogenital infection are diphtheria, listeriosis,[77] Mimeae conjunctivitis[14,78] and chancroid *(Haemophilus ducreyi).*

It is most important in any of these oculogenital infections to examine the patient's sexual part-ner.

Table 6-5 lists the classification and therapeutic measures for treating the preceding oculogenital infections.

REFERENCES

1. Torrey JC and Reese MK: Initial aerobic flora of new-born infants: selective tolerance of the upper respiratory tract for bacteria, Am J Dis Child 69:208, 1945.
2. Prentice MJ, Hutchinson GR, and Taylor-Robinson D: A microbiological study of neonatal conjunctivae and conjunctivitis, Br J Ophthalmol 61:601, 1977.
3. Molgaard IL, Nielsen PB, and Kaern J: A study of the incidence of neonatal conjunctivitis and of its bacterial causes including *Chlamydia trachomatis:* clinical exam-ination, culture and cytology of tear fluid, Acta Oph-thalmol (Copenh) 62:461, 1984.
4. Pierce JM, Ward ME, and Seal V: Ophthalmia neonato-rum in the 1980's: incidence, aetiology and treatment, Br J Ophthalmol 66:728, 1982.
5. Crede CSF: Die verhutung der augenentzundung der neugeborenen, Arch Gynak 21:179, 1881.
6. American Academy of Pediatrics: Prophylaxis and treat-ment of neonatal gonococcal infections, Pediatrics 65:1047, 1980.
7. Rothenberg R: Ophthalmia neonatorum due to *Neisseria gonorrhoeae:* prevention and treatment, Sex Transm Dis 6(suppl):187, 1979.
8. Laga M et al: Prophylaxis of gonococcal and chlamydial

ophthalmia neonatorum: a comparison of silver nitrate and tetracycline, N Engl J Med 318:653, 1988.
9. Jones BR: Laboratory tests for chlamydial infection, Br J Ophthalmol 58:438, 1974.
10. Wang S and Grayston JT: Immunologic relationship be-tween genital TRIC, lymphogranuloma venereum, and related organisms in a new microtiter indirect immuno-fluorescent test, Am J Ophthalmol 70:367, 1970.
11. Schachter J: Reply to letter to editor, JAMA 234:592, 1975.
12. Tabbara KF and Babb AA: Lacrimal system complica-tions in trachoma, Ophthalmology 87:298, 1980.
13. Thygeson P and Stone W Jr: Epidemiology of inclusion conjunctivitis, Arch Ophthalmol 27:91, 1942.
14. Burns RP and Florey MJ: Conjunctivitis caused by Mimeae, Am J Ophthalmol 56:386, 1963.
15. Hansman D: Inclusion conjunctivitis, Med J Aust 1:151, 1969.
16. Chandler JW et al: Ophthalmia neonatorum associated with maternal neonatal chlamydial infection, Trans Am Acad Ophthalmol Otolaryngol 83:OP302, 1971.
17. Alexander ER et al: Prospective study of perinatal *Chlamydia trachomatis* infection. In Hobson D and

CORNEAL INVOLVEMENT	OTHER SIGNS	TREATMENT
May have severe corneal scarring, inflammation and vascularization (usually superior) Sclerokeratitis	Preauricular adenopathy Elephantiasis of lids Optic neuritis Uveitis Episcleritis Sclerokeratitis	Tetracycline 1 to 1.5 g orally every day for 3 to 4 weeks
Negative	Preauricular adenopathy Lid edema	Benzathine penicillin G, 2.4 million units IM

Holmes KK, editors: Nongonococcal urethritis and related infections, Washington, DC, 1977, American Society for Microbiology.

18. Schachter J: Chlamydial infections, N Engl J Med 298:428, 1978.

19. Schachter J et al: Prospective study of perinatal transmission of *Chlamydia trachomatis,* JAMA 255:3374, 1986.

20. Hammerschlag MR et al: Prospective study of maternal and infantile infection with *Chlamydia trachomatis,* Pediatrics 64:142, 1979.

21. Armstrong JH, Zacarias F, and Rein MF: Ophthalmia neonatorum: a chart review, Pediatrics 57:884, 1976.

22. Ostler HB: Oculogenital disease, Surv Ophthalmol 20:233, 1976.

23. Hobson D, Rees E, and Viswalingam ND: Chlamydial infections in neonates and older children, Br Med Bull 39:128, 1983.

24. Forster RK, Dawson CR, and Schachter J: Late follow-up of patients with neonatal inclusion conjunctivitis, Am J Ophthalmol 69:467, 1970.

25. Mordhorst CH and Dawson C: Sequelae of inclusion conjunctivitis and associated disease in parents, Am J Ophthalmol 71:861, 1971.

26. Persson K et al: Neonatal chlamydial eye infection: an epidemiological and clinical study, Br J Ophthalmol 67:700, 1983.

27. Schachter J et al: Pneumonitis following inclusion blennorrhea, J Pediatr 87:779, 1975.

28. Schacter J and Dawson C: Is trachoma an ocular component of a more generalized chlamydial infection? Lancet 1:702, 1979.

29. Beem MO and Saxon EM: Respiratory tract colonization and a distinctive pneumonia syndrome in infants infected with *Chlamydia trachomatis,* N Engl J Med 296:306, 1977.

30. Harrison JR et al: *Chlamydia trachomatis* infant pneumonitis, N Engl J Med 298:702, 1978.

31. Gow JA, Ostler HB, and Schachter J: Inclusion conjunctivitis with hearing loss, JAMA 229:519, 1974.

32. Rapoza PA et al: Epidemiology of neonatal conjunctivitis, Ophthalmology 93:456, 1986.

33. Duke-Elder S and Leigh AG: System of ophthalmology, vol 8, Diseases of the outer eye, St Louis, 1965, Mosby–Year Book, Inc.

34. Lepage P et al: Single-dose cefotaxime intramuscularly cures gonococcal ophthalmia neonatorum, Br J Ophthalmol 72:518, 1988.

35. Haimovici R and Roussel TJ: Treatment of gonococcal conjunctivitis with single-dose intramuscular ceftriaxone, Am J Ophthalmol 107:511, 1989.

36. Ullman S, Roussell TJ, and Forster RK: Gonococcal keratoconjunctivitis, Surv Ophthalmol 32:199, 1987.

37. Burns RP and Rhodes DH: *Pseudomonas* eye infection as a cause of death in premature infants, Arch Ophthalmol 65:517, 1961.

38. Hagler WS, Walters PV, and Nahmias AJ: Ocular involvement in neonatal herpes simplex virus infection, Arch Ophthalmol 82:169, 1969.

39. Nahmias AJ and Hagler WS: Ocular manifestations of herpes simplex in the newborn (neonatal ocular herpes), Int Ophthalmol Clin 12:191, 1972.

40. Hutchinson DS, Smith RE, and Haughton PB: Congenital herpetic keratitis, Arch Ophthalmol 93:70, 1975.

41. Cibis A and Burde RM: Herpes simplex virus–induced congenital cataracts, Arch Ophthalmol 85:220, 1971.

42. Whitley RJ et al: Vidarabine therapy of neonatal herpes simplex virus infection, Pediatrics 66:495, 1980.

43. Bron AJ and Seal DV: The defenses of the ocular surface, Trans Ophthalmol Soc UK 105:18, 1986.

44. Fredrickson AB: Behavior of mixed culture of microorganisms, Annu Rev Microbiol 31:63, 1977.

45. Locatcher-Khorazo D, Sullivan N, and Gutierrez E: *Staphylococcus aureus* isolated from normal and infected eyes: phage types and sensitivity to antibacterial agents, Arch Ophthalmol 77:370, 1967.

46. Watt PJ: Pathogenic mechanism of organisms virulent to the eye, Trans Ophthalmol Soc UK 105:26, 1986.

47. Wilson LA: Bacterial conjunctivitis. In Duane T and Jaeger E, editors: Clinical ophthalmology, vol 4, Philadelphia, 1988, Harper & Row, Publishers, Inc.

48. Londer L and Nelson DL: Orbital cellulitis due to *Hemophilus influenzae,* Arch Ophthalmol 91:89, 1974.

49. Feingold M and Gellis SS: Cellulitis due to *Hemophilus influenzae* type B, N Engl J Med 272:788, 1965.

50. Steere AC et al: Lyme arthritis: an epidemic of oligoarticular arthritis in children and adults in three Connecticut communities, Arthritis Rheum 20:7, 1977.

51. Bruhn FW: Lyme disease, Am J Dis Child 138:467, 1984.

52. Wan WL et al: The clinical characteristics and course of adult gonococcal conjunctivitis, Am J Ophthlamol 102:575, 1986.

53. Ullman S et al: *Neisseria gonorrhoeae* keratoconjunctivitis, Ophthalmology 94:525, 1987.

54. Thygeson P and Kimura S: Chronic conjunctivitis, Trans Am Acad Ophthalmol Otolaryngol 67:494, 1963.

55. Rosenthal RL and Blackman A: Bone marrow hypoplasia following use of chloramphenicol eye drops, JAMA 191:136, 1965.

56. Centers for Disease Control: 1985 STD treatment guidelines, MMWR 34:75S, 1985.

57. Kestelyn P et al: Treatment of adult gonococcal keratoconjunctivitis with oral norfloxacin, Am J Ophthalmology 108:516, 1989.

58. Parinaud H: Conjonctivite infectieuse paraissant transmise a l'homme par les animaux, Recueil Ophthalmol 11:176, 1889.

59. Verhoeff FH and King MJ: Parinaud's conjunctivitis: a mycotic disease due to a hitherto undescribed filamentous organism, Arch Ophthalmol 42:345, 1913.

60. Verhoeff FH and King MJ: Leptotrichosis conjunctivae (Parinaud's conjunctivitis): artificial cultivation of the leptotriches in three of four cases, Arch Ophthalmol 9:701, 1933.

61. Carithers HA: Cat-scratch disease: an overview based on a study of 1200 patients, Am J Dis Child 139:1124, 1985.

62. English CK et al: Cat-scratch disease: isolation and culture of the bacterial agent, JAMA 259:1347, 1988.

63. Wear DJ et al: Cat-scratch disease bacilli in the conjunctiva of patients with Parinaud's syndrome, Ophthalmology 92:1282, 1985.

64. Wear DJ et al: Cat-scratch disease: a bacterial infection, Science 221:1403, 1983.

65. Luna LB: Manual of histologic staining methods of the Armed Forces Institute of Pathology, ed 3, New York, 1968, McGraw-Hill, Inc.

66. Bogue C et al: Antibiotic therapy for cat-scratch disease? JAMA 262:813, 1989.

67. Francis E: Oculoglandular tularemia, Arch Ophthalmol 28:711, 1942.

68. Kaye D: Tularemia. In Braunwald E et al, editors: Harrison's principles of internal medicine, ed 11, New York, 1987, McGraw-Hill, Inc.

69. Gordon DM: Ocular sporotrichosis, Arch Ophthalmol 37:56, 1947.

70. McGrath H and Singer JI: Ocular sporotrichosis, Am J Ophthalmol 35:102, 1952.

71. Bennett JE: Fungal infections. In Braunwald E et al, editors: Harrison's principles of internal medicine, ed 11, New York, 1987, McGraw-Hill, Inc.

72. Chandler AC and Locatcher-Khorazo D: Primary tuberculosis of the conjunctiva, Arch Ophthalmol 71:202, 1964.

73. Archer D and Bird A: Primary tuberculosis of the conjunctiva, Br J Ophthalmol 51:679, 1967.

74. Anhalt EF, Chang G, and Byron HM: Conjunctival tuberculosis, Am J Ophthalmol 50:265, 1965.

75. Maxey EE: Primary syphilis of the palpebral conjunctiva, Am J Ophthalmol 65:13, 1965.

76. Cubbold RJD and MacDonald A: Molluscum contagiosum as a sexually transmitted disease, Practitioner 204:416, 1970.

77. Burdin JC, Weber M, and Martin F: Epidemiological study of human listeriosis in France: considerations of about 62 cases observed in Lorraine, Rev Epidemiol Sante Publique 22:279, 1974.

78. DeBord GG: Species of the tribes *Mimeae, Neisseriaceae,* and *Streptococceae* which confuse the diagnosis of gonorrhea by smears, J Lab Clin Med 28:710, 1943.

CONJUNCTIVITIS II:
NONINFECTIOUS CAUSES

NONINFECTIOUS CAUSES OF CONJUNCTIVAL INFLAMMATION

A number of noninfectious disorders can cause conjunctival inflammation, and these should be considered in the differential diagnosis, particularly in chronic or recurrent disease. A partial list follows and some specific entities are discussed below.

Immunologic
  Hay fever
  Vernal catarrh
  Atopic keratoconjunctivitis
  Contact dermatoconjunctivitis
Other primary conjunctival diseases
  Superior limbic keratoconjunctivitis
  Masquerade syndrome (carcinoma)
  Floppy eyelid syndrome
  Limbal dyskeratosis

Ocular disease
  Blepharitis
  Meibomitis
  Episcleritis
  Scleritis
  Intraocular inflammation
  Angle-closure glaucoma
Medications—toxic effects of many drugs,
particularly:
  Gentamicin
  Idoxuridine
  Neomycin
  Preservatives

133

Dermatologic disorders (in part)
  Acne rosacea
  Psoriasis
  Atopic dermatitis
  Discoid lupus erythematosus
  Cicatricial pemphigoid
  Erythema multiforme
  Other mucous membrane diseases
Other systemic diseases
  Gout
  Lymphoma
  Thyroid disease
  Kawasaki disease
  Reiter's syndrome
  Toxic shock syndrome
  Ataxia telangiectasia
  Arteriovenous fistulae
  Blood dyscrasias: polycythemia, leukemia,
    multiple myeloma, dysproteinemia

Environmental and irritative
  Ultraviolet radiation
  Therapeutic radiation
  Foreign particles (for example, fiberglass)
  Ophthalmia nodosa (caterpillar hairs)
  Burdock (thistle)
  Diffenbachia plant

FLOPPY EYELID SYNDROME

Floppy eyelid syndrome, a noninfectious cause of chronic conjunctivitis, is characterized by the presence of a lax, easily everted upper lid. The syndrome was first described by Culbertson and Ostler in 1981,[1] and many other cases have been described since,[2-8] indicating that this is a relatively common disorder.

CLINICAL MANIFESTATIONS

Patients complain of redness, irritation, foreign body sensation, and mucoid discharge. The symptoms usually are worse in the morning and improve over the day. Intermittent blurring of vision and mild itching may also be present.

One or both eyes can be affected, and this appears to relate to which side the patient sleeps on; if he or she consistently sleeps on one side, the ipsilateral eye is the one affected; otherwise both lids are affected. Most patients with this disorder have been obese, but obesity is not necessarily present.

On examination the most prominent feature is the laxity of the upper lid. This must be tested for to be appreciated. By pulling the eyelid skin upward, the lid everts (Fig. 7-1). Spontaneous eversion can also occur upon squeezing the lids closed (Fig. 7-2). When pulling upward on the lashes, as in standard lid eversion, the lid rolls upward, with no resistance from the tarsus. The tarsus feels soft and rubbery and is easily folded.

A papillary response is evident in the superior tarsal conjunctiva, and mucus strands can be seen. A coarse punctate keratopathy, diffuse or primarily superior, superior corneal pannus,[1,7] filaments,[7] and mild ptosis may also be present. Schirmer testing has indicated decreased tear flow in some patients.

ASSOCIATED FINDINGS

Scrapings have yielded primarily polymorphonuclear leukocytes, with some lymphocytes. In rare cases eosinophils also are present.[3] Histologic specimens of the superior tarsus show a dense chronic inflammatory infiltrate in the substantia propria, with a normal tarsus.[1,3,5,6] Occasionally keratinization of the surface epithelium[1] and subepithelial scarring[3] are present.

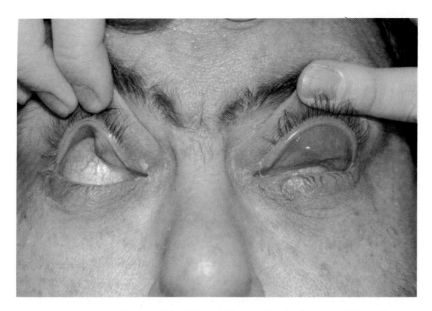

Fig. 7-1. Eversion of upper lids with superior traction in floppy eyelid syndrome.

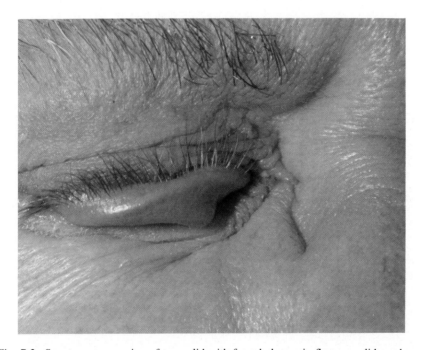

Fig. 7-2. Spontaneous eversion of upper lid with forced closure in floppy eyelid syndrome.

Floppy eyelid syndrome has been noted in association with several diseases (keratoconus,[2] hyperglycinemia,[4] blepharochalasis,[6] and keratotorus[8]) but in none is there a clear relationship.

ETIOLOGY

The cause of floppy eyelid syndrome is unknown, except that it is often related to obesity. However, no endocrinologic abnormalities have been identified in these patients.[1,2] Culbertson and Ostler proposed that lid eversion occurred during sleep, resulting in contact of the upper lid and cornea with the pillow, and this has been reported by some of the patients' spouses. Although this may often be the case, the underlying cause for the laxity of the upper lids is unknown.

TREATMENT

Treatment is aimed at eliminating lid eversion or contact with bedclothes. The simplest methods are taping the lids shut at night and using an eye shield. These measures provide at least temporary relief in most patients and can be used to confirm the diagnosis. Permanent relief can be obtained with horizontal lid shortening procedures.[4,5,7]

Lubricants, cromolyn sodium, and contact lenses have not been very useful.

MASQUERADE SYNDROME

Occasionally conjunctival tumors grow in a diffuse, minimally elevated manner and appear as a chronic conjunctivitis.[9-12] Squamous cell carcinoma is the most common type to manifest itself in this manner, but sebaceous carcinoma also may do so.[10,13,14] The conjunctivitis is unilateral and may have persisted for years. The involved conjunctiva is diffusely inflamed, mildly thickened, and may contain vascular tufts or subepithelial scarring (Fig. 7-3). A mucoid discharge may be present. The cornea frequently displays a diffuse, nonspecific, punctate keratitis. Cytologic examination of conjunctival scrapings may suggest malignancy by the presence of atypical and pleomorphic cells and multinucleated cells. A biopsy should be performed whenever the disease is suspected and probably in all cases of idiopathic chronic conjunctivitis unresponsive to therapy. It is important to obtain specimens from several sites and to take a wedge specimen from the lid if sebaceous carcinoma is suspected.

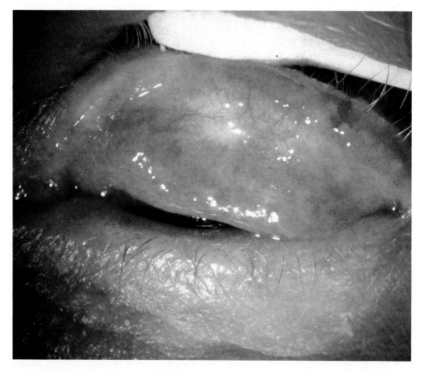

Fig. 7-3. Masquerade syndrome. Abnormal surface and scarring of superior tarsus caused by superficially spreading sebaceous cell carcinoma.

MUCUS FISHING SYNDROME

Mucus fishing is a behavior that contributes to inflammation and mucus production in some patients with conjunctivitis. Described by McCulley, Moore, and Matoba in 1985,[15] this syndrome is brought about by self-induced mechanical trauma to the conjunctiva during removal of mucous filaments from the eye. The patients have underlying conditions that cause mucous production, most commonly keratoconjunctivitis sicca, but they induce further irritation and mucous production by using their fingers, cotton swabs, tissues, cotton balls, or washcloths to remove the mucus. When patients are asked to demonstrate this behavior, it is evident that conjunctival contact occurs, most commonly in the medial interpalpebral conjunctiva. Rose bengal staining is usually present in the traumatized area.

Once the diagnosis is made, the patient can be educated about avoiding contact with the eye. Cessation of mucus fishing, combined with treatment of the underlying disorder, leads to resolution of signs and symptoms.

REITER'S SYNDROME

Reiter's syndrome consists of conjunctivitis, urethritis, arthritis, circinate balanitis, shallow ulcerations of the buccal mucosa, and a characteristic dermatitis, keratoderma blennorrhagica. Young men are primarily affected; the disease is extremely rare in women and children. It is seen worldwide and is the most common cause of arthritis in young men. It is strongly correlated with HLA-B27; more than 76% of patients with Reiter's syndrome have HLA-B27, versus an incidence of less than 10% in the general population. Infectious origins have been proposed, but the evidence is contradictory and inconclusive. Some cases occur after diarrheal illness, including epidemics of bacillary dysentery,[16] *Campylobacter jejuni,*[17] and *Salmonella* enteritis.[18] Other cases appear to relate to venereal disease, particularly nongonococcal urethritis, which is most commonly caused by chlamydial infection[19,20] or *Mycoplasma (Ureaplasma urealyticum).* Therefore in at least some patients the disease appears to be triggered by an infectious process in the urogenital tract or gut, coupled with a specific genetic background.[21]

Usually the gastrointestinal or genitourinary symptoms precede the onset of other symptoms by days to weeks. The most common manifestation of Reiter's syndrome is arthritis, which occurs in more than 90% of patients. It is typically an acute, oligoarticular, and asymmetric arthritis most frequently affecting the lower extremities. Mucocutaneous lesions, mainly oral and genital, are also seen in a high percentage of patients. These lesions are painless red macules that can be easily overlooked. The lesions of keratoderma blennorrhagica consist of painless hyperkeratotic papules that occur most often on the palms and soles but may also appear elsewhere. Some individuals have pleuritis, pericarditis, aortic insufficiency, or neurologic manifestations.

The diagnosis is made clinically, since no specific laboratory findings are present. The presence of oligoarticular, seronegative, asymmetric arthritis lasting longer than 1 month and found in association with urethritis or cervicitis, is sufficient for diagnosis of Reiter's syndrome.[22-24]

Reiter's syndrome is usually self-limited, subsiding in 6 weeks to 6 months, and complete remission with full recovery of the joints is the rule. However, relapses can occur and may be precipitated by sexual exposure. Skin and mucous membrane lesions heal without a trace. In a minority of patients the arthritis persists and can be disabling. In rare cases patients with clinical features of Reiter's syndrome develop typical psoriatic arthritis.

Ocular Manifestations

Conjunctivitis is the most common ophthalmic manifestation of Reiter's syndrome.[24] Iridocyclitis, episcleritis, scleritis, and keratitis may also be seen.[25,26] The conjunctivitis is papillary in nature, with mucopurulent discharge (Fig. 7-4). Conjunctival scarring occurs in rare cases.[24] The iridocyclitis

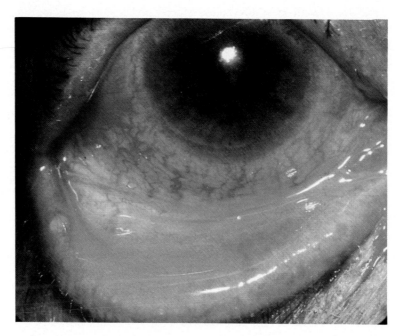

Fig. 7-4. Mucopurulent discharge and papillary conjunctival response in Reiter's syndrome.

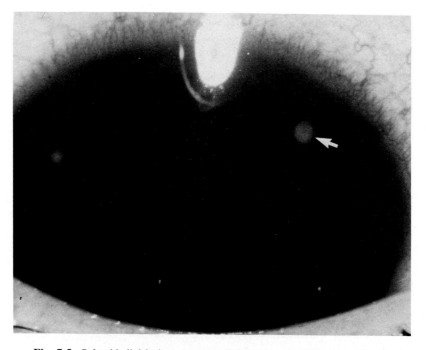

Fig. 7-5. Subepithelial lesions *(arrow)* of the cornea in Reiter's syndrome.

is nongranulomatous, and posterior synechiae are rare. The corneal complications consist of punctate epithelial lesions, central erosive corneal lesions, and peripheral subepithelial opacities (Fig. 7-5).[25,27]

As with the systemic disease, ocular involvement is usually self-limited. Topical corticosteroids may be necessary for keratitis or iritis. Systemic steroids should be avoided, since they can aggravate the skin disease. Patients should be tested for chlamydial infection which, if present, should be treated with systemic tetracycline or erythromycin.

KAWASAKI DISEASE (MUCOCUTANEOUS LYMPH NODE SYNDROME)

Kawasaki disease is an acute multisystem disease of children consisting of fever, characteristic mucous membrane and skin findings, and lymphadenopathy. A widespread arteritis is present that can affect the coronary arteries. There is reddening of the palms and soles, membranous fingertip desquamation, a polymorphous exanthem of the trunk without crust or vesicles, and reddening of the lips, tongue, and oral mucosae.

Most affected children have bilateral conjunctival injection.[28] Exudative conjunctivitis,[29] subconjunctival hemorrhage, superficial punctate keratopathy, and anterior uveitis[30] also can be seen.[31]

SUPERIOR LIMBIC KERATOCONJUNCTIVITIS

Superior limbic keratoconjunctivitis (SLK) is a frequently unrecognized cause of chronic, recurrent keratoconjunctivitis. Because it is a distinct clinical entity, SLK usually can be diagnosed readily if the clinician is familiar with the condition. Accurate diagnosis, in turn, enables initiation of the proper therapy and avoidance of harmful or ineffective measures. Often the patient has been using topical antibiotic, antiviral, or corticosteroid medications, which achieve little or no response. In fact, such medications are likely to produce toxic or allergic reactions that can obscure the signs of the original disease. Therefore a high index of suspicion must be maintained by the ophthalmologist to diagnosis all cases of SLK.

Since the disorder was first recognized in the early 1960s by Theodore[32,33] and Thygeson,[34-36] little has been added to the description. Superior limbic keratoconjunctivitis is a chronic, inflammatory condition of the eye that can cause considerable ocular irritation.[37] It occurs most commonly between 20 and 60 years of age.[38] Cases have been reported in patients from 4 to 81 years of age, with a mean age of 49 years. At least 75% of the cases occur in females,[38-40] and there appears to be no racial predilection. The disease occurs nationwide in the United States; the cases occur sporadically and are nonfamilial. There is no seasonal variation.

Superior limbic keratoconjunctivitis most commonly is bilateral, but often one eye is more severely involved. Exacerbations may affect one eye and then the other.

Abnormal thyroid function, most commonly hypothyroidism, has been reported in 26% to 50% of patients with SLK.[39,41-44]

The disease is quite unpredictable in duration and recurrence. Periods of remission and exacerbation occur, with individual attacks lasting for a few days to longer than a year. The disease may persist for several weeks to 10 years or perhaps even longer, but most cases eventually resolve spontaneously. Visual loss does not occur except through inappropriate treatment.

CLINICAL MANIFESTATIONS

The symptoms of SLK are usually more severe than objective findings would suggest. One of the foremost complaints is a burning sensation. In addition, patients may experience irritation, foreign body sensation, pain, photophobia, ptosis, and blepharospasm. Visual impairment, discharge, or itching of the eyes are not usually encountered.

Papillary hypertrophy and marked inflammation occur on the superior tarsal conjunctiva (Fig. 7-6). In severe cases this area may have a diffuse velvety appearance, but medium or giant papillae do not form. The severity of disease on the superior tarsus usually parallels that of the superior limbus. In extremely severe cases, a pseudomembrane can be seen on the superior tarsus.[38] The conjunctiva of the lower lid is not involved.

The superior limbus is almost always involved by papillary hypertrophy and hyperemia. A fleshy, gray thickening of epithelium occurs in the superior limbal area (Fig. 7-7). A boggy apron of conjunctiva, folding over the superior limbus, is occasionally seen. Fine epithelial keratitis is often present in the upper fifth of the cornea. In severe cases edema or even bullous keratopathy can affect the superior cornea. A micropannus occasionally is noted.

Filaments in the area of the superior limbus are present in a third of the cases (Fig. 7-8) and may also occur on the bulbar and tarsal conjunctiva.[33] The appearance of filaments usually is accompanied by an acute worsening of the symptoms; desquamation of filaments can lead to epithelial loss. When filaments occur, they may overshadow the picture of the underlying disease, and the condition may be misdiagnosed simply as filamentary keratitis.

Hyperemia of the superior bulbar conjunctiva arranged in a "corridor" fashion is a constant finding and is most evident when the patient's gaze is directed downward (Fig. 7-9). This injection is most intense at the limbal area and fades as it approaches the superior fornix. The conjunctiva is thickened and often lusterless because of keratinization of the surface. The remaining conjunctiva exhibits a mild hyperemia.

Other possible findings include increased mucus, pseudoptosis, and edema of the superior bulbar conjunctiva. Decreased corneal sensation and decreased vision caused by induced astigmatism occur in rare cases.[39]

The instillation of rose bengal reveals rather characteristic involvement of the cornea, limbus, and conjunctiva.[45] Fine and uniform areas of epithelial staining are found immediately above and below

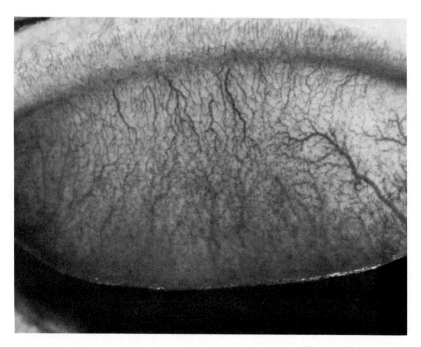

Fig. 7-6. Papillary response of superior tarsal conjunctiva in superior limbic keratoconjunctivitis. (From Grayson M: Perspectives in ophthalmology, vol 1, Hagerstown, Md, 1976, Ankho International Co.)

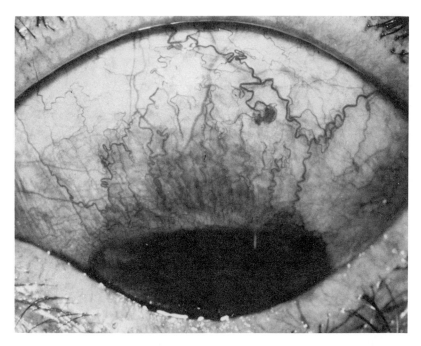

Fig. 7-7. SLK. Thickening and graying of epithelium in superior limbal area, associated with characteristic vascular injection of bulbar conjunctiva. (From Grayson M: Perspectives in ophthalmology, vol 1, Hagerstown, Md, 1976, Ankho International Co.)

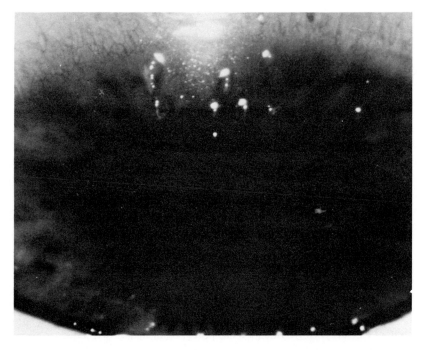

Fig. 7-8. Filaments on the superior limbal cornea in SLK. (From Grayson M: Perspectives in ophthalmology, vol 1, Hagerstown, Md, 1976, Ankho International Co.)

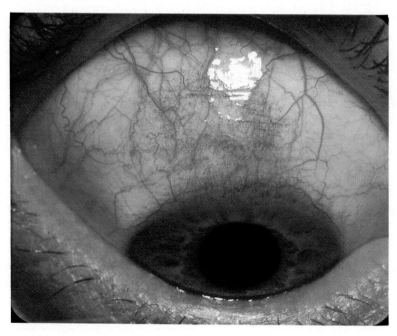

Fig. 7-9. Superior bulbar conjunctiva in SLK showing corridor of injection and staining with rose bengal red.

the superior limbus. Superficial, punctate staining of the bulbar conjunctiva usually involves the 10:30 to 1:30 area and extends about 4 to 5 mm above the limbus (see Fig. 7-9). Corneal staining often is seen extending 1 to 2 mm centrally from the limbus. Similar but less extensive staining may be seen with fluorescein.

Areas of localized dryness of the involved superior bulbar conjunctiva may be present, but tear production usually is normal. However, in the occasional cases with decreased tear production, inferior filaments and interpalpebral conjunctival staining may be present, as well as the typical superior changes. It is best to treat the dry eye state first (with lubricants, punctal occlusion, and so on) before treating the SLK.

LABORATORY EVALUATION

Giemsa-stained scrapings from the superior bulbar conjunctiva show keratinization of the epithelial cells (see Fig. 4-6).[46] The keratinized epithelial cells contain keratohyalin granules. With further keratinization the cytoplasm decreases in volume and takes on a purplish hue. Some epithelial cells may demonstrate degenerated nuclei that appear pyknotic and shrunken. Scrapings of the palpebral conjunctiva may be normal or may reveal similar changes. A mild inflammatory reaction, with polymorphonuclear cells predominating, may be present. It has been reported that in Papanicolaou-stained scrapings of the superior bulbar conjunctiva, the nuclear chromatin may be condensed into unusual figures such as an S shape, bar, or coil.[47] The significance of these findings is not clear.

Biopsy specimens of the bulbar conjunctival epithelium exhibit keratinization, acanthosis, and mild dyskeratosis. Cytoplasmic edema, nuclear pyknosis, and intracellular accumulation of glycogen are seen.[39,46,48,49] Electron microscopy shows that the keratinization characteristics of the conjunctival epithelium are similar to those occurring in normal skin.[48] Also, nuclear changes similar to those reported in conjunctival scraping specimens were observed: an abnormal aggregation of the nuclear chromatin, with formation of multilobed nuclei and multinucleated cells.[47,50]

Biopsy specimens of the epithelium and stroma of the palpebral conjunctiva demonstrate an inflammatory infiltration consisting of neutrophils, lymphocytes, and plasma cells with a preponderance of neutrophils. An inflammatory exudate of similar cellular makeup may be present, overlying the thickened conjunctiva.[46] Staining with the periodic acid-Schiff or alcian blue stain does not occur. The laboratory test of consistent value seems to be the finding of keratinized cells.

DIFFERENTIAL DIAGNOSIS

Differential diagnosis can be approached by considering the following conditions with or without filaments:

Conditions without filaments
   Trachoma
   Marginal infiltrates at superior corneal location
   Limbal vernal keratoconjunctivitis
   Phylctenulosis
   Giant papillary conjunctivitis
   Contact lens–induced keratoconjunctivitis (CLIK)
Conditions with filaments
   Keratoconjunctivitis sicca
   Masquerade syndrome

In none of the nonfilamentous conditions listed is there significant bulbar conjunctival staining. Corneal staining, follicles, and scarring on the upper tarsal conjunctiva, Herbert pits, and gross pannus help differentiate trachoma. The presence of basophilic intracytoplasmic inclusions and response to specific treatment for trachoma aid in the differentiation. Limbal vernal disease may be differentiated by the presence of fragmented eosinophils on scrapings, the gelatinous appearance of the limbal lesions, with overlying Trantas dots, and giant papillae on the upper tarsal plate. In addition, the seasonal nature and response of vernal disease to steroids and cromolyn sodium are important clues. The limbal phlyctenule has a characteristic clinical picture. This raised yellow-white, self-limited, conjunctival limbal lesion is primarily associated with a sensitivity to staphylococci. Other causes of phlyctenular disease such as candidiasis and tuberculosis should be kept in mind.

The corneal and conjunctival staining of keratoconjunctivitis sicca is mainly in the interpalpebral zone. If the eye is dry enough to cause filament formation, Schirmer testing is usually markedly abnormal, and the precorneal tear film is filled with debris. A loss of luster occurs on the corneal surface. Scrapings may reveal goblet cells.

The differentiation of contact lens–induced keratoconjunctivitis and superior limbic keratoconjunctivitis may be difficult in contact lens wearers. This is discussed in the section on contact lens–induced keratoconjunctivitis. As with any case of chronic conjunctivitis, masquerade syndrome should be suspected, and if the conjunctiva appears dysplastic, a biopsy should be performed. Misdiagnosis of sebaceous cell carcinoma as SLK was reported in one case.[14]

ETIOLOGY

The cause of SLK is unknown. Viral and fungal cultures have been negative. Bacterial cultures have yielded normal flora, including *Staphylococcus epidermidis* and diphtheroids. Eosinophils, basophils, and inclusions have not been found. The frequent association with thyroid disease may suggest some immunologic connection, but no evidence exists that the disease occurs on an immunologic basis.[51]

Wright has suggested that the initial pathologic process occurs in the superior tarsal conjunctiva, with development of chronic inflammation and tightness of the lid against the globe.[44] He proposed that this interfered with the normal removal of surface cells from the epithelium of the bulbar conjunctiva.

The hypothesis proposed by Wilson and Ostler[52,53] best explains all the findings in this disease. According to this hypothesis, SLK results from a combination of increased tension of the upper lid against the globe and increased mobility of the upper bulbar conjunctiva. The increased tension of the upper lid may be caused by edema or exophthalmos, which may be related to thyroid disease or chronic inflammation from other causes. Laxity or edema of the superior bulbar conjunctiva may arise from hypothyroidism or aging or may be congenital. The movement of the lid against the conjunctiva and of the conjunctiva against the globe results in chronic mechanical irritation. The response of the eye to this is injection, papillary hypertrophy, cellular infiltration, and abnormal epithelial maturation, with surface keratinization.

Silver nitrate treatment removes the abnormal conjunctival epithelium and temporarily improves symptoms, until the process again results in an abnormal surface. Scarring of the bulbar conjunctiva to the globe, which may occur with prolonged inflammation, multiple silver nitrate treatments, or with cautery or conjunctival resection, prevents the abnormal movement of the conjunctiva.

It is interesting to note that SLK occurred in the superior temporal conjunctiva in a patient with esotropia,[52] and that thyroid patients with lid retraction seem not to develop SLK.[44]

TREATMENT

Topical application of silver nitrate solution improves the condition in most patients, and in some cases complete remission is achieved.[33,38] Filaments often disappear, and the symptoms and clinical findings usually are reduced by the next day. Limbal staining is most resistant to treatment and may take several weeks to disappear. Two or three treatments at least 2 days apart may be required before relief is obtained. As mentioned, however, recurrences are frequent after 4 to 6 weeks, and retreatment is required.

A cotton-tipped applicator that has been impregnated with a 0.5% to 1% solution of silver nitrate is used. Ampules marketed for Credé prophylaxis contain 1% silver nitrate and may be diluted with sterile water (not sodium chloride) for use. My practice has been to treat both the upper tarsal and bulbar conjunctiva. The silver nitrate–moistened applicator is rubbed vigorously over both surfaces. Afterward the eye is irrigated with normal saline.

Strong concentrations of silver nitrate cause chemical burns and silver staining of the cornea. Solid-tipped silver nitrate applicators must be avoided, since their use may result in a severe burn and opacification of the cornea that may necessitate penetrating keratoplasty.[54,55]

Simple mechanical scraping of the involved conjunctiva with a platinum spatula may be effective.[44,56] Pressure patching and bandage soft contact lens wear provide relief in some patients.[44,49,56] Cromolyn sodium was found effective by some researchers[57] but not by others.[44] In a few cases topical decongestants, zinc salts, and artificial tears may bring about temporary, symptomatic relief but will have no effect on the progress of the disease. Cryotherapy also has been advocated but does not appear to be as effective as silver nitrate treatment.

Thermocauterization of the superior bulbar conjunctiva often is effective, even in cases that do not respond to silver nitrate.[58] To perform this procedure, the superior bulbar conjunctiva is ballooned up with injection of local anesthetic, and small burns are created in an even distribution throughout the affected area.

Recession or resection of the superior bulbar conjunctiva usually is effective in cases that do not respond to other treatments.[49,59,60] The superior conjunctiva and Tenon's layer are dissected off the limbus and sclera from the 10:30 to 1:30 positions and for 5 to 8 mm posteriorly. The conjunctiva may be excised or recessed with the edges sutured to the globe with 7-0 chromic sutures. In the rare case that symptoms recur after this procedure, silver nitrate treatment or repeat resection are still effective.[60]

CONTACT LENS–INDUCED KERATOCONJUNCTIVITIS

In 1981 Wilson became the first to recognize that contact lens wear could cause a condition simulating SLK.[61] Since then several authors have reported series of patients with this syndrome, which can be called contact lens–induced keratoconjunctivitis (CLIK).[62-65]

CLINICAL MANIFESTATIONS

The symptoms of CLIK include redness, irritation, burning, itching, photophobia, crusting, and tearing. The vision often is mildly reduced, and wearing contact lenses may exacerbate the symptoms.

Superior conjunctival injection and limbal papillary hypertrophy usually are present. The superior corneal epithelium usually is irregular, thickened, and gray, with punctate fluorescein staining. This may extend down from the limbus in a V pattern toward the visual axis (Fig. 7-10). Subepithelial opacities often are present. Pannus may be present beneath the abnormal epithelium and may extend several millimeters onto the cornea. The superior tarsal conjunctiva may be normal or may display a mild to moderate papillary response. Filaments are present in a minority of cases. A summary of the differentiating features of CLIK and SLK is given in Table 7-1.

If untreated, progressive corneal involvement occurs (Fig. 7-11).[66] The epithelium becomes thicker and grayer and a greater area is involved. The pannus progresses centrally, and deep stromal vascularization can occur. In severe cases resolution may not occur after the patient stops wearing contact lenses, in which case keratoplasty is required.

In conjunctival scrapings early keratinization of the epithelium, a moderate polymorphonuclear response, and occasional lymphocytes are seen.[63,64] Eosinophils may be present in some patients. Biopsy specimens exhibit keratinization, acanthosis, and intracellular edema of the epithelium.[65] A chronic inflammatory infiltrate is present in the conjunctival stroma, with polymorphonuclear cells, plasma cells, and mononuclear cells.

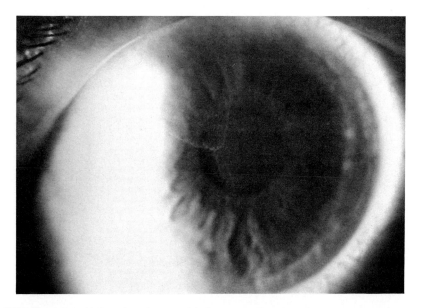

Fig. 7-10. CLIK. Irregular, thickened, and gray epithelium extending down from the superior limbus toward the visual axis.

TABLE 7-1. Differentiating Features of CLIK and SLK

CLINICAL FEATURES	CLIK	SLK
Age (most common)	15 to 35	40 to 60
Decreased vision (from keratopathy)	Common	No
Exacerbations and remissions unrelated to contact lens wear	No	Yes
Thyroid disease	No	Common
Response to contact lens wear	Worsens	Can improve
Itching	Common	No
More than minimal hyperemia of nasal temporal and inferior bulbar conjunctiva	Common	No
Keratopathy extending more than 3 mm below upper limbus	Common	No
Gelatinous papillary hypertrophy of limbus	Common	No
Gross pannus (more than 2 mm)	Occasionally	No
Subepithelial opacification	Common	No
Corneal filaments	Occasionally	Common
Eosinophils in conjunctival scrapings	Occasionally	No
Response to cessation of contact lens wear	Yes	No

Adapted from Wilson FM II: Differential diagnosis of superior limbic keratoconjunctivitis and papillary keratoconjunctivitis associated with contact lenses. In Hughes WF editor: The year book of ophthalmology 1981, Chicago, 1981, Mosby–Year Book, Inc.

ETIOLOGY

In many cases CLIK appears to be related to thimerosal exposure. Thimerosal was present in lens care solutions in most of the reported cases, but only a small minority of patients exhibited reactions to thimerosal on patch testing.[62,64,65] Mechanical factors have also been implicated.[67]

Most likely several factors can play a role: mechanical irritation of the superior limbus, exposure to preservatives and other chemicals in lens solutions, proteins, organisms and other materials deposited on contact lenses, and hypoxia of the epithelium beneath the lens, which would be expected to be greatest under the superior lid.

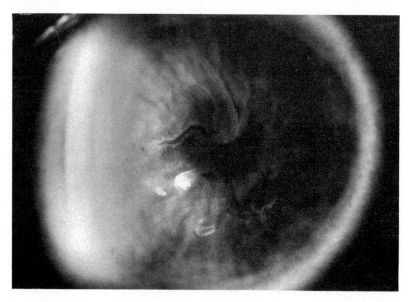

Fig. 7-11. Diffuse irregularity, opacification, and thickening of corneal epithelium related to contact lens wear (CLIK). (Courtesy of Richard A. Thoft, Pittsburgh.)

TREATMENT

Cessation of lens wear is the main treatment. Resolution of signs and symptoms occurs in most cases and takes several weeks to more than a year. Silver nitrate treatment or conjunctival resection, as used for SLK, may be helpful.[64] Lens wear often can be reinstituted, with refitting, switching to gas permeable hard contact lenses, or avoidance of thimerosal-containing solutions.[63,65]

LIGNEOUS CONJUNCTIVITIS

Ligneous conjunctivitis is a bilateral membranous conjunctivitis seen in childhood.[68-73] It is most common in children but can occur at any age and can even begin at birth. It is more frequent in females and is equally likely to be bilateral or unilateral. In several reports two siblings have developed ligneous conjunctivitis, and in one case two generations were affected.

Immediately preceding or concomitant with the development of conjunctivitis, many patients have signs and symptoms of acute systemic disease, including upper respiratory infections, tonsillitis, otitis media, sinusitis, vulvovaginitis, cervicitis, and fever. One case followed excision of pinguecu-lae.[74]

The eyes are often injected, and mucoid discharge may be present. The membranes are thick, yellow-white or red, and exhibit a hard, boardlike appearance (Figs. 7-12 and 7-13). They may be sessile or pedunculated and arise from the tarsal and/or bulbar conjunctiva. If the membranes are removed, the area beneath bleeds and the membrane regrows, usually in a few days. Occasionally corneal involvement occurs, and it can lead to perforation and loss of the globe. The course usually is chronic, lasting 4 to 44 years. Spontaneous resolution may occur after many recurrences.

Ligneous conjunctivitis may be associated with similar lesions affecting other mucous membranes[70] or the middle ear.[75] Tracheal involvement may be life threatening.[76]

Histopathologic sections of the membrane have revealed subepithelial deposits of eosinophilic amorphous material, granulation tissue, and chronic inflammatory cells. The amorphous material is composed of fibrin, albumin, and immunoglobulins.[70,74,75,77] Eosinophils (Fig. 7-14), mononuclear cells, neutrophils, and mast cells may be present.

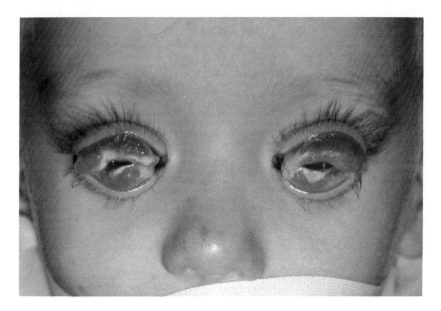

Fig. 7-12. Ligneous conjunctivitis involving all four lids. (Courtesy of Eugene Helveston and Forrest D. Ellis, Indianapolis.)

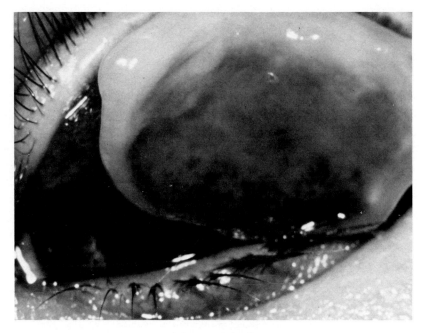

Fig. 7-13. Thick, boardlike conjunctival membrane in ligneous conjunctivitis.

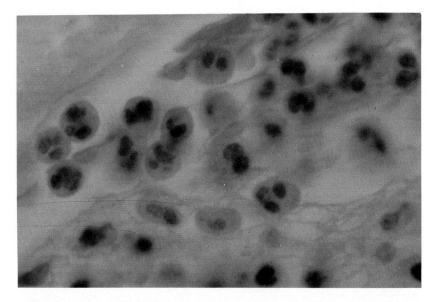

Fig. 7-14. Eosinophils noted in scraping from patient with ligneous conjunctivitis.

Ligneous conjunctivitis has generally been resistant to treatment. Numerous treatments have been proposed, with case reports illustrating success in some patients but failures in subsequent ones. Hyaluronidase,[68,78] fibrinolysin,[79] alpha-chymotrypsin,[74] cryotherapy,[79] and cromolyn sodium[76] have all been recommended. Azathiaprine was effective in one case,[70] and excision combined with topical cyclosporine was effective in two cases.[77] Total excision of the membrane, combined with excision of the tarsus and conjunctiva, and replacement with donor sclera was effective in another case.[80] Antibiotics, steroids, antiviral agents, cautery, and beta and x-ray irradiation have been ineffective.[70]

The cause of ligneous conjunctivitis is unclear. Hidayat and Riddle[70] suggested that the disorder was related to an abnormal hyperpermeability of blood vessels, but this may be a secondary phenomenon. Bateman and colleagues[81] felt that ligneous conjunctivitis is genetic and most likely inherited in an autosomal recessive pattern.

REFERENCES

1. Culbertson WW and Ostler HB: The floppy lid syndrome, Am J Ophthalmol 92:568, 1981.

2. Parunovic A: Floppy eyelid syndrome, Br J Ophthalmol 67:264, 1983.

3. Schwartz LK, Gelender H, and Forster RK: Chronic conjunctivitis associated with "floppy eyelids," Arch Ophthalmol 101:1884, 1983.

4. Gerner EW and Hughes SM: Floppy eyelid with hyperglycinemia, Am J Ophthalmol 98:614, 1984.

5. Dutton JJ: Surgical management of floppy eyelid syndrome, Am J Ophthalmol 99:557, 1985.

6. Goldberg R et al: Floppy eyelid syndrome and blepharochalasis, Am J Ophthalmol 102:376, 1986.

7. Moore MB, Harrington J, and McCulley JP: Floppy eyelid syndrome: management including surgery, Ophthalmology 93:184, 1986.

8. Parunovic A and Bozidar I: Floppy eyelid syndrome associated with keratotorus, Br J Ophthalmol 72:634, 1988.

9. Theodore FH: Conjunctival carcinoma masquerading as chronic conjunctivitis, Eye Ear Nose Throat Monthly 46:1419, 1967.

10. Brownstein S, Codere F, and Jackson WB: Masquerade syndrome, Ophthalmology 87:259, 1980.

11. Irvine AR: Diffuse epibulbar squamous cell epithelioma, Am J Ophthalmol 64:550, 1967.

12. Wolfe JT et al: Sebaceous carcinoma of the eyelid: errors in clinical and pathologic diagnosis, Am J Surg Pathol 8:597, 1984.

13. Foster CD and Allansmith MR: Chronic unilateral blepharoconjunctivitis caused by sebaceous carcinoma, Am J Ophthalmol 86:218, 1978.

14. Condon GP, Brownstein S, and Codere F: Sebaceous cell carcinoma of the eyelid masquerading as superior limbic keratoconjunctivitis, Arch Ophthalmol 103:1525, 1985.

15. McCulley JP, Moore MB, and Matoba AY: Mucus fishing syndrome, Ophthalmology 92:1262, 1985.

16. Paronia I: Reiter's disease, Acta Med Scand 131(suppl 213):1, 1948.

17. Saari KM and Kaurenen O: Ocular inflammation in Reiter's syndrome associated with *Campylobacter jejuni* enteritis, Am J Ophthalmol 90:572, 1980.

18. Saari KM et al: Ocular inflammation in Reiter's disease after *Salmonella* enteritis, Am J Ophthalmol 90:63, 1980.

19. Week LA et al: Urethritis associated with *Chlamydia:* clinical and laboratory diagnosis, Minn Med 59:288, 1976.

20. Martin DH et al: *Chlamydia trachomatis* infections in men with Reiter's syndrome, Ann Intern Med 100:207, 1984.

21. Calin A and Fries JF: An "experimental" epidemic of Reiter's syndrome revisited: follow-up evidence of genetic and environmental factors, Arthritis Rheum 84:564, 1976.

22. Willkens RF et al: Reiter's syndrome: evaluation of preliminary criteria for definite disease, Arthritis Rheum 24:844, 1981.

23. Keat A: Reiter's syndrome and reactive arthritis in perspective, N Engl J Med 309:1606, 1983.

24. Lee DA et al: The clinical diagnosis of Reiter's syndrome: ophthalmic and nonophthalmic aspects, Ophthalmology 93:350, 1986.

25. Ostler HB et al: Reiter's syndrome, Am J Ophthalmol 71:986, 1971.

26. Mills RP and Kalina RE: Reiter's keratitis, Arch Ophthalmol 87:447, 1972.

27. Wiggins RE, Steinkuller PG, and Hamill MB: Reiter's keratoconjunctivitis, Arch Ophthalmol 108:280, 1990.

28. Meade R and Brandt L: Manifestations of Kawasaki disease in New England outbreak of 1980, J Pediatr 100:558, 1982.

29. Ammerman S et al: Diagnostic uncertainty in atypical Kawasaki disease, and a new finding: exudative conjunctivitis, Pediatr Infect Dis 4:210, 1985.

30. Burns J et al: Anterior uveitis associated with Kawasaki syndrome, Pediatr Infect Dis 4:258, 1985.

31. Ohno S et al: Ocular manifestations of Kawasaki's disease (mucocutaneous lymph node syndrome), Am J Ophthalmol 93:713, 1982.

32. Theodore FH: The collected letters of the International Correspondence Society of Ophthalmologists and Otolaryngologists, Series 6, June 30, 1961, p 89.

33. Theodore FH: Superior limbic keratoconjunctivitis, Eye Ear Nose Throat Monthly 442:25, 1963.

34. Thygeson P: Further observations on superficial punctate keratitis, Arch Ophthalmol 66:158, 1961.

35. Thygeson P: Observations on filamentary keratitis. Transactions of the 102nd annual meeting of the American Medical Association, Section of Ophthalmology, 1963.

36. Thygeson P and Kimura SJ: Chronic conjunctivitis, Trans Am Acad Ophthalmol Otolaryngol 67:494, 1963.

37. Grayson M and Wilson FM II: Superior limbic keratoconjunctivitis, Perspect Ophthalmol 1:234, 1977.
38. Theodore FH: Further observations on superior limbic keratoconjunctivitis, Trans Am Acad Ophthalmol Otolaryngol 71:341, 1967.
39. Cher I: Clinical features of superior limbic keratoconjunctivitis in Australia: a probable association with thyrotoxicosis, Arch Ophthalmol 82:580, 1969.
40. Corwin ME: Superior limbic keratoconjunctivitis, Am J Ophthalmol 66:338, 1968.
41. Sutherland AL: Superior limbic keratoconjunctivitis, Trans Ophthalmol Soc N Z 21:89, 1969.
42. Tenzel RR: Comments on superior limbic filamentous keratitis, Arch Ophthalmol 79:508, 1968.
43. Theodore FH: Comments on findings of elevated protein bound iodine in superior limbic keratoconjunctivitis, Arch Ophthalmol 79:508, 1968.
44. Wright P: Superior limbic keratoconjunctivitis, Trans Ophthalmol Soc UK 92:555, 1972.
45. Theodore FH: Diagnostic dyes in superior limbic keratoconjunctivitis and other superficial entities. In Turtz AI, editor: Proceedings of the Centennial Symposium: Manhattan Eye, Ear and Throat Hospital, vol 1: Ophthalmology, St Louis, 1969, Mosby–Year Book, Inc.
46. Theodore FH and Ferry AP: Superior limbic keratoconjunctivitis: clinical and pathological correlations, Arch Ophthalmol 84:481, 1970.
47. Wander AH and Musukawa T: Unusual appearance of condensed chromatin in conjunctival cells in superior limbic keratoconjunctivitis, Lancet 2:42, 1981.
48. Collin HB et al: Keratinization of the bulbar conjunctival epithelium in superior limbic keratoconjunctivitis: an electron microscopic study, Acta Ophthalmol (Copenh) 56:531, 1978.
49. Donshik PC et al: Conjunctival resection treatment and ultrastructural histopathology of superior limbic keratoconjunctivitis, Am J Ophthalmol 85:101, 1978.
50. Collin HB et al: The fine structure of nuclear changes in superior limbic keratoconjunctivitis, Invest Ophthalmol Vis Sci 17:79, 1978.
51. Eiferman RA and Wilkins EL: Immunologic aspects of superior limbic keratoconjunctivitis, Can J Ophthalmol 14:85, 1979.
52. Wilson FM and Ostler HB: Superior limbic keratoconjunctivitis, Int Ophthalmol Clin 26:99, 1986.
53. Ostler HB: Superior limbic keratoconjunctivitis. In Smolin G and Thoft RA, editors: The cornea: scientific foundations and clinical practice, Boston, 1987, Little, Brown & Co, Inc.
54. Grayson M and Pieroni D: Severe silver nitrate injury to the eye, Am J Ophthalmol 70:227, 1970.
55. Laughrea PA, Arentsen JJ, and Laibson PR: Iatrogenic ocular silver nitrate burn, Cornea 4:47, 1985.
56. Mondino BJ, Zaidman GW, and Salamon SW: Use of pressure patching and soft contact lenses in superior limbic keratoconjunctivitis, Arch Ophthalmol 100:1932, 1982.
57. Confino J and Brown SI: Treatment of superior limbic keratoconjunctivitis with topical cromolyn sodium, Ann Ophthalmol 19:129, 1987.
58. Udell IJ et al: Treatment of superior limbic keratoconjunctivitis by thermocauterization of the superior bulbar conjunctiva, Ophthalmology 93:162, 1986.
59. Tenzel K: Resistant superior limbic keratoconjunctivitis, Arch Ophthalmol 89:439, 1973.
60. Passons GA and Wood TO: Conjunctival resection for superior limbic keratoconjunctivitis, Ophthalmology 91:966, 1984.
61. Wilson FM: Differential diagnosis of superior limbic keratoconjunctivitis and papillary keratoconjunctivitis associated with contact lenses. In Hughes WF, editor: Year Book of Ophthalmology 1981, Chicago, 1981, Mosby–Year Book, Inc.
62. Miller RA, Brightbill FS, and Slama SL: Superior limbic keratoconjunctivitis in soft contact lens wearers, Cornea 1:293, 1982.
63. Stenson S: Superior limbic keratoconjunctivitis associated with soft contact lens wear, Arch Ophthalmol 101:402, 1983.
64. Fuerst DJ, Sugar J, and Worobec S: Superior limbic keratoconjunctivitis associated with cosmetic soft contact lens wear, Arch Ophthalmol 101:1214, 1983.
65. Sendele DD et al: Superior limbic keratoconjunctivitis in contact lens wearers, Ophthalmology 90:616, 1983.
66. Bloomfield SE, Jakobiec FA, and Theodore FH: Contact lens induced keratopathy: a severe complication extending the spectrum of keratoconjunctivitis in contact lens wearers, Ophthalmology 91:290, 1984.
67. Carpel EF: Superior limbic conjunctivitis, Arch Ophthalmol 102:662, 1984 (letter).
68. Firat T: Ligneous conjunctivitis, Am J Ophthalmol 78:679, 1974.
69. Firat T and Tinaztepe B: Histochemical investigations on ligneous conjunctivitis and a new method of treatment, Acta Ophthalmol (Copenh) 48:3, 1970.
70. Hidayat AA and Riddle PJ: Ligneous conjunctivitis: a clinicopathologic study of 17 cases, Ophthalmology 94:949, 1987.
71. McGrand JC, Rees DM, and Garry J: Ligneous conjunctivitis, Br J Ophthalmol 53:373, 1969.
72. Spaeth GL: Chronic membranous conjunctivitis: a persisting problem, Am J Ophthalmol 64:300, 1967.
73. Spencer LM, Straatsma BR, and Foos RY: Ligneous conjunctivitis, Am J Ophthalmol 80:365, 1968.
74. Girard LJ, Veselinovic A, and Font RL: Ligneous conjunctivitis after pingueculae removal in an adult, Cornea 8:7, 1989.
75. Marcus DM et al: Ligneous conjunctivitis with ear involvement, Arch Ophthalmol 108:514, 1990.
76. Cooper TJ, Kazdan JJ, and Cutz E: Ligneous conjunctivitis with tracheal obstruction: a case report, with electron microscopy findings, Can J Ophthalmol 14:57, 1979.
77. Holland EJ et al: Immunohistochemical findings and results of treatment with cyclosporine in ligneous conjunctivitis, Am J Ophthalmol 107:160, 1989.
78. Francois J and Victoria-Troncoso V: Treatment of ligneous conjunctivitis, Am J Ophthalmol 65:674, 1968.
79. Melikian HE: Treatment of ligneous conjunctivitis, Ann Ophthalmol 17:763, 1985.
80. Berlin AJ et al: Scleral grafting in the management of ligneous conjunctivitis, Ophthalmic Surg 13:288, 1982.
81. Bateman JB et al: Ligneous conjunctivitis: an autosomal recessive disorder, J Pediatr Ophthalmol Strabismus 23:137, 1986.

CHLAMYDIAL INFECTIONS

Chlamydial infections (Table 8-1) are some of the most common diseases affecting humans. A chlamydial ocular disease, trachoma, affects approximately one seventh of the world's population and is the greatest cause of preventable loss of vision. Trachoma is rare in the United States, but adult and neonatal inclusion conjunctivitis are commonly seen. In adults chlamydial conjunctivitis is commonly misdiagnosed; suspicion of the disease and awareness of its clinical features are necessary for recognition.

THE ORGANISM

The chlamydiae have been classified in a separate section, as members of the order Chlamydiales. Like bacteria, they contain both DNA and RNA, divide by binary fission, are inhibited by sulfonamides and other antibiotics, and contain muramic acid in their cell walls; like true viruses, they are obligate, intracellular parasites. The family is called Chlamydiaceae, the genus, *Chlamydia*. The genus comprises two species, *C. trachomatis,* which causes eye disease, and *C. psittaci,* which infects primarily nonhuman species, particularly birds. *C. trachomatis* strains contain glycogen, produce io-

TABLE 8-1. Features of Chlamydial Conjunctivitis

FEATURE	ACUTE TRACHOMA	ADULT CHLAMYDIAL KERATOCONJUNCTIVITIS	LYMPHOGRANULOMA VENEREUM	C. PSITTACI
Incidence	Regional, endemic	Common	Uncommon	Rare
Onset	Insidious in children, acute in adults	Acute or subacute	Subacute	Acute or subacute
Duration (untreated)	Months to years	3 to 12 months	Usually 3 to 4 weeks, rarely years	?3 months
Laterality	Bilateral	Unilateral more common	Unilateral	?Unilateral
Adenopathy	Small, usually nontender	Small, usually nontender	Large	Small
Conjunctival response	Follicular, mainly superior; Limbal follicles common; Follicles can be expressed	Follicular, mainly inferior	Follicular; Granulomatous	Follicular
Pannus	Superior 1 to 3 mm; Common early	Superior 1 to 2 mm; Occasionally	Uncommon but can be severe	No
Epithelial lesions	Superior punctate keratitis	Punctate keratitis; Focal epithelial keratitis; More common peripherally, especially superiorly	Minimal	Diffuse, fine keratitis
Subepithelial infiltrates	Occasional; Superior	Occasional	Superior infiltration, can lead to diffuse vascularization	Can occur; Superior
Sequelae	With chronic disease, reinfection, corneal and conjunctival scarring develop	None	Can lead to severe corneal and conjunctival scarring	None
Transmission	Eye to eye	Genital to eye	Genital to eye	Cat to human

dine-staining intracytoplasmic inclusions, and are sensitive to sulfonamides, whereas *C. psittaci* strains do not contain glycogen, do not produce iodine-staining inclusions, and are not sensitive to sulfonamides. Fifteen serotypes of *C. trachomatis* have been identified. Strains A, B, Ba, and C are usually associated with trachoma, strains D through F with venereal disease and inclusion conjunctivitis, and strains L1, L2, and L3 with lymphogranuloma venereum.

Chlamydiae have a unique developmental cycle. The infectious organism exists in a form called an elementary body (EB). This is approximately 300 nm in diameter and has a rigid cell wall. The EB attaches to and is phagocytosed by an epithelial cell. Once in the cell it transforms into a larger particle, approximately 1000 nm, which is called a reticulate or initial body (RB). Over the next 48 hours the RB multiplies by binary fission to produce an aggregate of elementary bodies. These are located in the cytoplasm, usually near the nucleus, and can be seen in cytology as an inclusion body. The new EBs are released to infect other epithelial cells.

Chlamydial infection in the newborn is covered in Chapter 6.

ADULT CHLAMYDIAL KERATOCONJUNCTIVITIS (ACK)
EPIDEMIOLOGY

Ocular infection after the newborn period results from venereal disease. Chlamydia is a common venereal disease, with 3 to 5 million new cases a year in the United States.[1,2] It accounts for 35% to 50% of cases of nongonococcal urethritis in men and is recovered from the cervix in 20% to 33% of women in clinics for sexually transmitted diseases.[1,3-5] Ocular inoculation may occur by spread from the genitalia to the fingers to the eye, from the genitalia directly to the eye, or from the genitalia to fomites to the eye. Autoinoculation is most common; eye-to-eye transmission is unusual. Inclusion conjunctivitis can also be transmitted in swimming pools with inadequately prepared chlorination.[6] (Most conjunctivitis from swimming pools is caused by the chlorine-resistant adenoviruses.)

CLINICAL MANIFESTATIONS

The incubation period averages 5 days, but ranges from 2 to 19 days. Unilateral disease is more common than bilateral. The onset is typically subacute but may be acute. The patient complains of foreign body sensation, tearing, photophobia, redness, and lid swelling. The eye is mildly irritated and injected, and a scant mucopurulent discharge is present. Follicular hypertrophy is more marked in the lower tarsal conjunctiva (Fig. 8-1), in contrast to trachoma, and may take 2 to 3 weeks to appear. No pseudomembranes are present, but a small, preauricular, tender node may develop. A pseudoptosis is often seen. Epithelial keratitis can be present, consisting of small, focal epithelial lesions that stain with fluorescein and tend to be more common in the periphery. Subepithelial infiltrates can occur, usually 2 to 3 weeks after the onset of the conjunctivitis; they tend to be smaller than those seen in adenovirus (Fig. 8-2). A superior corneal micropannus can be seen (see Fig. 6-3). Small marginal corneal abscesses also can occur.[7]

Otitis media has been reported to occur on the same side as the involved eye in as many as 14% of cases.[8] A mild iritis also can be seen.

Untreated, inclusion conjunctivitis can persist for 6 to 18 months. When a conjunctivitis persists for longer than 6 weeks in a person of the sexually active age group, one should be suspicious of the possibility of inclusion conjunctivitis.

A comparison of the features of ACK and adenoviral epidemic keratoconjunctivitis is given in Table 8-2.

DIAGNOSIS

Scrapings of the conjunctival epithelium with Giemsa or Wright stain can be of immense value.[9] The predominant inflammatory cells are polymorphonuclear leukocytes. Inclusions can be seen with

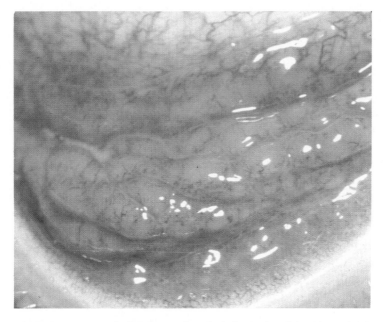

Fig. 8-1. Marked follicular response in inferior conjunctival fornix in adult chlamydial keratoconjunctivitis. (Courtesy F Wilson II, Indianapolis, Ind.)

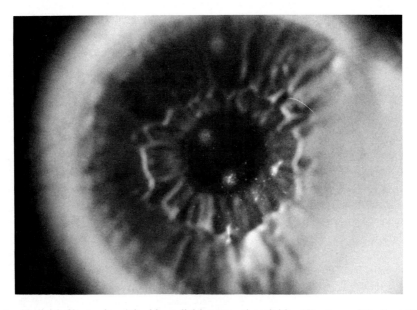

Fig. 8-2. Subepithelial infiltrates in adult chlamydial keratoconjunctivitis. (Courtesy of Bartly J Mondino, Los Angeles, Calif.)

TABLE 8-2. Comparison of Adult Chlamydial Keratoconjunctivitis (ACK) and Adenoviral Epidemic Keratoconjunctivitis (EKC)

FEATURE	ACK	EKC
Laterality	Unilateral more common	Bilateral more common
Discharge	Mucopurulent	Watery
Follicles	+	+
Adenopathy	Small, sometimes tender node	Prominent, tender node
Membranes	No	Occasionally
Focal epithelial keratitis	Occasionally, more common peripherally and superiorly	Usually, more common centrally
Subepithelial infiltrates	Occasionally, smaller than in EKC	Common
Associated findings	Otitis media, urethritis	None
Duration	Can last longer than a year	Conjunctivitis lasts 2 to 3 weeks
Cytology	Mixed mononuclear and polymorphonuclear cells; occasionally inclusions	Mononuclear cells (polymorphonuclear cells if membranes present)

Giemsa stain or with fluorescent antibody-staining of conjunctival scrapings. The inclusions, which are basophilic and are located in the cytoplasm of the epithelial cells (Fig. 8-3), are similar to the inclusions (Halberstaedter-Prowazek bodies) found in trachoma. The inclusion bodies are located immediately above the nucleus and form a small cap that sits on the nucleus. The inclusion consists of infectious elementary bodies. The elementary bodies are round, appear to be equal in size, have sharp-edged cell walls, and are light purple when stained with Giemsa stain. One must make sure when viewing the slide that true inclusion bodies are not mistaken for pseudoinclusions such as bacteria, extrusions of nuclear chromatin granules, or pigment granules. In addition to the elementary bodies, initial bodies may be found. The initial body is larger than the elementary body and stains dark blue, often in a bipolar fashion. Inclusion bodies are seen much more frequently in the chlamydial oculoglandular infection of infancy; they may be difficult to find in adults.

McCoy cell tissue culture is the definitive means of diagnosis but is not widely available. It also can be negative in up to half of cases and is impaired by antibiotic treatment.[10,11]

Because of the difficulties with these traditional tests, immunologic tests recently have been developed for diagnosing chlamydial infection. Both direct tests (examination of ocular specimens for chlamydial antigen) and indirect tests (testing of serum for antichlamydial antibodies) have been devised. A fluorescein-conjugated monoclonal antibody direct test is commercially available and has been reported to be highly sensitive and specific.[11-14] In our experience this test is difficult to interpret and should be read only by those with a great deal of experience. An enzyme immunosorbent assay (Chlamydiazyme, Abbott Laboratories, North Chicago, IL) was found to be fairly sensitive and specific (71% and 97%, respectively).[14]

Serum titers also can be useful. Commercial tests for antichlamydial IgG and IgA antibody titers are available and are relatively easy to perform.[13,15-17] Repeated tests showing a rising titer are diagnostic for recent infection, but single highly elevated titers suggest acute infection. Of course, antibodies can be present as a result of previous or nonocular infection.

TREATMENT

Topical treatment is not sufficient, because it is not curative, and frequently extraocular infection is also present. The treatment of choice is tetracycline, 250 mg orally four times daily for 3 weeks. The tetracycline should be taken on an empty stomach, and the patient should avoid milk products

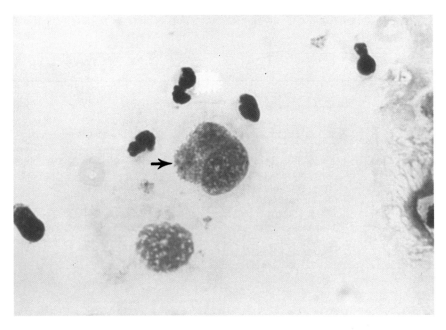

Fig. 8-3. Intracytoplasmic inclusion *(arrow)* in chlamydial conjunctivitis. (Courtesy of Regis P Kowalski, Pittsburgh, Pa.)

and antacids, which can prevent absorption of the drug. Pregnant women or children under 7 years of age should not be given tetracycline. Doxycycline, 300 mg initially followed by 100 mg per day for 2 weeks, is a simpler regimen that appears to be as effective. Erythromycin, 250 mg four times daily for 3 weeks, or sulfisoxazole, 0.5 to 1 g four times daily for 3 weeks, can be used if tetracycline is contraindicated or not tolerated. It is crucial to treat the patient's sexual partner to prevent reinfection.

TRACHOMA
EPIDEMIOLOGY

Trachoma has been around for 3000 years, if not longer, and has ravaged a good part of the world. Even today it is a major cause of preventable blindness. Around the world, 700 million cases are estimated, about 200 million of which involve blindness or significantly decreased visual acuity.

Trachoma is prevalent among the American Indians of the southwestern United States. Many cases are found in the "trachoma belt" of Arkansas, Missouri, Oklahoma, West Virginia, and Kentucky.

The disease is spread from eye to eye by way of fingers, fomites, water, and occasionally by flies. Its highest incidence is in unhealthy, dirty, crowded conditions, primarily in the low socioeconomic stratum of society. Even in endemic areas, the disease is associated with poorer personal hygiene, particularly decreased face washing, and improved hygiene has dramatically lowered the prevalence of disease.[18,19] It is the childhood form that is important in the spread of disease in both the family and the community. In endemic areas preschool children serve as a reservoir of acute infection. Virtually all children are infected by 2 years of age, and acute infection is uncommon in adults. A failure to induce immunity in trachoma may occur and may account for the long duration of the disease and for the reinfections that are so common among schoolchildren who have been treated successfully during the school year.

Repeated inoculation with the chlamydia is probably necessary for development of trachoma.[20] Bacterial conjunctivitis is also very common in these populations and can play an important role in the pathogenesis of the scarring and blinding complications. Jones described the situation in which trachoma arises as one of "ocular promiscuity," which entails "conditions that favor the frequent, unrestricted, and indiscriminate mixing of ocular contacts or of ocular discharges."[21]

Although serotypes A through C usually are associated with trachoma, clinically typical cases of trachoma can develop from venereal infection with serotypes D through K.

CLINICAL MANIFESTATIONS

Acute infection with trachoma can be seen in children or can be mild and go unrecognized. Approximately 5 days after inoculation, the child develops bilateral conjunctival injection, tearing, photophobia, and mucopurulent discharge. A tender preauricular node may be present. About 3 weeks later follicles may develop in the upper tarsal conjunctiva and sometimes at the limbus.

MacCallan[22] has divided the clinical features of trachoma into four stages. This system describes the course of trachoma but is not useful in estimating the intensity of disease, which is important in determining the outcome.[23] Therefore another classification has been developed to score the intensity of inflammation.[23,24]

In the MacCallan classification, *stage I* is called incipient trachoma, and the signs and symptoms are similar to those of acute infection. This stage is characterized by the presence of immature follicles in the upper tarsal conjunctiva. These follicles are soft and easily expressible, unlike those of nontrachomatous follicular conjunctivitis. Follicles may also be seen at the limbus and on the caruncle. A minimal exudate usually occurs; however, if a secondary infection is present, greater exudation is seen. Intense cellular infiltration of the conjunctiva can occur; the subepithelial tissue of the conjunctiva is edematous and infiltrated with round inflammatory cells, mainly lymphocytes and plasma cells. Papillary hypertrophy also occurs, and the follicles may be buried as a result. In this stage of early formation of conjunctival follicles, one may see a diffuse punctate keratitis and early formation of a superior corneal pannus. Fibrovascular tissue may grow into the cornea underneath the epithelium and destroy Bowman's layer.

MacCallan's *stage II* is considered established trachoma and is characterized by mature follicles and more advanced keratitis. This stage is divided into IIa, in which the follicular response is predominant (Fig. 8-4), and IIb, in which follicles are seen but are largely obscured by a rather intense papillary response. Stage IIb is primarily a florid inflammation of the upper tarsal conjunctiva, with more acute inflammation and cellular infiltration. The mature follicles have the appearance of "sago" grains and can undergo central necrosis. The corneal pannus as well as the subepithelial edema and round cell infiltration may increase. Large macrophages with phagocytosed debris (Leber's cells) appear in the conjunctival substantia propria (see Fig. 4-10). At this stage the follicles cannot be differentiated histologically from lymphoid follicles secondary to other causes.

Stage III brings about variable amounts of scarring and cicatrization (Fig. 8-5). The limbal corneal follicles, if present, cicatrize, and the area is covered with thickened transparent epithelium (*Herbert's pits*) (Fig. 8-6). These pits are pathognomonic of trachoma. Scarring also occurs in the palpebral conjunctiva and is manifested clinically by the appearance of fine linear scars on the tarsal conjunctiva and sometimes in the bulbar conjunctiva. The horizontal linear scars that are noted in the upper tarsal conjunctiva are known as *Arlt's line*. Cicatrization of the lids, symblepharon, trichiasis, and other lid distortions begin to develop.

Each of the first three stages may last for months or years. In *stage IV*, or healed trachoma, the conjunctival and corneal inflammation has subsided. Follicles and papillae are no longer present, and there is no inflammatory infiltration of the cornea. The amount of residual scarring is determined by the severity of the inflammation in the previous stages.[23] The scarring produces dry eyes, entropion,

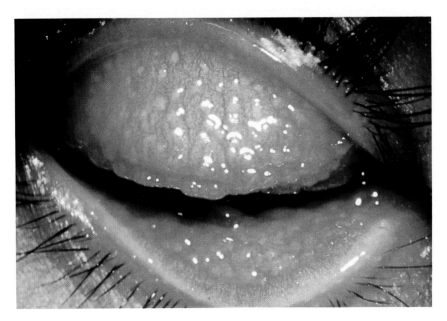

Fig. 8-4. Stage IIa trachoma.

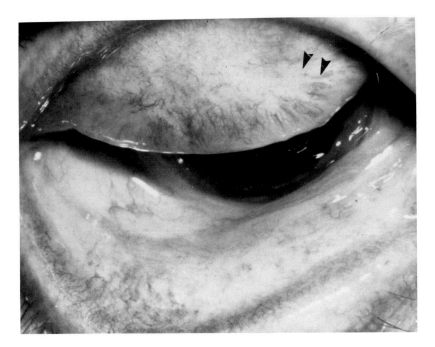

Fig. 8-5. Scarring of conjunctiva of upper tarsus *(double arrow)* in stage III trachoma.

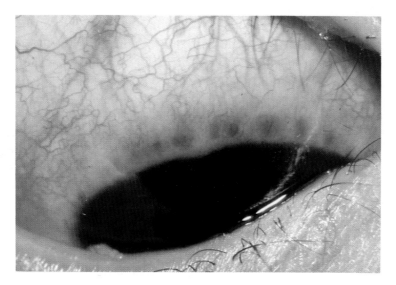

Fig. 8-6. Herbert's pits in stage III trachoma.

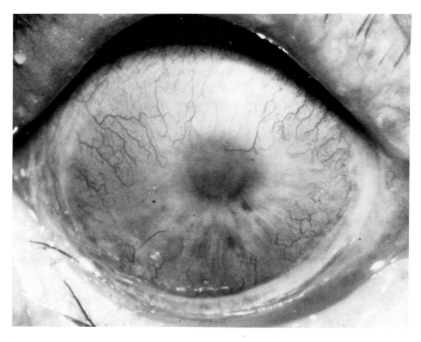

Fig. 8-7. Scarring, vascularization, and corneal opacification in stage IV trachoma.

and trichiasis. It is the complications of these disorders, including subsequent bacterial keratitis, that lead to blindness.

Corneal findings can include gross pannus of the upper portion of the cornea, epithelial and subepithelial keratitis, and corneal ulceration. Corneal scarring, opacification, and vascularization can be so severe that vision is markedly impaired (Fig. 8-7). The corneal findings are more prominent in the superior cornea.

Lacrimal complications such as punctal phimosis, punctal occlusion, canalicular occlusion, naso-lacrimal obstruction, dacryocystitis, and fistulae in the skin have been reported in trachoma.[25]

DIAGNOSIS

The primary inflammatory reaction may be a polymorphonuclear response with a mucopurulent discharge and preauricular adenopathy; however, lymphocytes, plasma cells, lymphoblasts, necrotic epithelial cells, and multinucleated giant epithelial cells may be seen. Basophilic, intracytoplasmic, epithelial inclusion bodies (Halberstaedter-Prowazek bodies) similar to those described in inclusion conjunctivitis are seen in this disease. The frequency of their presence depends on the stage of the trachoma, with up to 40% of smears positive in moderate cases.[26,27]

Fluorescent monoclonal antibody (FMA) staining of conjunctival smears is slightly less specific but more sensitive than Giemsa staining of smears.[26,28] In one study an enzyme immunoassay was found to be more specific than FMA or Giemsa staining.[29]

TREATMENT

The ideal treatment is with a full, oral dose of tetracycline, sulfonamide, or erythromycin for at least 3 weeks. If tetracycline is the drug given, the dosage should be 500 mg orally three times a day for at least 3 weeks. This medication should be taken 1 hour before or 2 hours after meals with water or juice but no milk. Tetracycline is not to be used in pregnant women or in children younger than 7 years of age.

Trisulfapyrimidines (triple sulfa) may be used. In adults the dose is 2 to 4 g immediately followed by a maintenance dosage of 2 to 4 g daily in three or four divided doses for at least 3 weeks. In children a loading dose of half of the 24-hour dose is followed by a maintenance dosage of 150 mg/kg per 24 hours in three or four dosages for at least 3 weeks. Trisulfapyrimidines are not to be used in pregnant women, nursing mothers, or infants younger than 2 months of age.

This systemic treatment is most effective in sporadic cases in nonendemic areas. In hyperendemic areas in which half or more of the children have active disease and seasonal epidemics of bacterial conjunctivitis are present, reinfection and recurrent bacterial infection prevent elimination of the disease. Elimination of the reservoir of the organism by mass treatment with systemic antibiotics is not practical. Therefore the aim of the therapy instead is to avoid blinding complications. Topical tetracycline twice a day, given as a continuous 6-week course, appears to reduce or eliminate blinding complications. Similar results were achieved with a 5-day course of topical tetracycline repeated once monthly for 6 months.[30,31] Topical medication may act by reducing the intensity of the disease, the rate of transmission, and the bacterial flora and seasonal conjunctivitis that contribute to the gravity of trachoma in these areas. Oral antibiotic therapy is recommended as an adjunct in children with moderate to severe trachoma to improve the outcome.[32] Surgical treatment is also important to correct entropion, trichiasis, and lacrimal disorders.

OTHER CHLAMYDIAL INFECTIONS

CHLAMYDIA PSITTACI

Chlamydia psittaci produces an infection of birds, with occasional transmission to humans. Its name comes from the Greek word for parrot *(psittakos),* which was the vector for the first recognized cases in humans. It can cause an asymptomatic infection, mild influenza-like illness, or serious pneumonia. Rare cases of conjunctivitis have been reported.[33,34] An acute or chronic follicular conjunctivitis can occur that may be similar to adult inclusion conjunctivitis. A diffuse follicular response, mild preauricular adenopathy, and mucopurulent discharge can be seen. There is no scarring of the conjunctiva. A diffuse epithelial keratitis and subepithelial infiltration can occur; however, no pannus is noted. No inclusions can be found on scrapings. The same organism can be isolated from the patient's cats, who may have a similar conjunctivitis. There are no sequelae of any importance, and the disease apparently responds to tetracycline.

LYMPHOGRANULOMA VENEREUM

Lymphogranuloma venereum is transmitted venereally and usually is manifested by genital lesions followed by lymphadenitis and febrile systemic illness. A follicular conjunctivitis or granulomatous reaction associated with periauricular adenopathy (Parinaud's oculoglandular syndrome) can occur.[35] The conjunctivitis usually resolves after 3 to 4 weeks but can persist for years. Elephantiasis of the lids can occur in chronic cases as a result of blockage of lymphatic drainage. Corneal involvement is uncommon but can be severe. Spotty marginal corneal infiltration, usually superior, becomes deep and confluent and spreads centrally. Superficial vascularization can ensue and may become so profuse that it resembles an epaulet.[36] Episcleritis, sclerokeratitis, and interstitial keratitis also have been seen. Chlamydial inclusions often are found on conjunctival scrapings. The Frei test is positive in half of these patients. Optic neuritis and anterior uveitis occasionally are seen,[36] and the orbit also may be involved.[37]

REFERENCES

1. Judson FN: Assessing the number of genital chlamydial infections in the United States, J Reprod Med 30:269, 1985.
2. Schachter J et al: Are chlamydia infections the most prevalent venereal disease? JAMA 231:1252, 1975.
3. Schachter J: Chlamydial infections, N Engl J Med 298:428, 1978.
4. Schachter J, Causse G, and Tarizzo ML: Chlamydiae as agents of sexually transmitted diseases, Bull WHO 54:245, 1976.
5. Thompson SE and Washington AE: Epidemiology of sexually transmitted *Chlamydia trachomatis* infections, Epidemiol Rev 5:96, 1983.
6. Morax V: Les conjonctivites folliculaires, Paris, 1933, Masson et Cie.
7. Darougar S and Viswalingam ND: Marginal corneal abscess associated with adult chlamydia ophthalmia, Br J Ophthalmol 72:774, 1988.
8. Dawson C et al: Experimental inclusion conjunctivitis in man. III. Keratitis and other complications, Arch Ophthalmol 78:341, 1967.
9. Yoneda C et al: Cytology as a guide to the presence of chlamydial inclusions in Giemsa-stained conjunctival smears in severe endemic trachoma, Br J Ophthalmol 59:116, 1975.
10. Schachter J et al: Evaluation of laboratory methods for detecting acute TRIC agent infection, Am J Ophthalmol 70:377, 1970.
11. Taylor HR, Agarwala N, and Johnson SL: Detection of experimental *Chlamydia trachomatis* eye infection in conjunctival smears and in tissue culture by use of fluorescein-conjugated monoclonal antibody, J Clin Microbiol 20:391, 1984.

12. Hawkins DA et al: Rapid, reliable diagnosis of chlamydial ophthalmia by means of monoclonal antibodies, Br J Ophthalmol 69:640, 1985.
13. Bialasiewicz AA and Jahn GJ: Evaluation of diagnostic tools for adult chlamydial keratoconjunctivitis, Ophthalmology 94:532, 1987.
14. Sheppard JD et al: Immunology of adult chlamydial conjunctivitis, Ophthalmology 95:434, 1988.
15. Darougar S et al: Rapid serological test for diagnosis of chlamydial ocular infections, Br J Ophthalmol 62:503, 1978.
16. Wang S and Grayston J: Immunologic relationship between genital TRIC, lymphogranuloma venereum, and related organisms in a new microtiter indirect immunofluorescence test, Am J Ophthalmol 70:367, 1970.
17. Arffa RC, Kowalski RP, and Springer DS: The value of serology in the diagnosis of adult chlamydial keratoconjunctivitis, Ophthalmology 95(suppl):145, 1988.
18. Marx R: Sociomedical aspects of trachoma, Acta Ophthalmol (Copenh) 66(suppl 183):1, 1988.
19. Taylor HR et al: Hygiene factors and increased risk of trachoma in central Tanzania, Arch Ophthalmol 107:1821, 1989.
20. Taylor HR et al: An animal model of trachoma II. The importance of repeated infection, Invest Ophthalmol Vis Sci 23:507, 1982.
21. Jones BR: The prevention of blindness from trachoma, Trans Ophthalmol Soc UK 95:19, 1975.
22. MacCallan A: The epidemiology of trachoma, Br J Ophthalmol 15:369, 1931.
23. Dawson C, Jones B, and Darougar S: Blinding and nonblinding trachoma: assessment of intensity of upper tarsal inflammatory disease and disabling lesions, Bull WHO 52:279, 1975.

24. Darougar S and Jones BR: Trachoma, Br Med Bull 39:117, 1983.

25. Tabbara KF and Babb AA: Lacrimal system complications in trachoma, Ophthalmology 87:298, 1980.

26. Taylor PB, Burd EM, and Tabbara KF: Comparison of diagnostic laboratory techniques in the various stages of trachoma, Ophthalmology 94(suppl):123, 1987.

27. Bettman JW Jr et al: Inclusion conjunctivitis in American Indians of the Southwest, Am J Ophthalmol 70:363, 1970.

28. Rapoza PA et al: Direct immunofluorescence monoclonal antibody staining of conjunctival smears for trachoma. Paper presented at the annual meeting of the Ocular Microbiology and Immunology Group, Dallas, Nov 1987.

29. Tabbara KF and Rahi A: Enzyme immunoassay in the detection of chlamydial antigens in patients with trachoma, Ophthalmology 94(suppl):123, 1987.

30. Dawson CR et al: Intermittent trachoma chemotherapy: a controlled trial of topical tetracycline or erythromycin, Bull WHO 59:91, 1981.

31. Dawson CR, Jones BR, and Tarisso ML: Guide to trachoma control. In Programmes for the Prevention of Blindness, World Health Organization, Geneva, 1981.

32. Dawson CR and Schachter J: Strategies for treatment and control of blinding trachoma: cost-effectiveness of topical or systemic antibiotics, Rev Infect Dis 7:768, 1985.

33. Ostler B, Schachter J, and Dawson C: Acute follicular conjunctivitis of epizootic origin, Arch Ophthalmol 82:587, 1969.

34. Viswalingam ND, Wishart MS, and Woodland RM: Adult chlamydial ophthalmia (paratrachoma), Br Med Bull 39:123, 1983.

35. Duke-Elder S and Leigh AG: System of ophthalmology, vol 8, Diseases of the outer eye, St Louis, 1965, Mosby–Year Book, Inc.

36. Scheie HG, Crandall AS, and Henle W: Keratitis associated with lymphogranuloma venereum, JAMA 135:333, 1947.

37. Endicott JN, Kirconnel WS, and Beam D: Granuloma inguinale of the orbit with bony involvement, Arch Otolaryngol 96:457, 1972.

INFECTIOUS ULCERATIVE KERATITIS: BACTERIAL

Infectious corneal ulcers can be caused by viruses, bacteria, fungi, or parasites. In the developed countries of the world herpes simplex is by far the most common cause of corneal infection. Herpes simplex infections are discussed in Chapter 11. Bacterial corneal ulcers are less common, and fungal and parasitic corneal ulcers are the least common, although they have become more important numerically in the past two decades. A central corneal infection is a threat to vision and to the eye; it is a true ocular emergency. Therefore it is important to learn to differentiate infectious from noninfectious infiltrates and ulcers. Whenever a corneal infection is suspected, immediate laboratory studies and therapy should be instituted. Frequent and careful follow-up and adjustment of therapy are necessary to ensure the best outcome. Bacterial keratitis will be covered in this chapter; fungal and parasitic infections are discussed in Chapter 10.

PATHOGENESIS

Several mechanisms protect the surface of the eye from infectious agents, some of which were discussed in Chapter 6. The lids physically block organisms from entering the eye and remove them from the corneal surface. The mechanical flushing action of the tears is important as a defense against infection, as is the presence of lysozyme, lactoferrin, beta-lysin, and natural antibodies, principally

IgA, in the tears. Mucus can trap and remove organisms. Intact epithelial surfaces are an important line of defense against infection. The adherent glycocalyx and mucin layers on the corneal surface may inhibit microbial attachment and penetration. The normal flora of the ocular surface help prevent overgrowth of indigenous organisms or invasion by pathogens.

In addition the eye's acute, nonspecific inflammatory reaction to injury, through phagocytosis of the invaders by neutrophils and, later, macrophages, helps the uncompromised host to control or destroy invading organisms. Specific humoral and cellular reactions also counteract opportunists but require 5 to 8 days to develop, unless there has been previous exposure to the invading agent. The nonspecific inflammatory reaction ordinarily takes care of all opportunists that have breached the conjunctival epithelium; the specific humoral and cellular reactions are needed by the uncompromised host only if the microbic inoculum is overwhelming.

Interference with any of these defense mechanisms predisposes the host to corneal infection. Lid abnormalities such as exposure, trichiasis, entropion, or lagophthalmos are frequently associated with infection. Dry eyes and lacrimal drainage obstruction reduce the flushing of organisms from the surface and the availability of antibacterial proteins. Antibiotics often play a role in the development of opportunistic infections of the cornea. Abuse of antibiotics can contribute to a compromising situation by shifting the normal, relatively benign flora of the conjunctival sac to allow growth of more pathogenic bacteria.

Other conditions that reduce the integrity of the corneal epithelium include bullous keratopathy, medication toxicity (for example, antibiotics, antiviral drugs, or anesthetics), corneal anesthesia, recurrent erosions, chemical or physical injury, viral infection, and contact lenses. Contact lenses have become increasingly associated with corneal infections.[1-3] Soft lenses, particularly those worn as extended wear (overnight wear), are associated with the highest risk.[4,5] Contact lenses deprive the cornea of oxygen, serve as a source of microbes, damage the corneal epithelium, and interfere with protective tear flow. Patients who do not care for their lenses properly are more likely to develop an infection, but infections also occur in people without obvious breaks in technique.[6,7]

Localized or systemic impairment of immune response frequently contributes to corneal infections. The use of topical corticosteroids is the most common cause of localized immunosuppression. The following systemic conditions can result in a compromised host and thus facilitate the development of corneal infection[8-10]:

1. Immunosuppressive drugs
2. Extensive body burns
3. Pregnancy (last trimester)
4. Chronic alcoholism
5. Severe malnutrition
6. Infancy
7. Old age
8. Immunodeficiency syndromes such as Wiskott-Aldrich syndrome and acquired immunodeficiency syndrome (AIDS)
9. Drug addiction
10. Malignancy

The most common precipitating event in microbial keratitis is the development of an epithelial defect. Thus an abrasion, foreign body, erosion, or rupture of an epithelial bulla often precedes a central corneal ulcer. In individuals with decreased systemic resistance, such as debilitated, elderly, alcoholic, or diabetic individuals or patients with decreased local defenses such as those with keratoconjunctivitis sicca, organisms normally present in the tear film can produce infections. Alternatively, pathogenic bacteria can be introduced in foreign bodies, through poor hygiene, in contact lenses, or in topical medications. Gram-negative bacteria, including *Pseudomonas, Serratia,* and *Proteus,* have been isolated from ocular medications used by patients who developed infectious keratitis.[11]

Only a few organisms can penetrate intact epithelium: *Neisseria gonorrhoeae, Corynebacterium diphtheriae, Haemophilus aegyptius* and *Listeria.* In rare cases organisms reach the corneal stroma through hematogenous spread; in those cases they typically cause perilimbal infection.

The physician should recognize the eye's natural defense mechanisms, using them to advantage and refraining from thwarting them. It is also important to diagnose underlying conditions that may have led to the infection and to correct or ameliorate them if possible.

ORGANISMS

Bacterial organisms that may cause keratitis can be classified according to type, Gram stain, and desire for oxygen, as outlined below.

I. Gram-positive organisms
  A. Aerobes
    1. Micrococci
      a. *Staphylococcus aureus*
      b. *Staphylococcus epidermidis*
    2. Streptococci
      a. Alpha-hemolytic streptococci
      b. Beta-hemolytic streptococci
      c. nonhemolytic streptococci
      d. *Streptococcus pneumoniae*
    3. Bacilli
      a. Spore-forming
        (1) *Bacillus*
        (2) Clostridium
      b. Non-spore forming
        (1) *Corynebacterium*
        (2) Listeria
  B. Anaerobes
    1. Cocci
      a. *Peptostreptococcus*
      b. *Peptococcus*
    2. Bacilli
      a. Spore forming: *Clostridium*
      b. Non-spore forming
        (1) *Actinomyces*
        (2) Propionibacterium
  C. Acid-fast bacilli
    1. *Mycobacterium*
    2. *Nocardia*
II. Gram-negative organisms
  A. Aerobes
    1. Diplococci: *Neisseria*
    2. Rods
      a. Enterobacteriaceae
        (1) *Escherichia*
        (2) *Klebsiella*
        (3) *Enterobacter*
        (4) *Proteus*
        (5) *Serratia*
        (6) *Citrobacter*

    b. Others
      (1) *Pseudomonas*
      (2) *Azotobacter*
      (3) *Acinetobacter*
  3. Diplobacillus: *Moraxella*
  4. Coccobacillus: *Haemophilus*
B. Anaerobes
  1. Rods (non-spore forming)
    a. *Fusobacterium*
    b. *Bacteroides*

The relative frequency of different bacterial ulcers differs geographically within the United States. It appears that staphylococcal infections are seen more frequently in the eastern and northeastern areas of the United States, whereas *Pseudomonas* infections are found more often in the more temperate climates of the country. *Streptococcus pneumoniae* was previously the most common corneal pathogen, particularly in the eastern and western portions of the country, but its relative incidence has declined.[12-14] Now *Pseudomonas* and staphylococcal infections are more common.

As with any bacterial disease, the manifestations and the severity of corneal infections depend on the organism and the host's response.[15] The virulence of an organism is determined by its ability to adhere to the corneal surface, to penetrate the epithelium, to multiply and spread within the corneal tissue, and to resist the host's defenses, as well as its elaboration of toxins. Less virulent organisms can cause disease only in compromised corneas, whereas the most virulent organisms can cause severe disease in relatively intact corneas.

Following are the bacteria that most commonly cause corneal ulcers in an uncompromised cornea:
1. *Pseudomonas aeruginosa*
2. *Streptococcus pneumoniae*
3. *Moraxella*
4. Beta-hemolytic streptococcus
5. *Klebsiella pneumoniae*

Many other organisms are less frequently seen (for example, *Escherichia coli*, *Proteus*, *Mycobacterium fortuitum*, and *Nocardia*).

Opportunistic pathogens are microbic agents that have been regarded as contaminants or harmless inhabitants but that, in the compromised host, can multiply and produce corneal disease.[16] In the compromised cornea *Staphylococcus aureus* is the most common cause of central corneal ulcers; however, a wide range of microorganisms can produce serious disease:
1. *Staphylococcus aureus*
2. Staphylococcus epidermidis
3. Alpha-hemolytic streptococci
4. Beta-hemolytic streptococci
5. *Pseudomonas aeruginosa*
6. *Proteus*
7. *Enterobacter aerogenes*
8. Others, such as *Escherichia* and *Nocardia*

The following organisms are particularly frequent in contact lens wearers:
1. *Pseudomonas aeruginosa*
2. *Staphylococcus aureus*
3. *Staphylococcus epidermidis*
4. *Serratia marcescens*
5. Other Enterobacteriaceae: *E. coli, Klebsiella, Proteus*

In children over 3 years of age, the organisms that cause keratitis are similar to those seen in adults; however, under 3 years of age, *Pseudomonas aeruginosa* and streptococcal species account for the large majority of infections.[17]

CLINICAL MANIFESTATIONS

When a bacterial corneal ulcer develops, conjunctival injection and chemosis, lid edema, decreased vision, pain, tearing, photophobia, and purulent discharge usually are present. The conjunctival reaction is nonspecific, with a mainly papillary response, and injection is greatest near the limbus. The corneal epithelium becomes ulcerated, and the stroma exhibits infiltration and may be gray-white and necrotic. Infiltration and edema of the cornea may even be observed in areas away from the site of the ulcer. Stromal abscesses may be evident as small, deep infiltrates beneath relatively clear stroma and intact epithelium. An anterior chamber reaction often is present, and in more severe cases fibrin plaques may be observed on the endothelium, and a fibrinoid aqueous or hypopyon may be seen.

The hypopyon is caused by the toxic effects of the infection on the vessels of the iris and ciliary body, with resultant outpouring of fibrin and polymorphonuclear leukocytes. Usually the hypopyon is sterile as long as Descemet's membrane is intact. A hypopyon can be seen with any bacterial infection (Fig. 9-1), but it is relatively more common in ulcers caused by *Streptococcus pneumoniae* (Fig. 9-2) and *Pseudomonas* (Fig. 9-3). It should be remembered that hypopyons are also seen with viral and fungal corneal ulcers. Noninfectious causes of hypopyon include Behçet's syndrome, abuse of topical anesthetic agents, severe lye burns, and therapeutic contact lenses (particularly in anesthetic corneas).

The clinical signs and symptoms of bacterial corneal ulcers vary with the virulence of the organism, the previous status of the cornea, the duration of infection, the immune status of the host, and previous antibiotic and corticosteroid use. More virulent organisms cause greater stromal destruction and elicit a more marked host response, hence the sign and symptoms of infection are more pronounced. In immunosuppressed patients, or with corticosteroid use, the signs of inflammation, in-

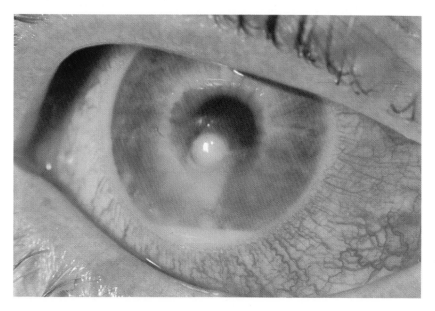

Fig. 9-1. Hypopyon ulcer resulting from staphylococcal infection. Infiltrate is round and localized, with more or less distinct borders.

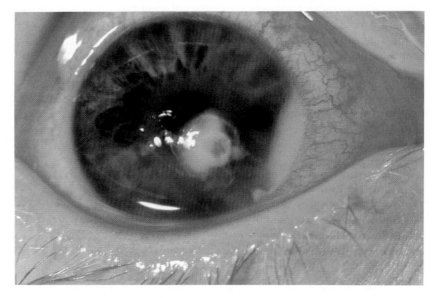

Fig. 9-2. Central corneal ulcer caused by *Streptococcus pneumoniae*. Eccentric location of hypopyon was caused by patient lying on side.

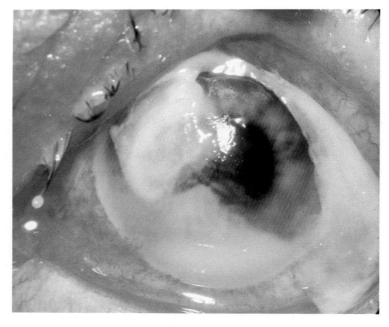

Fig. 9-3. Hypopyon ulcer caused by *Pseudomonas aeruginosa* infection. Extensive lysis of collagen structure has occurred.

cluding redness, pain, infiltration, and anterior chamber reaction, are relatively reduced, and greater ulceration and extension of infection can occur before presentation.

The use of hydrophilic contact lenses can alter the presentation of bacterial ulcers. Infections associated with contact lenses are often multifocal, and the epithelial and stromal infiltration is more diffuse. Contact lens wearers who present with corneal abrasions may have early bacterial infections. Often a patient whose eye is patched for a contact lens–associated abrasion, without any sign of infiltration, returns with a well-developed corneal ulcer the following day.[18] It probably is best not to use an eye patch on contact lens wearers with abrasions, but rather to take cultures, begin antibiotic therapy, and reevaluate the patient's condition the following day.

DIFFERENTIAL DIAGNOSIS

It is most important to quickly recognize and treat bacterial corneal infections, but in doing so herpes simplex ulceration, noninfectious marginal infiltrative and ulcerative keratitis, trophic ulceration, and toxic keratopathy should be kept in mind as differential diagnostic conditions. In a recent review of patients hospitalized for corneal ulceration, 65% of the patients had nonbacterial ulcers.[19]

Various aids can be used to differentiate herpetic keratitis from a bacterial ulcer. Most commonly stromal herpes manifests itself as an epithelial dendrite, subepithelial scarring, or disciform edema, and these are usually relatively easy to differentiate from bacterial keratitis. Less often a necrotizing, infiltrative keratitis occurs, probably caused by active viral proliferation in the stroma, and this presents more of a diagnostic dilemma. A history of previous herpetic keratitis or of recurrent ocular disease may be elicited. In herpetic infection corneal sensitivity is usually decreased, and this can be a helpful feature. However, bacterial and herpetic ulcers can be indistinguishable clinically, and bacterial infection often occurs in patients with corneas scarred by previous herpetic infection. Therefore laboratory diagnosis often is required. In herpetic keratitis scrapings may contain multinucleated giant cells and no bacteria, and viral culture or immunologic tests may confirm the diagnosis.

Both infectious and immunologic infiltrates can occur in the limbal cornea. Catarrhal infiltrates, related to staphylococcal blepharitis, are probably most common. These are typically 0.5 to 2 mm long, located approximately 1 mm central to the limbal vessels, and are associated with an epithelial defect (see Chapter 18). However, infectious infiltrates can have the same appearance. For instance, *Alternaria* organisms can cause marginal infiltrates that resemble an immune infiltrate, and occasionally gram-negative organisms are isolated from marginal corneal ulcers in cicatricial pemphigoid. One helpful differentiating feature is that catarrhal infiltrates are often multiple, while infectious ulcers are rarely so. The presence of blepharitis and/or meibomitis and evidence of previous marginal inflammation suggests catarrhal ulceration.

Sterile infiltrates often occur in contact lens wearers, and it can be very difficult to differentiate these from infectious infiltrates. Sterile infiltrates tend to be smaller (less than 1 mm), multiple or arcuate in shape, and tend not to be associated with significant pain, discharge, epithelial defect, or anterior chamber reaction (Fig. 9-4).[20] In some cases these infiltrates appear to be reactions to thimerosal (Fig. 9-5). However, it is not possible to be certain that any infiltrate is sterile. Therefore for any infiltrate associated with lens wear, it is best to discontinue lens wear, scrape and culture, forgo patching the eye, and follow the patient closely. Depending on the degree of suspicion of infection and the severity of the infiltrate, regular strength or fortified antibiotics are administered.

Noninfectious ulceration can occur in the presence of a chronic epithelial defect, especially when it is associated with keratitis sicca. Stromal lysis and even perforation can occur. Usually cellular infiltration is absent, in contrast to bacterial infections. These ulcers are located in the interpalpebral space, where the cornea is more prone to the effects of drying. Topical corticosteroid use often contributes to the stromal ulceration.

Peripheral corneal ulceration can occur in autoimmune diseases, particularly rheumatoid arthritis, or in Mooren's ulceration. These ulcers typically develop in a concentric shape near the limbus and may be associated with adjacent scleritis. Usually cellular infiltration is minimal or absent, but marked infiltration can occur. Differentiation from infectious ulceration can be difficult, and often cultures need to be taken and antibiotic treatment initiated because the possibility of infection cannot be eliminated.

Toxic keratopathy is often seen from overuse of such drugs as amphotericin B, idoxuridine, neo-

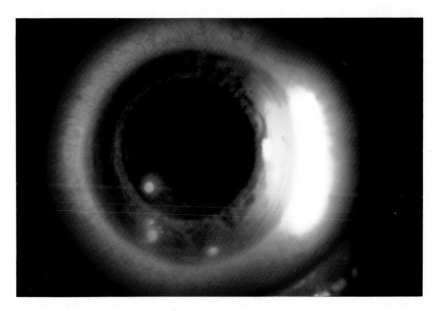

Fig. 9-4. Sterile corneal infiltrates associated with contact lens wear.

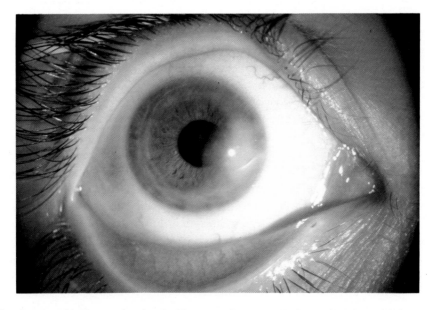

Fig. 9-5. Sterile corneal infiltrates associated with contact lens wear. Patient exhibited reaction to thimerosal on patch testing. (Courtesy of Bartly J Mondino, Los Angeles.)

mycin, gentamicin, and topical anesthetics. If these drugs are used for 10 days or longer, multifocal stromal infiltration may be seen.

SPECIFIC BACTERIAL ULCERS

In some cases the appearance of an ulcer can suggest a particular bacterial agent or group of agents. The characteristic features of infections produced by some agents are discussed below. However, it should be kept in mind that the clinical appearance is never diagnostic; isolation and identification of the causative organism or organisms are essential in all cases.

RING ULCERS

Ring abscess of the cornea is an uncommon finding in ocular infectious disease. Its occurrence is an indication of the devastating nature of the inflammatory reaction and usually foretells a grave prognosis for the eye. This condition can result from hematogenous spread of the bacteria or penetrating injury at the limbus. Although a variety of microorganisms, including *Pseudomonas aeruginosa* (Fig. 9-6), *Streptococcus, Listeria,* and *Proteus* species, have been implicated in causing ring abscesses, *Bacillus* species have been isolated most frequently.[21]

INFECTIOUS CRYSTALLINE KERATOPATHY

Infectious crystalline keratopathy is an uncommon form of corneal bacterial infection.[22-25] The stromal opacity is crystalline in appearance, resembling a snowflake, and is not associated with a cellular infiltrate or other signs of ocular inflammation. The infection usually occurs within a corneal graft, lying within the midstroma with clear stroma superficial to it. The epithelium often is intact (Fig. 9-7). Most cases have been caused by *Streptococcus viridans,* but *Haemophilus aphrophilus*[26] and *Peptostreptococcus* have also been isolated. Also, fungal infection was found in two cases, and in one case only calcium was seen.[27] Therefore biopsy often is necessary for diagnosis. Antibiotic treatment often has been unsuccessful, and keratoplasty has been required.

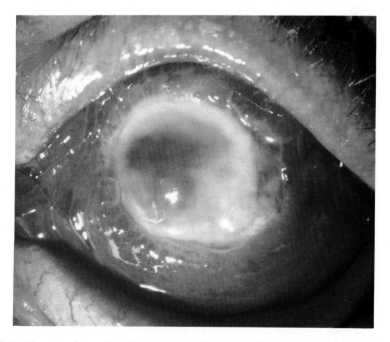

Fig. 9-6. Ring ulcer caused by *Pseudomonas.* (Courtesy of Y. Jerold Gordon, Pittsburgh.)

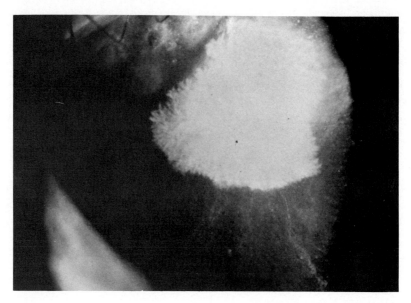

Fig. 9-7. Infectious crystalline keratopathy, caused by *Streptococcus sanguis,* in a graft. (Courtesy of Massimo Busin, Bonn, Germany.)

STAPHYLOCOCCI

S. aureus is often found on normal skin and conjunctiva and is an opportunistic corneal pathogen. *S. aureus* species produce coagulase, whereas *S. epidermidis* and other non-*aureus* species do not. Most *S. aureus* ferment mannitol, whereas most non-*aureus* species do not. Mannitol fermentation has been thought to be a predictor of pathogenicity of non-*aureus* strains[28]; however, more recently this was not supported.[29]

The corneal ulcer resulting from *S. aureus* tends to be round or oval and often remains localized with distinct borders (see Fig. 9-1); however, on occasion the ulcer may be diffuse, demonstrating microabscesses in the anterior stroma that are connected by stromal infiltrates. *S. aureus* ulcers tend to develop more in depth than width and often are associated with hypopyon and endothelial plaques. Staphylococcal blepharitis often is present.

Non-*aureus* staphylococci, such as *S. epidermidis,* can be isolated from most normal eyes, and it is an equally frequent cause of keratitis. These staphylococci are opportunists, affecting compromised corneas, and are unlikely to be the cause of infection in a healthy cornea. *S. aureus* is more virulent, but antibiotic resistance is more common among non-*aureus* strains.[29]

Corneal ulcers produced by non-*aureus* staphylococci appear similar to those caused by *S. aureus,* except they tend to be more indolent, with less infiltration and anterior chamber reaction. However, severe ulcers can occur.

STREPTOCOCCI

S. pneumoniae is found in the upper respiratory tract in half of the population; its proximity to the eye may account for the frequency of problems associated with it. Pneumococcal ulcers frequently occur after corneal trauma and often have been associated with chronic dacryocystitis. Most pneumococci are surrounded by a polysaccharide capsule, which protects them against phagocytosis. They tend to produce acute, purulent infections.

The keratitis may be localized or may have a tendency to spread in one direction, usually centrally. The edge may be undermined and covered by overhanging tissue. Pneumococcal ulcers have a

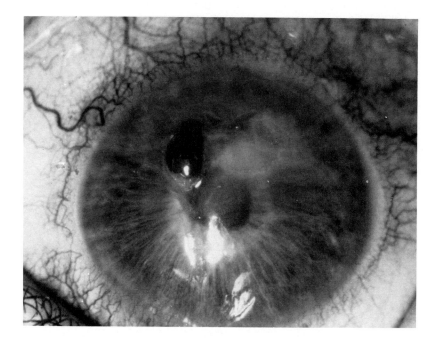

Fig. 9-8. Perforated corneal ulcer with iris prolapse.

tendency to be accompanied by marked anterior chamber reaction, including hypopyon (see Fig. 9-2), and perforation is more common (Fig. 9-8).[30]

S. pyogenes (beta-hemolytic streptococcus) is an infrequent cause of corneal infections, and the ulcers tend to be severe. Marginal corneal ulcers resulting from this organism also may be associated with dacryocystitis.[31] Alpha-hemolytic streptococci are present in the upper respiratory tract and the mouth. This organism is relatively nonvirulent and causes infections (for example, infectious crystalline keratopathy) mainly in corneas with previous chronic disease. *S. faecalis* can cause an ulcer of the cornea in the presence of severely impaired host resistance or after epithelial injury.

OTHER GRAM-POSITIVE ORGANISMS

Gram-positive rods, an infrequent cause of keratitis, usually involve the cornea only when host resistance is impaired. *Bacillus cereus* has emerged as an important ocular pathogen, possibly one of the most destructive organisms to affect the eye.[21] Most cases of *B. cereus* infection have occurred as a result of hematogenous dissemination, usually in intravenous drug abusers. Cases also have occurred after penetrating injury, particularly with soil-contaminated foreign bodies. Characteristically severe pain develops within 24 hours of the injury and is followed rapidly by chemosis, periorbital swelling, and extreme proptosis. Shortly thereafter, low-grade fever may occur, accompanied by a moderate leukocytosis. Invariably a ring of edema forms in the peripheral cornea followed by the rapid development of a circumferential corneal abscess.

Listeria[32,33] and *Corynebacteria* are uncommon causes of corneal infection. Anaerobic gram-positive bacteria often reside in the skin and mucous membranes and are seen in the fecal flora. In rare cases peptostreptococci, *Propionibacterium acnes,*[34] *Clostridium,*[35] and other gram-positive species have been recovered from corneal ulcers.[36,37] *Clostridium* can produce gas that can be seen in the anterior chamber, stroma, or under the epithelium.[35]

PSEUDOMONAS AERUGINOSA

P. aeruginosa is one of the most important corneal pathogens and is the most common gram-negative organism causing corneal ulcers.[38-40] *P. aeruginosa* is found on skin, in saliva, and in the gastrointestinal tract and occurs ubiquitously in the environment. It has been found as a contaminant in hospitals, in fluorescein solutions,[41] eye mascara,[42] and poorly cared for contact lens cases. It has become the most common cause of corneal infection in contact lens wearers.[1,2,3,43] It also frequently causes keratitis in comatose patients[44] and has been cultured from patients with tracheostomies.

Surface tissue damage must be present for *Pseudomonas* adherence and infection.[45,46] The virulence of *Pseudomonas* organisms is related to their elaboration of lipases, proteases, and exotoxins and the presence of a surface glycocalyx.[47,48] The surface glycocalyx enhances resistance to phagocytosis and antibody-mediated complement killing; exotoxin A, similar to diphtheria toxin, inhibits protein synthesis in human cells, particularly macrophages; lipases attack cell membranes; and proteases digest the proteoglycan ground substance and can destroy small blood vessels. Host enzymes, released in response to *Pseudomonas* infection, also play a large role in the destructive effect.[49] The relative importance of bacterial and host factors in the destructiveness of *Pseudomonas* corneal infections is unclear. In experimental models, immunization against endotoxin,[50] slime capsule,[51] or outer membrane proteins[52] significantly decreased the severity of *Pseudomonas* ulcers, but immunization against proteases and exotoxin A did not.[53]

P. aeruginosa can cause a rapidly spreading ulcer; in 24 hours the ulcer may extend to twice its size (see Fig. 9-3), and perforation can occur in 2 to 5 days. The ulcer can be central or paracentral, and dense stromal infiltrates and necrosis are characteristic. Edema of the surrounding cornea, posterior corneal stromal folds, and endothelial plaques are seen. Diffuse epithelial graying, or "ground glass" appearance, often is noted in the nonulcerated portion of the cornea. A copious mucopurulent discharge that may have a greenish color often adheres to the ulcer surface. The greenish color is caused by a fluorescent pigment produced by some strains, and it causes the exudate to fluoresce when exposed to ultraviolent light.[54] Hypopyon usually is present (see Fig. 9-3).

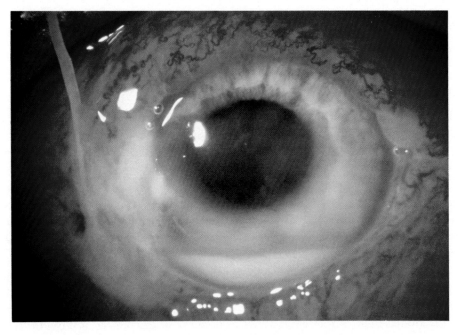

Fig. 9-9. *Pseudomonas* corneoscleritis. (Courtesy of Edward Alfonso, Miami.)

Early descemetocele formation, melting, and perforation are not infrequent. Circumferential progression of the ulceration is common, and a ring ulcer can form (see Fig. 9-6). *Pseudomonas* corneal infection can extend into the sclera, worsening the prognosis (Fig. 9-9).[55] This infection can smolder for a long time after treatment is initiated and can recur many days after therapy has been discontinued, particularly if steroids are administered.[56-58] Thus therapy should be continued for several weeks after apparent clinical cure, and steroids should be used cautiously.

Contact lens–associated *Pseudomonas* infections can also manifest themselves as several elevated granular opacities.[59] Less virulent *Pseudomonas* strains can produce more indolent infections, similar to those caused by other bacteria. These strains may lack the enzymes or toxins found in more virulent strains.

MORAXELLA

Moraxella organisms commonly are found in the nasopharynx and genitourinary tract. They can cause corneal infection in compromised hosts, particularly alcoholics, diabetics, and malnourished and other debilitated patients. The corneal ulcer is an indolent paracentral or peripheral one that usually is oval in shape and localized with an undermined necrotic edge. It progresses deep into the stroma over days or weeks, and untreated ulcers may perforate. Hypopyon may or may not be present. The organism is present in the depths of the crater. The anterior segment is highly inflamed, and the host's resistance usually is low.

FAMILY ENTEROBACTERIACEAE

Enterobacteriaceae species such as *Escherichia coli, Serratia, Klebsiella,* and *Proteus*[37] used to be relatively uncommon causes of bacterial keratitis, but such infections are becoming more frequent, particularly in association with contact lens wear. Otherwise, they are seen primarily in compromised eyes. In compromised eyes *Proteus vulgaris* is probably most common. *Proteus* species can cause a severe keratitis, similar to *Pseudomonas* (Fig. 9-10), and perforation and ring ulcer have been seen.

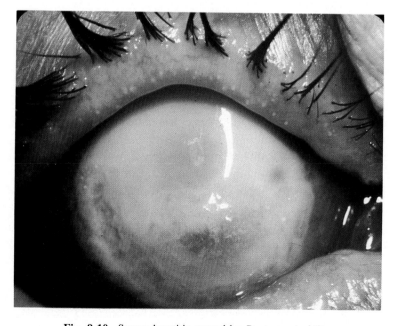

Fig. 9-10. Severe keratitis caused by *Proteus mirabilis.*

Serratia marcescens appears to the member of this group most commonly involved in contact lens–related infections. It contains an endotoxin and protease and can cause a severe ulcer, resulting in perforation.[60,61] Peripheral infiltrates and paracentral ulcers also can occur.

NEISSERIA

The gram-negative cocci *N. gonorrhoeae* and *N. meningitidis* can invade the cornea after conjunctivitis, through an intact epithelium, and cause an ulcer. These ulcers are extremely dangerous, particularly in the newborn, since they can rapidly lead to corneal perforation (see Fig. 6-6). Marked purulent discharge, injection, and chemosis usually are present. Systemic treatment is required. Further discussion of gonococcal infection and the current treatment recommendations can be found in Chapter 6.

ATYPICAL MYCOBACTERIA

Atypical mycobacteria are acid-fast organisms that are harbored in the soil. *M. fortuitum,*[62,63] *M. chelonei,*[64] *M. avium-intracellulare,*[65] and *M. gordonae*[66] have produced corneal ulcers, most commonly after trauma. The corneal ulcers are similar to those produced by *Moraxella* and *Nocardia* in that they are indolent, progressing slowly over weeks or months.[63,64,67] The bed of the ulcer can have a "cracked windshield" appearance. Often anterior chamber reaction is minimal. Any recalcitrant ulcer should prompt suspicion of a *Mycobacterium* species, and an acid-fast stain and culture on Lowenstein-Jensen medium should be obtained. Medical treatment often is unsuccessful, and the lesion may need to be removed surgically.

OTHER BACTERIAL ULCERS

Corneal ulcers caused by *Nocardia* and *Actinomyces* are usually indolent and may simulate the indolent ulcers caused by *Moraxella* and *M. fortuitum*. In these cases anterior chamber reaction usually is minimal. *Nocardia* and *Actinomyces* ulcers also may simulate mycotic corneal ulcers because of the presence of "hyphate edges" and satellite lesions, and they may be elevated.[68-72] One case presented as chronic epithelial defect with "calcareous" bodies at the epithelial edge.[73] Sulfonamides, including trimethoprim-sulfamethoxazole,[73,74] and ampicillin are recommended for treatment of *Nocardia* keratitis; penicillin is recommended for *Actinomyces* infections.

LABORATORY WORK

An etiologic diagnosis is important in dealing with bacterial keratitis to guide antibiotic therapy.[75] The mere clinical appearance of the ulcer is not enough to warrant a specific etiologic diagnosis, and "shotgun" therapy often is ineffective. Every ophthalmologist should be equipped to take adequate scrapings of the ulcer and should know how to interpret the findings. The techniques of obtaining corneal specimens, staining, and culture media are discussed in Chapter 4. Briefly, corneal smears should be obtained for Gram and Giemsa staining, and specimens should be inoculated onto blood agar, chocolate agar, and thioglycolate broth. If fungal infection is suspected, a smear should be examined with a fungal stain (for example, PAS or GMS), and a fungal medium such as Sabouraud's dextrose agar should be inoculated.

If the patient has been wearing contact lenses, the lens case and lens care solutions should be cultured. In some cases these will indicate the causative organism or organisms when corneal cultures do not. Similarly, if a patient has been taking ocular medications, specimens from each should be taken for culture.

Rapid detection tests are becoming available for some bacteria. The limulus lysate test uses horseshoe crab cells to detect endotoxin-producing gram-negative bacteria (see Chapter 4). An enzyme immunoassay for detecting group A streptococci is available and appears to be useful in corneal infections.[76]

TREATMENT

ANTIBIOTIC THERAPY

Initial antibiotic therapy. In any case in which a bacterial keratitis is suspected, antibiotic treatment should be given until a more definitive diagnosis can be made. The initial treatment is based on the interpretation of the corneal smears and a clinical assessment of the severity of the keratitis. There is disagreement over whether to begin with broad-spectrum coverage or to tailor initial therapy based on the smear morphology. In previous editions of this text, Jones' method of specifically tailored initial therapy was recommended.[77,78] However, most cornea specialists, including myself, now prefer to use combined broad-spectrum therapy in most cases. Gram stain results do not correlate that highly with culture results, particularly if the observer is inexperienced or if a number of organisms or no organisms are seen. In the best of circumstances, in experienced hands and if a single organism is seen in the Gram stain, the culture results are consistent approximately 70% to 80% of the time.[77,78] Since the consequences of not covering for the causative organism can be very serious and smears often are inaccurate, most now recommend administering broad-spectrum antibiotics.[13,79,80] The objection to broad-spectrum coverage is that it increases the risk of antibiotic side effects and antagonism and that no broad-spectrum coverage can treat all possible organisms.[78]

Broad-spectrum coverage is best obtained with an aminoglycoside and a cephalosporin (Table 9-1); currently I use cefazolin and tobramycin. This combination is effective against approximately 95% of all ocular bacterial isolates and all common bacteria. However, this treatment is modified if gonococcal keratoconjunctivitis is suspected, if there is a hyperpurulent conjunctivitis and gram-negative cocci are present in smears, or in some cases of severe keratitis when smears contain gram-negative rods, causing suspicion of *Pseudomonas* involvement. In those unusual cases in which acid-fast mycobacteria, fungi, or *Acanthamoeba* are seen in smears, specific therapy for these agents is administered.

The cephalosporin antibiotics generally are more active in vitro against penicillinase-producing staphylococci and streptococci than bacitracin, erythromycin, and lincomycin. Cefazolin (50 mg/ml) is less toxic topically than bacitracin (10,000 U/ml) and less irritating than methicillin or other semi-synthetic penicillins.

TABLE 9-1. Broad-Spectrum Initial Antibiotic Therapy in Treating Bacterial Keratitis

	SELECTION OF AGENTS	
RESULTS OF SMEARS	**TOPICAL**	**INTRAVENOUS**
One bacterium Two or more types of bacteria No microorganisms	Cefazolin (50 mg/ml) and Tobramycin (14 mg/ml) (vanco- mycin 50 mg/ml or bacitra- cin 10,000 U/ml in penicillin-allergic patients)	
Exceptions		
Hyperacute conjunctivitis with gram-negative cocci on smear	Penicillin G or bacitracin	Penicillin G, ceftriaxone, or spectinomycin (if penicillin sensitive)
Severe keratitis with gram- negative rods, consider adding	Polymyxin B or piperacillin	
Hyphae	Natamycin*	
Yeasts	Amphotericin B*	
Acid-fast bacilli	Amikacin	
Perforation or scleral exten- sion, add		Cefazolin and gentamicin

*See Table 10-4.

Gentamicin and tobramycin remain the initial antibiotics of choice for coverage against gram-negative rods. This is based on their stability, good corneal and intraocular penetration, and broad bactericidal activity, which includes *Pseudomonas, Enterobacter,* and *Klebsiella* and other aerobic gram-negative organisms. Tobramycin is two to four times more active than gentamicin, by weight, against *Klebsiella, Enterobacter, Serratia,* and *Proteus* and, in our laboratory, tobramycin has been active against a significantly higher percentage of *Pseudomonas* isolates (84% vs. 60%). Tobramycin also may be less nephrotoxic than gentamicin.

However, many rarer bacterial causes of keratitis are not adequately treated by the combination of a cephalosporin and an aminoglycoside; the most important of these rarer causes is *Neisseria.* Therefore if *Neisseria* infection is suspected, topical bacitracin or penicillin, saline lavage, and intravenous penicillin G or ceftriaxone should be administered. Using two effective agents often is advantageous in cases of *Pseudomonas* infection, particularly before sensitivity is determined. This is because the need for treatment is urgent, because no one agent is effective against all isolates, and because experimentally using two agents appeared to be more effective than using only one.[81] I use a combination of tobramycin and either polymyxin B or piperacillin in these cases, but ticarcillin and carbenicillin are also good choices.

Grading the severity of infection is useful in estimating the urgency of appropriate treatment and the risk of perforation and in predicting the causative organism or organisms (Table 9-2). If an infection is judged to be mild, standard strength topical antibiotics probably will be effective, and the risk of initially ineffective therapy is reduced. In some mild cases, when the patient has already received antibiotics, corneal scrapings can be delayed for 12 to 24 hours to increase the likelihood of isolating the responsible organism.

Routes

Topical. In nearly all cases, fortified topical antibiotic preparations are used. Experimentally, very high concentrations have been more effective than the concentrations provided in commercially prepared solutions[81-85]; however, clinically the advantage is less evident.[86] Since there does not appear to be an increase in the adverse effects of these medications when the fortified doses are used, it is probably best to use the higher concentrations. The methods of preparation of fortified antibiotic solutions are given in Table 9-3. Two antibiotics should not be mixed together in the same container, and the antibiotic solution should be replaced every 5 to 7 days. The antibiotic remains effective for at least 4 weeks,[87,88] but the preservative concentration is reduced, and contamination can occur.

Increasing the frequency of antibiotic drop administration, up to every 30 minutes, has been demonstrated to increase its effectiveness.[81] Part of the benefit frequent administration of drops may be by washing away bacteria and inflammatory products from the ocular surface. Some authors recommend

TABLE 9-2. Severity Grade of Microbial Keratitis

	SEVERITY GRADE	
FEATURE	NONSEVERE	SEVERE*
Rate of progression	Slow, moderate	Rapid
Suppuration		
Area	Less than 6 mm diameter	Larger than 6 mm diameter
Depth	Superficial two thirds	Inner one third
Depth of ulceration	Superficial one third	Inner one third
Perforation	Unlikely to occur	Present, imminent
Scleral suppuration	Absent	Present

From Jones DB: Ophthalmology 88:814, 1981.
*An ulcer is considered severe if it meets three or more of these criteria.

TABLE 9-3. Preparation of Topical Antibiotics Commonly Used to Treat Bacterial Corneal Ulcers

ANTIBIOTIC	REMOVE	ADD	PLACE	CONTENT	FINAL CONCENTRATION
Bacitracin	9 ml from 15 ml tear substitute bottle	3 ml tears to each of three vials (50,000 U/vial)	All 3 ml from each of three vials (total 9 ml) in original tear substitute bottle	9 ml reconstituted bacitracin and 6 ml tears	10,000 U/ml
Kanamycin		1 vial (500 mg in 2 ml) kanamycin to tear bottle		2 ml kanamycin and 15 ml tears	30 mg/ml
Penicillin G	3 ml tears from 15 ml tear substitute bottle	3 ml tears to one vial penicillin G (5 megaunits)	1 ml reconstituted penicillin in new tear bottle	1 ml penicillin G and 5 ml tears	100,000 U/ml
Carbenicillin		1 ml carbenicillin (100 mg) to 15 ml tear substitute bottle		1 ml carbenicillin and 15 ml tears	6 mg/ml
Vancomycin	2 ml tears from 15 ml tear substitute bottle	2 ml tears to one vial vancomycin (500 mg)	2 ml reconstituted vancomycin in tear bottle	2 ml vancomycin and 13 ml tears	33 mg/ml
Gentamicin		2 ml parenteral solution (40 mg/ml) to 5 ml bottle ophthalmic gentamicin			14 mg/ml
Cefazolin		5 ml of sterile water to 1 g vial of cefazolin	5 ml reconstituted cefazolin in 15 ml tear bottle	5 ml cefazolin and 15 ml artificial tears	50 mg/ml
Tobramycin		2 ml of tobramycin (40 mg/ml) to 5 ml bottle ophthalmic preparation		2 ml tobramycin parenteral and 5 ml tobramycin ophthalmic	14 mg/ml
Amikacin	2 ml tears from 15 ml tear substitute bottle	2 ml of amikacin (100 mg/ml) to tear bottle		2 ml amikacin and 13 ml artificial tears	13 mg/ml
Ticarcillin	1 ml tears from 15 ml tear substitute bottle	1 ml ticarcillin (100 mg/ml) to 15 ml tear substitute		1 ml ticarcillin 15 ml tears	6 mg/ml
Piperacillin	5.3 ml from 15 ml tear substitute	9 ml of sterile saline to 2 gm vial of piperacillin	0.3 ml reconstituted piperacillin in tear bottle	0.3 ml piperacillin and 9.7 ml tears	7 mg/ml
Polymyxin B	6 ml from 15 ml tear substitute	5 ml to Polymyxin B (500,000 U/vial)	1 ml reconstituted polymyxin B in tear bottle	1 ml polymyxin B and 9 ml tears	10,000 U/ml

administering drops every 15 minutes around the clock in every case, but this appears to be excessive. Even in the worst cases, administration every 30 minutes is sufficient, and in many cases hourly medication is used. If two antibiotics are used, they can be alternated (for example, every 30 minutes) or given together (5 minutes apart, every hour). An initial loading dose, such as 1 drop every minute for 5 minutes, may also increase the stromal antibiotic concentration.[89]

Subconjunctival. The use of subconjunctival antibiotics is controversial. They can rapidly produce high corneal drug levels, but this is short lasting, with subtherapeutic levels reached by 9 hours.[85,90] In animal models, fortified topical antibiotics are equally as effective as subconjunctival injections,[81,82,85,90-93] and subconjunctival injections do not provide additional effect when fortified antibiotic solutions are administered.[40,93,94] Since similarly high concentrations of antibiotics can be obtained in the infected eye by the less traumatic means of frequent topical drops, topical medication seems more logical and just as effective a form of therapy as subconjunctival antibiotics. This is important, especially since subconjunctival antibiotic therapy has certain disadvantages: patient apprehension, more ocular inflammation, more pain than topical therapy, and a risk of intraocular administration (although rare, important).

Therefore I recommend subconjunctival antibiotics in only a few situations: when frequent topical administration is not possible, when fortified antibiotic solutions are not available, or to initiate treatment when topical administration will be delayed. In children topical administration usually is limited, so subconjunctival injections are performed every 12 to 24 hours. Chloral hydrate sedation (100 mg/kg), topical anesthesia, and physical restraint often are sufficient and are preferable to general anesthesia.[17] The antibiotic injection should be placed adjacent to the site of infection, and if two different antibiotics are given, they should be injected at different sites. The methods of preparation of subconjunctival antibiotic injections are given in Table 9-4.

TABLE 9-4. Preparation and Dosage of Subconjunctival Antibiotics Commonly Used to Treat Bacterial Corneal Ulcers

ANTIBIOTIC	DOSE PER VIAL	DILUENT VOLUME	CONCENTRATION	INJECTION	TOTAL DOSE
Carbenicillin	1 g	5 ml	200 mg/ml	0.5 ml	100 mg
Colistin*	150 mg	2 ml	75 mg/ml	0.3 ml	25 mg
Gentamicin	80 mg	—	40 mg/ml	0.5 to 1 ml	20 to 40 mg
Methicillin	1 g	5 ml	200 mg/ml	0.5 ml	100 mg
Ampicillin	1 g	5 ml	200 mg/ml	0.5 ml	100 mg
Cephaloridine	500 mg	2.5 ml	200 mg/ml	0.5 ml	100 mg
Cefazolin	500 mg	2.5 ml	200 mg/ml	0.5 ml	100 mg
Neomycin	500 mg	1 ml	500 mg/ml	0.5 to 1 ml	250 to 500 mg
Penicillin G*	5 megaunits	2.5 ml	2 megaunits/ml	0.25 to 0.5 ml	0.5 to 1 megaunit
Vancomycin	500 mg	5 ml	100 mg/ml	0.25 ml	25 mg
Polymyxin B	50 mg	5 ml	10 mg/ml	0.5 ml	5 mg
Erythromycin	1 g	5 ml	200 mg/ml	0.5 ml	100 mg
Tobramycin	80 mg	—	80 mg/ml	0.25 ml	20 mg
Ticarcillin	1 g	10 ml	100 mg/ml	1 ml	100 mg
Piperacillin	2 g	10 ml	200 mg/ml	0.5 ml	100 mg
Amikacin	100 mg	—	50 mg/ml	0.5 ml	25 mg
Clindamycin	600 mg/4 ml	4 ml	75 mg/ml	0.5 ml	38 mg

*Painful subconjunctival injection can be avoided if tetracaine is applied topically before injection. To reenforce this, one may apply 4% cocaine with a cotton type of applicator to the area of the intended injection. Use a tuberculin syringe with a 27-gauge needle and inject 0.5 ml 1% lidocaine. This may be given before the injection of the drug or with the drug. Colistimethate sodium (Coly-Mycin M) parenteral is the generic name for colistin to be used for subconjunctival injection.

Other routes. Systemic antibiotics are not routinely recommended in treating infected corneal ulcers. Even in inflamed eyes, only low concentrations of antibiotics usually can be achieved in the cornea and aqueous after systemic administration, and using these systemic drugs does not appear to add to the effect of topical or subconjunctival antibiotics.[94] Systemic antibiotics are used if there is actual or imminent corneal perforation, for corneal ulcers with associated scleral infiltration or endophthalmitis, and in some cases as adjunctive therapy when an ideal local antibiotic regimen cannot be used. Systemic treatment is also given for infections in which noncorneal tissues are frequently involved, for infection caused by *Neisseria,* to infants with *Pseudomonas* keratitis, or when *Haemophilus* keratitis is accompanied by cellulitis.

Other techniques of antibiotic administration have been proposed. Continuous irrigation can be achieved through a small plastic catheter passed through the lid[95,96] or by means of a cannulated contact lens, such as the Mediflow lens. These devices require partial patient immobilization and are relatively impractical. Hydrophilic contact lenses, plastic polymer or collagen, can serve as a reservoir of antibiotic and produce high corneal concentrations.[97-100] These can reduce the necessity for frequent administration of drops; however, they also reduce removal of mucopurulent material and accompanying destructive enzymes from the corneal surface.

Temporary canalicular occlusion is another method of increasing the efficacy of topical antibiotics. In rabbits intracanalicular collagen implants prolonged the retention of antibiotic in tears, increased stromal concentration, and increased bacterial killing.[101] Iontophoresis can deliver high doses of antibiotics to the corneal stroma,[102,103] but this has not been tested clinically.

Antibiotic treatment can be given at home if the patient is able to comply with the taxing regimen and can return for daily examinations[104]; however, this often is not possible. Certainly any outpatient who is not responding to treatment should be admitted to the hospital, and incorrect technique or poor compliance with treatment should be suspected.

Specific antibiotics. The following section contains information about antibiotics used to treat corneal ulcers. Tables 9-5 and 9-6 give a general survey of microbial organisms and antibiotic agents suitable for treatment. Table 9-7 compiles facts concerning the most-used antibiotic agents and classifies them according to their effectiveness and penetration into the eye. As mentioned before, Tables 9-3 and 9-4 list the dosages and methods of preparation for fortified topical and subconjunctival antibiotics commonly used to treat bacterial keratitis, and the dosages are summarized in Table 9-8.

Penicillin G. Penicillins are bactericidal antibiotics that inhibit the biosynthesis of cell wall mucopeptide by sensitive bacteria. All of the penicillins contain a 6-aminopenicillanic acid nucleus, which consists of a beta-lactam ring and a thiazolidine ring, and differ in the side chains attached to this nucleus. Penicillin G (benzylpenicillin), one of the first penicillins, is effective against gram-positive cocci and *Neisseria, Moraxella,* and many *Klebsiella pneumoniae* isolates. It is not effective against most staphylococci, since they produce a penicillinase, which breaks down the beta-lactam ring. Penicillin G is the most active agent against most gram-positive and gram-negative anaerobes, except for *Bacteroides fragilis.*[77]

Although the penicillins are considered bactericidal drugs, the presence of penicillin in the medium is not directly lethal to the organism. If the bacterial protoplast is protected against osmotic destruction by an artificial hypertonic medium or is in a loculated accumulation of protein-rich exudate (abscess), renewed growth of bacteria occurs when penicillin is removed from the environment.[105] The penicillins are effective only against active, growing bacteria and have little effect on vegetating organisms not synthesizing new cell wall material.

When given systemically penicillin penetrates into the aqueous humor of the normal eye. Intraocular inflammation reduces the effect of the blood−aqueous humor barrier; thus high levels of penicillin are found in the intraocular fluids of inflamed eyes. Penicillin G is absorbed poorly from the gas-

Text continued on p. 186.

TABLE 9-5. General Survey of Antimicrobial Coverage

ORGANISM	EFFECTIVE ANTIBIOTIC
GRAM-POSITIVE COCCI	
Staphylococcus aureus	Cefazolin
	Methicillin if penicillinase producer
	Penicillin G if nonpenicillinase producer
Staphylococcus epidermidis	Cefazolin
	Vancomycin
	Gentamicin
Streptococcus sp.	Penicillin G
S. pneumoniae	Penicillin G
	Erythromycin
Anaerobic streptococci	Penicillin G
GRAM-NEGATIVE COCCI	
Neisseria gonorrhoeae	Aqueous penicillin (with probenecid)
	Ceftriaxone
	Ampicillin (with probenecid)
	Tetracycline
	Spectinomycin
	Bacitracin (topically)
GRAM-POSITIVE BACILLI	
Clostridium sp.	Penicillin G
Bacillus sp.	Gentamicin
Corynebacterium diphtheriae	Bacitracin
	Penicillin G
Listeria monocytogenes	Ampicillin
GRAM-NEGATIVE BACILLI	
Escherichia coli	Gentamicin
Klebsiella pneumoniae	Gentamicin
	Cephalosporin
Proteus mirabilis	Gentamicin
	Ampicillin
Serratia marcescens	Gentamicin
Haemophilus influenzae	Chloramphenicol
	Gentamicin
	Polymyxin B
Pseudomonas aeruginosa	Tobramycin
	Gentamicin
	Ticarcillin
	Carbenicillin
	Piperacillin
	Polymyxin B
	Amikacin
Moraxella sp.	Gentamicin
	Cefazolin
	Chloramphenicol
Acinetobacter sp. (formerly Mimeae)	Gentamicin
	Amikacin
MISCELLANEOUS ORGANISMS	
Actinomyces israelii	Penicillin G
	Tetracycline
Nocardia sp.	Sulfonamides
Mycobacteria	Amikacin
	Rifampin

TABLE 9-6. Antibiotic Sensitivities of Common Bacteria

	AMPICILLIN	BACITRACIN*	CEFAMANDOLE	CEFAZOLIN*	CHLORAMPHENICOL*	ERYTHROMYCIN*	GENTAMICIN*	METHICILLIN*	NEOMYCIN*	PENICILLIN G*	PIPERACILLIN	POLYMIXIN B*	SULFONAMIDES*	TETRACYCLINES*	TOBRAMYCIN*	TRIMETHOPRIM-SULFAMETHOXAZOLE	VANCOMYCIN
GRAM-POSITIVE COCCI																	
Staphylococcus epidermidis*	±	±	+	⊕	+	±	+	+	+	−	±	−	+	±	+	+	+
Staphyloccus aureus*	−	+	+	⊕	+	+	+	+	+	−	±	−	+	+	+	+	+
alpha-Hemolytic streptococci*	+	⊕	+	+	+	+	±	+	−	⊕	+	−	+	±	−	+	+
beta-Hemolytic streptococci*	+	+	+	⊕	+	+	±	+	−	⊕	+	−	±	±	±	+	+
nonhemolytic streptococci*	⊕	±	−	−	+	±	±	±	−	±	+	−	±	±	±	±	+
Streptococcus pneumoniae*	+	+	+	⊕	+	⊕	−	+	−	⊕	+	−	+	+	−	+	+
Anaerobic Streptococcus sp.*	±	+	+	+	+	+	−	±	−	⊕	+			±	−		
GRAM-POSITIVE BACILLI																	
Bacillus sp.*		−		±	+	±	⊕	−	+	−		−	+	±	+		
Clostridium sp.		±	±	±	±	±	−			−	⊕	+	−	±	−		+
Corynebacterium sp.*	±	⊕	+	±	+	±	+	±	+	±			+	+	+	+	+
Listeria monocytogenes	⊕			−	+	+				±		−		+			
GRAM-NEGATIVE COCCI																	
Neisseria sp.*	⊕	+	±	+	±	+	+	±	±	⊕	+	±	+	±	+		−
GRAM-NEGATIVE BACILLI																	
Acinetobacter sp.*	−	−	−	−	−	−	⊕	−	⊕	−	+	+	+	+	+	+	−
Bacteroides fragilis*	−		−	−	+	−	−	−	−	−	±	−		−	−	−	−
Bacteroides sp.*	±		±	−	⊕	+	−	−	−	⊕	±	−		±	−	−	−
Citrobacter sp.*		−	±	±	+	−	±	−	±	−	+	+	⊕	±	±	+	−
Enterobacter sp.*	±	−	±	−	+	−	⊕	−	⊕	−	+	+	⊕	+	⊕	+	−
Escherichia coli*	±	−	+	±	+	−	⊕	−	±	−	+	⊕	±	±	⊕	+	−
Haemophilus influenzae*	±	−	±	−	⊕	±	+	±	±	±	±	+	+	+	+	+	−
Klebsiella sp.*	−	−	+	±	+	−	⊕	−	+	±	+	±	±	±	⊕	+	−
Moraxella sp.*	+	+	±	+	+	+	⊕	+	+	⊕	+	+	+	+	+	+	−
Proteus mirabilis*	±	−	±	±	±	−	⊕	−	+	−	+	−	+	−	⊕	+	−
Proteus sp. (indole positive)*	−	−	±	−	±	−	⊕	−	+	−	+	−	+	+	+	+	−
Pseudomonas sp.*	−	−	−	−	−	−	±	−	−	−	+	+	−	−	+	−	−
Salmonella sp.*	⊕	−		−	⊕	−	+	−		±	+	+	−		+	+	−
Serratia sp.*	−	−	−	−	+	−	⊕	−	⊕	−	+	−	+	−	⊕	+	−
Shigella sp.	⊕	−		−	+	−		−		±	+	+	−	±		+	−
OTHERS																	
Actinomyces sp.*	+	+	±	±	+		−		−	⊕			±	+	−		+

+ = 80% to 100% of isolates sensitive.
± = 40% to 79% of isolates sensitive.
− = less than 40% of isolates sensitive.
*Data from Campbell Laboratory, Pittsburgh.
⊕Drug of choice or commonly used drug.

TABLE 9-7. Spectrum, Penetration, and Action of Principal Antibiotics Used to Treat Bacterial Corneal Ulcers

DRUG	SPECTRUM GRAM-POSITIVE ORGANISMS	SPECTRUM GRAM-NEGATIVE ORGANISMS	PENETRATION	ACTION	IMPORTANT FACTS
Amikacin	−	+		Bactericidal	Active against large number of gram-negative bacteria resistant to gentamicin, kanamycin, and tobramycin Active against mycobacteria Cochlear toxicity
Ampicillin	+	±|	Good	Bactericidal	Not effective against penicillinase-producing staphylococci, indole-positive *Proteus* or *Pseudomonas*
Bacitracin	+	−		Bactericidal	Allergy is rare; not to be given systemically because of toxicity
Carbenicillin	+	+	Fair	Bactericidal	May be synergistic with gentamicin in severe *Pseudomonas*, *Proteus*, and *E. coli* infections; not effective against penicillinase-producing staphylococci, *Klebsiella*, or *Serratia*
Cephalosporins (similar in action to penicillins)	+	±|	Good	Bactericidal	Effective against penicillinase-producing staphylococci and streptococci (except enterococci) and isolates of *E. coli*, *Klebsiella*, and *Proteus mirabilis*; not good against *Pseudomonas*, indole-positive *Proteus*, or *H. influenzae*
Chloramphenicol	+	+	Good	Bacteriostatic	Serious blood dyscrasias
Cloxacillin	+	−		Bactericidal	Penicillinase resistant

			Penetration		Comments
Dicloxacillin	+	−		Bactericidal	Penicillinase resistant
Erythromycin	+	−	Good	Bacteriostatic	Topical ointment is used, subconjunctival injection is also given; may be employed when patient is allergic to penicillin
Gentamicin	±	+	Poor	Bactericidal	Effective against *Pseudomonas* and some staphylococci Nephrotoxic, ototoxic
Methicillin	+	−	Poor	Bactericidal	Effective against penicillinase-producing staphylococci Nephrotoxic; depresses bone marrow
Neomycin	±	+	?Good	Bactericidal	For topical and subconjunctival use only Hypersensitivity
Oxacillin	+	−	Poor	Bactericidal	Penicillinase resistant
Penicillin G	+	−	Good in inflamed eye	Bactericidal	Hypersensitivity
Piperacillin	+	+	Poor	Bactericidal	Particularly useful against *Pseudomonas*
Polymyxin B	−	+		Bactericidal	Effective against *Pseudomonas* but not against *Proteus vulgaris* Nephrotoxic
Sulfonamides	+	+	Good	Bacteriostatic	Hypersensitivity
Tetracyclines	+	+		Bacteriostatic	Effective against *Chlamydia*; not for pregnant women or children under 8; take on an empty stomach
Tobramycin	±	+		Bactericidal	Effective against most penicillinase-producing staphylococci, as well as *Pseudomonas, Enterobacter, Klebsiella, Serratia,* and *E. coli* Ototoxic and nephrotoxic, with some neuromuscular toxicity

TABLE 9-8. Dosages for Principal Antibiotics Used to Treat Bacterial Keratitis

DRUG	TOPICAL (FORTIFIED)	SUBCONJUNCTIVAL	PARENTERAL
Amikacin	50 mg/ml	25 mg	15 mg/kg/day IM or slow IV in two or three divided doses
Ampicillin	—	100 mg	2 to 4 g every 4 hours IV
Amoxicillin	—	—	500 mg to 1 g every 8 hours orally
Bacitracin	10,000 U/ml	—	—
Carbenicillin	4 mg/ml	100 mg	2 to 6 g every 4 hours IV with 0.5 g probenecid orally four times a day
Cefazolin	50 mg/ml	100 mg	0.5 to 1.5 g every 6 hours IV
Cephaloridine	50 mg/ml	100 mg	1 g every 4 hours IV (maximum is 4 g every 24 hours
Chloramphenicol	5 mg/ml	100 mg	
Clindamycin	—	40 mg	1 g every 8 hours IV
Colistimethate sodium	—	25 mg	5 mg/kg/day IM in two to four doses
Erythromycin	5 mg/g ointment*	100 mg	2 to 4 g daily orally in four divided doses or 1 g every 6 hours IV
Gentamicin	14 mg/ml	20 to 40 mg	3 to 5 mg/kg/day IM or IV
Kanamycin	—	30 mg	—
Methicillin	—	75 to 100 mg	200 mg/kg/day
Neomycin	5 mg/g ointment* 3.5 mg/ml solution	250 to 500 mg	—
Oxacillin	—	75 to 100 mg	2 to 2.5 g every 4 hours IV with 0.5 g probenecid orally four times a day
Penicillin G	100,000 U/ml	500,000 to 1 million U (300 to 600 mg)	2 to 6 megaunits every 4 hours IV with 0.5 g probenecid orally four times a day
Polymyxin B	10,000 U	10 mg	—
Piperacillin	6.7 mg/ml	100 mg	3 to 4 g every 4 to 6 hours IV
Spectinomycin	—	—	2 g IM
Sulfacetamide	30%	—	—
Ticarcillin	6.7 mg/ml	100 mg	200 mg/kg IV in three divided doses
Tobramycin	14 mg/ml	20 to 40 mg	3 to 5 mg/kg/day IM or IV
Vancomycin	50 mg/ml	25 mg	1 g every 12 hours IV

*Not fortified.

trointestinal tract; thus the drug is given intravenously or intramuscularly. The systemic dose is 2 to 6 megaunits every 4 hours, to be given intravenously. The rapid secretory mechanism from the kidney and clearance of the drug can be blocked by probenecid, 500 mg orally every 6 hours. If this is given, the level of penicillin will be raised twofold to fourfold. The dose for subconjunctival injection is 0.5 to 1 megaunit.[36,106,107]

Adverse reactions to penicillin G occur in approximately 10% of patients and include hypersensitivity reactions such as skin rash, drug fever, urticaria, and occasionally an anaphylactic reaction that may be fatal.

Ampicillin. Ampicillin is effective against a wider spectrum of gram-negative organisms than is penicillin G but is less active against streptococci, staphylococci, and pneumococci. Like penicillin G, it is destroyed by bacterial penicillinase. The spectrum of action against gram-negative organisms includes *Haemophilus influenzae, Proteus mirabilis,* and many strains of *Escherichia coli, Salmonella, Shigella,* and *Moraxella.* Ampicillin is not effective against *Pseudomonas aeruginosa.*[77,105]

A systemic dose of 2 to 4 g every 4 hours intravenously and a subconjunctival dose of 100 mg in 0.33 ml of sterile water are advised.[77,106] Ampicillin is used against *N. gonorrhoeae* at a dose of 3.5 g orally with probenecid (0.5 to 1 g).

Allergic phenomena occurring with ampicillin are similar to those reported with penicillin G, but there also may be a transient increase in the serum glutamic-oxaloacetic transaminase (SGOT) level.[105]

Amoxicillin. Amoxicillin is similar to ampicillin in structure and spectrum of activity. It is effective against nonpenicillinase-producing staphylococci, streptococci, and most isolates of *H. influenzae, E. coli,* and *P. mirabilis.* Its main advantage over ampicillin is its greater absorption from the gastrointestinal tract and the lack of interference of absorption by meals. Blood levels usually are higher than those with ampicillin. Oral doses produce high levels (500 mg to 1 g every 8 hours is recommended).

Penicillinase-resistant penicillins. This group of semisynthetic penicillins includes oxacillin, cloxacillin, dicloxacillin, methicillin, and nafcillin. These drugs are strongly resistant to destruction by bacterial penicillinase but are less effective against nonpenicillinase-producing gram-positive microorganisms than is penicillin G. They should be reserved to treat infections known to be caused by penicillinase-producing staphylococci.[77,105] Like other penicillins, they are bactericidal.

Compared with the other penicillinase-resistant penicillins, methicillin is less active by weight against penicillinase-producing staphylococci, but this difference is compensated for by differences in serum protein binding. Methicillin has relatively low serum binding, with theoretically greater availability for antimicrobial action, whereas the others are highly protein bound. Methicillin cannot be given orally, whereas oxacillin, dicloxacillin, cloxacillin, and nafcillin can.

The adult dose of methicillin is 2 g intravenously every 4 hours. Pulse-dose injection of the proper dose of methicillin dissolved in a small amount of fluid is the best method of administration. A subconjunctival injection of 100 mg of methicillin or oxacillin can be given.[77,106-108]

With the use of methicillin, one may see skin rashes, urticaria, and bone marrow depression with reversible neutropenia. Renal function is impaired in some individuals.

Carbenicillin. Carbenicillin is a semisynthetic penicillin with decreased activity against gram-positive organisms but a wider spectrum of activity against gram-negative organisms.[75,77,109,110] It is useful against *Pseudomonas aeruginosa,* indole-positive *Proteus,* and *Enterobacter.* Carbenicillin is not useful in managing corneal ulcers caused by gram-positive cocci, since it is not penicillinase resistant. Some evidence suggests that carbenicillin is synergistic with gentamicin against *Pseudomonas* organisms, but there is also evidence that carbenicillin antagonizes the effect of gentamicin.[111] Carbenicillin should not be used if the patient has a history of sensitivity to penicillin. The subconjunctival dose is 100 to 125 mg; the systemic dose is 2 to 6 g every 4 hours intravenously.

Ticarcillin. Ticarcillin is similar to carbenicillin in structure and antimicrobial activity. It exhibits broad activity against indole-positive and indole-negative *Proteus, E. coli,* and *Enterobacter* species. It is not active against penicillinase-producing staphylococci. The in vitro synergism with gentamicin is similar to that of carbenicillin. Subconjunctival injection of 100 mg produces high concentrations. Intravenous injection of 200 to 300 mg/kg in three divided doses for systemic administration is recommended. The main indication for parenteral ticarcillin would be in combination with gentamicin or tobramycin in keratitis and endophthalmitis caused by *Pseudomonas.* Use for other gram-negative infections is guided by sensitivity testing.

Bacitracin. Bacitracin acts similarly to penicillin G by interfering with cell wall synthesis and binding to cell membranes to produce false pores and flux of ions. Bacitracin is bactericidal and is effective against *Neisseria,* gram-positive cocci, and some gram-positive bacilli, including *Corynebacte-*

rium diphtheriae, Clostridium, and *Actinomyces.* Bacitracin is effective against penicillinase-producing staphylococci.[77,108]

The use of bacitracin in ophthalmology should be restricted to topical administration and subconjunctival injection; it is too toxic for systemic use. In severe infections the concentration can be increased so that the dose of ophthalmic drops is 10,000 U/ml.[108] Fortified bacitracin is irritating to the ocular surface and can cause a keratopathy. Allergic sensitization is rare.

Gentamicin. The aminoglycosides gentamicin and tobramycin have proven effective in the treatment of *P. aeruginosa* keratitis and have replaced polymyxin B and colistin in its initial management.

Gentamicin is bactericidal,[112] achieving this by binding to bacterial RNA polymerase and blocking protein synthesis. It is effective against most gram-negative bacteria, including *Pseudomonas aeruginosa, E. coli, Serratia marcescens, Proteus, Klebsiella,* and *Moraxella.* Gentamicin is active against staphylococci[113] and some streptococci but not against pneumococci. As mentioned previously, although carbenicillin may act synergistically with gentamicin in vitro, there is also some evidence that in vivo the combination may be antagonistic.

As with other aminoglycosides, gentamicin is ototoxic and nephrotoxic. If gentamicin is given systemically, renal function should be tested so that the dose can be adjusted if renal function is reduced and to monitor for renal toxicity. Gentamicin should not be given concurrently with other ototoxic agents.[77] Gentamicin inhibits epithelial wound healing[114] and can cause punctate keratopathy or pseudomembranous conjunctivitis.

Gentamicin can be given subconjunctivally 20 mg/ml or topically at concentrations of 8 to 18 mg/ml. If it is found necessary to give gentamicin systemically, it may be given intravenously or intramuscularly, 3 to 5 mg/kg daily in three divided doses; careful monitoring of kidney function is necessary.

Tobramycin. Tobramycin is similar to gentamicin in antimicrobial activity and toxicity, however it is reported to be two to four times more active in vitro, by weight, against *P. aeruginosa.*[115] It is also effective against many gentamicin-resistant strains. In our laboratory 84% of *Pseudomonas aeruginosa* isolates were sensitive to tobramycin and only 62% were sensitive to gentamicin. However, gentamicin was effective against a greater percentage of streptococcal isolates. For keratitis caused by sensitive organisms, there has been no evidence to date that tobramycin is superior clinically to gentamicin. The toxicity of the two drugs is similar.

Doses for tobramycin are as follows: topical, 8 to 18 mg/ml (most commonly 14 mg/ml); subconjunctival, 10 to 20 mg; intramuscular or intravenous, 3 to 5 mg/kg in three divided doses.

Amikacin. Some strains of *Pseudomonas* resistant to gentamicin are also resistant to tobramycin. For these strains amikacin, a semisynthetic aminoglycoside, often is effective. Most acquired resistance to aminoglycosides involves microbial enzymatic inactivation of the drugs in the bacterial membrane or near the site of drug transport. Amikacin is resistant to inactivation by most bacterial enzymes and is effective in cases of *P. aeruginosa* keratitis resistant to tobramycin and gentamicin. (Colistin or polymyxin B are other therapeutic alternatives.) On the other hand, organisms resistant to amikacin usually are resistant to gentamicin, tobramycin, and kanamycin. Like other aminoglycosides, amikacin can be toxic to the cochleovestibular apparatus.

The systemic dose is 15 mg/kg/day by slow intravenous drip. Amikacin is a second-order drug reserved for infections caused by susceptible strains of *P. aeruginosa;* by other gram-negative organisms known to be resistant to kanamycin, gentamicin, and tobramycin; and by mycobacteria.

Erythromycin. Bacteriostatic in low concentrations and bactericidal in high concentrations, erythromycin is effective against gram-positive cocci, gram-positive bacilli, *Neisseria,* and *Moraxella.* It is also effective against chlamydia and mycoplasma. Erythromycin is used as either a topical solution or an ointment in a concentration of 5 mg/ml. It is well tolerated by the conjunctiva and the cornea but penetrates the cornea poorly. Subconjunctival injections of 5 to 10 mg in a small volume of distilled water may be used. Erythromycin can be given orally, at a dose of 1 to 2 g per day in two to four divided doses, but it commonly causes gastrointestinal symptoms. The drug frequently is used when a patient is allergic to the penicillins or cephalosporins.

Cephalosporins. The cephalosporins are semisynthetic compounds, similar to penicillin, derived from a naturally occurring antibiotic produced by the fungus *Cephalosporium.*[116,117] Like penicillin, they are bactericidal and exert their effect by interfering with cell wall synthesis. All of these drugs are effective against nonpenicillinase-producing staphylococci, pneumococci, and streptococci and some strains of gram-negative bacilli, particularly *E. coli, Proteus mirabilis,* and *Klebsiella*. The second-generation cephalosporins (for example, cefamandole, cefoxitin, and cefuroxime) have a wider gram-negative spectrum than the first-generation cephalosporins (cephalothin, cephaloridine, cefazolin, and cephalexin), but none of these are effective against *Pseudomonas*. However, some of the third- and fourth-generation drugs, particularly ceftazidime and cefoperazone, are effective against *Pseudomonas*. None of the cephalosporins are very effective against methicillin-resistant staphylococci or enterococcal streptococci.[118]

Cephalosporins have been proposed as an alternative antibiotic for use when a patient is known to be allergic to penicillin.[107,119] Approximately 8% of patients known to be sensitive to penicillin will have a reaction to a cephalosporin, so the drug should be administered with caution.[107]

Cephalothin is less sensitive to staphylococcal penicillinase than others of this group and is preferred for staphylococcal infections. It may be given in doses of 1 g in 10 ml of sterile water injection intravenously over a 5-minute period, with the dose to be repeated every 4 to 6 hours.[77,108] Cephalothin is painful on intramuscular injection. A subconjunctival injection of 50 mg is used and may be repeated daily as needed.[108]

Cefazolin is another first-generation cephalosporin that is commonly used to treat keratitis. Its systemic dose is 1 g intravenously four times a day. It is less painful than others on intramuscular injection and is therefore preferred for this method. It can be given topically (50 mg/ml) or subconjunctivally (100 mg/ml). It is relatively nontoxic to the corneal epithelium. As discussed previously, it often is used with an aminoglycoside in initial broad-spectrum treatment of bacterial keratitis.

Experience with the newer generation cephalosporins in keratitis is limited.

Chloramphenicol. Chloramphenicol is bacteriostatic and acts by inhibiting protein synthesis. It is active against a wide range of gram-positive and gram-negative organisms (Table 9-6) and is most useful against ampicillin-resistant *Haemophilus influenzae*. Chloramphenicol penetrates well into aqueous and vitreous after parenteral or oral administration. Its wide spectrum, excellent penetration, and convenience of use should have made this a desirable drug; however, its adverse effects limit its use.

The most serious adverse reaction is bone marrow suppression, which can be severe and irreversible.[75,77] Other adverse reactions include skin rash, optic neuritis, "gray" illness, and gastrointestinal inflammation. The reactions may be idiosyncratic, not dose related, or toxic and dose related. Systemic administration of chloramphenicol should be reserved for severe infections in which the causative organism is known to be sensitive to chloramphenicol and to no other drug. Otherwise, it is better to use other, safer antibiotics such as penicillin G, semisynthetic penicillins, and cephalosporins. Patients given systemic chloramphenicol should have a reticulocyte count and complete blood count every 2 days. Treatment should be discontinued if granulocyte, platelet, red cell, or reticulocyte counts decline. The oral dose is 50 mg/kg given daily in a divided dose.

Only one well-documented case of bone marrow suppression has been reported after topical use of chloramphenicol, and prolonged treatment with large doses was given.[120] However, it is probably wise to avoid topical use of this drug unless it is absolutely necessary, mainly for medicolegal reasons.

Polymyxin B. Polymyxin B is effective against gram-negative bacteria, is bactericidal, and penetrates the cornea poorly. It binds to plasma membranes and alters cell permeability. Organisms resistant to polymyxin are also resistant to colistin. Polymyxin B is used in *Pseudomonas* and Enterobacteriaceae infections but not in *Proteus* or *Serratia* infections.

Polymyxin B is nephrotoxic at systemic doses exceeding 2.2 mg/kg daily; in view of this, it should be used only topically.

Colistin. In structure and spectrum of activity, colistin is similar to polymyxin. Colistin is bactericidal and is active against gram-negative bacilli, including *Pseudomonas* and *Moraxella*.[75,77,108] Some strains of *Proteus* are resistant to colistin, as are most gram-positive organisms. Colistin may be obtained as a sulphate or a methane sulphate salt. For subconjunctival and topical use in ophthalmology, the sulphate is the preparation of choice.[77] These preparations are nephrotoxic when given systemically.

Tetracycline. Tetracyclines are bacteriostatic antibiotics that interfere with bacterial protein synthesis by blocking attachment of transfer RNA to ribosomes. Tetracyclines are effective against a broad spectrum of gram-positive and gram-negative organisms, as well as against *Actinomyces, Chlamydia,* mycobacteria, and *Treponema pallidum*. However, many bacterial isolates are resistant, so its use should be guided by sensitivity testing. Oral tetracycline has also been shown to reduce corneal ulceration after alkali burns in experimental animals.[121]

For topical use tetracycline is now available in both solution and ointment forms. It has good corneal penetration and rarely causes adverse reactions. Absorption of oral tetracyclines is inhibited by iron, antacids, dairy products, and other calcium-containing products. It is best to take it on an empty stomach. Systemic side effects include gastrointestinal upset, phototoxicity, pseudotumor cerebri, renal toxicity, and hepatic dysfunction. Tetracyclines cause bone and tooth discoloration and enamel hypoplasia and should not be given to pregnant women or to children under 8 years of age.

Sulfonamides. The sulfonamides are bacteriostatic agents that inhibit bacterial synthesis of folic acid. They are active against a variety of gram-positive and gram-negative bacteria, as well as chlamydia. They are not first-line drugs for most causes of keratitis but are the treatment of choice for *Nocardia*. Penetration of topical preparations is good, and these drugs are well tolerated, including fortified solutions (30%). After systemic administration, allergic reactions, even Stevens-Johnson syndrome, can occur, as well as blood dyscrasias and gastrointestinal upset.

Vancomycin. Vancomycin has been used with increasing frequency because many strains of *Staphylococcus epidermidis* are resistant to other antibiotics. Vancomycin is bactericidal and acts by inhibiting cell wall synthesis. It is effective against most gram-positive bacteria, including methicillin-resistant staphylococci and nonhemolytic streptococci. The systemic use of vancomycin is limited by nephrotoxicity and ototoxicity, and subconjunctival injections (25 mg) can cause sloughing. However, topical use (50 mg/ml) and intravitreal use appear to be well tolerated.

Neomycin. Neomycin is a bactericidal antibiotic that is effective against a wide spectrum of gram-negative bacteria, as well as staphylococci. Neomycin may be given topically or subconjunctivally (Table 9-8). Commercially it is most commonly available in combination with polymyxin B and bacitracin. Hypersensitivity reactions and punctate keratitis occasionally occur. Neomycin does not inhibit epithelial healing.[114] Since subconjunctival injections may be quite painful, it is advisable to instill a topical anesthetic agent, followed by an injection of 0.5 ml of 1% lidocaine. The lidocaine should be allowed to diffuse; then the neomycin should be injected slowly and carefully.

Rifampin. Rifampin is effective against mycobacteria, chlamydia, and some gram-positive and gram-negative bacteria.[122] Rifampin inhibits bacterial growth by blocking RNA-polymerase activity. Clinically, it is used orally in the treatment of mycobacterial infections.

Spectinomycin. Spectinomycin is related to the aminoglycosides but is different in structure and action from the other drugs. It has a broad in vitro action against gram-positive and gram-negative aerobic organisms. Spectinomycin is primarily used in gonorrheal infection to treat penicillin-sensitive individuals. The recommended dose is 2 to 4 g by intramuscular injection.

New antibiotics. Quinolones are a new class of antibiotics that inhibit DNA replication. One of these, ciprofloxacin, has a broad spectrum of activity that includes *Pseudomonas,* gram-positive cocci, anaerobes, chlamydia and mycobacteria. Ciprofloxacin penetrates the cornea well, and a topical solution of 3 mg/ml was found to be effective against *Pseudomonas* keratitis in an animal model.[123] In a comparative study of treatment of methicillin-resistant *S. epidermidis,* ciprofloxacin was more effective than cefazolin or tobramycin and equally as effective as vancomycin.[124] Enoxacin, another quinolone with broad-spectrum activity, also has been found effective in an animal model.[125]

Imipenem, another new antibiotic, is a member of the carbapenem class of beta-lactam antibiotics, which are resistant to bacterial beta-lactamase. Imipenem is active against most bacteria, including *Pseudomonas,* streptococci, and staphylococci, including methicillin-resistant strains. A 5 mg/ml topical solution has been found to be effective against an aminoglycoside-resistant *Pseudomonas* strain in a rabbit model.[126] Aztreonam, another new beta-lactam antibiotic (a monobactam), also has broad gram-negative activity but is not active against gram-positive organisms.

Fusidic acid has been used since the 1960s to treat severe systemic staphylococcal infections, but it just recently became available in Europe commercially as a topical ophthalmic preparation (Fucithalmic). It is a bactericidal drug with good corneal penetration even when the epithelium is intact, and it is effective against beta-lactamase–producing and methicillin-resistant staphylococci. In one clinical study fusidic acid proved safe and effective in the treatment of staphylococcal keratitis.[127]

Adjunctive Therapy

Cycloplegics should be used to increase comfort and to decrease formation of posterior synechiae. Mucopurulent and necrotic debris should be removed daily. Factors that contributed to the development of the infection or that could impair healing should be eliminated, if possible. Entropion, trichiasis, or lagophthalmos should be corrected. Punctal occlusion or lateral tarsorrhaphy should be considered in patients with keratitis sicca.

Collagenase inhibitors such as EDTA, acetylcysteine, or heparin have been proposed, on a theoretic basis, to decrease stromal ulceration by bacterial and host enzymes. However, such agents have not been found beneficial clinically. Tuftsin, a naturally occurring protein that enhances the phagocytic and bactericidal activity of PMNs, potentiated the effect of gentamicin against *Pseudomonas* keratitis in rabbits,[128] but it has not been tested clinically.

Corticosteroids. The use of corticosteroids in the management of microbial keratitis is controversial. Corticosteroids are effective agents for suppression of the harmful effects of the host inflammatory response, but they also impair the phagocytosis and intracellular killing of bacteria by host effector cells. In experimental studies of *S. aureus* and *P. aeruginosa* keratitis, topical corticosteroids have not interfered with bacterial killing by appropriate antibiotics.[129-131] The course was no different from that seen when the antibiotics were used alone. Clinically, corticosteroid use has appeared to promote recurrence of *Pseudomonas* keratitis.[56,57]

In summary, the safety or the efficacy of corticosteroids in human microbial keratitis has not been established.[34] I recommend that corticosteroids not be used in most cases of bacterial keratitis. They may be used to decrease scarring under certain conditions: after at least 4 to 5 days of antibiotic therapy, if the infectious process appears to be resolving, if concurrent bactericidal antibiotic treatment is given, and if reduction of scarring will improve visual outcome. In addition, it is preferable that the epithelium be intact and that the infection not be caused by *Pseudomonas.*

Course

It is most important to follow carefully the progress of the corneal ulcer.[77,108] At each examination the area and density of infiltration, the size and depth of ulceration, the size of the epithelial defect, the amount of stromal edema, the extent of scleral involvement, and the anterior chamber reaction should be recorded. Measurements can be made with the continuous beam adjustment on a Haag-Streit slit-lamp microscope.

Untreated corneal ulcers, whether peripheral or central at the onset, tend to progress toward the central cornea away from the vascularized limbus. Early signs of improvement include a decrease in the infiltrate's "fluffiness," a blunting of the perimeter, decreased discharge, increased comfort, and decreased anterior chamber reaction. Later, a decrease in density and size of the infiltrate, reepithelialization, and vascularization are seen. The most helpful signs of improvement are the blunting of the perimeter of the stromal suppuration, reduction in the cellular infiltrate, reduction of the edema in the adjacent stroma, and progressive epithelialization. Fibrin exudate on the endothelium and hypopyon may resolve slowly and do not necessarily reflect the degree of improvement of the corneal process. In general, during the first 24 to 48 hours a lack of progression indicates that the treatment is effective. However, early progression of the keratitis can occur despite appropriate antibiotic treatment, particularly in *Pseudomonas* infections.

Many danger signs point to further trouble, such as increases in pain, the surface area of the ulcer, cellular stromal infiltration, suppuration, or anterior chamber reaction; or lysis of corneal stroma (see Fig. 9-3) or, at times, sclera.

Modification of therapy after 24 to 48 hours depends on the progress of the keratitis and culture results (Fig. 9-11). If the keratitis is improving, usually the initial regimen should be continued regardless of culture results. Often organisms that are not sensitive to an agent in vitro are sensitive at the high stromal levels achieved with topical administration of fortified antibiotics. If two agents were initiated and the isolate is sensitive to only one of them, the second agent can be discontinued or replaced with a more appropriate antibiotic.

If the keratitis is worsening and preliminary identification suggests that the initial antibiotic regimen is ineffective, a more appropriate antibiotic should be given. Tables 9-5, 9-6, and 9-9 can be used as guides for modified antibiotic therapy. More definitive identification and sensitivity determination can be used to further refine therapy when this information becomes available.

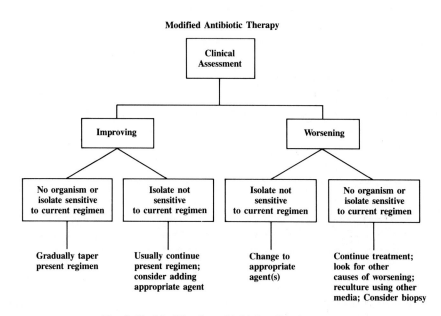

Fig. 9-11. Modification of initial antibiotic therapy.

TABLE 9-9. Modified Antibiotic Therapy Based on Preliminary Identification of Selected Organisms

| | ANTIBIOTIC | | |
ORGANISM	TOPICAL	SUBCONJUNCTIVAL	INTRAVENOUS*
Micrococcaceae sensitivities unknown	Cefazolin (50 mg/ml)	Cefazolin (100 mg)	Nafcillin (200 mg/kg/day)
Micrococcus, Staphylococcus; penicillin-resistant	Cefazolin (50 mg/ml)	Cefazolin (100 mg)	Nafcillin (200 mg/kg/day)
Micrococcus, Staphylococcus; penicillin-sensitive	Penicillin G (100,000 U/ml)	Penicillin G (500,000 U)	Penicillin G (2 to 6 megaunits/4 hours)
Streptococcus,† Pneumococcus	Penicillin G (100,000 U/ml)	Penicillin G (500,000 U)	Penicillin G (2 to 6 megaunits/4 hours)
Anaerobic gram-positive cocci	Penicillin G (100,000 U/ml)	Penicillin G (500,000 U)	Penicillin G (2 to 6 megaunits/4 hours)
Corynebacterium sp.	Bacitracin (10,000 U/ml)	Penicillin G (500,000 U)	Penicillin G (2 to 6 megaunits/4 hours)
Azotobacter sp.	Gentamicin (14 mg/ml)	Gentamicin (20 mg)	Gentamicin (3 to 5 mg/kg/day)
Mycobacterium sp.	Amikacin (50 mg/ml)	Amikacin (25 mg)	Amikacin (5 mg/kg/day)
Neiserria gonorrhoeae *N. meningitidis*	Penicillin G (100,000 U/ml)	Penicillin G (500,000 U)	Penicillin G (2 to 6 megaunits/4 hours)
Enterobacteriaceae	Gentamicin (14 mg/ml)	Gentamicin (20 mg)	Gentamicin (3 to 5 mg/kg/day)
Pseudomonas sp.	Tobramycin and polymyxin B (2 mg/ml) or piperacillin (7 mg/ml)	Tobramycin (20 mg)	Tobramycin (3 to 5 mg/kg/day)
Moraxella sp.	Gentamicin (14 mg/ml)	Gentamicin (20 mg)	Gentamicin (3 to 5 mg/kg/day)
Haemophilus influenzae	Ampicillin (0.5-1 g/6 hours)	Chloramphenicol (100 mg)	Chloramphenicol (50 mg/kg/day)
Other aerobic, gram-negative rod	Gentamicin (14 mg/ml)	Gentamicin (20 mg)	Gentamicin (3 to 5 mg/kg/day)
Anaerobic gram-negative rod	Penicillin G (100,000 U/ml)	Penicillin G (500,000 U)	Penicillin G (2 to 6 megaunits/4 hours)

Modified from Jones DB: Ophthalmology 88:814, 1981.

*Reserve for scleral suppuration or corneal perforation (impending or existing).

†Excludes *S. faecalis;* requires combined therapy (for example, penicillin G and gentamicin).

If no organism is isolated or if the isolated organism is sensitive to the current regimen and the keratitis continues to worsen beyond 1 or 2 days, other infectious and noninfectious causes for the keratitis must be considered. The patient should be examined for keratitis sicca, trichiasis, entropion, or other conditions that could contribute to the keratitis. Also, noninfectious causes of infiltrative ulcerative keratitis should be considered, such as those discussed previously under differential diagnosis.

Tissue may be destroyed through mechanisms other than replication of microorganisms. For example, if extensive tissue damage has occurred, corneal ulceration will progress despite elimination of viable bacteria because of white cell infiltration and dissolution of necrotic stroma. The objectives at this stage of management are to halt additional structural alteration, promote stromal healing and reepithelialization, and prevent drug toxicity.[36] Corneal ring-shaped infiltrates can occur with infections caused by gram-negative bacteria, particularly *Pseudomonas* (Fig. 9-12).[57,132] These infiltrates appear to be an immunologic reaction to bacterial endotoxin,[133,134] and respond to corticosteroids.

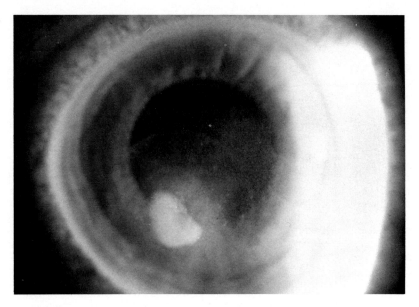

Fig. 9-12. Immunologic ring infiltrate around bacterial keratitis.

They generally are seen 10 to 14 days after the onset of the infection. It is important to differentiate these infiltrates from worsening or recurrence of infection.

Herpetic keratitis, atypical bacteria, fungi, and parasites may be present, and repeat corneal specimens should be obtained and examined for these agents. If the keratitis is indolent, antibiotic therapy can be discontinued for 1 to 2 days before reculture. Also, a corneal biopsy should be considered, since it is more likely to be diagnostic than a scraping.

Strict guidelines cannot be provided for the reduction or termination of antibiotics in keratitis that is improving with therapy. The duration of viable organisms in the cornea can vary according to the responsible bacteria, duration of infection, severity of the suppuration, depth of involvement, and other factors. Repeat corneal cultures during therapy are not reliable. Epithelialization alone can not be used to indicate the resolution of infection, because any of these antibiotics can deter epithelial healing and produce other toxic and allergic reactions.

In general, if clinical improvement is seen, antibiotic drops can be reduced in frequency after 48 to 72 hours of therapy. Usually the interval between drops is doubled every 3 to 4 days. During tapering, treatment can be switched to commercial strength drops. I do this when the frequency of administration has been decreased to 4 to 6 times per day. Treatment usually is continued at least until the epithelium is healed and, particularly for *Pseudomonas* infections, often is continued for 1 to 2 weeks longer. If the patient has been hospitalized, he or she can be discharged once the keratitis is improving and the regimen is reduced to one the individual can follow without assistance. The patient should be alert to the danger signs of resurgent keratitis and should promptly report increased pain, decreased vision, or purulent discharge.

The severe inflammatory reaction from virulent bacterial ulcers of the cornea can lead to permanent changes such as anterior polar cataracts, posterior and anterior synechiae, increased intraocular pressure, descemetocele or perforation (see Fig. 9-8),[108] stromal scars, and edema of the cornea.

SURGICAL TREATMENT

Tissue adhesive (cyanoacrylate) is useful in treating or preventing corneal perforation (see Fig. 19-26). With progressive stromal necrosis or descemetocele formation, applying tissue adhesive can reduce the likelihood of perforation. The adhesive is also bacteriostatic.[135] Perforations of up to 2 mm in diameter can be sealed with tissue adhesive, restoring integrity to the globe. Iris can be left in the wound, or the anterior chamber can be restored with air or viscoelastic material. A stromal or scleral plug can be used in conjunction with adhesive to close larger perforations. Necrotic stroma, epithelium, and other debris must be removed from the ulcer bed before the adhesive is applied. Usually a bandage contact lens must be put in place afterward. The adhesive is left in place until it loosens spontaneously, the bed becomes vascularized, or keratoplasty is performed.

A patch graft or penetrating keratoplasty are other alternatives for corneal perforation.

Conjunctival flaps can be used to treat ulcers unresponsive to medical therapy.[136,137] The flap brings blood vessels to the infected area to facilitate removal of bacteria, to promote healing, and to provide a stable surface. Conjunctival flaps are particularly useful in peripheral keratitis, where a partial flap can be placed without compromising vision. All necrotic material should be removed before placement of the flap, or the flap itself may necrose. Also, a flap alone is not sufficient treatment for a perforation.

Keratoplasty also can be considered when ulceration and necrosis progress despite medical treatment, particularly if all the involved tissue can be removed. The results of keratoplasty in acutely infected or inflamed eyes vary; the surgery is more complicated, intraocular inflammation and scarring are increased, and the risk of rejection and glaucoma are greater, especially in larger grafts.[138-140] The chance of a clear graft is fairly good if the graft's diameter is 8 mm or less, and in one report the results were equal to those cases in which surgery was delayed until the keratitis had resolved.[140] Certainly the globe and the potential for vision can be preserved by this type of surgery, even if the risk for rejection is high. It is best to treat with antibiotics for 24 to 36 hours before surgery, even if perforation is present, and to remove all the infected tissue. Culture and histologic examination of the removed tissue should be performed.

Various other treatments have been used to kill bacteria or remove infected stroma. Since *Pseudomonas* organisms seem to be susceptible to cryotherapy in vivo,[141] this may be considered as an adjunct to medical and surgical treatment of severe *Pseudomonas* infections.[142] *Pseudomonas* corneal ulcers with scleral extension have been treated successfully with combined keratoplasty and cryotherapy.[143]

Carbon dioxide[144] and excimer lasers[145] have proved capable of removing infected stroma.

REFERENCES

1. Weissman OD et al: Corneal ulcers associated with extended-wear soft contact lenses, Am J Ophthalmol 97:476, 1984.
2. Galentine PG et al: Corneal ulcers associated with contact lens wear, Arch Ophthalmol 102:891, 1984.
3. Wilhelmus KR: Review of clinical experience with microbial keratitis associated with contact lenses, CLAO J 13:211, 1987.
4. Schein OD et al: The relative risk of ulcerative keratitis among users of daily-wear and extended-wear soft contact lenses, N Engl J Med 321:773, 1989.
5. Poggio EC et al: The incidence of ulcerative keratitis among users of daily-wear and extended wear soft contact lenses, N Engl J Med 321:779, 1989.
6. Cohen EJ et al: Corneal ulcers associated with cosmetic extended wear soft contact lenses, Ophthalmology 94:109, 1987.
7. Bowden FW et al: Patterns of lens care practices and lens product contamination in contact lens associated microbial keratitis, CLAO J 15:49, 1989.
8. Allen HF: Current status of prevention, diagnosis, and management of bacterial corneal ulcers, Ann Ophthalmol 3:235, 1971.
9. Allen JC: Infection and the compromised host, Baltimore, 1976, Williams & Wilkins.
10. Ostler HB and Okumoto M: Anaerobic streptococcal corneal ulcer, Am J Ophthalmol 81:518, 1976.
11. Schein OD et al: Microbial keratitis associated with contaminated ocular medications, Am J Ophthalmol 105:361, 1988.
12. Ostler HB, Okumoto M, and Wilkey C: The changing pattern of the etiology of central bacterial corneal (hypopyon) ulcer, Trans Pac Coast Otoophthalmol Soc 55:237, 1974.
13. Hyndiuk RA: Bacterial keratitis. In Smolin G and Thoft RA, editors: The cornea: scientific foundations and clinical practice, Boston, 1983, Little, Brown & Co.
14. Asbell P and Stenson S: Ulcerative keratitis: survey of 30 years' laboratory experience, Arch Ophthalmol 100:77, 1982.
15. Jones DB: Pathogenesis of bacterial and fungal keratitis, Trans Ophthalmol Soc UK 98:367, 1978.
16. Prier JE: Opportunistic pathogens, Baltimore, 1974, University Park Press.

17. Ormerod LD et al: Microbial keratitis in children, Ophthalmology 93:449, 1986.

18. Clemons CS et al: *Pseudomonas* ulcers following patching of corneal abrasions associated with contact lens wear, CLAO J 13:161, 1987.

19. Musch DC, Sugar A, and Meyer RF: Demographic and predisposing factors in corneal ulceration, Arch Ophthalmol 101:1545, 1983.

20. Stein RM et al: Infected vs sterile corneal infiltrates in contact lens wearers, Am J Ophthalmol 105:632, 1988.

21. O'Day DM et al: The problem of *Bacillus species* infection with special emphasis on the virulence of *Bacillus cereus,* Ophthalmology 88:833, 1981.

22. Meisler DM et al: Infectious crystalline keratopathy, Am J Ophthalmol 97:337, 1984.

23. Gorovoy MS et al: Intrastromal noninflammatory bacterial colonization of a corneal graft, Arch Ophthalmol 101:1749, 1983.

24. Samples JR, Baumgartner SD, and Binder PS: Infectious crystalline keratopathy: an electron microscopic analysis, Cornea 4:118, 1985.

25. Reiss GR, Campbell RJ, and Bourne WM: Infectious crystalline keratopathy, Surv Ophthalmol 31:69, 1986.

26. Groden LR, Pascucci SE, and Brinser JH: *Haemophilus aphrophilus* as a cause of crystalline keratopathy, Am J Ophthalmol 104:89, 1987.

27. Weisenthal RW et al: Postkeratoplasty crystalline deposits mimicking bacterial infectious crystalline keratopathy, Am J Ophthalmol 105:70, 1988.

28. Thygeson P: Mannitol fermentation as an indicator of conjunctival pathogenicity of staphylococci, Arch Ophthalmol 20:274, 1938.

29. Bowers R et al: Non-aureus staphylococcus in corneal disease, Invest Ophthalmol Vis Sci 30(suppl):380, 1989.

30. Okumoto M and Smolin G: Pneumococcal infections of the eye, Am J Ophthalmol 77:346, 1974.

31. Kim HB and Ostler HB: Marginal corneal ulcer due to beta-streptococcus, Arch Ophthalmol 95:454, 1977.

32. Holland S et al: Corneal ulcer due to *Listeria monocytogenes,* Cornea 6:144, 1987.

33. Holbach LM, Bialasiewicz AA, and Boltze HJ: Necrotizing ring ulcer of the cornea caused by exogenous *Listeria monocytogenes* serotype IVb infection, Am J Ophthalmol 106:105, 1988.

34. Jones DB: Decision-making in the management of microbial keratitis, Ophthalmology 88:814, 1981.

35. Stern GA, Hodes BL, and Stock EL: *Clostridium perfringens* corneal ulcer, Arch Ophthalmol 97:661, 1979.

36. Jones DB and Robinson NM: Anaerobic ocular infections, Trans Am Acad Ophthalmol Otolaryngol 83:309, 1977.

37. Okumoto M et al: *Proteus* species isolated from human eyes, Am J Ophthalmol 81:495, 1976.

38. Bohigian GM and Escapini H: Corneal ulcer due to *Pseudomonas aeruginosa:* a comparison of the disease in California and El Salvador, Arch Ophthalmol 85:405, 1971.

39. Burns RP: Laboratory methods in diagnosis of eye infections. In Infectious diseases of the conjunctiva and cornea: Symposium of the New Orleans Academy of Ophthalmology, St Louis, 1963, Mosby – Year Book, Inc.

40. Hyndiuk RA: Experimental *Pseudomonas* keratitis, Trans Am Ophthalmol Soc 79:541, 1981.

41. Vaughan DG: Contamination of fluorescein solutions, Am J Ophthalmol 39:55, 1955.

42. Wilson LA and Ahearn DC: *Pseudomonas*-induced corneal ulcers associated with contaminated eye mascara, Am J Ophthalmol 84:112, 1977.

43. Golden B, Fingerman L, and Allen HF: *Pseudomonas* corneal ulcers in contact lens wearers: epidemiology and treatment, Arch Ophthalmol 85:543, 1971.

44. Hutton WL and Sexton RR: Atypical *Pseudomonas* corneal ulcers in semicomatose patients, Am J Ophthalmol 73:37, 1972.

45. Stern GA, Weitzenkorn D, and Valenti J: Adherence of *Pseudomonas aeruginosa* to the mouse cornea: epithelial versus stromal adherence, Arch Ophthalmol 100:1956, 1982.

46. Stern GA, Lubniewski A, and Allen C: The interaction between *P. aeruginosa* and the corneal epithelium, Arch Ophthalmol 103:1221, 1985.

47. Watt PJ: Pathogenic mechanisms of organisms virulent to the eye, Trans Ophthalmol Soc UK 105:26, 1986.

48. Dart JKG and Seal DV: Pathogenesis and therapy of *Pseudomonas aeruginosa* keratitis, Eye 2(suppl):S46, 1988.

49. Kessler E, Mondino B, and Brown SI: The corneal response to *Pseudomonas aeruginosa:* histopathological and enzymatic characterization, Invest Ophthalmol Vis Sci 16:116, 1977.

50. Kreger AS et al: Immunization against experimental *Pseudomonas aeruginosa* and *Serratia marcescens* keratitis. Vaccination with lipopolysaccharide endotoxins and proteases, Invest Ophthalmol Vis Sci 27:932, 1986.

51. Maresz-Babczyszyn J and Sokalska M: Immunity to *Pseudomonas* keratitis in rabbits vaccinated with extracellular slime from mucoid *Pseudomonas aeruginosa* strains producing proteases, Arch Immunol Ther Exp (Warsz) 29:653, 1981.

52. Moon MM et al: Monoclonal antibodies provide protection against ocular *Pseudomonas aeruginosa* infection, Invest Ophthalmol Vis Sci 29:1277, 1988.

53. Steuhl KP et al: Relevance of host-derived and bacterial factors in *Pseudomonas aeruginosa* corneal infections, Invest Ophthalmol Vis Sci 28:1559, 1987.

54. Burns RB: *Pseudomonas aeruginosa* keratitis: mixed infections of the eye, Am J Ophthalmol 67:257, 1969.

55. Raber IM et al: *Pseudomonas* corneal-scleral ulcers. Paper presented at the annual meeting of the Ocular Microbiology and Immunology Group, San Francisco, Nov 3, 1970.

56. Harbin T: Recurrence of a corneal *Pseudomonas* infection after topical steroid therapy: report of a case, Am J Ophthalmol 58:670, 1964.

57. Laibson PR: Cornea and sclera, Arch Ophthalmol 88:553, 1972.

58. Alfonso E et al: *Pseudomonas* corneoscleritis, Am J Ophthalmol 103:90, 1987.

59. Rosenfeld SI et al: Granular epithelial keratopathy as an unusual manifestation of *Pseudomonas* keratitis as-

sociated with extended-wear soft contact lenses, Am J Ophthalmol 109:17, 1990.

60. Kreger AS and Griffin QK: Corneal damaging proteases of *Serratia marcescens,* Invest Ophthalmol Vis Sci 14:190, 1975.

61. Lass JF et al: Visual outcome in eight cases of *Serratia marcescens* keratitis, Am J Ophthalmol 92:384, 1981.

62. Dugel PU et al: *Mycobacterium fortuitum* keratitis, Am J Ophthalmol 105:661, 1988.

63. Lazar M et al: *Mycobacterium fortuitum* keratitis, Am J Ophthalmol 78:530, 1974.

64. Newman PE et al: A cluster of cases of *Mycobacterium chelonei* keratitis associated with outpatient office procedures, Am J Ophthalmol 97:344, 1984.

65. Knapp A, Stern GA, and Hood CI: *Mycobacterium avium-intracellulare* corneal ulcer, Cornea 6:175, 1987.

66. Moore MB, Newton C, and Kaufman HE: Chronic keratitis caused by *Mycobacterium gordonae,* Am J Ophthalmol 102:516, 1986.

67. Ostler HB, Thygeson P, and Okumoto M: Infectious diseases of the eye. III. Infections of the cornea, J C E Ophthalmol 39:113, 1978.

68. Ralph RA, Lemp MA, and Liss G: *Nocardia asteroides* keratitis: a case report, Br J Ophthalmol 60:104, 1976.

69. Climenhaga DB, Tokarewicz AC, and Willis NR: *Nocardia* keratitis, Can J Ophthalmol 19:284, 1984.

70. Srinivasan M and Sharma S: *Nocardia asteroides* as a cause of corneal ulcer: case report, Arch Ophthalmol 105:464, 1987

71. Hirst L et al: *Nocardia asteroides* keratitis, Br J Ophthalmol 63:449, 1979.

72. Hirst LW, Merz WC, and Green WR: *Nocardia asteroides* corneal ulcer, Am J Ophthalmol 94:123, 1982.

73. Perry HD, Nauheim JS, and Donnenfeld ED: *Nocardia asteroides* keratitis presenting as a persistent epithelial defect, Cornea 8:41, 1989.

74. Donnenfeld ED et al: Treatment of *Nocardia* keratitis with topical trimethoprim-sulfamethoxazole, Am J Ophthalmol 99:601, 1985.

75. Herman PE: General principles of antimicrobial therapy, Mayo Clin Proc 52:603, 1977.

76. Sobol WM et al: Rapid streptococcal antigen detection in experimental keratitis, Am J Ophthalmol 107:60, 1989.

77. Jones DB: A plan for antimicrobial therapy in bacterial keratitis, Trans Am Acad Ophthalmol Otolaryngol 79:95, 1975.

78. Jones DB: Initial therapy of suspected microbial corneal ulcers. II. Specific antibiotic therapy based on corneal smears, Surv Ophthalmol 24:97, 1979.

79. Baum J: Initial therapy of suspected microbial corneal ulcers. I. Broad spectrum antibiotic therapy based on prevalence of organisms, Surv Ophthalmol 24:97, 1979.

80. Baum J: Therapy for ocular bacterial infection, Trans Ophthalmol Soc UK 105:69, 1986.

81. Davis SD, Sarff LD, and Hyndiuk RA: Antibiotic therapy of experimental *Pseudomonas* in guinea pigs, Arch Ophthalmol 95:1638, 1977.

82. Davis SD, Sarff LD, and Hyndiuk RA: Topical tobramycin therapy of experimental *Pseudomonas* kerati-

tis: an evaluation of some factors that potentially enhance efficacy, Arch Ophthalmol 96:123, 1978.

83. Kupferman A and Leibowitz HM: Topical antibiotic therapy of *Pseudomonas aeruginosa* keratitis in guinea pigs, Arch Ophthalmol 97:1699, 1977.

84. Davis SD, Sarff LD, and Hyndiuk RA: Relative efficacy of the topical use of amikacin, gentamicin and tobramycin in experimental *Pseudomonas* keratitis, Can J Ophthalmol 15:28, 1980.

85. Baum J and Barza M: Topical vs subconjunctival treatment of bacterial corneal ulcers, Ophthalmology 90:162, 1983.

86. Stern GA and Driebe WT: The effect of fortified antibiotic therapy on the visual outcome of severe bacterial corneal ulcers, Cornea 1:341, 1982.

87. Osborn E et al: The stability of 10 antibiotics in artificial tears, Am J Ophthalmol 82:775, 1976.

88. Bowe BE, Snyder JW, and Eiferman RA: Fortified ophthalmic antibiotic preparations: an in-vitro study of potency and storage mechanisms, Invest Ophthalmol Vis Sci 30(suppl):199, 1989.

89. Glasser DB et al: Loading doses and extended dosing intervals in topical gentamicin therapy, Am J Ophthalmol 99:329, 1985.

90. Baum JL et al: Concentration of gentamicin in experimental corneal ulcers: topical vs subconjunctival therapy, Arch Ophthalmol 92:315, 1974.

91. Davis SD, Sarff LD, and Hyndiuk RA: Comparison of therapeutic routes in experimental *Pseudomonas* keratitis, Am J Ophthalmol 87:710, 1979.

92. Davis SD, Sarff LD, and Hyndiuk RA: Experimental *Pseudomonas* keratitis in guinea pigs: therapy of moderately severe infections, Br J Ophthalmol 63:436, 1979.

93. Leibowitz HM, Ryan WJ, and Kupferman A: Route of antibiotic administration in bacterial keratitis, Arch Ophthalmol 99:1420, 1981.

94. Baum J: Treatment of bacterial ulcers of the cornea in the rabbit: a comparison of administration by eye drops and subconjunctival injections, Trans Am Ophthalmol Soc 80:369, 1982.

95. Hessburg PC: Management of *Pseudomonas* keratitis, Surv Ophthalmol 14:43, 1969.

96. Burris TE, Newsome DI, and Rowsey JJ: Hessburg subpalpebral antibiotic lavage of *Pseudomonas* corneal and corneoscleral ulcers, Cornea 1:347, 1982.

97. Matoba AY and McCulley JP: The effect of therapeutic soft contact lenses on antibiotic delivery to the cornea, Ophthalmology 92:97, 1985.

98. Busin M, Goebbels M, and Spitznas M: Medicated bandage lenses for sustained gentamicin release, Ophthalmology 94(suppl):124, 1987.

99. O'Brien TP et al: Use of collagen corneal shields versus soft contact lenses to enhance penetration of topical tobramycin, J Cataract Refract Surg 14:505, 1988.

100. Unterman SR et al: Collagen shield drug delivery: therapeutic concentrations of tobramycin in the rabbit cornea and aqueous humor, J Cataract Refract Surg 14:500, 1988.

101. Gilbert ML, Wilhelmus KR, and Osato MS: Intracanalicular collagen implants enhance topical antibiotic bioavailability, Cornea 5:167, 1986.

102. Hobden JA et al: Iontophoretic application of tobramy-

cin to uninfected and *Pseudomonas aeruginosa*–infected rabbit corneas, Antimicrob Agents Chemother 32:978, 1988.

103. Rootman DS et al: Iontophoresis of tobramycin for the treatment of experimental *Pseudomonas* keratitis in the rabbit, Am J Ophthalmol 106:262, 1988.

104. Groden LR and Brinser JH: Outpatient treatment of microbial corneal ulcers, Arch Ophthalmol 104:84, 1986.

105. Wilkowske CJ: The penicillins, Mayo Clin Proc 52:616, 1977.

106. Baum JL, Barza M, and Weinstein L: Preferred routes of antibiotic administration in treatment of bacterial ulcers of the cornea, Int Ophthalmol Clin 13:31, 1973.

107. Records RE: Antimicrobial therapy in ophthalmology, Int Ophthalmol Clin 10:473, 1970.

108. Jones DB: Early diagnosis and therapy of bacterial corneal ulcers, Int Ophthalmol Clin 13:1, 1973.

109. Bodey GP et al: Carbenicillin therapy for *Pseudomonas* infection, JAMA 218:62, 1971.

110. Hoffman TA and Bulloch WE: Carbenicillin therapy of *Pseudomonas* and other gram-negative bacillary infections, Ann Intern Med 73:165, 1970.

111. McLoughlin JE and Reeves DS: Clinical and laboratory evidence for inactivations of gentamicin by carbenicillin, Lancet 1:261, 1971.

112. Sloan SH, Pettit TH, and Letwach KD: Gentamicin penetration in aqueous humor of eyes with corneal ulcers, Am J Ophthalmol 73:750, 1972.

113. Richards F, McCall D, and Cox C: Gentamicin treatment of staphylococcal infections, JAMA 215:1297, 1971.

114. Stern GA et al: Effect of topical antibiotic solutions on corneal epithelial wound healing, Arch Ophthalmol 101:644, 1983.

115. Neu HC: Tobramycin: an overview, J Infect Dis 134(suppl):1, 1976.

116. Moellering RC Jr and Swartz MN: The newer cephalosporins, N Engl J Med 294:24, 1976.

117. Thompson RL: The cephalosporins, Mayo Clin Proc 52:625, 1977.

118. Thornsberry C: Review of in vitro activity of third-generation cephalosporins and other newer beta-lactam antibiotics against clinically important bacteria, Am J Med 79(suppl 2A):14, 1985.

119. Kaplan K, Reisberg B, and Weinstein L: Cephaloridine: studies of therapeutic activity and untoward effects, Arch Intern Med 121:17, 1968.

120. Rosenthal RL and Blackman A: Bone marrow hypoplasia following use of chloramphenicol eye drops, JAMA 191:136, 1965.

121. Seedor JA et al: Systemic tetracycline treatment of alkali-induced corneal ulceration in rabbits, Arch Ophthalmol 105:268, 1987.

122. Wilkie J, Smolin G, and Okumoto M: The effect of rifampicin on *Pseudomonas* keratitis, Can J Ophthalmol 7:309, 1972.

123. O'Brien TP et al: Topical ciprofloxacin treatment of *Pseudomonas* keratitis in rabbits, Arch Ophthalmol 106:1444, 1988.

124. O'Brien TP et al: Comparative topical treatment of methicillin resistant *Staphylococcus epidermidis* keratitis in rabbits. Paper Presented at the annual meeting of the Ocular Microbiology and Immunology Group, Las Vegas, Oct 7, 1988.

125. Sugar A et al: Treatment of experimental *Pseudomonas* corneal ulcers with enoxacin, a quinolone antibiotic, Arch Ophthalmol 104:1230, 1988.

126. Sawusch MR et al: Topical imipenem therapy of aminoglycoside-resistant *Pseudomonas* keratitis in rabbits, Am J Ophthalmol 106:77, 1988.

127. Tabbara K, Antonios S, and Alvarez H: Effects of fusidic acid on staphylococcal keratitis, Br J Ophthalmol 73:136, 1989.

128. Smith PC, Zam S, and Stern GA: The effect of tuftsin in the treatment of experimental *Pseudomonas* keratitis, Cornea 5:181, 1986.

129. Leibowitz HM and Kupferman A: Topically administered corticosteroids: effect on antibiotic-treated bacterial keratitis, Arch Ophthalmol 98:1287, 1980.

130. Davis SD, Sarff LD, and Hyndiuk RA: Corticosteroid in experimentally induced *Pseudomonas* keratitis: failure of prednisolone to impair the efficacy of tobramycin and carbenicillin therapy, Arch Ophthalmol 96:126, 1978.

131. Smolin G, Okumoto M, and Leong-Sit L: Combined gentamicin-tobramycin-corticosteroid treatment. II. Effect on gentamicin-resistant *Pseudomonas* keratitis, Arch Ophthalmol 98:473, 1980.

132. Duke-Elder S and Leigh AG: System of ophthalmology, vol 8, Diseases of the outer eye, St Louis, 1965, Mosby–Year Book, Inc.

133. Mondino BJ et al: Corneal rings with gram-negative bacteria, Arch Ophthalmol 95:2222, 1977.

134. Belmont JB et al: Noninfectious ring-shaped keratitis associated with *Pseudomonas aeruginosa,* Am J Ophthalmol 93:338, 1982.

135. Eiferman RA and Snyder JW: Antibacterial effect of cyanoacrylate glue, Arch Ophthalmol 101:958, 1983.

136. Gundersen T: Conjunctival flaps in the treatment of corneal disease with reference to a new technique of application, Arch Ophthalmol 60:880, 1958.

137. Buxton JN and Fox ML: Conjunctival flaps in the treatment of refractory *Pseudomonas* corneal abscess, Ann Ophthalmol 18:315, 1986.

138. Malik SRK and Singh G: Therapeutic keratoplasty in *Pseudomonas pyocyaneus* corneal ulcers, Br J Ophthalmol 55:326, 1971.

139. Zu DN et al: Therapeutic keratoplasty in the management of purulent corneal ulceration: report of 100 cases, Jpn J Ophthalmol 23:412, 1979.

140. Hill JC: Use of penetrating keratoplasty in acute bacterial keratitis, Br J Ophthalmol 70:502, 1986.

141. Alpren TVP et al: Cryotherapy for experimental *Pseudomonas* keratitis, Arch Ophthalmol 97:711, 1979.

142. Codere F, Brownstein S, and Jackson B: *Pseudomonas aeruginosa* scleritis, Am J Ophthalmol 91:706, 1981.

143. Eiferman RA: Cryotherapy of *Pseudomonas* keratitis and scleritis, Arch Ophthalmol 97:1637, 1979.

144. Sarno EM et al: Carbon dioxide laser therapy of *Pseudomonas aeruginosa* keratitis, Am J Ophthalmol 97:791, 1984.

145. Serdarevic O et al: Excimer laser therapy for experimental *Candida* keratitis, Am J Ophthalmol 99:534, 1985.

INFECTIOUS KERATITIS: FUNGAL AND PARASITIC

FUNGAL KERATITIS

The number of cases of fungal keratitis has increased over the past 20 to 30 years because of improved diagnosis as well as increased incidence.[1-9] Despite advances in both diagnostic techniques and antifungal agents, diagnosis and management continue to be a challenge for the ophthalmologist. The morbidity of fungal infections tends to be greater than that of bacterial keratitis because the diagnosis is often delayed and because available drugs are not as effective. It is necessary, therefore, to be aware of the clinical presentation of fungal keratitis, to promptly suspect its presence, and to implement proper laboratory investigation to establish the diagnosis. Management, both medical and surgical, is not as well defined as in bacterial keratitis and depends more on clinical judgment. An informed, reasoned approach is essential.

CLASSIFICATION OF FUNGI

Taxonomists use a complex classification of fungi based primarily on sexual reproduction; however, a simpler, morphologic classification is sufficient for fungi important in ocular disease. These fungi can be divided into filamentous, yeast, and diphasic forms.[10]
Filamentous fungi. The hyphae of these multicellular fungi branch, forming a tangled mass on the culture medium called a *mycelium* (Fig. 10-1).

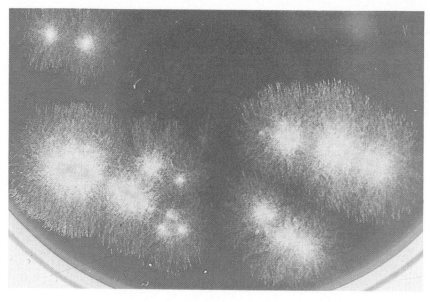

Fig. 10-1. Blood agar plate incubated at room temperature showing *Aspergillus fumigatus* mycelia.

Septate organisms. The hyphae are divided by cell walls into cellular compartments that contain one or more nuclei (Fig. 10-2). The following fungi are most often associated with ocular disease:

1. *Fusarium*
2. *Cephalosporium*
3. *Aspergillus*
4. *Cladosporium*
5. *Penicillium*
6. *Paecilomyces*
7. *Phialophora*
8. *Curvularia*
9. *Alternaria*

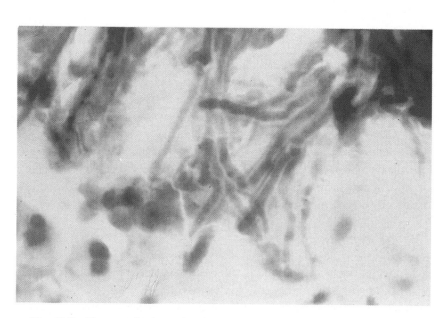

Fig. 10-2. Giemsa-stained scraping from corneal ulcer exhibiting septate hyphae.

These filamentous organisms predominantly affect normal eyes after corneal abrasion or trauma involving some kind of vegetable matter. The fungi are ubiquitous, found both outside and inside the home, and mainly on organic matter. Infections occur more frequently in the temperate zones of the country. *Fusarium* species are the most common corneal fungal pathogens in the southern United States,[11] and probably in the Western hemisphere. They are primarily plant pathogens, and *Fusarium* keratitis often occurs in agricultural workers.

Nonseptate organisms. There is no regular division of the hyphae by septae; the filaments exist as long tubes with numerous nuclei scattered throughout. The fungi in this group rarely cause corneal disease but can cause hematogenous endophthalmitis and sinus and orbital infections. The most common pathogens are as follows:

1. *Mucor*
2. *Rhizopus*
3. *Absidia*

Yeasts. Yeasts are fungi with usual and dominant growth as unicellular organisms. They often produce pseudohyphae and buds, and occasionally true hyphae, depending on the environment. The following organisms are most significant:

1. *Candida*
2. *Cryptococcus*
3. *Rhodotorula*

Candida species are opportunistic pathogens that are part of the normal flora of the skin; respiratory, gastrointestinal, and vaginal mucosa; and occasionally conjunctiva. Corneal ulcers caused by *Candida* usually occur in eyes where there is some predisposing factor. Agricultural exposure and trauma occurring outdoors usually are not factors in the pathogenesis of yeast keratitis. Infections also can occur in the lacrimal passages, lids, and conjunctiva.

Yeast do not form a mycelium in culture. They form white, opaque, smooth colonies on Sabouraud media, which may be mistaken for staphylococcal colonies (Fig. 10-3).

Diphasic fungi. Diphasic fungi possess two distinct morphologic forms: the yeast phase, which occur in tissues, and a mycelial phase, which occur on media and natural surfaces. Diphasic fungi rarely cause keratitis but are important pathogens. The following are most commonly seen:

1. *Blastomyces*[12]
2. *Coccidioides*
3. *Histoplasma*
4. *Sporothrix*

PATHOGENESIS

In general, fungal keratitis is more prevalent in warmer climates, such as the southern and southwestern parts of the United States. In these areas there is a marked seasonal variation in the incidence of fungal keratitis, particularly the forms caused by filamentous fungi; the variation is most likely a result of environmental factors. For instance, in Florida the incidence of fungal keratitis is highest between November and March, when it is cool, dry, and windy[11]; in India the incidence is greatest in September and October during harvesting.[13] In cooler climates, infection with yeasts is more common than infection with filamentous fungi, and there is less seasonal variation.

Many corneal ulcers are caused by fungi commonly considered to be saprophytes (that is, fungi that live on dead or decaying organic matter). About 7% of normal healthy eyes have fungi on the lids or conjunctiva at one time or other, probably as transient inhabitants. The most virulent fungal infections occur in persons with no apparent deficiency in resistance. These cases usually are associated with injury to the cornea from twigs or other plant matter. Less virulent organisms, such as *Candida albicans,* are seen more in compromised hosts, such as those with Sjögren's syndrome, erythema multiforme, endocrinopathy,[3] immunodeficiency, diabetes, alcoholism, or hypovitaminosis A.[14] Corneal disease, such as persistent epithelial defect, stromal ulceration, herpes simplex infec-

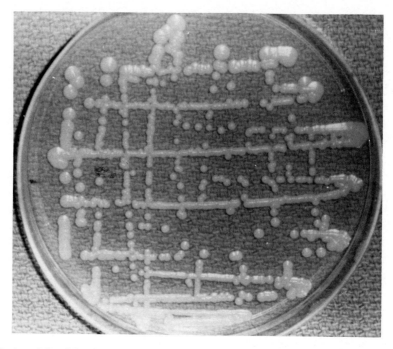

Fig. 10-3. Colonies of *Candida albicans* growing on Sabouraud medium can be mistaken for colonies of staphylococci.

tion, topical steroid use, and contact lens wear, also appears to predispose an eye to fungal infection, particularly yeast infection.

Corneal infections are relatively difficult to establish in experimental animals, even after intrastromal injection, and the mechanisms underlying development of human disease are unclear. These fungi do elaborate proteases and toxins, such as the trichthecenes, cytotoxins produced by some species of *Fusarium* and *Acremonium,* and aflatoxin, a liver carcinogen produced by *Aspergillus.*[15] However, the role of these substances in corneal disease is unknown. Some filamentous fungi appear to be relatively nonimmunogenic; they can proliferate extensively in the cornea without eliciting much inflammatory response. In addition, their large size inhibits phagocytosis. Topical steroids may enhance their replication.

A number of *Candida* virulence factors have been identified. *Candida* species produce proteolytic enzymes and lipases, which aid host invasion. A surface protein aids epithelial adherence, and an unidentified secreted substance inhibits digestion of pseudohyphae by neutrophils.[16] The large size of the pseudohyphae also inhibits phagocytosis. Resistance to *Candida* infection appears to depend on the location: resistance to mucocutaneous infection is mainly T-cell dependent, but resistance to disseminated disease depends more on other innate defenses, such as neutrophils.[17]

Fungi can contaminate contact lens solutions, as well as the lens itself,[18-20] and lead to keratitis. Filamentous fungi are more likely to cause keratitis in cosmetic or aphakic soft contact lens wearers, and yeasts more likely in therapeutic lens wearers.[21] Good contact lens hygiene and heat disinfection are the best methods for preventing fungal contamination.

CLINICAL MANIFESTATIONS

In most infections symptoms and signs occur within 1 to 2 days. Symptoms are similar to those caused by bacterial ulcers, except that fungal ulcers are more often indolent. In some cases days or weeks may elapse before the patient seeks medical care.

The corneal ulcer caused by filamentous fungi often has grayish white infiltration, with rough-textured surface areas elevated above the plane of the uninvolved cornea (Fig. 10-4). The margins, which are irregular and extend into the adjacent stroma (Fig. 10-5), may exhibit a feathery outline. Foci of infiltration can be seen several millimeters away from the main area of involvement (Fig. 10-6); these are called satellite lesions. The epithelium can be intact over the infiltrate. An endothelial plaque may be seen paralleling the ulcer. A ring infiltrate may surround the primary lesion, most likely representing an antibody response to fungal antigen. In addition, a hypopyon and purulent discharge may occur, even when the infiltrate appears minimal (Fig. 10-4). Conjunctival injection and anterior chamber reaction may be quite severe.

The clinical appearance of filamentous fungal keratitis is quite variable, and often indistinguishable from bacterial, viral, or parasitic infection. Early infections may resemble staphylococcal infection, especially if near the limbus, or herpes simplex keratitis. *Nocardia, Actinomyces, Streptomyces,* mycobacteria, and other bacteria can present similarly. Infection that occurs beneath an intact epithelium also can occur with herpes viruses, *Acanthamoeba,* and some avirulent bacteria (for example, *Streptococcus viridans*). Ring infiltrates also occur with keratitis due to herpes viruses, *Acanthamoeba,* and gram-negative rods.

Yeast infections tend to present a different picture. They usually exhibit an oval, plaquelike, elevated lesion that is reasonably well outlined and is often widely surrounded by stromal edema. These more closely resemble a bacterial keratitis (Fig. 10-7). The differences between filamentous and yeast fungal keratitis are as follows:

FILAMENTOUS FUNGI	YEASTS
Occurs more frequently in young people (occupational and outdoor activity)	Usually occurs in compromised host; preexisting corneal disease or steroid treatment
Signs may be present 24 to 48 hours after injury	Usually more focal and suppurative, resembling bacterial keratitis
Usually no predisposing factor	
Area involved can be localized and often is elevated; epithelial defect may or may not be present; often has feathery edges and satellite lesions	Edges not feathery, and satellitism not usually seen; often elevated
Inflammation can be mild or severe, with hypopyon and endothelial plaque	

Histopathology

Severe inflammation of the cornea can result from fungal infection due to replicating and nonreplicating fungi, mycotoxins, proteolytic enzymes, and soluble fungal antigens.[22] These agents can result in necrosis of the corneal lamellae, acute inflammation, antigenic response with immune ring formation, hypopyon, and severe uveitis.[23] In general, the virulence of the filamentous fungi ranges from the more destructive *Fusarium solanae,* through many species, including those of *Cephalosporium, Aspergillus,* and *Penicillium,* to the more leisurely pathogens, such as *Phialophora,* which may grow indolently in the cornea over a period of months.

The inflammatory response tends to be less marked than in bacterial keratitis, and the epithelium is frequently intact over the infection. Multiple microabscesses may surround the main lesion of central ulceration and infiltration. Limbal infiltration with lymphocytes and plasma cells increases with progressive keratitis and can result in a ring abscess. The infection tends to become deeper with time. In more advanced disease, fungi may be absent from the surface and the superficial stroma, which may explain the difficulty in recovering the organisms in scrapings. The hyphae can penetrate through the stromal lamellae (Fig. 10-8) and Descemet's membrane and spread into the anterior chamber. When this occurs, it is usually seen as a retrocorneal or anterior chamber inflammatory mass adjacent

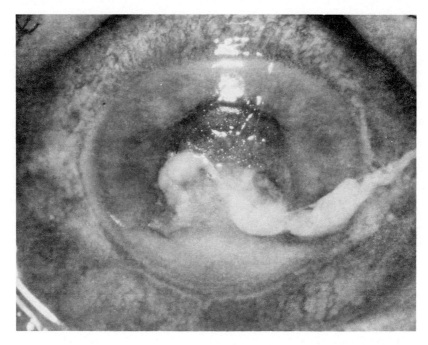

Fig. 10-4. Fungal keratitis with stromal infiltration and hypopyon. Note raised edge and extensive purulent discharge.

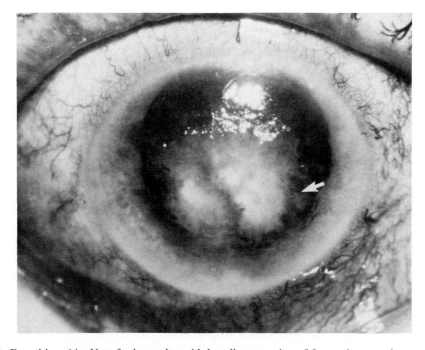

Fig. 10-5. Fungal keratitis. Note feathery edge with lamellar extension of fungus in corneal stroma *(arrow)*.

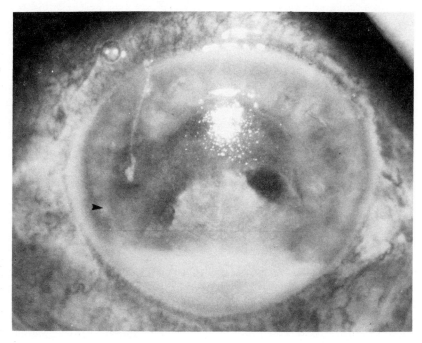

Fig. 10-6. Satellite lesion *(arrow)* in fungal ulcer with large hypopyon and extensive stromal necrosis.

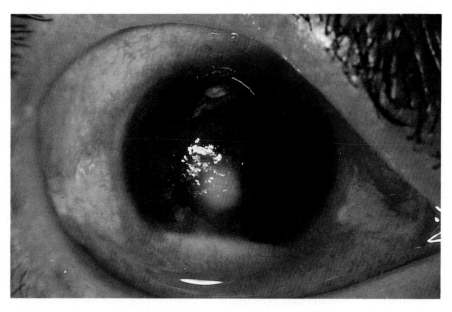

Fig. 10-7. *Candida albicans* corneal infection.

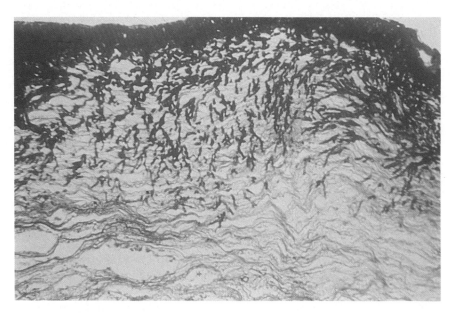

Fig. 10-8. Fungus makes its way through corneal lamellae and may penetrate Descemet's membrane. (PAS.)

to an area of deep keratitis.[24] Some *Fusarium* species infections appear to have a predilection for the posterior chamber, where their accumulation can cause a severe glaucoma.[25]

DIAGNOSIS

Although the clinical history and appearance may be suggestive of fungal keratitis, definite diagnosis requires laboratory confirmation. As discussed earlier, infection with herpes simplex, *Nocardia, Actinomyces, Streptomyces,* mycobacteria, other bacteria, and *Acanthamoeba* can result in a similar picture.

Multiple scrapings (four to eight) should be taken from the ulcer under slit-lamp microscope magnification and examined. The smears are air dried or fixed with methanol and stained with Giemsa stain, Gram stain, and with one or two special fungal stains (see Chapter 4).[26-28] All staining material and all media should be fresh. Gram stain will darken the fungus walls; the Giemsa stain will highlight the cytoplasm, but the walls are seen only by contrast (Fig. 10-2). Probably the best stain for fungi is the Gomori methenamine silver technique; however, it is relatively difficult and time consuming to perform. PAS stain, calcofluor, Ink-KOH, or acridine orange are other options.

The next step is to inoculate the proper media. At least one medium appropriate for fungi should be inoculated whenever fungal keratitis is a possibility, such as one of the following:

1. Blood agar plate incubated at room temperature and 37° C. (*Fusarium* grows well at 37° C.)
2. Sabouraud medium incubated at room temperature (no additives) is probably the most sensitive.
3. Beef heart infusion broth at room temperature (gentamicin added) kept on a platform shaker.

Most fungal isolates grow out within 2 to 3 days, but some can take 3 weeks or more.

The frequency of identification of fungal elements in smears depends on the quality of the specimen, the experience of the observer, the stain, and the duration of infection. Even with experienced observers, Gram- and Giemsa-stained smears are positive in only two thirds to three fourths of cases.[11,29] Nevertheless, it is important to examine smears because they often contain fungi even though no growth is obtained in culture.[30] Specific fungal identification is not possible, but yeasts and filamentous fungi usually can be differentiated. Biopsy may be necessary for diagnosis, particularly in long-standing infection.[31]

TREATMENT

Antimicrobial therapy for fungal keratitis is currently not as well developed as therapy for bacterial keratitis. No ideal agent—one which would be fungicidal and lack toxicity and which could penetrate the cornea well—is available. The available agents tend only to inhibit growth and allow the host to eradicate the infection. Penetration of most agents is limited, and many are irritating or toxic to the ocular surface.

Antifungal agents. Following are the main drugs used for treatment of filamentous and yeast infection of the cornea:

1. Amphotericin B
2. Natamycin
3. Imidazole compounds (clotrimazole, miconazole, and ketoconazole)
4. Flucytosine

Tables 10-1 through 10-4 summarize the spectrum of activity, dosages, and other characteristics of these drugs.

Amphotericin B. Amphotericin B, a heptaene polyene, is active against *Candida, Cryptococcus,* and *Aspergillus* species; but is variably active against *Fusarium* species. In one animal study, amphotericin B was found to be the most effective agent against two strains of *Candida albicans.*[32] It was the most frequently used agent before the development of natamycin and was effective in many cases, but resistance was common and toxicity limited its use.[1,33]

Amphotericin B is fungistatic, insoluble, and relatively toxic, and it can not penetrate intact epithelium.[34,35] Stromal penetration of denuded, inflamed stroma is better, but only a small percentage of the drug present is active.[36] It is unstable in light, water, heat, and pH extremes.[37] Like other polyenes, it binds to sterols in the cell membrane of fungi and increases its permeability. To a lesser extent, it also binds sterols present in human cell membranes, which is one of the reasons for its toxicity.

The adverse effects of topical amphotericin include burning, chemosis, epithelial clouding, greenish discoloration, and punctate keratopathy. These effects are partly caused by the bile salt used to stabilize the drug in solution. Dilute preparations (0.05% to 0.15%) are less toxic and appear to be as

TABLE 10-1. Activity of Antifungal Agents*

	AMPHOTER-ICIN B	NATAMYCIN	MICONAZOLE	CLOTRIMA-ZOLE	KETOCONAZOLE	FLUCYTO-SINE
YEASTS						
Candida	+	±	±	+	+	+
Torulopsis	+	+	+	+		+
FILAMENTOUS FUNGI						
Fusarium	±	+	±	±	−	−
Aspergillus	+	+	+	+	−	±
Paecilomyces	−	−	+	±	+	−
Curvularia	+	+	+		+	−
Cladosporium	+	+	+	±		+
Penicillium	+	+				±

*Based on limited experimental and human data. Susceptibility in individual cases can vary greatly.

TABLE 10-2. Review of Antifungal Agents

DRUG	TYPE	ROUTES	TOPICAL PENETRATION*	TOPICAL TOXICITY	COMMENTS
Amphotericin B	Polyene	Topical Systemic†	Poor	+	Unstable in light, water, heat, and pH extremes. Systemic use causes damage to erythrocytes and renal tubules
Natamycin	Polyene	Topical	Fair	+	Insoluble and unstable
Miconazole	Imidazole	Topical Subconjunctival Systemic (IV)	Good	−	Unstable in solution; must be reformed weekly
Clotrimazole	Imidazole	Topical Subconjunctival	?	+ (especially commercial preparations)	
Ketoconazole	Imidazole	Topical Systemic (oral)	Good	−	Systemic administration generally well tolerated, but hepatoxicity can occur
Flucytosine	Pyrimidine	Topical Systemic (oral)	?	−	Best used in combination with amphotericin B. Systemic administration is generally well tolerated, but bone marrow and liver toxicity can occur

*Deepithelialized cornea.
†Not effective for keratitis and very toxic.

effective.[38] Systemic administration is toxic and ineffective for keratitis. The toxicity is related to membrane damage in erythrocytes and renal tubular cells.[39]

Current recommendations are to use a concentration of 0.05%, with an initial application every 5 minutes for 1 hour, and then one drop hourly. Amphotericin B should be prepared in distilled water for eye drops because it precipitates in sodium chloride solution. Amphotericin B should not be given as a subconjunctival injection because it is painful and can lead to local necrosis.

Natamycin. Natamycin (pimaricin 5%), a tetraene polyene antibiotic, is the only antifungal agent commercially available for ophthalmic use. Like amphotericin B, it alters the permeability of fungal cell membranes, is insoluble, and lacks stability, but it is less toxic.[40] It penetrates the deepithelialized cornea well, and to a much lesser extent also penetrates intact epithelium.[36] As with amphotericin B, only a small percentage of the intrastromal drug is bioactive.[41] It appears to be effective only

TABLE 10-3. Dosages of Antifungal Agents

DRUG	TOPICAL	INITIAL TOPICAL FREQUENCY	SUBCONJUNCTIVAL	SYSTEMIC
Amphotericin B	0.05% (.5 mg/ml)	Every 5 minutes for 1 hour, then hourly	—	*
Natamycin	5% (50 mg/ml)	Every 30 minutes for the first 3 to 4 days then 6 to 8 times daily	—	—
Miconazole	1% (10 mg/ml)	Hourly	5-10 mg	30 mg/kg/day IV
Clotrimazole	1% (10 mg/ml)	Hourly?	5-10 mg	—
Ketoconazole	1%-2% (10-20 mg/ml)	Hourly?	—	200 to 400 mg/day orally in one dose
Flucytosine	1% (10 mg/ml)	Hourly?	—	150 mg/kg/day orally in four divided doses

*Not effective in keratitis. If contemplated, obtain infectious disease consultation.

TABLE 10-4. Initial Therapy of Fungal Keratitis

FUNGUS	TOPICAL	SUBCONJUNCTIVAL*	SYSTEMIC*
Filamentous	Natamycin	Miconazole	Miconazole
Yeast	Amphotericin B	Miconazole	Flucytosine

*May be added to topical use, depending on severity of keratitis.

against relatively superficial infections. Natamycin has a broad spectrum of activity against filamentous fungi and is the drug of choice for these organisms.[5,41-44] It is also effective against yeasts, including *Candida albicans*. In South Florida, Forster and Rebell[45] found natamycin to be effective in 85% of *Fusarium solani* infections, 60% of those caused by other nonpigmented filamentous fungi, 90% of those caused by pigmented filamentous fungi, and 75% of yeast infections.

A 5% suspension is applied topically, and it usually "adheres" to the ulcer site. It also forms a ropelike strand in the inferior fornix, which may serve as a reservoir for the drug. For the first 3 to 4 days, drops should be given every half hour,[46] and then decreased to six to eight times per day. With frequent or prolonged use, it can cause epithelial toxicity.

Imidazole compounds. The imidazole compounds inhibit synthesis of ergosterol, which is needed for fungal cell membranes, and at higher concentrations can directly damage the fungal cell wall.[47,48] In vitro they are fungistatic at low concentrations and fungicidal at high concentrations, but it is unlikely that these higher concentrations can be achieved in the cornea.

Miconazole can be used topically, subconjunctivally, or systemically. Good stromal levels occur after subconjunctival injection and after topical administration if the epithelium is removed.[49] Aqueous levels are high after intravenous administration. Miconazole is relatively unstable in solution and must be reformulated weekly. Miconazole is active against most yeasts and many filamentous fungi but is variably active against *Fusarium* and *Aspergillus* species.[50] With limited experience, topical,[51] combined topical and subconjunctival (with oral ketoconazole),[52] and intravenous miconazole[53] have been effective in most human cases. Both topical and subconjunctival administration have been well tolerated.

Clotrimazole also has broad antifungal activity and appears to be of most value in treatment of *Aspergillus*.[54] Too toxic for systemic use, it is well tolerated when given topically in a 1% concentration in arachis oil or dermatologic cream.

Ketoconazole is more water soluble and is better absorbed after systemic administration than other imidazoles. Good corneal levels are obtained after topical, subconjunctival, or oral administration.[55] In both experimental models and limited human trials, oral or topical ketoconazole has been effective in every case,[56-59] except in one animal study in which neither oral nor topical ketoconazole was effective against one strain of *Aspergillus fumigatus*.[60] Topical preparations (1% to 2%) have been well tolerated, as has systemic administration, although hepatotoxicity can occur.

Flucytosine. Flucytosine[61,62] (5-fluorocytosine, or Ancobon) is a fluorinated pyrimidine and is fungistatic.[63,64] Flucytosine is selectively taken up by susceptible fungi and deaminated to fluorouracil, which blocks thymidine synthesis.[41] It is not metabolized by human cells; up to 95% of the dose is excreted. However, gastrointestinal flora can convert flucytosine to fluorouracil, which is then absorbed. Flucytosine is effective against *Candida* and *Cryptococcus* and certain strains of *Aspergillus*, *Penicillium*, and *Cladosporium*, but is not effective against *Fusarium* or *Cephalosporium*. Some yeast strains are resistant, and resistance can develop during therapy, both of which reduce its usefulness. In general, the results have been disappointing when flucytosine is used alone. Combined treatment, particularly with amphotericin B, is probably best because the combination appears to be more effective and the chance for resistance is reduced.

Topically flucytosine is used as drops in a 1% solution (10 mg/ml) every hour and appears to be well tolerated. The combination of flucytosine and amphotericin B may be of particular value in systemic candidiasis. The suggested oral dose is 50 to 150 mg/kg/day in four divided doses. Systemic administration is relatively risk-free, but bone marrow and liver toxicity can occur. These complications are dose-related and reversible if the drug is withdrawn. Therefore, regular hematologic and liver function evaluation should be performed. Gastrointestinal upset and skin rashes can also occur.

Selection of therapy. Several factors limit the determination of efficacy of antifungal agents: (1) The number of cases of fungal keratitis is small; (2) in vitro susceptibility testing has not been standardized and has not correlated well with clinical results; and (3) testing in laboratory animals has been limited. Therefore, precise guidelines for drug therapy cannot be given. Because the greatest cumulative experience has been with natamycin and has shown it to be relatively effective and nontoxic, there is some bias toward its continued use. However, the newer agents have some potential benefits, and as more experience is accumulated they may supplant natamycin as the drug of choice.

Antifungal therapy should not be initiated without laboratory evidence of fungal keratitis for these reasons: the clinical history and appearance are not diagnostic; prolonged therapy is required; the response is slow and easily confused with the normal resolution of many nonfungal processes; and the agents are often toxic. If necessary, repeated scrapings and cultures or biopsy should be performed to make the diagnosis.

In fungal keratitis, selection of the proper antifungal agent is based mainly on clinical response. Identification of the fungus in smears or culture media may be useful in initial selection, but the susceptibility of different strains of the same species can vary greatly. Sensitivity determinations can be useful, but they are not performed by many laboratories and are unreliable even when available.[65] If testing is performed, the broth dilution method appears to be the most reliable method. Certainly, if the patient is doing well on one drug, treatment should not be changed unless toxicity to the drug develops. Tables 10-1 through 10-4 summarize the selection of antifungal agents for treatment.

The response to treatment is usually extremely slow. Often, improvement is not seen until an effective agent has been given for weeks. Signs of improvement of a fungal ulcer are decreased size of the central corneal infiltrate, disappearance of the satellite lesions, and rounding out of the feathery margins. Persistent epithelial staining may be noticed, but this often indicates toxicity from medications. Conjunctival injection and chemosis often result from antifungal agents, so their presence or absence cannot be used as an indication of the success of therapy.

Severe corneal damage can occur rapidly as a result of replicating fungi, mycotoxins, and enzymes, and the battle may be lost, particularly if treatment is delayed or a more virulent fungus is present. If there is no response to medication, the corneal infiltration and ulceration expand and a descemetocele (Fig. 10-9) or perforation can occur. This may happen despite effective microbial therapy; the host response to the infection, including difficulty with phagocytosis and removal of nonviable fungi, may itself cause progressive inflammation and ulceration.

As in bacterial keratitis, whenever the keratitis appears to be worsening despite therapy, repeat scrapings and cultures should be obtained. Another pathogen may be present, the initial diagnosis may have been incorrect, or there may be toxicity from medications. Reinfection from contaminated ocular medications or intravenous drug abuse also should be considered. If, in fact, the fungus appears to be resistant to the current regimen, another agent should be selected (Table 10-1).

Treatment should be continued long enough to allow the normal body defenses to cope with the remaining organisms. Long-term therapy, at least 6 weeks, should be anticipated. Negative scrapings or cultures during treatment are not sufficient to indicate eradication of the fungal agent, and great care should be exercised in discontinuing treatment. After medication is discontinued, the patient should be closely followed for evidence of recrudescence.

When infection extends into the anterior chamber, intraocular antifungal therapy is required. Often keratoplasty, lensectomy, excision of involved iris, and vitrectomy are also necessary.[24] Amphotericin B (10 µg) appears to be the best intraocular agent; miconazole (40 µg) also may be effective and appears to be well tolerated.[66]

Corticosteroids. In fungal infections, invasion of the cornea is aided by alteration of the host. One of the ways to impair host defenses at the time of inoculation of the fungal organism is through steroid use. Steroids aid growth of many fungi in the cornea and impair their elimination by the host.

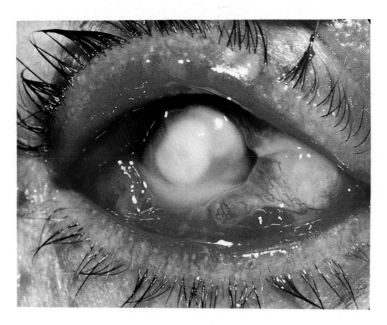

Fig. 10-9. Perforated *Fusarium solani* corneal ulcer.

The aim of giving corticosteroids in conjunction with the proper antifungal agent[67,68] is the control of active inflammation to minimize or eliminate structural alteration. If steroids are given for this reason, they should be given only after antifungal treatment has resulted in clinical improvement. Systemic steroids should not be given, effective antifungal agents should be given before topical steroids are introduced, and the patient must be immunologically competent and should be followed carefully. One must be prepared for the possibility of rapid worsening, including ulceration and perforation, which require surgical intervention.

If fungal infection is diagnosed in a patient who has been treated with topical corticosteroids, the medication should be decreased gradually. Abrupt cessation of steroids can be dangerous because a rebound response can arise and perforation can follow. Corticosteroids reduce inflammatory cell response to the infection, and, when the treatment is stopped, an exuberant response, with great release of destructive enzymes, can occur. Under these circumstances the cornea can perforate.

Surgical treatment. Regular debridement of the base of the ulcer is useful to remove organisms, necrotic stroma, and other inflammatory debris. This procedure can be performed with a scalpel blade or Kimura spatula. If the infection is superficial and localized, lamellar keratectomy can be useful.[69] However, this procedure usually is mainly a "debulking" of the infection; the infection often extends further than it appears clinically, so such surgery often results in incomplete removal. Treatment should be continued and the patient carefully monitored.

A conjunctival flap, the main treatment before development of antifungal agents, can still be useful in unresponsive cases. Bringing host vessels to the site of infection often improves killing and removal of the fungi and can prevent perforation. A deep lamellar keratectomy should be performed first and all necrotic stroma removed. Conjunctival flaps are particularly useful in localized peripheral infections; a partial inlay flap can treat the infection, greatly shortening the course and reducing morbidity while preserving vision.

If perforation occurs, tissue adhesive can be used to restore integrity. Penetrating keratoplasty can be useful if progressive ulceration or perforation occurs or if the infection does not respond to medi-

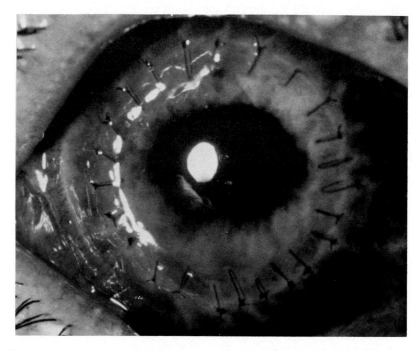

Fig. 10-10. Penetrating keratoplasty, 8.5 mm, for perforated fungal ulcer in Fig. 10-6.

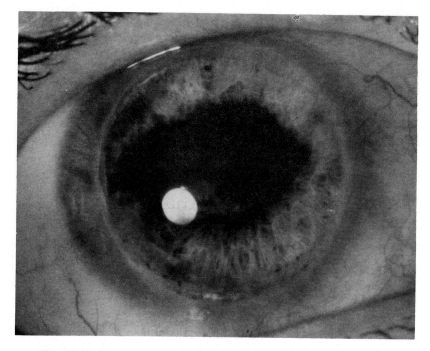

Fig. 10-11. Final result of clear corneal graft in case shown in Fig. 10-6.

cal treatment[70-75] (Figs. 10-10 and 10-11). Lamellar grafts should be avoided because of the frequent presence of fungi in the residual cornea, even if it is clear clinically, leading to recurrence of infection. The graft should encompass all clinically involved cornea, but incomplete removal should be expected. Antifungal therapy should be continued and steroid use minimized. Despite the likelihood that fungi are already present in the anterior chamber or are introduced during surgery, endophthalmitis rarely occurs.[24,76] Medical therapy is successful in the majority of cases and usually should be exhausted before resorting to keratoplasty. If a large residual corneal scar results from the ravages of the disease, a corneal transplant, which offers a better prognosis, can be performed at a later date. Forster and Rebell[45] reported that some form of early therapeutic surgery was required in 11 of 61 cases of fungal keratitis at their institution, penetrating keratoplasty being performed in nine cases. Patients most likely to require keratoplasty were those with deep seated infections and those who received corticosteroids before diagnosis.

PARASITES

Parasitic infections of the cornea are rare in the United States but are a major cause of morbidity and blindness in other parts of the world. Onchocerciasis is one of the four leading causes of blindness worldwide, affecting 40 to 50 million people in Africa and Central America, approximately 1 million of which develop blindness.[77] Interest in parasitic infections in the United States has increased recently because of the emergence of *Acanthamoeba* as an important pathogen. Although still rare, it has been recognized with increasing frequency, and treatment options are limited, often inadequate, and controversial.

ACANTHAMOEBA

Acanthamoeba is a genus of free-living protozoa of the subphyla Sarcodina. Like other protozoa, they are unicellular and can exist in two forms, active trophozoite and dormant cyst. The trophozoite form (16 to 47 μm long) is motile, proliferates, and feeds on bacteria, fungi, and other unicellular organisms. In adverse conditions the trophozoites encyst, forming a double wall containing cellulose. The cyst form (10 to 25 μm in diameter) is much more resistant to extreme environments, as well as to chlorine and other antimicrobial agents.

Acanthamoeba are ubiquitous, having been found in all types of liquid media, including tap water, bottled water, swimming pools, hot tubs, and contact lens solutions, as well as soil and air.[78] Their prevalence appears to peak during warmer weather. *Acanthamoeba* can be isolated from the mouth and pharynx of some asymptomatic adults and children,[79,80] and humoral immunity appears to be common in the general population.[81] Thus, although we are probably constantly exposed to these organisms, clinical infections rarely result. The reasons for the development of clinical infections are not known. It is likely that a break in the epithelial surface is necessary for entry of the organism, and repeated exposure, or inoculation into an immunoprivileged site, such as the cornea, may also be required. Concomitant infection with bacteria, fungi, or viruses may be necessary initially to provide the *Acanthamoeba* organism with food.[82,83] Like fungi, *Acanthamoeba* can be relatively nonimmunogenic; they often exist in the cornea without surrounding inflammatory cell infiltration. They release enzymes, including phospholipases, lysozyme, and cellulase. Some species are more pathogenic than others, but the factors that determine virulence have not been identified.

Clinical infections elsewhere in the body also have been rare. The most common is a granulomatous encephalitis, which is usually fatal. Single cases of ear, mandible, orbit, and skin infection have been reported, as well as one case of intraocular extension of a meningeal infection.

The first case report of *Acanthamoeba* keratitis appeared in 1974[84]; since then numerous cases have been diagnosed.[85-91] It appears that it is not just that cases are more likely to be recognized, but that the incidence of the disease is increasing rapidly. The majority of recent cases have been related to contact lens wear, most commonly soft contact lenses, and the use of contaminated solutions, including tap water, well water, homemade saline solutions, and saliva. In these cases, *Acanthamoeba* is usually isolated from one or more of the sources cited earlier, as well as bacteria and fungi, which may serve as a food source for the *Acanthamoeba*.[92,93] Those cases not associated with contact lens wear have followed corneal trauma, but the source of the *Acanthamoeba* is often unclear. Although patients of any age can be affected, *Acanthamoeba* keratitis is most common in young adults. They are usually in good health and are immunocompetent.

Clinical manifestations. The clinical features of *Acanthamoeba* keratitis are given in Table 10-5.[94,95] Symptoms include pain, photophobia, irritation, foreign body sensation, tearing, and de-

TABLE 10-5. Clinical Features of *Acanthamoeba* Keratitis

FEATURE	FREQUENCY	WHEN PRESENT
Pain	+ + + +	E,L*
Ring infiltrate	+ + +	L
Central stromal infiltrate	+ + +	L
Epithelial haze, punctate staining, pseudodendrites, elevated lines	+ +	E,L
Recurrent epithelial breakdown	+ +	E,L
Decreased corneal sensation	+ +	E,L
Radial keratoneuritis	+	E
Scleritis	+	L
Adenopathy	+	
Hypopyon	+	L
Increased intraocular pressure	+	L

*E, Early; L, late.

creased vision. The pain is often severe and out of proportion to the signs of inflammation. In the earliest stages of infection, signs may be limited to the epithelium. Epithelial defects, pseudodendrites (Fig. 10-12), punctate staining, haze, elevated epithelial lines, and microcysts may be present. In early stromal involvement, edema is more prominent than infiltration (Fig. 10-13). The pattern of stromal infiltration varies, but it is generally most dense in the midperiphery, sometimes forming a complete ring (Fig. 10-14). Usually there is a central infiltrate, but the cornea within the ring can be relatively clear. A double ring, or a central infiltrate alone, can also be observed. Satellite infiltrates,

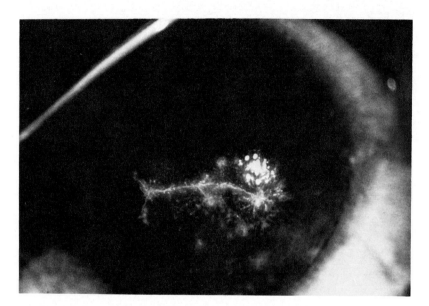

Fig. 10-12. Pseudodendritic epithelial staining in *Acanthamoeba* keratitis.

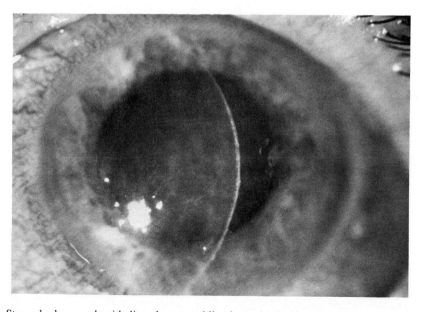

Fig. 10-13. Stromal edema and epitheliopathy, resembling herpetic disciform keratitis, in *Acanthamoeba* infection.

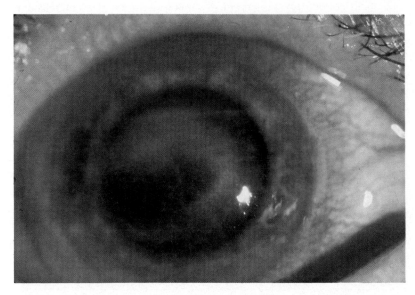

Fig. 10-14. Ring infiltrate in *Acanthamoeba* keratitis. (Courtesy Y. Jerold Gordon, Pittsburgh.)

which may appear granular, may be present outside the ring. The epithelium overlying the infiltrates can be intact, but often there is recurrent epithelial breakdown.

Radial keratoneuritis occurs in a minority of cases but seems to be pathognomonic (Fig. 10-15). Fluffy infiltrates are observed along the course of one or more corneal nerves. These infiltrates may involve the central or peripheral portions of the nerves; they are often transient and can precede other forms of stromal infiltration.[89] Neural inflammation may be responsible for the unusually intense pain that many of these patients experience. It also can explain why decreased corneal sensation is frequently observed.

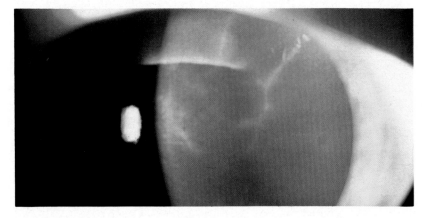

Fig. 10-15. Radial keratoneuritis in *Acanthamoeba* keratitis. (Courtesy Scott Portnoy, Pittsburgh.)

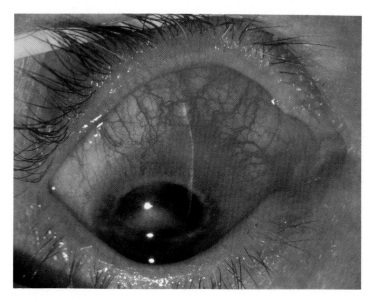

Fig. 10-16. Nodular scleritis in *Acanthamoeba* keratitis. (Courtesy Y. Jerold Gordon, Pittsburgh.)

Nodular or diffuse scleritis may be associated with the keratitis, usually adjacent to the limbus (Fig. 10-16). Anterior chamber reaction is usually present and can be severe enough to produce an hypopyon or increased intraocular pressure. Adenopathy has been present in some cases.

Diagnosis. As can be inferred form the previous description, the clinical presentation of *Acanthamoeba* keratitis is rarely diagnostic. However, some features should make one suspect *Acanthamoeba,* and this suspicion is most important in making the diagnosis. Specimens should be inoculated onto nonnutrient agar, which has been overlayed with *Escherichia coli* or *Enterobacter aerogenes,* although growth on blood or chocolate agar has occurred in some cases. Most standard stains, including Gram, Giemsa, or Wright, will indicate the organism when it is present in smears, but often a careful search by an experienced observer is required. Calcofluor white and acridine orange can facilitate detection.

These tests are often unsuccessful, however, particularly early in the course. Removal and examination of intact but abnormal epithelium may be helpful, but corneal biopsy is often required for diagnosis. If the patient has worn contact lenses, the lenses and all solutions should be cultured. Isolation of the organism is suggestive and may be sufficient to initiate therapy, providing the clinical presentation is consistent.

Treatment. Overall, the treatment for *Acanthamoeba* keratitis has been disappointing, to some extent because the infection was usually well advanced before diagnosis; however, available treatment is also suboptimum. A few drugs kill trophozoites in vitro, but it is unclear whether any are cysticidal. Evaluation of the drugs has been restricted by the small number of cases treated, the varying stages at which treatment was initiated, the natural waxing and waning of the disease, and the differences among *Acanthamoeba* strains. Improvement is slow with any of these agents, and unless medical treatment is initiated very early in the course of an infection, prolonged therapy is necessary. It is likely that excystation or host removal of remaining organisms is required to eliminate the infection.

Early penetrating keratoplasty has been advocated by some to remove or debulk the resistant infection. Although this procedure can be successful, in many cases the organism is present in the remaining tissue, and infection recurs in the graft. *Acanthamoeba* infection frequently extends into apparently clear stroma, and its limits cannot be appreciated without tissue examination. Recurrent infections in the corneal graft tend to be even more difficult to treat than primary infections.

In general, medical therapy should be pursued if the condition is responsive. Penetrating keratoplasty is best performed after prolonged medical treatment; in reported cases, recurrences were less common if medical treatment had been given for at least 4 months before surgery.[94] Penetrating keratoplasty can be considered earlier, however, if the diagnosis is made early in the course of infection and it is felt that all involved tissue can be excised. Certainly, if perforation occurs, keratoplasty may be necessary to preserve the globe.

Antiamebic agents. The following drugs have been effective against *Acanthamoeba* in vitro:

Diamidines
1. Propamidine (Brolene eye drops)
2. Dibromopropamidine (Brolene ointment)
3. Others (for example, stilbamidine, pentamidine)

Imidazoles
4. Ketoconazole
5. Miconazole
6. Clotrimazole

Aminoglycosides
7. Neomycin
8. Paromomycin

Pyridones
9. Ciclopirox olamine

The following were less consistency effective and required higher concentrations than the previous agents:

Polypeptides
10. Polymyxin B

Polyenes
11. Amphotericin B
12. Natamycin

Pyrimidine
13. 5-Flucytosine

Diamidines. To date the experience with propamidine has been the most extensive, and some medical cures have been achieved, mainly in combined use with polymyxin B-neomycin-gramicidin drops (Neosporin).[96,97] Propamidine has antibacterial and antifungal activity and is sold over the counter in Britain but is not available in the United States. The recommended treatment regimen is as follows (The Brolene Study Group, Coordinated by Bausch & Lomb Pharmaceuticals): Initially propamidine and polymyxin B-neomycin-gramicidin drops are alternated every 30 to 60 minutes around the clock, for 3 days. For the remainder of the first week, drops are given hourly during the day and every 2 hours at night. Administration is then gradually tapered to four times/day. Dibromopropamidine ointment can be given at bedtime. Treatment should be continued for at least 1 year in most cases.

Propamidine is toxic to the epithelial surface, often causing conjunctival injection and chemosis, corneal epithelial microcysts, and punctate keratopathy.[98]

Imidazoles. Miconazole, clotrimazole, and ketoconazole were effective in vitro against some strains of *Acanthamoeba*. Topical miconazole, topical clotrimazole 1% to 2%, and oral ketoconazole (200 to 400 mg/day) were effective in some patients but not in others. Probably the most promising of the imidazoles is clotrimazole, which has been used successfully in several cases in conjunction with propamidine or after unsuccessful treatment with propamidine.[99] In some of these cases, clotrimazole was the most effective agent in vitro. In some cases the 1% dermatologic cream (commercially available) is tolerated, but in others clotrimazole powder must be obtained from Schering Laboratories (Kenilworth, NJ) and a 1% to 2% suspension formulated in artificial tears. Miconazole may be effective, but also can be irritating, and must be reformulated weekly because it is unstable in solution. Although oral ketoconazole may be useful, it carries a small risk of hepatotoxicity.

Others. The aminoglycosides neomycin and paromomycin appear to be less effective than the previous two groups, but they may be useful in combination with other agents. Neomycin is somewhat toxic and can induce hypersensitivity reactions.

Other treatment. In *Acanthamoeba* keratitis, as in other forms of infectious keratitis, the use of corticosteroids is controversial. Corticosteroids reduce inflammation and increase comfort but also reduce the host's capacity to eradicate the infection. In *Acanthamoeba* keratitis the antimicrobial agents currently available cannot kill all the organisms in the cornea, particularly the cyst forms, and the host response appears to be particularly important. In addition, corticosteroids inhibit excystation of the organism into the more susceptible trophozoite form, at least in vitro.[100] Clinically the effect of corticosteroids on outcome is not clear, but results seem to be better if corticosteroid use is avoided or kept to a minimum.

The usefulness of cryotherapy of infected corneas is not clear. It did not prevent recurrence of *Acanthamoeba* after keratoplasty in one case,[101] but it appeared to be useful in five others.[102] In two in vitro studies, the cysts were resistant to cryotherapy in one[103] and sensitive to it in another[104]; the combination of cryotherapy and antibiotics was more effective than antibiotics alone.

Relief of the pain associated with these infections can be difficult. Success with sulindac (Clinoril), a nonsteroidal antiinflammatory agent, has been reported in some patients. In resistant cases retrobulbar injections of alcohol may be used. A 1-ml injection, consisting of ⅓ ml absolute alcohol and ⅔ ml 2% lidocaine will give anesthesia for 2 to 4 weeks, with full recovery. Temporary ptosis and other nerve palsies can also occur.

Prevention. Proper contact lens hygiene probably can prevent the development of *Acanthamoeba* keratitis. Homemade saline solutions, tap water, and saliva should be avoided. Patients should not swim while wearing their lenses. Avoidance of bacterial and fungal contamination of lenses, lens cases, and solutions will probably also help prevent *Acanthamoeba* infection. Heat disinfection is effective in killing *Acanthamoeba* cysts and trophozoites. Hydrogen peroxide disinfection systems were effective if they did not contain a metal catalyst and exposure was for at least 2 hours.[105] Chlorhexidine and benzalkonium have variable effect: They appear to kill both trophozoites and cysts of some isolates, but in other cases they were not effective against either.[105-109] Thimerosal, sorbic acid, ethylenediaminetetraacetic acid (EDTA), and quarternary ammonium compounds are generally ineffective.

OTHER PROTOZOA

Leishmania are flagellated obligate intracellular protozoa that are members of the subphylum Mastigophora. They are found in Africa, Central America, the Middle East, India, and South America. The reservoir of the organisms is in rodents and dogs, and infection is transmitted to humans by infected sandflies. Involvement of the conjunctiva or cornea is more commonly seen in the Americas. It usually occurs by autoinoculation from a nearby infection or direct extension. Corneal involvement begins as a phlyctenule-like process but quickly progresses to deep infiltration and abscess formation.[110,111] Perforation can occur after 3 to 4 weeks. Treatment is with meglumine antimoniate and sodium stibogluconate, either intravenously or intramuscularly.

Microsporida are small obligate intracellular protozoa that rarely cause keratitis.[112,113] Infection may be more commonly seen in patients with acquired immune deficiency syndrome (AIDS), where it causes mainly epithelial rather than stromal disease.[114] No effective treatment is known.

ONCHOCERCIASIS

Onchocerca volvulus is a filarial nematode (threadworm) that is an endemic cause of infection (river blindness) in Central and Western Africa, Central America, and the northernmost portions of South America. Larvae are transmitted to humans via the *Simulium* black fly. These develop into adults in the subcutaneous tissue, and the females release microfilaria that migrate through the skin and subcutaneous tissue. The microfilariae are 0.22 to 0.36 mm long and 5 to 10 μm in diameter. They can migrate into any portion of the globe, including the conjunctiva, cornea, and anterior chamber, either by direct invasion or via the blood.

In endemic areas most individuals are infected in the first few years of life. The living organism tends to be well tolerated, but upon its death a reaction ensues. The more severe complications usually occur after many years of chronic infestation or with microfilaricidal treatment.

The earliest evidence of ocular involvement is the presence of live organisms. The living microfilaria can be seen easily in the anterior chamber, and this is facilitated by having the patient sit with the head between the knees for 2 minutes before examination to concentrate the organisms in the central anterior aqueous. Detection of live microfilariae in the corneal stroma is more difficult because they are transparent, immobile, and often coiled.

The signs of conjunctival involvement include injection, chemosis, swelling of the lids, limbitis, and phlyctenules. *Limbitis* is seen as small, pale, yellow globules at the limbus, which often form acutely, either spontaneously or after initiation of antifilarial treatment. The lesions are thought to represent eosinophilic granuloma formation around dead microfilariae.

The earliest corneal inflammatory lesions occur near the limbus as a localized transient reaction around a dead worm. The cellular infiltrate consists of lymphocytes and eosinophils.[115] Later, other "snowflake" or "nummular" infiltrates can occur throughout the stroma and are also transient. All of these localized infiltrates are referred to as *punctate keratitis.* A more severe reaction, *sclerosing keratitis,* is a diffuse infiltrative process that begins inferiorly and can progress upward to involve the entire cornea, leaving permanent scarring and vascularization in its wake.[116,117]

In addition to the aforementioned findings, anterior uveitis, optic neuritis, optic atrophy, and chorioretinitis may occur in onchocerciasis. Ivermectin, 150 mg/kg orally, repeated annually, appears

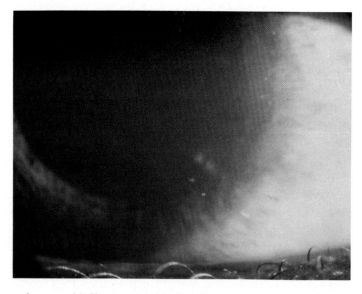

Fig. 10-17. Nummular corneal infiltrates caused by *Loa loa*. (Courtesy Massimo Busin, Bonn, Germany.)

to be the most effective treatment and is less likely than diethylcarbamazine to cause exacerbation of ocular inflammation.[118,119]

OTHER PARASITES

A number of other parasites can cause corneal inflammation, including *Loa loa* (Fig. 10-17), *Trypanosoma* and *Multiceps*.[120,121]

REFERENCES

1. Jones DB, Sexton RR, and Rebell G: Mycotic keratitis in South Florida: a review of thirty-eight cases, Trans Ophthalmol Soc UK 89:781, 1969.
2. Forster RK and Rebell G: The diagnosis and management of keratomycoses. I. Cause and diagnosis, Arch Ophthalmol 93:975, 1975.
3. Richman RA et al: Candidiasis and multiple endocrinopathy with oral squamous cell carcinoma complications, Arch Dermatol 111:625, 1975.
4. Forster RK, Rebell G, and Wilson LA: Dermatiaceous fungal keratitis: clinical isolates and management, Br J Ophthalmol 59:372, 1975.
5. Jones BR: Principles in the management of oculomycosis: XXXI Edward Jackson Memorial Lecture, Am J Ophthalmol 79:15, 1975.
6. Naumann G, Green WR, and Zimmerman LE: Mycotic keratitis, Am J Ophthalmol 64:668, 1969.
7. Kaufman HE and Wood RM: Mycotic keratitis, Am J Ophthalmol 59:993, 1965.
8. Jones BR, Richards AB, and Morgan G: Direct fungal infection of the eye in Britain, Trans Ophthalmol Soc UK 89:727, 1969.
9. Doughman DJ et al: Fungal keratitis at the University of Minnesota 1971-1981, Trans Am Ophthalmol Soc 80:235, 1982.
10. Rippon JW: Medical mycology: the pathogenic fungi and actinomycetes, Philadelphia, 1974, WB Saunders.
11. Liesegang TJ and Forster RF: Spectrum of microbial keratitis in South Florida, Am J Ophthalmol 90:38, 1980.
12. Rodrigues MM and Laibson P: Exogenous mycotic keratitis caused by *Blastomyces dermatitidis*, Am J Ophthalmol 75:782, 1973.
13. Poria VC et al: Study of mycotic keratitis, Indian J Ophthalmol 33:229, 1985.
14. Montes LF, Krumdiek C, and Cornwell PE: Hypovitaminosis in patients with mucocutaneous candidiasis, J Infect Dis 128:227, 1973.
15. Burda CD and Fisher E: Corneal destruction by extracts of *Cephalosporium mycelium*, Am J Ophthalmol 50:926, 1960.
16. Okumoto M: Infectious agents: fungi. In Smolin G and Thoft RA, editors: The cornea: scientific foundations and clinical practice, Boston, 1983, Little, Brown & Co.
17. Rogers TJ and Balish E: Immunity to *Candida albicans*, Microbiol Rev 44:660, 1980.
18. Donzis PB et al: Microbial contamination of contact lens care systems, Am J Ophthalmol 104:325, 1987.
19. Simmons RB et al: Morphology and ultrastructure of fungi in extended-wear soft contact lenses, J Clin Microbiol 24:21, 1986.
20. Yamaguchi T et al: Fungus growth on soft contact lenses with different water contents, CLAO J 10:166, 1984.
21. Wilhelmus KR et al: Fungal keratitis in contact lens wearers, Am J Ophthalmol 106:708, 1988.
22. Aronson SB and Elliot JH: Ocular inflammation, St Louis, 1972, Mosby–Year Book, Inc.
23. Dudley MA and Chick EW: Corneal lesions produced in rabbits by an extract of *Fusarium moniliforme*, Arch Ophthalmol 72:346, 1964.
24. Pflugfelder SC et al: Exogenous fungal endophthalmitis, Ophthalmology 95:19, 1988.
25. Jones BR et al: Corneal and intraocular infection due to *Fusarium solani*, Trans Ophthalmol Soc UK 89:757, 1969.
26. Jones DB et al: Early diagnosis of mycotic keratitis, Trans Ophthalmol Soc UK 89:805, 1969.
27. Wilson LA and Sexton RR: Laboratory diagnosis in fungal keratitis, Am J Ophthalmol 66:646, 1968.
28. Wilson LA and Sexton RR: Laboratory aids in diagnosis. In Duane T and Jaeger E, editors: Clinical ophthalmology, vol. 4, Philadelphia, 1988, Harper & Row.
29. Jones DB: Strategy for the initial management of suspected microbial keratitis. In New Orleans Academy of Ophthalmology. Symposium on medical and surgical diseases of the cornea, St Louis, 1980, Mosby–Year Book, Inc.
30. Ishibashi Y, Hommura S, and Matsumoto Y: Direct examination vs culture of biopsy specimens for the diagnosis of keratomycosis, Am J Ophthalmol 103:636, 1987.
31. Ishibashi Y and Kaufman HE: Corneal biopsy in the diagnosis of keratomycosis, Am J Ophthalmol 101:288, 1986.
32. O'Day DN, Robinson RD, and Head WS: Efficacy of antifungal agents in the cornea. I. A comparative study, Invest Ophthalmol Vis Sci 24:1098, 1983.
33. Anderson B and Chick EW: Treatment of corneal fungal ulcers with amphotericin B and mechanical debridement, South Med J 56:270, 1963.
34. Green WR, Bennett JE, and Goos RD: Ocular penetration of amphotericin B, Arch Ophthalmol 73:769, 1965.
35. O'Day DM et al: Corneal penetration of amphotericin B and natamycin, Curr Eye Res 5:877, 1986.
36. O'Day DM et al: Bioavailability and penetration of topical amphotericin B in the anterior segment of the rabbit eye, J Ocul Pharmacol 2:371, 1986.
37. Bindschadler DO and Bennett JE: A pharmacologic guide to the clinical use of amphotericin B, J Infect Dis 170:427, 1969.
38. Wood TO, Tuberville AW, and Monnett R: Keratomy-

cosis and amphotericin B, Trans Am Ophthalmol Soc 83:397, 1985.

39. Medoff G and Kobayaski GS: Strategies in the treatment of systemic fungal infections, N Engl J Med 302:145, 1980.
40. Raab WP: Natamycin (pimaricin): its properties and possibilities in medicine, Stuttgart, 1972, Georg Thieme Verlag.
41. Johns KJ and O'Day DM: Pharmacologic management of keratomycoses, Surv Ophthalmol 33:178, 1988.
42. Jones DB, Forster RL, and Rebell G: *Fusarium solani* keratitis treated with natamycin (pimaricin): 18 consecutive cases, Arch Ophthalmol 88:147, 1972.
43. Forster RK: Fungal diseases. In Smolin G and Thoft RA, editors: The cornea: scientific foundations and clinical practice, Boston, 1983, Little Brown.
44. Newmark E et al: Clinical experience with pimaricin therapy in fungal keratitis, South Med J 64:935, 1971.
45. Forster RK and Rebell G: The diagnosis and management of keratomycoses. II. Medical and surgical management, Arch Ophthalmol 93:1134, 1975.
46. O'Day DM et al: In vitro and in vivo susceptibility of *Candida* keratitis to topical polyenes, Curr Eye Res 6:363, 1987.
47. Sud IJ and Feingold DS: Mechanism of action of the antimycotic imidazoles, J Invest Dermatol 76:438, 1981.
48. Beggs WH and Hughes CE: Exploitation of the direct cell damaging action of antifungal azoles, Diag Microbiol Infect Dis 6:1, 1987.
49. Foster CS and Stefanyszyn M: Intraocular penetration of miconazole in rabbits, Arch Ophthalmol 97:1703, 1979.
50. Stevens DA, Levine HB, and Deresinski SC: Miconazole in coccidioidomycosis. II. Therapeutic and pharmacologic studies in man, Am J Ophthalmol 80:191, 1976.
51. Foster CS: Miconazole therapy for keratomycosis, Am J Ophthalmol 91:622, 1981.
52. Fitzsimons R and Peters AL: Miconazole and ketoconazole as a satisfactory first-line treatment for keratomycosis, Am J Ophthalmol 101:605, 1986.
53. Ishibashi Y, Matsumoto Y, and Takei K: The effects of intravenous miconazole on fungal keratitis, Am J Ophthalmol 98:433, 1984.
54. Jones DB, Jones BR, and Robinson NM: Clotrimazole (Canesten) therapy of fungal keratitis, Chemotherapy 6:189, 1975.
55. Chu W et al: Intraocular penetration of ketoconazole in rabbits, Invest Ophthalmol Vis Sci 18(suppl):133, 1979.
56. Torres MA et al: Topical ketoconazole for fungal keratitis, Am J Ophthalmol 100:293, 1985.
57. Ishibashi Y and Kaufman HE: Topical ketoconazole for experimental *Candida* keratitis in rabbits, Am J Ophthalmol 102:522, 1986.
58. Ishibashi Y: Oral ketoconazole therapy for keratomycosis, Am J Ophthalmol 95:342, 1983.
59. Ishibashi Y and Matsumoto Y: Oral ketoconazole therapy for experimental *Candida albicans* keratitis in rabbits, Sabouraudia 22:323, 1984.
60. Komadina TG et al: Treatment of *Aspergillus fumiga-*

tus keratitis in rabbits with oral and topical ketoconazole, Am J Ophthalmol 99:476, 1985.
61. Steer PL et al: 5-Fluorocytosine, an oral antifungal compound: a report on clinical and laboratory experience, Ann Intern Med 76:15, 1972.
62. Symoens J: Clinical and experimental evidence on miconazole for the treatment of systemic mycoses: a review, Proc R Soc Med 70:4, 1977.
63. Block E and Bennett J: Pharmacologic studies with 5-fluorocytosine, Antimicrob Agents Chemother 1:476, 1972.
64. Bennett JE: Flucytosine, Ann Intern Med 86:319, 1977.
65. O'Day DM et al: In vitro and in vivo susceptibility of *Candida* keratitis to topical polyenes, Invest Ophthalmol Vis Sci 28:874, 1987.
66. Tolentino FI et al: Toxicity of intravitreous miconazole, Arch Ophthalmol 100:1504, 1982.
67. Newmark E, Ellison AC, and Kaufman HE: Combined pimaricin and dexamethasone therapy of keratomycosis, Am J Ophthalmol 71:718, 1971.
68. O'Day DM, Moore T, and Aronson S: Deep fungal corneal abscess: combined corticosteroid therapy, Arch Ophthalmol 86:414, 1971.
69. Sanitato JJ, Kelly CG, and Kaufman HE: Surgical management of peripheral fungal keratitis, Arch Ophthalmol 102:1507, 1984.
70. Polack FM, Kaufman HE, and Newmark E: Keratomycosis, medical and surgical treatment, Arch Ophthalmol 85:410, 1971.
71. Singh G and Malik SR: Therapeutic keratoplasty in fungal corneal ulcers, Br J Ophthalmol 56:41, 1972.
72. Forster RK and Rebell G: Therapeutic surgery in failures of medical treatment of fungal keratitis, Br J Ophthalmol 59:366, 1975.
73. Sanders N: Penetrating keratoplasty in treatment of fungus keratitis, Am J Ophthalmol 70:24, 1970.
74. Jones BR, Jones DB, and Richards AB: Surgery in the management of keratomycosis, Trans Ophthalmol Soc UK 89:887, 1976.
75. Hill JC: Use of penetrating keratoplasty in acute bacterial keratitis, Br J Ophthalmol 70:502, 1986.
76. Wilson LA and Cavanagh HD: Penetrating keratoplasty for exogenous *Paecilomyces* keratitis followed by postoperative endophthalmitis, Am J Ophthalmol 98:552, 1984.
77. O'Day J and Mackenzie CD: Ocular onchocerciasis: diagnosis and current clinical approaches, Trop Doct 15:87, 1985.
78. Warhurst DC: Pathogenic free-living amoebae, Parasitol Today 1:24, 1985.
79. Wang SS and Feldman HA: Isolation of *Hartmanella* species from human throats, N Engl J Med 277:1174, 1967.
80. Rivera F et al: Pathogenic and free-living protozoa cultured from the nasopharyngeal and oral regions of dental patients, Environ Res 33:428, 1984.
81. Cursons RTM, Brown TJ, and Keys EA: Immunity to pathogenic free-living amoebae, Lancet 1:877, 1977.
82. Martinez AJ and Janitschke K: *Acanthamoeba,* an opportunistic microorganism: a review, Infection 13:251, 1985.

83. Jones DB: *Acanthamoeba*—the ultimate opportunist? Am J Ophthalmol 102:527, 1986.

84. Nagington J et al: Amoebic infection of the eye, Lancet 2:1547, 1974.

85. Hirst LW et al: Management of *Acanthamoeba* keratitis: a case report and review of the literature, Ophthalmology 91:1105, 1984.

86. Cohen EJ et al: Diagnosis and management of *Acanthamoeba* keratitis, Am J Ophthalmol 100:389, 1985.

87. Moore MB et al: *Acanthamoeba* keratitis associated with soft contact lenses, Am J Ophthalmol 100:396, 1985.

88. Theodore FH et al: The diagnostic value of a ring infiltrate in acanthamoebic keratitis, Ophthalmology 92:1471, 1985.

89. Moore MB et al: Radial keratoneuritis as a presenting sign in *Acanthamoeba* keratitis, Ophthalmology 93:1310, 1986.

90. Moore MB et al: *Acanthamoeba* keratitis: a growing problem in hard and soft contact lens wearers, Ophthalmology 94:1654, 1987.

91. Florakis GJ et al: Elevated epithelial lines in *Acanthamoeba* keratitis, Arch Ophthalmol 106:1202, 1988.

92. Donzis PB, Mondino BJ, and Weissman BA: Microbial contamination of contact lens care systems associated with *Acanthamoeba* keratitis, Presented at the OMIG meeting, Dallas, November 1987.

93. Larkin DFP, Kilvington S, and Easty DL: Contamination of contact lens storage cases by *Acanthamoeba* and bacteria, Br J Ophthalmol 74:133, 1990.

94. Auran JD, Starr MB, and Jakobiec FA: *Acanthamoeba* keratitis: a review of the literature, Cornea 6:2, 1987.

95. Moore MB: Parasitic infections. In Kaufman HE et al, editors: The cornea, New York, 1988, Churchill Livingstone.

96. Wright P, Warhurst D, and Jones BR: *Acanthamoeba* keratitis successfully treated medically, Br J Ophthalmol 69:778, 1985.

97. Moore MB and McCulley JP: *Acanthamoeba* keratitis associated with contact lenses: six cases of successful management, Br J Ophthalmol 73:271, 1989.

98. Johns K, Head S, and O'Day D: Corneal toxicity of propamidine, Arch Ophthalmol 106:68, 1988.

99. Driebe WT et al: *Acanthamoeba* keratitis: potential role for topical clotrimazole in combination chemotherapy, Arch Ophthalmol 106:1196, 1988.

100. Mathers WD et al: Immunopathology and electron microscopy of *Acanthamoeba* keratitis, Presented at OMIG, New Orleans, November 1986.

101. Samples JR et al: Management of *Acanthamoeba* keratitis possibly acquired from a hot tub, Arch Ophthalmol 105:707, 1984.

102. Binder PS: Cryotherapy for medically unresponsive *Acanthamoeba* keratitis, Cornea 8:106, 1989.

103. Meisler DM et al: Susceptibility of *Acanthamoeba* to cryotherapeutic method, Arch Ophthalmol 104:130, 1986.

104. Matoba AY et al: The effects of freezing and antibiotics on the viability of *Acanthamoeba* cysts, Arch Ophthalmol 107:439, 1989.

105. Silvany RE et al: The effect of currently available contact lens disinfection systems on *Acanthamoeba castellanii* and *Acanthamoeba polyphagia,* Ophthalmology 97:286, 1990.

106. Prasad NK: In vitro effect of drugs against pathogenic and non-pathogenic free-living amoebae and anaerobic amoebae, Indian J Exp Biol 10:43, 1972.

107. Ludwig IH et al: Susceptibility of *Acanthamoeba* in soft contact lens disinfecting systems, Invest Ophthalmol Vis Sci 27:626, 1986.

108. Penley CA, Willis SW, and Sickler SG: Comparative antimicrobial efficacy of soft and rigid gas permeable contact lens solutions against *Acanthamoeba,* CLAO J 15:257, 1989.

109. Brockman RJ et al: Survival of *Acanthamoeba* in contact lens rinse solutions, Invest Ophthalmol Vis Sci 28(suppl):370, 1987.

110. Duke-Elder S and Leigh AG: System of ophthalmology, vol VIII: diseases of the outer eye, St Louis, 1965, Mosby–Year Book, Inc.

111. Roizenblatt J: Interstitial keratitis caused by American (mucocutaneous) leishmaniasis, Am J Ophthalmol 87:175, 1979.

112. Pinnolis M et al: Nosematosis of the cornea. Case report, including electron microscopic studies, Arch Ophthalmol 99:1044, 1981.

113. Ashton N and Wirasinha P: Encephalitozoonosis (nosematosis) of the cornea, Br J Ophthalmol 57:669, 1973.

114. Friedberg DN et al: Microsporidal keratoconjunctivitis in acquired immunodeficiency syndrome, Arch Ophthalmol 108:504, 1990.

115. Garner A: Pathology of ocular onchocerciasis: human and experimental, Trans R Soc Trop Med Hyg 70:374, 1976.

116. Duke-Elder S and Leigh AG: System of ophthalmology, vol VIII: diseases of the outer eye, St Louis, 1965, Mosby–Year Book, Inc.

117. O'Day J and Mackenzie CD: Ocular onchocerciasis: diagnosis and current clinical approaches, Trop Doct 15:87, 1985.

118. Dadzie KY et al: Ocular findings in a double-blind study of ivermectin versus diethylcarbamazine versus placebo in the treatment of onchocerciasis, Br J Ophthalmol 71:78, 1987.

119. Taylor HR et al: Treatment of onchocerciasis: the ocular effects of ivermectin and diethylcarbamazine, Arch Ophthalmol 104:863, 1986.

120. Moore MB: Parasitic infections. In Kaufman HE et al, editors: The cornea, New York, 1988, Churchill Livingstone.

121. Duke-Elder S and Leigh AG: System of ophthalmology, vol VIII: diseases of the outer eye, St Louis, 1965, Mosby–Year Book, Inc.

INTERSTITIAL KERATITIS

The term "interstitial keratitis" refers to vascularization and nonsuppurative infiltration affecting the corneal stroma, usually associated with a systemic disease.

Nonsuppurative, nondisciform interstitial keratitis may be caused by the following pathologic conditions, the first 10 of which are the most common:

1. Congenital syphilis
2. Acquired syphilis
3. Tuberculosis
4. Leprosy
5. Onchocerciasis
6. Infectious mononucleosis
7. Lymphogranuloma venereum
8. Cogan's syndrome
9. Herpes zoster
10. Herpes simplex
11. Gold toxicity
12. Mumps
13. Rubeola
14. Vaccinia
15. Variola
16. Leishmaniasis[1]
17. Trypanosomiasis
18. Hodgkin's disease (rare)
19. Kaposi's sarcoma (rare)
20. Mycosis fungoides (rare)
21. Sarcoid (rare)
22. Incontinentia pigmenti (rare)
23. Toxicity to drugs such as arsenicals
24. Influenza (rare)

Nonsystemic conditions that may result in interstitial keratitis are chemical burns of the eye and chromium deficiency (in laboratory animals).[2]

Disciform keratitis is a circular area of corneal edema with intact epithelium and minimal infiltration. It is of variable size, and may be central or peripheral. Herpes simplex is the most common cause, but herpes zoster, early fungal or *Acanthamoeba* infection, mumps, varicella, variola, and vaccinia can also produce this picture.

Nondisciform interstitial keratitis may be diffuse, sectoral, focal, or multifocal (nummular). For purposes of discussion, interstitial keratitis will be divided into diffuse or sectoral types and nummular types.

DIFFUSE OR SECTORAL INTERSTITIAL KERATITIS
CONGENITAL AND ACQUIRED SYPHILIS

Approximately 90% of interstitial keratitis is caused by syphilis, with 87% resulting from congenital lues and 3% from acquired lues.

Based on the following indirect evidence, it appears that the host's immune response to the infection, rather than active bacterial proliferation, is responsible for the clinical disease:

1. Interstitial keratitis rarely develops in early congenital syphilis when *Treponema pallidum* abounds; it usually is delayed by many years.
2. Treponemes are rarely found in the corneas of patients with active interstitial keratitis.
3. Interstitial keratitis does not respond to penicillin or other antitreponemal agents and may actually worsen.
4. The cornea often shows prompt clinical improvement with corticosteroids.

Interstitial keratitis seems to have a higher incidence in females.[3] About two thirds of the cases resulting from congenital syphilis occur when patients are between 5 years and late teens; cases after age 30 are rare. The congenital form of disease is usually bilateral (80%), with the second eye becoming involved within a year in 75% of cases. As time passes, the second eye has less tendency to be affected, being involved after 5 years in only 2% of cases.

The interstitial keratitis secondary to acquired syphilis may occur within months after the onset of the infection but generally occurs 10 years later. The clinical course closely resembles that in congenital syphilis except that interstitial keratitis in acquired syphilis is usually uniocular (60% of cases), frequently milder, limited to a sector of cornea, and occasionally more amenable to treatment.

Clinical manifestations. The first signs of congenital luetic interstitial keratitis, which may precede symptoms by as much as several weeks, consist of an indistinct cellular infiltrate and edema in the endothelium followed by keratic precipitates and tiny opacities of the stroma. If untreated, the disease then passes through progressive, florid, and retrogressive stages.

The progressive stage, which usually lasts 1 to 2 weeks, begins with severe symptoms of pain, lacrimation, photophobia, and blepharospasm and is accompanied by circumcorneal vascular injection. The cornea becomes rapidly and extensively cloudy over a period of a few days, and then blood vessels begin to enter the peripheral cornea. Iridocyclitis and anterior choroiditis occur during this stage.

In the florid stage the changes that began in the progressive stage become more evident. The acute inflammation of the eye and heavy deep vascularization of the cornea persist for about 2 to 4 months. A wrinkling or folding of Descemet's membrane usually occurs.

The corneal cloudiness is a result of changes in all corneal layers. Stromal cellular infiltration usually appears as faint gray, soft-edged opacities that increase in number and coalesce to form a general haze. In other cases the process is generalized from the start, or clouding begins centrally. It imparts to the cornea a ground-glass appearance and can reduce vision to light perception. Epithelial edema occurs and may progress to vesicle and bullae formation.

Vascular invasion occurs in areas with stromal infiltration and starts from the periphery. Both superficial and deep vascularization can be seen. Superficial vessels, which can extend several millimeters onto the cornea, produce a crescentic elevation, which has been called an "epaulet" of vascularization. Deeper vessels run between the stromal lamellae in long, wavy, parallel lines. The extent of vascular invasion can vary widely. If the opacities begin in one sector, the vascularization is also sectoral. Extensive invasion of the deeper cornea by vessels can cause the cornea to appear a dull reddish pink, the so-called salmon patch.

Vascular invasion continues for 4 to 5 weeks, and usually the whole cornea becomes vascularized. Next, the retrogressive stage begins, the inflammation and symptoms begin to subside, and clearing starts. This stage lasts from 1 to 2 years. In most cases, clearing begins peripherally, proceeds centrally, and is accompanied by thinning of the cornea. The amount of clearing is remarkable, especially in young people; however, usually some opacity is left centrally as a diffuse haze (Fig. 11-1). These changes are usually most prominent posteriorly and in some cases are limited to the pre-Descemet's area (Fig. 11-2). The blood vessels, which tend to persist as fine opaque lines, are not obliterated, although thinner branches of larger vessels might become closed. In some the lumen is so small that a red blood cell is able only occasionally to pass through. These vessels were called "ghost vessels" in the past because they persisted but were not thought to carry blood.

In severe cases the corneal endothelium can be destroyed or damaged, resulting in permanent corneal edema. Linear formations of corneal guttae are seen. There may be splits in Descemet's membrane,[4] hyaline ridges and networks attached to the endothelium, band keratopathy, corneal thinning, lipid keratopathy, and Salzmann's degeneration.[5] Astigmatism can occur because of corneal irregularity and thinning. Late glaucoma may occur[6-9] as a result of hypertrophy of Descemet's membrane over the chamber angle,[4] inflammatory injury to the meshwork, synechiae, or narrow anterior chamber angles. The presentation may be acute or chronic.

There are many variations from the typical course of the disease. The disease may remain in the periphery of the cornea, be confined to one sector only, and be of short duration, or it may have more than one separate center of inflammation with its own vascular invasion existing simultaneously.

Generally, recurrences are transient and mild; they occur in about 9% of cases and may be associated with mild trauma (Fig. 11-3), laceration, or impairment of general health.

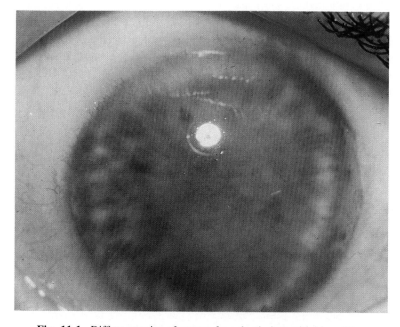

Fig. 11-1. Diffuse opacity of cornea from luetic interstitial keratitis.

Diagnosis. More than 90% of cases of interstitial keratitis are caused by syphilis, either congenital or acquired. The diagnosis of interstitial keratitis at any stage is predominantly clinical. Bilateral extensive edema and cellular infiltration of the stroma with deep vascularization should be considered as lues until proved otherwise. However, to see the acute attack today is rare; most cases now seen are in adults with residua of previous disease, which can be diagnosed by a careful history and examina-

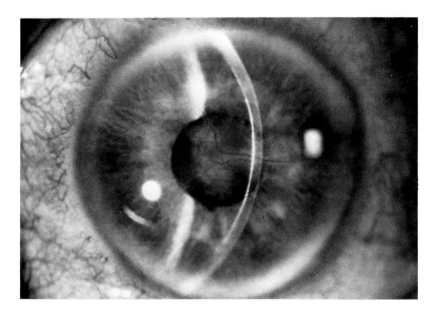

Fig. 11-2. Pre-Descemet's scarring from old luetic interstitial keratitis.

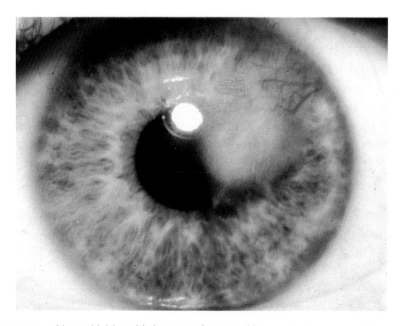

Fig. 11-3. Recurrence of interstitial keratitis because of trauma. Note sectoral response. (Courtesy of F. Wilson II, Indianapolis.)

tion. The hallmark is stromal scarring, opacification, and residual deep vascularization. In the late cases, deep stromal opacities, usually with a metallic sheen reflex in front of Descemet's membrane, are seen. Stromal "ghost" vessels become evident by direct illumination or retroillumination.

Iridocyclitis, chorioretinitis, optic neuritis, and sclerokeratitis can also occur in syphilis, and evidence of their occurrence can aid in the diagnosis. Findings of uveal involvement include atrophy of the iris stroma, posterior synechia, salt-pepper fundus, large patches of depigmentation and pigment proliferation, and a picture resembling retinitis pigmentosa, with vascular attenuation.

The patient's history is often helpful. A patient with congenital syphilis usually reports the occurrence of an ocular inflammation in childhood that lasted several months. There may be previous history of a positive serologic test or treatment for venereal disease or a family history of positive serology, venereal disease, abortions, or stillbirths.

Examination should be performed for other physical evidence of congenital lues, including frontal bossing, overgrowth of maxillary bones, Hutchinson's teeth, early loss of teeth, saddle nose, rhagades, and saber shins.[10] Other stigmata of congenital syphilis are scaphoid scapulae, high palatine arch, epiphyseal enlargement, congenital eighth nerve deafness, rhagades, and perforation of the palate or nasal septum. Hutchinson's teeth in congenital lues refers to small, barrel-shaped central permanent incisors, frequently with a central notch in the thickened biting edge. Hutchinson's triad is classic: characteristic appearance of the teeth, deafness, and interstitial keratitis. Neurosyphilis, such as general paresis and tabes dorsalis, can also occur.

Serologic testing is often useful. Reagin tests, such as the Venereal Disease Research Laboratory (VDRL) or rapid plasma reagin (RPR), are indicators of recent or active disease but also may be elevated in certain other diseases, such as lupus erythematosus, malaria, and heroin addiction. The fluorescent treponemal antibody absorption test (FTA-ABS) and microhemagglutination assay test (MHA-TP) detect patient serum antibodies against treponemes. The FTA-ABS and MHA-TP are more sensitive and specific and will remain positive even after treatment.[11,12]

Any patient with interstitial keratitis also should be questioned about vestibuloauditory symptoms and exposure to or history of tuberculosis, and an intermediate-strength purified protein derivative (PPD) skin test and control should be planted.

Treatment. Late burned-out interstitial keratitis needs no local treatment other than keratoplasty when indicated for decreased vision (Fig. 11-4).[13] In general results are good.

During the active disease topical steroids can be used to suppress inflammation. Although some ophthalmologists believe that interstitial keratitis should run its course without steroid treatment, it appears that the end result is better when steroids are administered; however, the disease may be prolonged. Without treatment or with heavy metal treatment, 25% to 50% of eyes recover to 20/30 or better vision, and 70% recover to 20/60 or better; with steroid treatment, 85% to 90% recover to 20/30 vision or better. Topical steroid drops are initially administered eight times/day and then gradually tapered after the acute process is controlled. Treatment may have to be continued for 18 months to 2 years.

Cycloplegia is also of benefit. If possible, the pupil should be kept moving,[14] but symptoms may necessitate use of atropine during the active stages of the disease.

Antimicrobial therapy should be given not for the eyes but for the presence of active systemic disease. If the patient has not received adequate systemic treatment in the past, if the treatment status is unknown, or if there are any signs or symptoms of neurosyphilis, the cerebrospinal fluid should be examined. Signs of neurosyphilis are pleocytosis, increased protein concentration, and VDRL reactivity. In primary, secondary, or early latent lues benzathine penicillin G (1.2 million units in each buttock) is sufficient. In late congenital syphilis 2.4 million units of aqueous procaine penicillin intramuscularly or intravenously is given daily for 10 days to prevent or treat cardiovascular, central nervous system, visceral, and osseous lesions.[11] If neurosyphilis is present, aqueous procaine penicil-

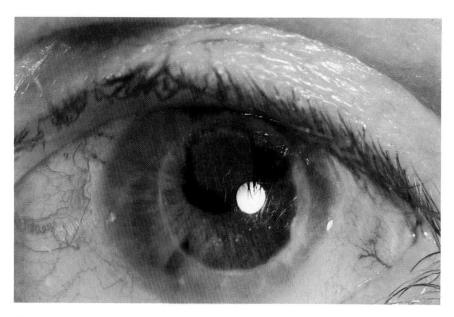

Fig. 11-4. When scarring from interstitial keratitis sufficiently impairs vision, good results are obtained with penetrating keratoplasty.

lin is administered as described earlier, with probenecid 500 mg, by mouth, four times daily, during the first 10 days, followed by benzathine penicillin G 2.4 million units intramuscularly weekly for three doses.

Treatment of the systemic disease does not seem to have any dramatic effect on the course of interstitial keratitis except that it may cause a flare-up, probably from liberation of antigen as in the systemic Herxheimer reaction. In addition, treatment of congenital syphilis does not prevent the onset of keratitis later, and penicillin treatment during the first attack of keratitis does not prevent subsequent involvement of the other eye.

COGAN'S SYNDROME

Cogan's syndrome of nonsyphilitic interstitial keratitis is bilateral and painful[15] and can occur at any age. Symptoms may include photophobia, fever, periorbital edema, and unilateral proptosis. The syndrome is associated with vestibuloauditory symptoms, which can be more severe than the ocular disease.[16] Cogan's syndrome is characterized by deep yellow nodular corneal stroma opacities (Fig. 11-5). Early in the disease, peripheral subepithelial nummular opacities are most commonly seen (Fig. 11-6)[17]; if these are treated with steroids, the classic picture may never develop. Deep corneal vascularization, mild uveitis, and episcleritis also may be noted.

The vestibuloauditory symptoms can precede or follow the ocular symptoms. Usually they are closely associated, but in some cases ocular disease develops as much as 2 years after the vestibuloauditory disease.[16] Typically, high-pitched unilateral tinnitus is followed rapidly by sensorineural deafness in the ipsilateral ear. Symptoms follow in the other ear within a few days. Balance symptoms are also present in most cases. In one study the majority of the patients ended up totally deaf and with no vestibular function; in some cases, however, complete resolution occurred after early corticosteroid treatment.[16] Nearly all other organ systems can be affected, with gastrointestinal hemorrhage and aortic insufficiency most common. The etiology is unknown but approximately 25% of patients with this syndrome have had clinical or tissue findings consistent with polyarteritis nodosa.[18,19]

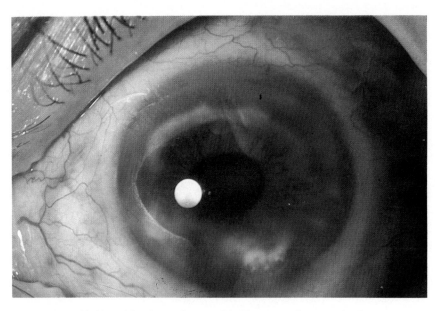

Fig. 11-5. Cogan's interstitial keratitis. (From Grayson M: The cornea in systemic disease. In Duane TD, editor: Clinical ophthalmology, vol 4, Hagerstown, MD, 1976, Harper & Row.)

Cogan's interstitial keratitis responds to topical corticosteroid therapy. Systemic corticosteroids are indicated for treatment of vestibuloauditory disease, or polyarteritis. It is important to consider this diagnosis, particularly when only subepithelial infiltrates are present. If the cause is assumed to be viral keratitis and no systemic treatment is given, permanent hearing loss can occur.

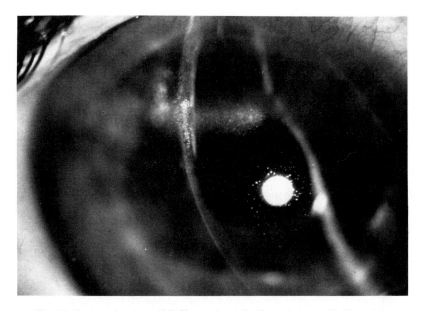

Fig. 11-6. Anterior stromal infiltrates in early Cogan's interstitial keratitis.

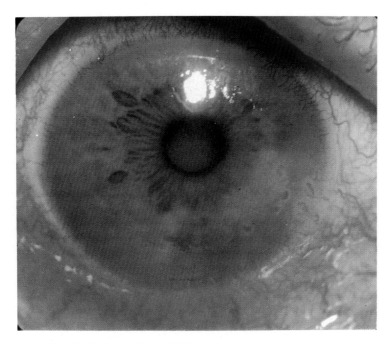

Fig. 11-7. Sectoral interstitial keratitis caused by tuberculosis.

TUBERCULOSIS

Tuberculosis interstitial keratitis is a rare disease in developed countries; even in the 1920s, when tuberculosis was much more prevalent than today, it accounted for less than 2.0% of cases of interstitial keratitis.[20] The keratitis may appear similar to luetic interstitial keratitis, but it is more often unilateral and sectoral. In tuberculosis the cornea is often involved in the peripheral inferior sector only (Fig. 11-7), where it forms a dense, abscesslike, nodular opacity, shaped like a ring. The infiltration is greatest in the middle and deeper layers of the cornea, and vascular ingrowth is mainly anterior; the central cornea is relatively spared. A sector-shaped sclerokeratitis or phlyctenulosis also may be seen. The clearing is less rapid and less complete than that of the syphilitic variety, leaving a dense, sectorlike scar. As in syphilitic interstitial keratitis, the host's response to bacterial antigens, and not active corneal infection, is probably responsible for the clinical disease. A focus of tuberculous disease lies elsewhere in the body. A positive tuberculin skin test and a negative FTA-ABS test aid in diagnosis. There may be a history of tuberculous disease or evidence of disease elsewhere in the body.

The systemic infection should be treated with antituberculous drugs such as isoniazid, streptomycin, or rifampin.[21] Topical steroids and cyloplegics are used for the corneal disease, as for syphilitic interstitial keratitis.

LEPROSY

Clinical manifestations. In leprosy, ocular involvement is more common and more severe in the lepromatous type. Corneal disease can take several forms. The most common finding is absent sensation due to fifth nerve involvement. Superficial punctate keratopathy, mainly interpalpebral, also is commonly seen and can be caused by corneal anesthesia, seventh nerve palsy, trichiasis, entropion, ectropion, or lagophthalmos.

Corneal inflammation occurs in three forms: superficial punctate keratitis, leprotic pannus, and

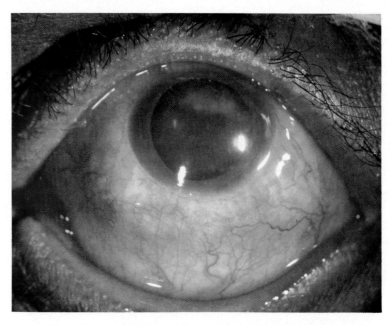

Fig. 11-8. Interstitial keratitis and punctate keratitis in leprosy.

interstitial keratitis[22-24] (Fig. 11-8). The superficial punctate keratitis begins in the superior temporal quadrant as discrete white superficial opacities near the limbus. These opacities resemble grains of chalk and lie in the epithelium and subepithelial stroma. They do not stain with fluorescein and are asymptomatic. They can spread inferiorly and centrally and with time can coalesce, resulting in a diffuse haze. More rarely they can become vascularized or lead to deeper stromal inflammation. Iritis frequently accompanies the keratitis. The chalk-dust opacities are composed of lepra bacilli surrounded by a polymorphonuclear infiltrate.

Nodular lepromata are frequently seen subconjunctivally, particularly at the temporal limbus (Fig. 11-9). Superficial vessels may grow out from them over the peripheral cornea, producing leprotic pannus.

Interstitial keratitis occurs in approximately 6% of cases and is seen late in the disease. Deep infiltration and vascularization begin in the periphery and move centrally, sometimes involving the visual axis. It is commonly bilateral, and most frequently affects the superotemporal quadrant. In contrast to luetic interstitial keratitis, vascularization is scant and late.

Multiple, small, creamy-white pearls may be present on the surface of the iris. Exposure keratitis, glaucoma, chronic conjunctivitis, lid nodules, thickened corneal nerves—sometimes with beading (beads on a string)—loss of eyebrows and eyelashes, distortion of the lids, seventh nerve palsy, and scleritis can also occur.

Pathogenesis. Lepromatous leprosy appears to develop in patients with reduced cell-mediated immunity and produces more severe clinical manifestations. Numerous nodular skin lesions and progressive thickening of the skin, particularly on the face and extensor surfaces of the extremities, produce the characteristic leonine facies. Diffuse involvement of peripheral nerves and lymph nodes occurs.

Primary leprous keratitis results from invasion of the cornea by lepra bacilli, via the corneal nerves, the limbal vessels, or by direct extension. Granulomatous inflammation occurs in the form of giant cells that contain the *Mycobacterium leprae* bacilli (lepra cells), large lipid-laden (foamy) macrophages, lymphocytes, and plasma cells. There is a predilection for involvement of nerve bundles,

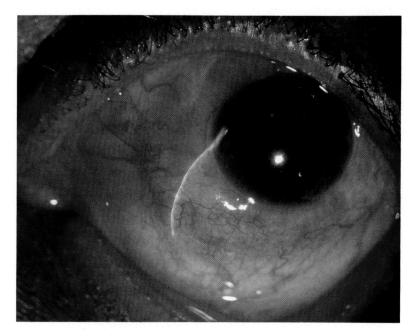

Fig. 11-9. Nodular conjunctival leproma in leprosy.

with such granulomatous lesions in and around the nerves. The predilection of leprosy for involvement of the anterior segment of the eye may be the result of its relatively low temperature.[25]

Diagnosis and treatment. The clinical appearance is often sufficient to make the diagnosis. The conjunctiva can be scraped and an acid-fast stain performed, but the yield is relatively low. Biopsies of conjunctival or cutaneous lesions are more likely to demonstrate the pleomorphic acid-fast bacilli, as well as the typical inflammatory lesions. The organism cannot be grown in vitro.

Systemic treatment involves long-term use of clofazimine, rifampin, and dapsone. Topical steroids are used to treat active keratitis or iritis.

VIRAL INTERSTITIAL KERATITIS

Although viral stromal keratitis is usually of a discoid type, it sometimes appears as a diffuse type of interstitial keratitis. This has been known to occur in mumps, lymphogranuloma venereum, influenza, herpes, measles, varicella, and vaccinia. In mumps, for example, the corneal involvement appears shortly after parotitis and is usually unilateral, consisting of a transient, mild, interstitial keratitis. Occasionally, severe keratitis profunda may develop, appearing as a gray opacity with white interlacing fibrillae; however, permanent vascularization is rarely seen.

Vaccinia keratitis may either be disciform or exhibit superficial ulcers. It has been reported to be recurrent in many cases.

PARASITIC INTERSTITIAL KERATITIS

Onchocerciasis, a filarial disease that is a major cause of blindness in central and western Africa and Central America, commonly produces interstitial keratitis. Two forms are seen: a multifocal, nummular "punctate" keratitis and a diffuse progressive sclerosing keratitis (see Chapter 10).

Trypanosomiasis occurs in both African and American variants and is caused by different species of *Trypanosoma,* a hemoflagellate. An interstitial keratitis, similar to luetic keratitis, can occur.[26] Conjunctivitis, palpebral and periorbital edema, and preauricular adenopathy also may be present.

DRUG-INDUCED INTERSTITIAL KERATITIS

Prolonged administration of certain systemic medications, such as arsenic and gold, has been associated with severe corneal infiltration and vascularization.

LYME DISEASE

Lyme disease is a multisystem disorder caused by infection with *Borrelia burgdorferi*, acquired through tick bites. Several cases of keratitis have been reported in patients with Lyme disease.[27-30] Multiple infiltrates were present at all levels of the stroma. Unilateral and bilateral cases occurred, and keratic precipitates were present in some cases. The infiltrates responded to topical steroid treatment.

NUMMULAR KERATITIS

The following conditions may be associated with subepithelial and nummular lesions:

1. Sarcoid
2. Tuberculosis
3. Adult chlamydial keratoconjunctivitis
4. Dimmer's nummular keratitis
5. Herpes zoster
6. Herpes simplex
7. Leprosy
8. Lues
9. Onchocerciasis
10. Epidemic keratoconjunctivitis
11. Brucellosis
12. Infectious mononucleosis
13. Varicella

Herpes simplex and herpes zoster may present with subepithelial lesions. Nebulous round or irregular subepithelial opacities can develop in the anterior stroma in the wake of epithelial infection. Stromal loss and vascularization can occur, particularly if steroid medications were administered. Other viral diseases in which subepithelial lesions can occur are epidemic keratoconjunctivitis and pharyngoconjunctival fever due to adenoviral infection. In these diseases the lesions are usually seen by the fifteenth day and may be present for 2 years. They are consistently coin-shaped, have no tendency to vascularize, and are limited to the superficial layers of the cornea. Development of facets or stromal loss is rare. In pharyngoconjunctival fever, the lesions tend to be smaller and more transitory, usually resolving by the sixth to eighth week.

Trachoma and adult chlamydial keratoconjunctivitis can exhibit subepithelial lesions and must be considered in the differential diagnosis. In trachoma a gross pannus and conjunctival scarring can be present. The subepithelial lesions in trachoma may be as large as 2 mm and may scar. They are usually superficial and affect the superior cornea. In adult chlamydial keratoconjunctivitis subepithelial infiltrates can affect any portion of the cornea and can appear identical to those seen in adenoviral infection, although they are usually smaller.

Brucellosis has also been reported as a cause of nummular keratitis.[31] In syphilis, subepithelial opacities can precede the interstitial keratitis and may be deep, round, and scattered. In onchocerciasis peripheral and central coin-shaped corneal infiltrates occur around dead microfilaria.

INFECTIOUS MONONUCLEOSIS

Bilateral interstitial and nummular keratitis can be associated with infectious mononucleosis.[32,33] Most of the opacities are coin-shaped, but they can coalesce to form broader lamellar infiltrates. The opacities are usually multiple and bilateral and are present in all levels of the stroma. They are more common in the peripheral cornea and can become vascularized or develop facets (Fig. 11-10). The epithelium is usually intact, and there is no anterior chamber reaction. The corneal sensation is normal. Infectious mononucleosis can be confirmed by a positive heterophil antibody test or serologic evidence of recent Epstein-Barr virus infection. Differentiation from herpes zoster and simplex and Lyme disease must be made. In most cases rapid improvement in signs and symptoms can be achieved with topical steroids.

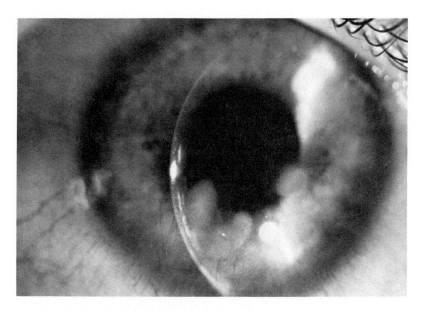

Fig. 11-10. Keratitis in Epstein-Barr virus infection consists of nummular infiltrates at multiple levels of stroma, which can become confluent or vascularized.

DIMMER'S NUMMULAR KERATITIS

Dimmer's nummular keratitis is a slowly developing, benign keratitis usually occurring unilaterally in young land workers. It is characterized by disc-shaped infiltrates in the superficial stroma, which later develop facets, and is not associated with conjunctivitis.[34-36] Related conditions have been described by Westhoff[37] and Lagraulet.[38] It was originally described in agricultural workers in Europe, but it appears to be more commonly seen in the Far East, where the disease has been called "padi keratitis" because it is usually seen in rice field workers. (Padi means "unhusked rice" in the Malayan language.) It also has been reported in South Africa and the United States.

Clinical manifestations. Dimmer's nummular keratitis presents with foreign body sensation, tearing, photophobia, blurred vision, and some degree of ciliary injection unassociated with any conjunctival discharge. Most patients have a history of trauma and exposure to irrigation water. The onset of symptoms has varied from 1 to 35 days after trauma. The keratitis is characterized by 10 to 50 subepithelial coin-shaped corneal opacities, 0.5 to 1.5 mm in diameter (Figs. 11-11 and 11-12). During the first few weeks of involvement the corneal infiltrates show a nondiscrete, round configuration, and a dull-white opacification that tends to spread and fade off into the surrounding cornea in edematous haze. With time they become more sharply demarcated. These lesions are usually in one plane of the cornea but can be seen at all levels. The epithelium over the discoid infiltrates remains smooth, but exhibits faint punctate staining with fluorescein, and edema may be present. Corneal sensation is intact in all these patients, and there is no iritis.

During the first 2 to 3 months, some of the nummular lesions may develop central dense nuclei. However, after about the fourth month the nuclei may resorb, resulting in annular forms with much clearer, slightly translucent centers and more opaque, dense rims. In some cases central depressions, or facets, form. Peripheral infiltrates can develop superficial vascularization and, rarely, proceed to ulceration.

The nummular infiltrates gradually resorb and scar, and the central facets become more pronounced. Symptoms typically persist for 9 to 12 months. The infiltrates regress over 6 to 8 years, but some faint scarring and peripheral vascularization can persist indefinitely.

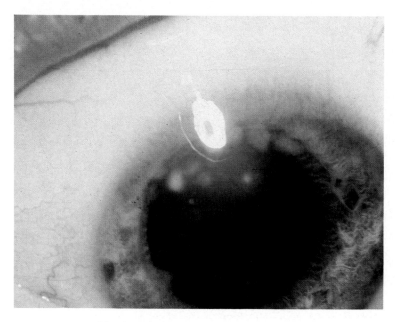

Fig. 11-11. Dimmer's nummular keratitis.

In some cases central lesions coalesce and form a disciform keratitis.[36] Deep stromal involvement with edema and infiltration of the stroma can also be seen. The deep central stromal infiltrate and edema usually start clearing during the fourth month, although some stromal haze may persist for a couple of years. Epithelial bullae may occur as a result of endothelial injury.

Etiology. The cause of Dimmer's nummular keratitis is unknown, but a viral agent is suspected. Cultures of the corneal lesions and serology have been unfruitful, except in one case in which an unidentified virus was isolated.[39] It has been suggested that the mechanism is similar to that seen in

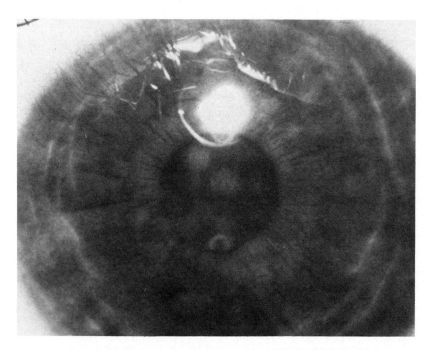

Fig. 11-12. Typical coin-shaped lesions in nummular keratitis.

adenoviral infection. The virus may replicate in the epithelial cells; antigens are liberated into the underlying stroma; stromal opacities probably are a reaction of the host to these viral antigens. The beneficial effect of steroids on these infiltrates further substantiates the possibility of an immunologic reaction. Of course, the inciting antigen may be another infectious agent, such as a parasite, or may be noninfectious; however, it is likely to be associated with the irrigation water in these regions.

Treatment. Topical corticosteroids can relieve discomfort and improve vision, but the final outcome appears to be the same. Once begun, treatment usually must be continued for 4 to 8 weeks to prevent recurrence of symptoms.

REFERENCES

1. Roizenblatt J: Interstitial keratitis caused by American (mucocutaneous) leishmaniasis, Am J Ophthalmol 87:175, 1979.
2. Martin GD, Stanley JA, and Davidson IW: Corneal lesions in squirrel monkeys maintained on a low chromium diet, Invest Ophthalmol 2:153, 1972.
3. Duke-Elder S and Leigh AG: System of ophthalmology, vol VIII, Diseases of the outer eye, St Louis, 1965, Mosby–Year Book, Inc.
4. Waring GO et al: Alterations of Descemet's membrane in interstitial keratitis, Am J Ophthalmol 81:773, 1976.
5. Vannas A, Hogan MJ, and Wood I: Salzmann's nodular degeneration of the cornea, Am J Ophthalmol 79:211, 1975.
6. Grant MW: Late glaucoma with interstitial keratitis, Am J Ophthalmol 79:87, 1975.
7. Knox DL: Glaucoma following inactive syphilitic interstitial keratitis, Arch Ophthalmol 66:18, 1961.
8. Lichter PR and Shaffer RN: Interstitial keratitis and glaucoma, Am J Ophthalmol 68:241, 1969.
9. Sugar HS: Late glaucoma associated with inactive syphilitic interstitial keratitis, Am J Ophthalmol 53:602, 1962.
10. Duke-Elder S and Leigh AG: System of ophthalmology, vol VIII, Diseases of the outer eye, St Louis, 1965, Mosby–Year Book, Inc.
11. Ryan SJ et al: Persistence of virulent *Treponema pallidum* despite penicillin therapy in congenital syphilis, Am J Ophthalmol 73:258, 1972.
12. Smith JL: Testing for congenital syphilis in interstitial keratitis, Am J Ophthalmol 72:816, 1971.
13. Rabb MF and Fine M: Penetrating keratoplasty in interstitial keratitis, Am J Ophthalmol 67:907, 1969.
14. Oksala A: Interstitial keratitis: its treatment by mydriatics and hydrocortisone and its recurrence, Am J Ophthalmol 44:217, 1957.
15. Cogan DG: Syndrome of nonsyphilitic interstitial keratitis and vestibuloauditory symptoms, Arch Ophthalmol 33:144, 1945.
16. McDonald TJ, Vollertsen RS, and Younge BR: Cogan's syndrome: audiovestibular involvement and prognosis in 18 patients, Laryngoscope 95:650, 1985.
17. Cobo LM and Haynes BF: Early corneal findings in Cogan's syndrome, Ophthalmology 91:903, 1984.
18. Char DH, Cogan DG, and Sullivan WR: Immunologic study of nonsyphilitic interstitial keratitis with vestibuloauditory symptoms, Am J Ophthalmol 80:491, 1975.
19. Cheson BD, Bluming AZ, and Alroy J: Cogan's syndrome: a systemic vasculitis, Am J Ophthalmol 60:549, 1976.
20. Duke-Elder S and Leigh AG: System of Ophthalmology, vol VIII: Diseases of the outer eye, St Louis, 1965, Mosby–Year Book, Inc.
21. Treatment of tuberculosis, Am Rev Respir Dis 127:790, 1983.
22. Duke-Elder S and Leigh AG: System of ophthalmology, vol VIII: Diseases of the outer eye, St Louis, 1965, Mosby–Year Book, Inc.
23. Spaide R et al: Ocular findings in leprosy in the United States, Am J Ophthalmol 100:411, 1985.
24. Shields JA, Waring GO, and Monte LG: Ocular findings in leprosy, Am J Ophthalmol 77:880, 1974.
25. Hobbs HE et al: Ocular histopathology in animals experimentally infected with *Mycobacterium leprae* and *M. lepraemurium*, Br J Ophthalmol 62:516, 1978.
26. Neame H: Parenchymatous keratitis in trypanosomiasis in cattle and in dogs and in man, Br J Ophthalmol 11:209, 1927.
27. Orlin SE and Lauffer JL: Lyme disease keratitis, Am J Ophthalmol 107:678, 1989.
28. Baum J et al: Bilateral keratitis as a manifestation of Lyme disease, Am J Ophthalmol 105:75, 1988.
29. Bertuch AW, Rocco E, and Schwartz WG: Lyme disease. Ocular manifestations, Ann Ophthalmol 20:376, 1988.
30. Kornmehl EW et al: Bilateral keratitis in Lyme disease, Ophthalmology 96:1194, 1989.
31. Woods AC: Nummular keratitis and ocular brucellosis, Arch Ophthalmol 34:490, 1946.
32. Pinnolis M, McCulley JP, and Urman JD: Keratitis associated with infectious mononucleosis, Am J Ophthalmol 89:791, 1980.
33. Matoba AY, Wilhelmus KR, and Jones DB: Epstein-Barr viral stromal keratitis, Ophthalmology 93:746, 1986.
34. Dimmer F: A type of corneal inflammation closely related to keratitis nummularis, Z Augenheilkd 13:621, 1905.
35. Pillat A: The differential diagnosis of nummular keratitis (Dimmer) and epidemic keratoconjunctivitis, Am J Ophthalmol 43:58, 1957.
36. Valenton MJ: Deep stromal involvement in Dimmer's nummular keratitis, Am J Ophthalmol 78:897, 1974.
37. Westhoff CHA: Keratitis punctata tropica (Sawah-keratitis), Geneesk T Ned Ind 52:419, 1912.
38. Lagraulet J: La keratite ponctuee "en volcan" des pays tropicaux, Arch Ophtalmol (Paris) 24:15, 1964.
39. Duke-Elder S and Leigh AG: System of ophthalmology, vol VIII: Diseases of the outer eye, St Louis, 1965, Mosby–Year Book, Inc.

VIRAL DISEASES

HERPES SIMPLEX

VIRUS

Herpes simplex virus (HSV) is a member of the family Herpesviridae, which also includes cytomegalovirus, varicella-zoster virus (VZV), and Epstein-Barr virus (EBV). Recently a new herpesvirus has been identified, human herpes virus 6, but its role in human disease has not been determined. All members of the group appear morphologically identical by electron microscopy. They are composed of a central DNA core and a protein capsid with 162 hollow, cylindric capsomeres (Table 12-1). This nucleocapsid is surrounded by an envelope of glycoprotein, lipid, and carbohydrate. The completely enveloped virus has a diameter of 130 to 180 μm.

The virus interacts with specific receptors on the surface of human cells (adsorption) and then enters the cell by pinocytosis (penetration). The DNA is released into the cell (uncoating) and travels to the nucleus, where it induces production of both host and virus specific enzymes, such as thymidine kinase and DNA polymerase. Viral proteins are synthesized in the cytoplasm and transported to the nucleus, where assembly of nucleocapsids takes place. Viral glycoproteins also become inserted into the host cell membrane.[1] The nucleocapsids bud through the nuclear membrane and are released from the cell. Cowdry type A eosinophilic intranuclear inclusion body is thought to be viral particles being assembled in the nucleus of an infected cell.

Latency and reactivation. Infection of some cells, however, does not follow this course and result in cell lysis. Herpes viruses have the rare ability to cause latent infections: EBV and cytomegalovirus become latent in lymphocytes, herpes zoster in dorsal root ganglia and trigeminal ganglia, and HSV in sensory (most commonly trigeminal), or autonomic ganglia, and the brain stem. After primary

TABLE 12-1. Properties of Herpes Simplex and VZV

PROPERTY	HERPES SIMPLEX	VARICELLA-ZOSTER
Morphology		
Core	DNA	DNA
Capsid	Icosahedron; 162 hollow cylindric capsomeres	Same
Envelope	Glycoprotein, lipid, carbohydrate	Same
Size	Core 75 μm Capsid 90-100 μm Enveloped particle 130-180 μm	Same
Inclusion body	Intranuclear, eosinophilic Cowdry type A	Same
Antigenic types	Type 1: labial herpes Type 2: genital herpes	One type only
Tissue tropism	Pantropic but prefers epithelium and nervous tissue	Pantropic but prefers epidermis, dermis and nervous tissue
Animal hosts	Most animals susceptible	Humans only
Tissue culture	Grows on a variety of cells	More fastidious; difficult to culture
Behavior in culture	Particles released into medium; produces diffuse CPE*	Extension occurs by direct passage between contiguous cells; CPE focal and slowly developing
Primary attack	Usually in childhood Stomatitis or keratoconjunctivitis Often inapparent	Usually in childhood Varicella Rarely inapparent
Latency	Sensory ganglia, most commonly gasserian and sacral, autonomic ganglia, and brain stem Possibly ocular sites	Dorsal root and trigeminal ganglia
Ganglionic localization	Neurons	Satellite cells
Triggers for recurrences	Fever, stress, ultraviolet light, trauma, menstruation, others	Immunosuppression, radiation, infection, others

*Cytopathic effect.

HSV infection at a peripheral site, the virus travels to the regional ganglia, where it can survive for decades in a relatively dormant state.[2] Under certain circumstances the state of infection alters, and viral production and shedding occurs. The virus travels down the nerve to the peripheral end organ and is released, where it can cause recurrent disease.

The site of latency for production of oral and corneal disease continues to be debated, but it is now clearly established that at least one site of latency is the trigeminal ganglion. Using sensitive methods of detection, latent infection with HSV had been demonstrated in 50% to 65% of human trigeminal ganglia obtained at autopsy.[2,3] Latency also has been shown to occur in sympathetic ganglia and, in mice, in the brain stem. Recent evidence also suggests that latent infection can occur at ocular sites, such as in endothelial cells or keratocytes.[4-8]

It is unclear whether mouth or nasopharyngeal primary infection can result in recurrent ocular disease, or whether patients with ocular disease all were inoculated in the conjunctiva at the time of primary infection. If oral infection alone can result in ocular disease, by what mechanism does the virus infect these neurons? It is possible that the virus can spread to adjacent neurons within the ganglion and set up latency there.[9-11] Productive viral infection has been demonstrated in neurons within ganglia, with release of virions capable of infecting of other neurons. Virus can be found in the eye of both rabbits and mice after inoculation of the snout.[11]

Infection of a ganglion by one HSV strain does not prevent future infection of that ganglion by another strain, at least in mice.[12] Clinically, in most people a single viral strain is responsible for each disease recurrence, but it appears that rarely a patient can harbor two or more different viruses, either of which can cause recurrent disease at the same location.[13-15] It is also possible that a person can harbor multiple strains of virus at different neurologic sites, for example, HSV-1 causing labial disease and HSV-2 causing genital disease.[16,17]

The mechanism by which the virus maintains latency and how this is altered to cause recurrent disease is not known. Recently it has been discovered that HSV does not lie dormant but actively produces a viral RNA, latency associated transcript (LAT), during latent infection.[18-22] LAT may inhibit further gene transcription and resultant production of infectious viral particles.

A wide variety of stimuli have been found to be able to stimulate recurrence, including febrile illnesses, stress, menstruation, trauma, sunlight, and heat. There also is some animal evidence that alteration of the adrenergic system (for example, by iontophoresis of the eye with epinephrine) can induce reactivation.[23,24] In general, immune status does not appear to play a significant role in herpetic reactivation or the severity of herpetic disease when it does occur. However, severe immunodeficiency can make the disease worse, and high doses of cyclophosphamide can stimulate reactivation.[25] Strain variations among HSV also appear to affect reactivation: Certain strains are associated with higher recurrence rates.[26]

It is apparent that viral shedding usually occurs without resultant clinical disease. What causes viral replication in host peripheral tissue, and subsequent clinical disease, is unclear. It may depend on the condition of the epithelium or local immunologic status; however, it is clear that recurrent clinical disease occurs despite systemic humoral and cell-mediated immunity against the virus. Serum antibody titers do not change with recurrent infections.

Virus and host factors. Genetic differences among strains appear to affect the manifestations of infection. The pattern of dendritic epithelial ulceration varies among different strains; each strain produces characteristically shaped ulcers.[27,28] Certain strains are more likely to produce stromal disease, and this is correlated with the amount of glycoproteins they produce during infection.[29,30] In addition, whether or not corticosteroids worsen the course of epithelial infection is strain related.[31]

Host response to the virus certainly plays a role in the disease process, but the relative importance of viral replication and its by-products and the host response to them remain to be elucidated. Most stromal disease appears to be largely immunologic, in that intact virus usually cannot be isolated from the stroma or found on electron microscopy.[32] The host response may be elicited by viral antigens that remain after epithelial infection or by viral proteins (but not intact virions) produced by persistent viral DNA (for example, in keratocytes).[33] Cell-mediated immunity is thought to be primarily responsible for disciform keratitis and antigen-antibody-complement responsible for interstitial keratitis, immune rings, and limbal vasculitis[34]; but the evidence is not very strong. Live virus appears to be present more often in necrotizing stromal keratitis, but host immune response also plays a large role.

The role of individual host differences in determining the course of infection appears to be relatively limited. For unknown reasons, herpetic infection does appear to be more frequent in patients with atopic disease. In some studies certain HLA types have been found to be more common in patients with recurrent disease, but other studies have not confirmed this finding.[35-37]

EPIDEMIOLOGY

Humans are the only natural reservoir of HSV, although experimental infection can be produced in rabbits, mice, primates, and other animals. In the United States, 70% of the population has been infected by 15 to 25 years of age, and 97% has been infected by 60 years of age, as demonstrated by serum-neutralizing antibody titers.[38] The initial infection is subclinical in 85% to 99% of the cases,[39] but these patients all become carriers. Approximately 1% of primary infections will lead to a severe acute systemic illness.[40]

Herpes simplex infection is the most common cause of corneal blindness in developed countries. Herpetic keratitis affects approximately 0.5 to 1.5/1000 population.[41,42] Both eyes are involved in approximately 12% of patients.[43,44] The rate of recurrence depends on the length of follow-up, which varies between 24% and 71% in different series.[41,45-47] In one 30-year study, the recurrence rates were 10% at 1 year, 23% at 2 years, and 63% at 20 years.[43] The time between recurrences is quite variable, ranging from a few weeks to decades. Approximately one in six patients with herpetic keratitis will have a marked reduction in vision, usually after multiple episodes over 3 to 15 years.[48,49]

Asymptomatic shedding can occur in the tears, as well as in saliva and respiratory and genital secretions; this finding appears more frequently than does clinical disease. The virus can be recovered from the oral and nasal secretions or stools in 20% of patients less than 2 years of age and from tears or saliva in 2% to 7% of older patients.

TYPES

There are two types of HSV: types 1 and 2. HSV-2 generally causes infection below the waist, and HSV-1 causes infections above the waist. HSV-2 is recovered principally from the genitals[50] but can also cause neonatal systemic infections,[51,52] localized skin lesions, aseptic meningitis, and chronic neurologic disease; it may be related to development of cervical cancer.[53] In disseminated neonatal infection, ocular involvement occurs in about 10% of cases (see Chapter 6). Most neonatal herpes keratitis and conjunctivitis is due to HSV-2; however, HSV-1 also can cause neonatal keratitis.[54] In adults, approximately 85% of ocular isolates are HSV-1.[55] HSV-2 corneal disease tends to be more severe.[55-57]

PRIMARY INFECTION

Systemic infection with HSV-1 usually occurs within the first few years of life, but cases can develop at any age. The young child is typically infected by salivary contamination from an adult with labial herpes; the characteristic clinical disease is an aphthous stomatitis. This primary infection is often unrecognized or entirely subclinical, but it can be severe. Primary infection outside the oral cavity is less common, but it can occur in other mucous membranes (for example, conjunctiva or in the skin).

The incubation period is 3 to 12 days. The most common manifestation of primary HSV ocular infection is an acute conjunctivitis with lymphadenopathy and malaise, usually unilateral (Fig. 12-1). The mild cases are follicular in nature; the more severe, pseudomembranous (50%). Dendrites can occasionally be seen on the bulbar conjunctiva. Keratitis accompanies the conjunctivitis in one third to one half of the cases, and there also may be vesicular or ulcerative skin lesions (75%). Corneal involvement usually follows the onset of skin lesions and conjunctivitis by 1 to 2 weeks and can be seen as diffuse superficial punctate keratitis (SPK), focal epithelial lesions, microdendrites, dendrites, or serpiginous ulcers. The skin eruption is similar to that arising elsewhere in the body, with edema and redness followed by vesicles or ulceration (Fig. 12-2). The number and location of vesicles varies, and confusion with herpes zoster can occur. The lesions can be limited to the lid margin, making it appear similar to staphylococcal and *Moraxella* ulcerative blepharitis (Fig. 12-3).

Conjunctivitis usually persists for about 2 weeks, but keratitis can last longer. Preauricular adenopathy, subepithelial scarring, fever, and gastroenteritis also can be seen. Stromal keratitis rarely occurs. Severe vesicular eruption associated with herpes, often referred to as Kaposi's varicelliform eruption, can occur and often is seen in patients who have an accompanying immune disease (for example, atopy). Progression to generalized infection or encephalitis can occur rarely. Involvement of the lacrimal canaliculi can result in permanent strictures and epiphora.[58]

Diagnosis. The diagnosis is based on (1) history, (2) clinical appearance, (3) cytologic characteristics, (4) virus isolation, and (5) serologic findings. A history of exposure to a parent or relative with labial herpes and a lack of previous herpetic disease are helpful. The clinical appearance can be highly suggestive; a young child with acute follicular or pseudomembranous conjunctivitis probably has primary herpetic disease. However, such a picture can be difficult to differentiate from epidemic keratoconjunctivitis,[59] vaccinia, chlamydia, or zoster. If vesicles appear on the lids (Fig. 12-2) the diagnosis is more likely, but vaccinia, herpes zoster, chickenpox, and bacterial blepharitis *(Staphylococcus* or *Moraxella)* also should be considered. Laboratory methods of diagnosis are discussed in the next section.

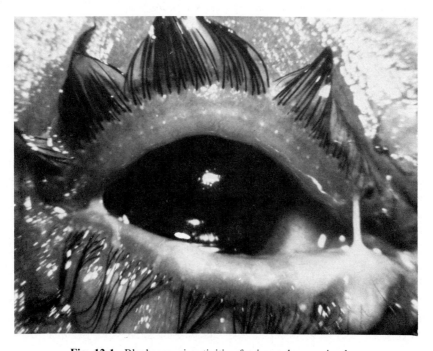

Fig. 12-1. Blepharoconjunctivitis of primary herpes simplex.

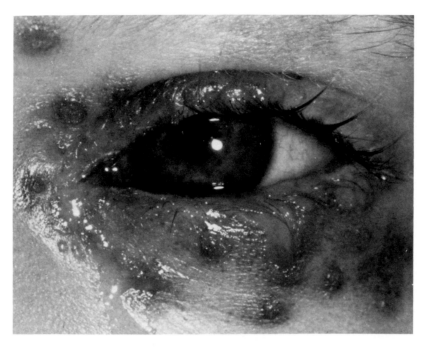

Fig. 12-2. Lid vesicles in primary herpes simplex.

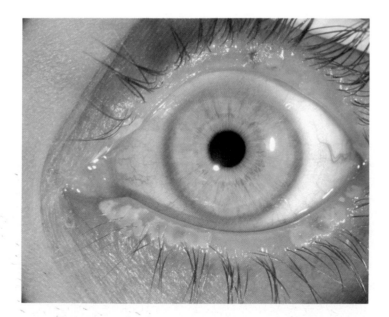

Fig. 12-3. Ulcerative blepharitis due to primary herpes simplex infection.

Treatment. Primary blepharoconjunctivitis will resolve without treatment. Although it has not been demonstrated, antiviral medication may shorten the course or decrease the risk of corneal complications. Therefore, an antiviral agent should be applied to eye and skin two to four times a day until the conjunctivitis and skin lesions resolve. Treatment of keratitis is the same as in recurrent disease: debridement and antiviral agents. The child may have to be restrained or anesthetized for debridement, which should be performed gently to prevent injury to Bowman's layer. Cycloplegia may be indicated for symptomatic relief.

RECURRENT HERPES

A general classification of recurrent herpes simplex infection with ocular involvement follows:
I. Vesicular eruption of the lids
II. Follicular conjunctivitis
III. Cornea
    A. Epithelial keratitis: active viral replication
        1. Dendritic
        2. Geographic (ameboid)
        3. Marginal (limbal)
    B. Indolent and trophic ulceration (postinfectious herpes): epithelial and stromal ulceration with or without active stromal inflammation
    C. Stromal keratitis
        1. Disciform keratitis
        2. Necrotizing, ulcerative keratitis
        3. Interstitial keratitis
        4. Stromal scarring
    D. Sclerokeratitis
    E. Endotheliitis
IV. Uveitis
        1. Endotheliitis
        2. Iritis
        3. Multifocal choroiditis

Recurrent lesions generally are localized, superficial, and self-limited (labial "fever blister" or "cold sore") (Fig. 12-4 and Table 12-2). Visual loss generally occurs from the cumulative effect of

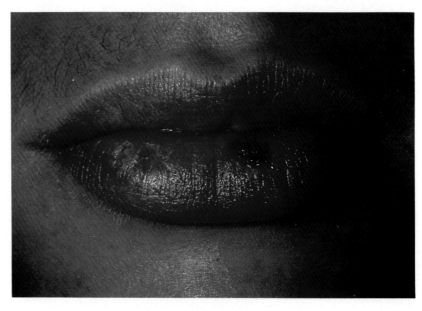

Fig. 12-4. Labial herpes simplex infection.

Table **12-2.** Recurrent Herpes Simplex Type 1

CHARACTERISTICS	DENDRITIC KERATITIS	HERPES LABIALIS
Latency	Gasserian ganglion	Gasserian ganglion
Trigger mechanisms	Fever most important; also sunburn, stress, menstruation, trauma, depression of cellular immunity by drugs, etc.	Fever most important; also sunburn, stress, menstruation, depression of cellular immunity by drugs, etc.
Premonitory symptoms	Foreign body sensation	Tingling and itching
Number of lesions	Varies from 1 to 10	Varies; often only 1
Intervals between recurrences	Vary with trigger mechanisms, especially with frequency of upper respiratory disease	Vary with trigger mechanisms, especially with frequency of upper respiratory disease
Subepithelial involvement	Varies from none to scar formation	No scarring
Secondary infection	Rare in immunocompetent individuals	Not seen in immunocompetent individuals *Note:* Skin vesicles on face may be superinfected with *S. aureus*
Duration (untreated)	50% or more heal within a week; remainder in 2 to 3 weeks	2 days to 3 weeks; average, 9 to 10 days
Disease in patients (immunosuppressed by kidney transplantation, Wiskott-Aldrich syndrome, etc.)	May have severe, chronic stromal disease, keratouveitis, secondary fungal or bacterial infection, perforation	May have deep cutaneous ulceration, dissemination to skin and viscera
Sensitivity	Corneal sensitivity is reduced	Skin area may be sensitive

multiple recurrences, each attack producing additional scarring, vascularization, and thinning. At any point severe necrotizing stromal disease, interstitial keratitis, or uveitis can occur, with more devastating consequences.

Blepharitis. Eyelid herpes is an uncommon form of recurrent disease. It may appear as isolated vesicles or a group of vesicles, which can be mistaken for herpes zoster; one must think of herpes simplex in any "recurrent zoster." As in primary disease, ulcerative blepharitis can occur and herpes simplex should be considered in the differential diagnosis of this condition.[60]

Conjunctivitis. Rarely, recurrent conjunctival herpes can occur without corneal lesions or with only SPK or subepithelial keratitis. The conjunctiva exhibits a moderate to severe papillary and follicular reaction and sometimes ulceration. The clinical features can be indistinguishable from those of adenovirus infection,[40] so it is important to consider herpes simplex in cases of acute follicular conjunctivitis, particularly those with recurrent disease, especially if corticosteroid administration is being considered.[61]

Corneal epithelial disease

Epithelial keratitis. Recurrent corneal epithelial disease usually occurs without accompanying conjunctivitis or lid lesions. The infection can appear as SPK, stellate epithelial lesions, dendritic ulcers, or geographic ulcers. The epithelial infection begins as fine punctate lesions that increase in size and later form white plaques of opaque epithelial cells 1 to 2 mm in diameter.[62] There can be a tendency toward palisading of epithelial cells at the periphery of each plaque. These plaques enlarge and develop into an easily recognized dendrite (Figs. 12-5 and 12-6). More than one dendrite can develop. As a dendrite grows, the central epithelium is lost; the peripheral, infected cells, stain with rose bengal, and the central area devoid of epithelium stains with fluorescein. The dendritic keratitis can occur at any location on the cornea, but recurrences tend to affect the same area as previous attacks. Stro-

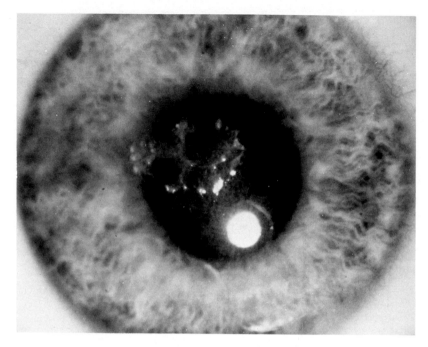

Fig. 12-5. Typical dendritic keratitis of herpes simplex.

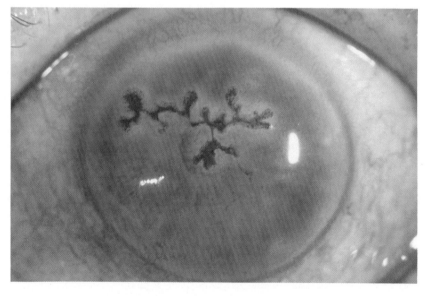

Fig. 12-6. Herpes simplex dendrite stained with rose bengal. (Courtesy of Y. Jerold Gordon, Pittsburgh.)

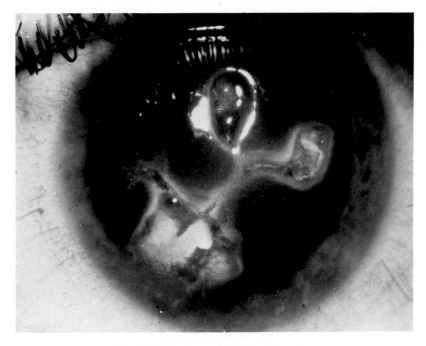

Fig. 12-7. Large ameboid dendritic ulcer.

mal infiltration can develop beneath the epithelial lesion. A mild iritis can be present, but keratic precipitates usually do not form.

The epithelial infection usually heals spontaneously in 5 to 12 days, but it can progress, particularly if topical steroids are administered, to form a geographic (also called ameboid) ulcer (Fig. 12-7) or spread to the stroma (3%). The geographic ulcers, like dendritic ulcers, have a margin of opaque, heaped-up cells, which stain with rose bengal. The edges may have a dendritic shape. With time, increasing stromal infiltration and anterior chamber reaction can develop. These ulcers tend to heal slowly, and epithelial ulceration can persist despite resolution of the active viral infection. When this happens the ulcers are called "metaherpetic", and these are discussed in the next section.

During early episodes the loss of corneal sensation is usually confined to the area of the lesion, but with repeated recurrences more generalized anesthesia occurs. It has been suggested that the greater the diminution of corneal sensitivity, the longer the healing period and the greater the tendency for recurrence.[63]

Peripheral nondendritic herpetic lesions can occur and can resemble staphylococcal marginal keratitis[64] (Fig. 12-8). These lesions tend to respond more slowly to treatment than more central infections and are predisposed to chronic trophic ulceration.[65,66] Fascicular ulcers resembling a fascicular phlyctenule also can occur (Fig. 12-9). These usually can be differentiated from phlyctenules by their association with dendritic scars and decreased corneal sensation.

In most cases healing occurs with little or no residual scarring. After more severe infections or after multiple attacks, however, superficial stromal scarring, loss of stroma, and vascularization occur.

Postinfectious (metaherpetic) ulcers. Sometimes epithelial defects persist or recur after viral epithelial and subepithelial disease. The ulcers can be dendritic, round, or oval, with sinuous or scalloped borders.[63] The edges of the ulcer are gray, appear rolled in, and do not stain with rose bengal.

By definition, virus cannot be cultured from these lesions. The corneal epithelium fails to cover

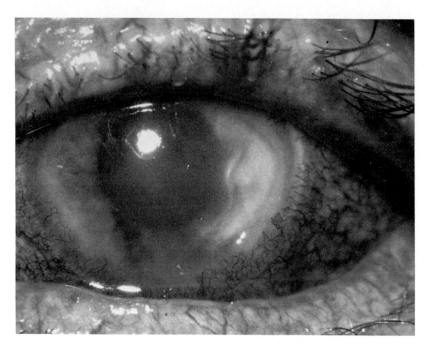

Fig. 12-8. Atypical marginal ulcer resulting from HSV type-2.

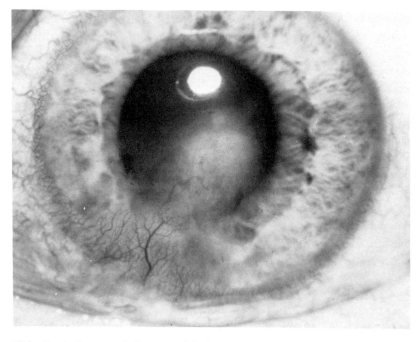

Fig. 12-9. Fascicular type of ulcer caused by herpes simplex, resembling phlyctenular lesion.

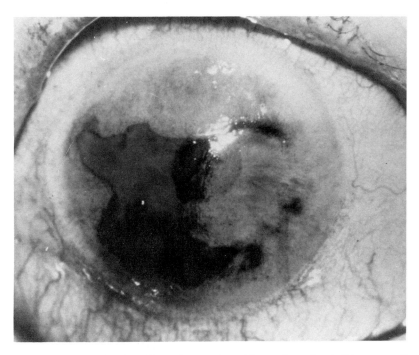

Fig. 12-10. Postinfectious herpetic ulcer. Large base stains with rose bengal red. Edges are rolled and heaped up.

the defect because of damage to its basement membrane, ongoing stromal inflammation, and the lack of trophic innervation.[67,68] The edges of the defect consist of piled-up epithelial cells that have failed to cover the ulcer base. The base of this lesion stains with rose bengal red (Fig. 12-10) and fluorescein, in contrast to the active dendritic lesion, in which the base stains only with fluorescein.

One should remember that live virus can remain for a long time. It can be difficult in some cases to distinguish between a recurring erosion or an active viral disease. In these doubtful instances it is advisable to take a viral culture or scraping of the lesion for fluorescent-antibody studies.

Stromal disease. The patterns of stromal involvement in herpetic keratitis are manifold. Edema, infiltration, vascularization, ulceration, endothelial inflammation, and uveitis all can occur, and their relative contributions vary considerably. However, it is possible to distinguish several common patterns, which can aid in making the diagnosis, guiding treatment, and estimating prognosis. If the stromal reaction is predominantly edema, with mild infiltration and uveitis, it is called *disciform edema;* if infiltration and necrosis dominate the picture, *necrotizing stromal keratitis;* if there is infiltration, edema, and vascularization, without ulceration, *interstitial keratitis;* if endothelial inflammation and destruction occur in relative isolation, *endotheliitis;* and if the uveitis is most pronounced, with mild stromal edema, infiltration or vascularization, *keratouveitis.*

Superficial stromal scarring. After epithelial infection residual opacities may be seen in the superficial stroma, most commonly "ghost" dendrites and small punctate granular lesions. The dendritic opacities are seen as areas of mild subepithelial edema, cellular infiltration, or scarring underlying the site of an epithelial dendrite. Peculiar subepithelial flecks that appear greasy or granular are frequently seen after herpetic keratitis; the pathogenesis of these whitish-yellow particles is uncertain.

Disciform keratitis. Disciform keratitis is characterized by stromal edema with some cellular infiltration in a circular or oval pattern beneath a dendritic lesion or under intact epithelium.[69] It can occur as a diffuse edematous keratitis (Fig. 12-11 and 12-12) or as an off-visual axis patch of disease. The

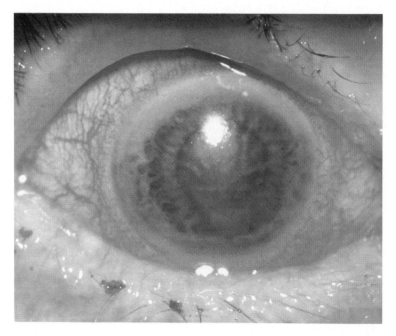

Fig. 12-11. Disciform keratitis.

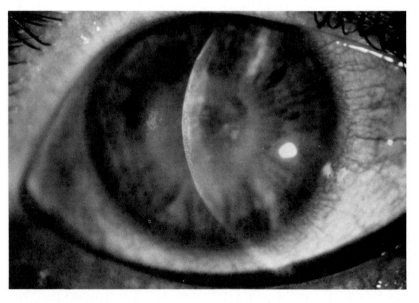

Fig. 12-12. Corneal swelling in disciform keratitis as seen with slit-lamp microscope beam. (Courtesy of Y. Jerold Gordon, Pittsburgh.)

patient reports photophobia, tearing, mild pain, and if central cornea is involved, reduced vision. There may be a history of previous herpetic disease. Disciform keratitis can appear as early as 5 to 10 days after the onset of a dendrite. The edema can involve the full thickness of the cornea or may just involve the area beneath the epithelium. Descemet's membrane is often wrinkled, and some degree of uveitis is usually present, especially with more severe corneal involvement. The endothelial cells under the disciform area are edematous and can give the appearance of guttae. Fine keratic precipitates may be present posterior to affected stroma.

The disciform keratitis can heal without complications or progress to an interstitial keratitis or necrotizing keratitis, with deep scarring.[63,70,71] Benign cases run a course of several months and heal with minimal scarring. In more severe cases immune rings, late corneal thinning, scar formation, and neovascularization can occur. Complications of the uveitis, particularly secondary glaucoma, can be seen.[39,72]

The pathogenesis of herpetic disciform keratitis is not known. The disciform lesion may represent an immunologic reaction to herpetic antigen.[1,73] Cell-mediated immunity is thought to be primarily responsible,[74] but antigen-antibody complexes also may be involved. The antigen may soak into the stroma during epithelial infection or may be produced in the stroma by viral DNA latent in keratocytes or other cells.[33,75] Alternatively, small amounts of live virus may be present, coming from epithelial infection, stromal nerves, or being produced in situ. Others have proposed that the main inflammatory reaction takes place in the endothelium; this reaction may be primarily immunologic or caused by active viral infection.[70,76-79]

Similar lesions can be seen with herpes zoster ophthalmicus, vaccinia, mumps, varicella, infectious mononucleosis, *Acanthamoeba,* chemical keratitis (for example, anesthetic abuse), and corneal trauma.[80]

Necrotizing keratitis. These complicated cases of viral keratitis usually occur in patients who have had previous attacks of herpetic keratitis. They may follow chronic or recurrent epithelial disease, disciform keratitis, superficial stromal disease, or recurrent disease of any type. In contrast to disciform keratitis, stromal infiltration and necrosis are predominant. In mild cases the infiltrates can be localized and lamellar. In severe cases a stromal abscess can develop, consisting of necrotic cheesy-white infiltration, which can occupy the entire thickness of the cornea (Fig. 12-13).[65] The epithelium can be intact, exhibit dendritic ulceration, or break down over stromal infiltration. Edema, ulceration, and vascularization often develop. A ring infiltrate can occasionally be seen surrounding the area of

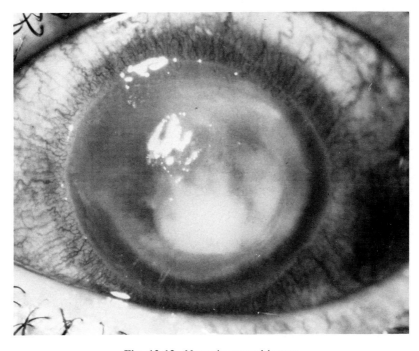

Fig. 12-13. Necrotic stromal herpes.

stromal disease (Fig. 12-14). The ring infiltrate consists of polymorphonuclear leukocytes brought forth by an interaction of viral antigen and circulating antibody, with fixation of complement. Uveitis is nearly always present and can be severe, with retrocorneal membrane, hypopyon, synechiae formation, secondary cataract and glaucoma. These cases can be indistinguishable from bacterial, fungal, or *Acanthamoeba* infection. In fact, the majority of *Acanthamoeba* infections are initially misdiagnosed as herpetic stromal keratitis.

Severe complications can occur in stromal herpetic keratitis. The stroma can perforate as a result of the disease or because of improper treatment (Fig. 12-15). The cornea is compromised and can become superinfected with fungi or bacteria. Fig. 12-16 demonstrates a case of *Paecilomyces* fungal superinfection of a herpetic stromal keratitis treated with steroid drops. Atopic individuals are especially prone to develop severe keratitis (Fig. 12-17).

Necrotizing stromal keratitis is most likely caused by direct viral infection of stroma and a subsequent host immune response. Virus has been observed in pathologic specimens[81] and has rarely been isolated from these corneas.[32,77,82,83] The relative importance of viral infection and the host's immune response in producing the clinical manifestations, especially the corneal destruction, is not known.

Interstitial keratitis. The term "interstitial keratitis" is used when infiltration, vascularization, and, sometimes, necrosis occur beneath intact stroma and epithelium. Single or multiple patches of dense infiltration can form and progress to necrosis and vascularization. They tend to be chronic and indolent, persisting for many months.

Sclerokeratitis. The sclera can become involved when there is peripheral interstitial or ulcerative keratitis. There is often scleral thinning and a great deal of pain, and treatment can be difficult.

Keratouveitis. Herpetic uveitis can be mild and incidental, compared with the corneal disease, or severe and a major source of complications. Disciform keratitis tends to be associated with mild anterior chamber reaction, and necrotizing keratitis with moderate to severe reaction. A common picture is one of diffuse keratitis, with stomal haze, edema, deep and superficial vascularization, and multi-

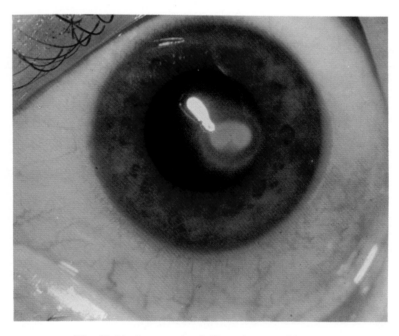

Fig. 12-14. Immune ring infiltrate in stromal herpes.

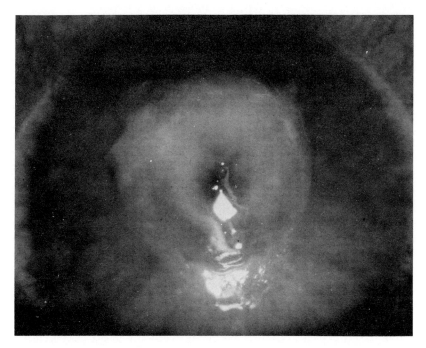

Fig. 12-15. Corneal perforation caused by severe stromal herpes.

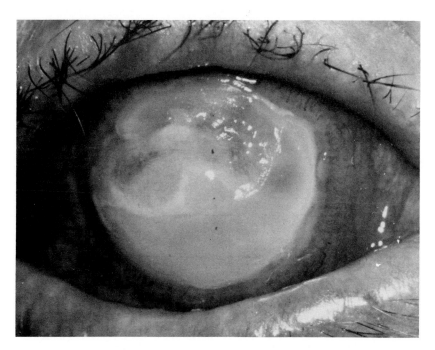

Fig. 12-16. *Paecilomyces* superinfection after prolonged treatment of herpes simplex keratitis with steroid drops.

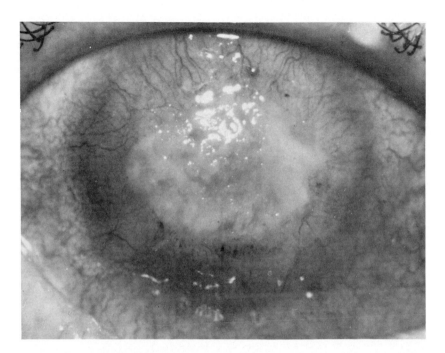

Fig. 12-17. Severe stromal herpes occurring in patient with atopic dermatitis.

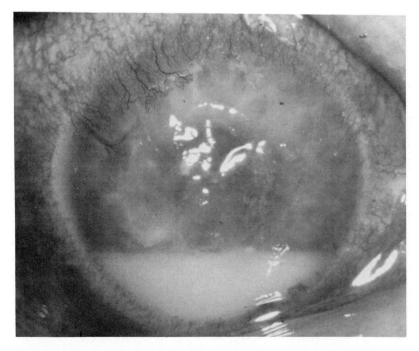

Fig. 12-18. Severe herpetic keratouveitis with hypopyon.

ple keratic precipitates. In more severe forms anterior chamber hemorrhage and hypopyon can result (Fig. 12-18). Ovoid sectoral iris atrophy can be seen.

In at least some of these cases, live virus is present in the anterior chamber, as well as possibly in the iris and endothelium. HSV has been obtained from aqueous in some cases[72,79,84] and identified histologically in others.[70,77,85] HSV can infect the superior cervical ganglion of the sympathetic chain and result in recurrent keratouveitis. However, in many cases live virus is not present, and the reaction is immunologic. Sundmacher and Neumann-Haefelin[79] found that two types of patients are likely to have live virus in the aqueous: those with serous focal iritis with heavy keratic precipitation and elevated intraocular pressure and those with endotheliitis and elevated pressure; therefore, these patients are more likely to benefit from antiviral therapy in addition to steroids.

Endotheliitis. In some cases endothelial dysfunction develops peripherally and progresses centrally across the cornea, as in endothelial rejection of a corneal graft.[86] In other cases plaques of endothelial inflammation and destruction can be seen.[87] These processes appear to involve active viral replication in the endothelium,[79,86] although subsequent immunologic reaction may also play a role. Some cases develop after epithelial disease.[87] I followed a patient who developed dendritic epithelial herpes simplex, followed 5 weeks later by multiple endothelial plaques. Five weeks after the plaques appeared the patient developed acute herpetic retinitis.

DIAGNOSIS

The diagnosis of herpes simplex keratitis often can be made clinically. The dendritic epithelial lesions are pathognomonic. A history of recurrent disease, decreased corneal sensation, involvement of multiple corneal layers, and disciform keratitis are all suggestive of herpes simplex.

Cytology examination typically shows a mononuclear exudate. Multinucleated giant epithelial cells, typically containing from two to ten nuclei (Fig. 12-19), may be seen in smears of epithelial scrapings and are fairly specific (also seen in varicella and zoster).[88] Intranuclear eosinophilic inclu-

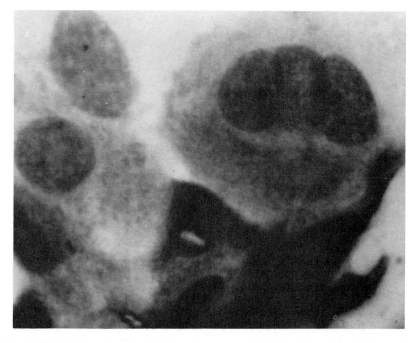

Fig. 12-19. Multinucleated epithelial cells seen in scraping of herpes simplex keratitis.

sion bodies, best seen with Papanicolaou stain, are helpful but infrequently found. Viral particles sometimes can be demonstrated with electron microscopy.[89]

Viral isolation in human cell culture is performed more often and can provide a definitive diagnosis, but it is still unavailable to many and is relatively expensive. Growth is usually observed in 2 to 4 days, but can take several weeks. Rose bengal should not be applied before obtaining a specimen because it can kill the virus.[90]

Viral antigens can be detected in specimens fairly rapidly using immunologic tests. Many types are available, including immunofluorescent,[73,91] immunoperoxidase, enzyme-linked immunoadsorbent assay (ELISA),[92] and immunofiltration methods.[93] The ELISA and immunofiltration methods appear to be most accurate.[94] An affinity membrane test has recently been described, whereby a membrane is touched to the cornea, and viral antigen adherent to the membrane is detected with peroxidase conjugated antibody.[95] This test appears to be simple and reliable, but more experience is required to assess its usefulness.

Some molecular biology techniques have been used to design potentially more sensitive diagnostic tests. Labeled herpes simplex DNA probes are used to detect viral DNA or RNA in specimens.[96-98] These tests appear to have great promise, but their clinical use has been limited.

Serologic testing may be useful in diagnosing primary infection. A sample should be obtained early in the disease, and again after 4 to 6 weeks, to document rising titers.

TABLE 12-3. Antiviral Agents

AGENT	MECHANISM OF ACTION	ADMINISTRATION	TOPICAL PENETRATION	VIRAL RESISTANCE	TOXICITY
Idoxuridine (IDU)	Pyrimidine analog Inhibits thymidine kinase, thymidylate kinase, and DNA polymerase Incorporated into viral DNA	Drop 0.1% Ointment 0.5%	Poor	+	+++
Vidarabine (Ara-A)	Pyrimidine analog Inhibits synthesis of viral DNA, mechanism unknown	Ointment 3% Intravenous		Less than IDU	++
Trifluorothymidine	Pyrimidine analog Inhibits thymidilate synthetase Incorporated into viral DNA	Drop 1%	Good	Rare	++
Acyclovir	Purine analog Activated by viral thymidine kinase Inhibits DNA polymerase	Ointment 3% Intravenous Oral	Good	+	+

TREATMENT

Antiherpetic drugs. Despite the prevalence of viral disease, the availability of antiviral agents has lagged behind that of other microbial agents. Most of the time the virus lies within human cells and utilizes many of the normal human enzymes for reproduction. Even after development of specific immunity to HSV, the virus persists in a relatively inaccessible site, central neural tissue, and in a relatively quiescent state.

Theoretically, viral disease can be treated by several mechanisms: (1) attachment to and entry into the cell, (2) inhibition of viral DNA synthesis, (3) inhibition of viral RNA or protein synthesis, (4) inhibition of viral assembly, (5) recognition and destruction of viral infected cells (by the presence of viral proteins in the cell membrane), (6) destruction of free viral particles, (7) prevention of latency, and (8) prevention of virus reactivation. Drugs marketed for use in herpetic keratitis use the second mechanism, inhibition of viral genome synthesis, but in the laboratory, potential agents that act by other mechanisms have been identified (Table 12-3).[99]

Idoxuridine. Idoxuridine (IDU), a pyrimidine analog similar to thymidine, was the first agent found to be clinically effective and eventually FDA approved.[100,101] It inhibits thymidine kinase, thymidylate kinase, and DNA polymerase and is incorporated into the viral DNA, thus producing a faulty DNA chain. IDU also can affect normal corneal epithelial cells, which also take up the drug[102-104]; however, human thymidine kinase does not use IDU as efficiently as viral thymidine kinase, accounting for the relative selectivity of the agent.

IDU is useful for epithelial infection,[105-108] but not for herpetic uveitis or deep stromal disease. With IDU treatment epithelial keratitis resolves within 10 days in about 55% to 70% of cases.[109-111] IDU is relatively unstable, penetrates the stroma poorly, and is quickly metabolized into an inactive form. Resistance to IDU may be encountered.

IDU can be toxic in repeated and long-term topical application and is even more toxic in "dry eye" patients.[109,112] In addition, it is topically sensitizing and can cause contact dermatitis (Fig. 12-20). In early toxicity the patient complains of burning or stinging on administration, and a diffuse punctate keratitis is seen. With continued administration, epithelial opacification and irregularity (Fig. 12-21), chronic epithelial defects, subepithelial infiltration, stromal ulceration, narrowing or oblitera-

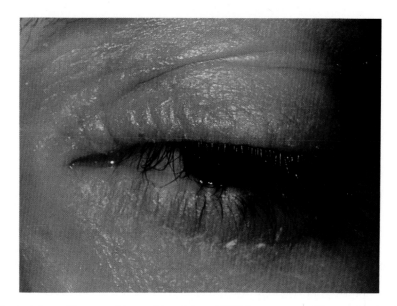

Fig. 12-20. Contact dermatitis caused by prolonged use of IDU in treatment of herpes simplex keratitis. (From Wilson FM II: Surv Ophthalmol 24:57, 1979.)

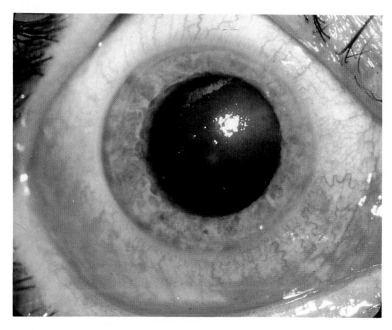

Fig. 12-21. Epithelial keratopathy and injection of inferior conjunctiva in toxic reaction to idoxuridine used to treat herpes simplex keratitis. (From Wilson FM II: Surv Ophthalmol 24:57, 1979.)

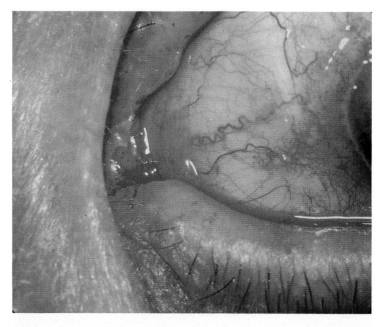

Fig. 12-22. Toxic follicular reaction and punctal occlusion secondary to IDU. (From Wilson FM II: Surv Ophthalmol 24:57, 1979.)

tion of the lacrimal puncta (Fig. 12-22), follicular conjunctivitis,[113] cicatricial conjunctivitis, or corneal pannus can develop. Experimentally, IDU inhibits keratocyte mitosis, corneal stromal repair,[104,114] and epithelial healing,[102] and teratogenicity has been reported in pregnant rabbits.[113] Use of IDU has largely been supplanted by newer agents that require less frequent administration and exhibit less toxicity and better penetration.

Vidarabine (adenine arabinoside). Adenine arabinoside (Ara-A) also inhibits synthesis of viral DNA, but the precise mechanism has not been determined. Ara-A is rapidly metabolized to arabinoside hypoxanthine, which, although it is more soluble and enters the stroma and aqueous, has only 20% of the antiviral activity of Ara-A. Due to its insolubility, Ara-A must be given in ointment form. Ara-A is effective against IDU-resistant strains,[80,115-117] but Ara-A–resistant strains also exist. Ara-A is equally as effective as IDU[111,118,119] and trifluorothymidine (F_3T)[120] in treatment of epithelial herpes, equal to IDU for stromal disease, but ineffective topically for herpes uveitis. Ara-A is generally better tolerated than IDU, but it can cause similar toxicity, particularly punctate keratopathy,[109,112,121] and can elicit hypersensitivity reactions. It is sufficiently tolerated to be given systemically and has been effective in herpetic encephalitis.[122] Ara-A impairs stromal healing, comparable to IDU, but was not teratogenic to rabbits.[123]

Overall, Ara-A is as effective as IDU in treating epithelial disease and can be used as an alternative in patients unable to use trifluridine because of toxicity or allergy.

Trifluridine (trifluorothymidine). Trifluridine (F_3T) is a halogenated pyrimidine that inhibits thymidylate synthetase and is incorporated into viral DNA, impairing transcription and translation of the viral genome. Trifluridine is twice as potent and 10 times more soluble than IDU in a 1% solution,[114,124,125] which greatly increases its ocular penetration. In the treatment of epithelial disease F_3T appears to be more effective than IDU[125-128] and about as effective as Ara-A,[120,129] although it appears to be more effective than Ara-A in healing steroid-treated ulcers.[125,130] Trifluridine is effective in some IDU- and Ara-A–resistant cases,[126,128,131] and resistance to F_3T is rare. Although as yet unproven, it may be of value for both deep stromal disease and uveitis because therapeutic levels of the drug can be obtained in the iris and anterior chamber.[132]

Toxicity can occur with the use of F_3T drops, especially with more prolonged use (more than 2 weeks).[112,133,134] Early signs of toxicity are punctate epithelial erosions and epithelial microcysts. Other complications include filaments, epithelial edema, stromal edema, punctal narrowing, and contact dermatitis. F_3T also tends to impair stromal wound healing. Overall, the toxicity of F_3T appears to be slightly less than that of IDU.

Trifluridine is currently the drug of choice in the United States. It is equal to or greater than other agents in effectiveness, resistance is rare, and penetration is good. Although acyclovir is of equal or superior value and is widely used in Europe, it is not available in the United States because its superiority to other agents has not been documented sufficiently for FDA approval.

Acyclovir. Acyclovir is an acyclic purine nucleoside analog with highly potent and specific activity against HSV types 1 and 2. Noninfected human cells are not affected because viral thymidine kinase is required for activation of the drug (by phosphorylation). Once in its active triphosphate form, it inhibits DNA polymerase. After topical application it penetrates the cornea and reaches the aqueous.[135] It appears to be approximately equal to F_3T and Ara-A in treatment of epithelial herpes.[136-140] In spite of initial optimism, it does not prevent the development of secondary stromal disease.[136,141]

Acyclovir is less toxic to the ocular surface than IDU, Ara-A, and F_3T. Experimentally, it has no significant detrimental effect on epithelial or stromal healing.[142] One of the drug's drawbacks is its greater potential for developing resistant strains. In vitro many mutant herpetic strains are found that do not produce thymidine kinase at all, or produce an altered thymidine kinase that does not phosphorylate the drug and are thus resistant.[143]

Systemic administration of acyclovir has been effective in treatment of genital herpes simplex[144] and herpes zoster.[145] Use of oral acyclovir in ocular herpes has been limited, but it may be beneficial in cases where live virus is suspected to be present in the cornea or anterior chamber.[146,147] It also appears to be as effective as topical acyclovir for herpes simplex epithelial keratitis[148-150] and appears to be useful in necrotizing stromal disease, endotheliitis, and keratouveitis.[146,147] It was not beneficial, however, for treating stromal herpes in one limited study.[151] Oral acyclovir reduces the frequency of genital[152-154] and cutaneous[155] recurrences as long as the drug is continued, and some evidence suggests that it can also reduce ocular recurrences.[147] Laboratory data are contradictory: In two studies, systemic acyclovir was not able to prevent recurrence of ocular herpes,[156,157] but in another it significantly lowered the incidence of ocular viral shedding, geographic ulceration, and stromal keratitis after penetrating keratoplasty.[158]

In those cases where it is likely that virus is present in the anterior chamber—those with focal serous iritis, marked keratic precipitates, and increased pressure and those with endotheliitis—acyclovir would probably be effective.

Interferons. Human cells infected with a virus produce interferon, a substance that inhibits viral infection of other cells. A number of different interferons are produced by different cells, but all appear to exert their effect by inhibiting translation of viral genes. Interferons do have an effect on herpetic keratitis; they are less effective than available agents,[159,160] but they do appear to potentiate the effect of other antiviral agents.[163,166] Despite an initial report,[159] they cannot prevent recurrences.[161,162] Whether the increase in efficacy is sufficient to warrant the combination of drugs remains to be determined.

Other agents. BVDU (5-[2-Bromovinyl]-2'-deoxyuridine), like acyclovir, is phosphorylated by viral thymidine kinase into the active form and therefore is relatively selective in its effect. More active against HSV-1 than HSV-2, it has been effective in clinical trials in treatment of epithelial herpes.[167]

Oligodeoxynucleotides are currently being investigated as antiviral agents. LAT analogs or other antisense nucleotides may be able to inhibit viral replication and suppress reactivation.

A variety of other agents have been found to be effective in treatment of herpetic keratitis in laboratory animals, including ribavirin and fluoro-deoxy-arabinofuranosyl-iosocytosine (FIAC), but have not been tested in humans.

Corticosteroids. The use of corticosteroids in herpetic keratitis remains controversial. Corticosteroids may be used judiciously in treating certain types of herpetic involvement of the cornea. In herpetic keratitis corticosteroids will reduce the immune response, decreasing edema, infiltration, inflammation, and neovascularization. On the other hand, corticosteroids slow epithelial and stromal healing, enhance collagenolytic enzyme production, increase the risk of microbial superinfection (Fig. 12-16), can induce glaucoma and cataract formation, decrease the host's elimination of viral antigens, and can exacerbate active viral infection. Corticosteroids do not appear to increase the risk of reactivation.[168] Corticosteroids are indicated in the treatment of herpetic diseases caused by the host's immunologic response, but not when there is active viral replication. Once corticosteroids are begun, it is often difficult to discontinue them; a rebound marked inflammatory response can occur.

Unfortunately, in many cases it is not possible to discern whether viral replication or host response is primarily responsible for the clinical disease. In general, corticosteroids are used for disciform keratitis and herpetic uveitis but not for epithelial disease. In necrotizing stromal keratitis corticosteroids are sometimes helpful, but the response is unpredictable and caution is indicated. Whenever the epithelium is ulcerated, even if virus is not present, the risk of complications, particularly stromal melting and superinfection, is greater. The risk of complications also seems greater in children. In all cases, the minimum necessary dose should be used, and antiviral medication should be given concomitantly. More specific recommendations are given later.

Specific treatment

Recurrent epithelial keratitis without stromal involvement. Debridement was the primary treatment for epithelial herpes for many years but has been relatively neglected since the development of anti-

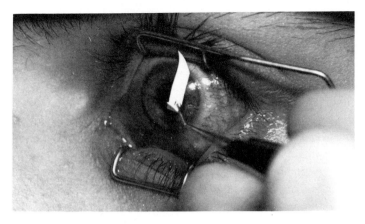

Fig. 12-23. Filter paper debridement of HSV epithelial keratitis. Dry cellulose acetate filter paper is gently applied to corneal surface.

viral agents. In fact, debridement may be equal or superior to antiviral treatment for epithelial herpes,[169] and the combination of debridement and antiviral treatment is more effective than antiviral treatment alone. Reepithelialization may be faster and the incidence of "ghost images" may be lower. One must perform epithelial debridement carefully, so as to avoid stromal injury. Use of a cotton-tipped applicator or cellulose acetate filter paper (Fig. 12-23)[170] is gentler and probably just as effective as scraping.

To improve the chances for eliminating the virus, it is best to administer antiviral medication in addition to debridement.

Antiviral Treatment of Epithelial Disease

DRUG	DOSE
Trifluridine drops 1% (Viroptic)	Nine times daily
Vidarabine ointment 3% (Vira-A)	Five times daily
Idoxuridine drops 0.1% (Stoxil, Herplex, Dendrid)	Every 1 hour by day
Idoxuridine ointment 0.5% (Stoxil)	Five times daily
Acyclovir, oral (Zovirax)	400 mg 5 times daily*
Acyclovir ointment† 3%	Five times daily

Trifluridine is administered nine times daily, and is continued until at least 3 to 5 days after epithelial healing, for up to 2 weeks. (Antiviral treatment is continued after epithelial healing because of experimental data indicating that virus titers rebound to high levels if antiviral therapy is discontinued too early.[171,172]) One should always be on guard for toxic effects of the drug if it is continued for more than 2 weeks. Cycloplegia may increase comfort.

If debridement alone is used, a cycloplegic agent is instilled and a pressure patch applied for 24 hours until the patient is reexamined. If the epithelial defect persists, pressure patching is repeated. If no improvement occurs in 5 to 6 days and the patient is known to be carrying out the proper instructions, debridement and patching may be employed again.

A very young child may need to be restrained before debridement is performed. If this is not possible, topical antiviral medication alone or in combination with oral acyclovir can be used.

---

*Approximate adult dose.
†Available from Burroughs Wellcome, 3030 Cornwallis Rd, Research Triangle Park, NC 27709.

Limbitis. Limbal inflammation or ulceration caused by herpes simplex can be extremely recalcitrant to treatment. Artificial tears are probably as effective as any other therapy. Fortunately, they tend to resolve spontaneously, over weeks to months, without much residual scarring. Antiviral agents may be useful and are recommended. Corticosteroids should be used only if the visual axis is involved or if symptoms are marked.

Disciform keratitis. Opinion varies about the use of corticosteroids in the treatment of disciform keratitis. Some prefer to treat only with cycloplegia and observation. They feel that corticosteroids prolong the disease course but do not affect the final outcome. Others believe that treatment with corticosteroids provides both short- and long-term visual benefits, and they treat all cases that involve the visual axis. I use corticosteroids when vision is significantly reduced, and in those rare cases where pain is marked. The minimum dose necessary to achieve the desired effect is the best course to follow. Once the keratitis has been treated with steroids, it is difficult to control the recurrent inflammation without again using steroids.[173] One must be certain that steroids are essential to treat the disease, as the patient may become committed to steroid use for many months.

Precise guidelines cannot be given, but disciform keratitis tends to be very responsive to steroids, and very dilute doses are often sufficient. Initially, prednisolone acetate .125% to 1% can be used two to four times daily; once the desired effect is achieved the dose is gradually tapered. Often doses as low as 0.005% daily, or 0.125% weekly are sufficient to prevent a resurgence of the disciform keratitis. It is possible either to increase the interval between drops, from daily to every 2 days up to weekly or to progressively dilute the steroid concentration. (This procedure can be performed by your pharmacist.)

Steroid use is more dangerous if an epithelial defect is present and, in most cases, should be avoided until healing occurs. If necessary, prednisone can be given orally (0.5 to 1.0 mg/kg/day). Cycloplegics are usually beneficial. Concurrent antiviral therapy is also indicated to lessen the risk should viral shedding or reinfection occur. One drop of antiviral medication is given for each steroid drop, up to four times per day.

Persistent epithelial defects. Persistent epithelial defects in patients with herpetic keratitis can occur for several reasons, and it is important to determine the exact cause. First, the existence of active viral infection, due to antiviral resistance, recurrence, or poor compliance, must be determined. Some clinical clues were discussed earlier. More commonly, failure of epithelial healing results from antiviral agent toxicity or persistent anterior stromal inflammation. Basement membrane and anterior stromal injury from repeated attacks of herpes can impair the epithelium's ability to cover the corneal surface. Secondary microbial infection is another common cause. Viral, bacterial, and fungal cultures are often useful to rule out active infection. If active viral replication is not present, antiviral medication should be reduced or discontinued. If bacterial infection is not present, antibiotics that interfere with epithelial healing should also be discontinued. Other conditions that impair epithelial healing may be present: dry eye, lagophthalmos, decreased corneal sensation, lid malposition, or trichiasis.

Topical or oral corticosteroids may be helpful to reduce stromal inflammation, but careful monitoring is essential because of the potential for stromal melting. If the surrounding epithelium is hypertrophic or loose it should be removed. Lubricating agents, patching, or a bandage lens will aid reepithelialization. If these measures are not successful a temporary tarsorrhaphy or a conjunctival flap may be necessary.

Stromal ulceration without infiltration. Stromal melting can occur in the presence of a persistent epithelial defect of any cause, even in the absence of active stromal infection. The possible causes and treatment are essentially the same as those discussed in the previous section. If progressive stromal loss is observed, corticosteroids should be avoided, and application of cyanoacrylate glue should be considered.

Stromal ulceration with infiltration (necrotizing stromal keratitis). This is the most difficult form of herpes simplex keratitis to manage. It appears that active viral infection is present in some cases, but most often the destructive process results from the host response in the absence of live virus. Viral culture is helpful, and samples should be taken to determine whether bacterial, fungal, or *Acanthamoeba* infection is present.

It is best to begin with antiviral treatment: drops five times daily, or ointment three times daily. After several days, if virus is not isolated in culture, topical corticosteroids can be added cautiously to reduce inflammation, infiltration, and patient discomfort. Low doses should be used initially, and the patient must be seen frequently. Oral prednisone (approximately 0.5 to 1.0 mg/kg) is often preferable to topical corticosteroids until the epithelium is healed. If ulceration progresses while the patient is on topical steroids, these drugs should be withheld and oral prednisone administered instead. With progressive stromal loss, placement of cyanoacrylate adhesive or a conjunctival flap or therapeutic keratoplasty may be necessary.

The role of oral acyclovir in these patients is currently being evaluated. I use oral acyclovir when patients are unresponsive to topical antiviral drugs and when steroids are ineffective or contraindicated.

Interstitial keratitis. If the epithelium is intact, topical corticosteroid use is less risky but should still be prescribed cautiously. Antiviral medication should be given concurrently (matched drop for drop up to four times daily). It has been hypothesized that limited production of viral proteins is occurring in many cases and complete viral replication in others[33]; therefore, antiviral medication, which blocks formation of viral gene products, may be beneficial. Clinically, however, topical antiviral drugs are rarely effective and are used primarily as prophylaxis, should viral shedding or infection recur.

When corticosteroids are administered, they should be gradually reduced, as discussed under treatment of disciform keratitis. Cycloplegic agents and topical lubricants are often helpful. Oral acyclovir may be useful.

Endotheliitis. Virus has been recovered from the anterior chamber in several cases, suggesting that active infection is present. Paracentesis and culture of aqueous can be performed to make this determination. Topical F_3T and acyclovir have been shown to produce adequate aqueous levels, and they may be effective when used alone; however, I have had success using oral acyclovir in addition. Therefore, I recommend oral acyclovir 200 mg four times daily and F_3T five times daily. Topical corticosteroid, for example, 1% prednisolone acetate, can be given in addition if the epithelium is intact. Acyclovir must be slowly tapered, and prolonged therapy is required in some cases.

Uveitis. In some cases the major site of inflammation is the anterior chamber. In most of these eyes, active viral infection is not present, so corticosteroids are the main treatment. If there is keratitis with a minimal iritis with no hypopyon and no sign of endothelial decompensation, it is best to use a strong cycloplegic agent and antivirals without steroids. In more severe cases, topical corticosteroids are administered (with antiviral prophylaxis), providing the epithelium is intact. If ulceration is present or the response to drops is insufficient, oral corticosteroids are given. As the ulcer epithelializes and stromal inflammation and uveitis improve, the systemic steroids should be stopped and topical steroids initiated, gradually tapering their application.

Oral acyclovir also can be effective, particularly in cases with marked anterior chamber reaction and elevated intraocular pressure, or if virus is isolated from the anterior chamber. If a patient is not responding to steroid and topical antiviral treatment, or if it is not possible to taper oral steroids without reactivation, oral acyclovir (200 to 400 mg four times a day) should be administered.

Prevention of recurrence. No treatment can prevent latency or eliminate latent infection. Chronic administration of low doses of antiviral drops does not prevent recurrent ocular infection; however, early treatment of recurrences does seem to lessen the severity and duration of the attack. Thus it is appropriate for patients to begin antiviral treatment as soon as they sense the onset of an attack. Many patients have prodromal symptoms or clear inciting events, such as fever, extreme stress, or menstruation, and treatment can be initiated at these times.

As was mentioned earlier, chronic administration of oral acyclovir prevents recurrence of genital and cutaneous herpes, but the efficacy of this practice for eye disease is yet to be determined.

Surgical treatment

Conjunctival flaps. Conjunctival flaps can provide a stable epithelial surface, stop ulceration, quiet inflammation, and provide comfort. They should be considered in eyes with persistent or recurrent epithelial defects, progressive ulceration, or marked inflammation unresponsive to therapy. They are particularly useful in chronic peripheral ulcers, where a partial flap can be placed without compromising vision.

Penetrating keratoplasty. If chronic stromal herpes leads to a descemetocele or perforation (see Fig. 12-15), keratoplasty may be necessary. A penetrating graft should be performed, rather than a lamellar graft, because the incidence of recurrence is much lower.[174,175] If possible, it is better to perform keratoplasty in a quiet eye because the success rate is higher.[176-179]

The extent of vascularization has been inversely related to graft success in some studies[176,177] but not in others.[179,180] The use of intensive postoperative steroid treatment appears to be beneficial.[176,181] Even in quiet eyes, however, recurrence of herpetic disease in the graft is common (Fig. 12-24), occurring in approximately 15% of eyes within 2 years.* In addition, there is a greater tendency for graft rejection and noninfectious epithelial defects. Oral acyclovir may be useful in reducing the risk of recurrence.[186]

Approximately 70% to 80% of grafts performed in quiet eyes are clear at 2 years and 50% to 60% at 5 years.[179] If graft failure occurs, the success rate for regrafts is about half that for the primary graft.

Oral corticosteroids are begun 1 to 2 days before keratoplasty, if possible, and are continued for approximately 2 weeks after surgery. Topical corticosteroids are begun the day after surgery and con-

---

*References 69, 133, 176, 178, 180, 182-185.

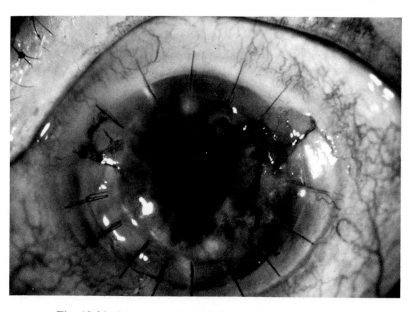

Fig. 12-24. Recurrence of HSV after penetrating keratoplasty.

tinued as long as necessary to control inflammation. Topical antiviral prophylaxis does not appear to be beneficial, except during rejection episodes when HSV recurrence is common.[179,184] I use oral acyclovir (1 to 2 g/day for 10 to 14 days), but its value has not been well demonstrated.

Epithelial recurrence is seen most commonly at the graft-host junction as nondendritic epithelial defects. It is impossible to differentiate clinically between noninfectious epithelial defects and herpetic recurrence, therefore the index of suspicion must be high, and cultures or immunologic testing should be performed. It is often difficult to differentiate between endothelial rejection and herpetic uveitis. If a typical rejection line is present, the diagnosis is clear; if not, the location of keratic precipitates (for example, graft vs. recipient) is not very helpful. In most cases both corticosteroid and antiviral agents are given.

VARICELLA-ZOSTER

VARICELLA-ZOSTER VIRUS

The varicella-zoster virus (VZV) is physically similar to the other herpesviruses: It has a DNA core, a protein coat, or capsid, and may have an envelope (Table 12-1). Like HSV, it replicates in the cell nucleus. Humans appear to be the only natural hosts of VZV. Until recently no animal model of VZV infection was available, limiting research efforts; a guinea pig model of ocular infection has now been developed.[187] The virus can be cultivated in vitro in human cell lines. However, cytopathogenic effects are focal and slow to develop. Extension of individual lesions occurs by direct passage of virus to contiguous cells. Multinucleated giant cells form, and eosinophilic inclusions are seen in the nucleus and occasionally in the cytoplasm of infected cells.

The virus causes both varicella (chickenpox) and herpes zoster (shingles).[188] The initial infection with VZV causes an acute exanthematous disease, chickenpox. The virus then becomes latent in the dorsal root ganglia of the spinal cord, or the trigeminal ganglia. Latency may actually occur in the satellite cells of the spinal column, not in the neurons.[189] Months to decades later, these patients can develop zoster, most likely caused by reactivation of endogenous latent virus.

VARICELLA

Epidemiology. Nearly everyone in the United States contracts varicella, usually before the age of 9 years. In less populous areas of the world (such as the tropics), infection is frequently delayed until adulthood. It is an epidemic disease and is highly contagious (80% to 90% of exposed susceptible individuals become infected). Transmission is through contact with respiratory secretions or cutaneous lesions. The incubation period is 10 to 21 days (average 14 to 17 days).

Clinical manifestations. The most common initial site of infection is the respiratory mucosa. Replication then occurs in the regional lymph nodes, and viruses are released into the bloodstream. The onset of clinical disease is abrupt, with development of a generalized rash, fever, and malaise. The rash occurs in crops, which appear successively over 2 to 5 days and follows a characteristic progression from macule to papule and vesicle, encrustation, and healing, usually without scarring. Complete recovery usually occurs in 1 to 2 weeks.

External ocular involvement occurs most commonly as a papillary conjunctivitis, but "pocks" (Fig. 12-25), dendritic keratitis, disciform keratitis, and interstitial keratitis have been reported.[190-192] Pocks can occur in the conjunctiva, appearing as vesicles with inflammatory cell infiltration and surrounding hyperemia and sometimes associated with focal ulceration or hemorrhage.[193,194] Localized corneal infiltrates, similar to phlyctenules, can also be seen. They usually occur at the time of systemic disease, when they most likely represent active viral infection, but they can also appear months later, possibly as an immunologic response to residual viral antigen. Both corneal and conjunctival lesions resolve spontaneously over 1 to 2 weeks, but the corneal lesions can cause scarring or vascularization (Fig. 12-26).

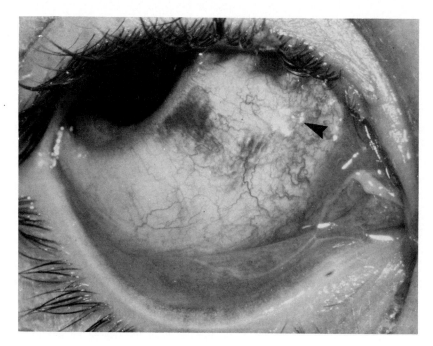

Fig. 12-25. Varicella vesicle of conjunctiva *(arrow)*.

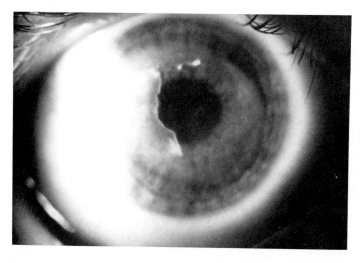

Fig. 12-26. Corneal scarring after varicella keratitis. (Courtesy of Stuart I. Brown, La Jolla, Calif.)

Punctate epithelial lesions can also occur during the acute systemic disease. Dendritic lesions have been reported several months after the systemic disease, sometimes occurring in eyes with disciform keratitis treated with topical steroids. The dendrites closely resemble zoster lesions.[193-196] Because they occurred long after the systemic disease, it is possible that they are local recurrences due to viral shedding. The disciform keratitis appears similar to that seen with HSV or zoster and can last for more than a year.[196-198]

Pocks or epithelial lesions may be treated with antiviral medications, although their efficacy has not been determined. Disciform keratitis will respond to corticosteroid treatment, but the same cautions apply as for HSV disciform disease.

HERPES ZOSTER

Epidemiology. Herpes zoster can occur at any age, in anyone who has had varicella. The incidence increases with age; the incidence of zoster is five times greater in individuals over 80 years of age than in adults between 20 and 40. At the other end of the spectrum, herpes zoster can occur in children several months of age.[199-201] Childhood development of zoster is much more likely if the mother has varicella during pregnancy or the child is infected during the first 2 months of life.[202,203] This phenomenon appears to be related to the infant's reduced immunologic reactivity during the primary attack and reduced immunologic memory against the virus.

An increase in the incidence and severity of zoster is seen in patients with impaired immunity, such as those with lymphoma or other malignancies,[204-206] with acquired immune deficiency syndrome (AIDS),[207,208] or on immunosuppressive therapy.[209,210] In most patients, however, no malignancy or immunologic defect can be found.[211-213] Approximately 2% of nonimmunosuppressed patients will develop a second episode of zoster.

Pathogenesis. Herpes zoster seems to be caused by a reactivation of the latent VZV in the dorsal root ganglion or trigeminal ganglion. After reactivation the virus spreads peripherally from the ganglion along the sensory nerve to the skin. The skin eruption is limited to the dermatomes corresponding to the involved sensory ganglion.

In addition to immunosuppression, radiation, syphilis, tuberculosis, malaria, carbon monoxide or arsenic poisoning, and trauma have been implicated in precipitating zoster.[192] Cases also can develop in patients who are exposed to someone with varicella or zoster.[192,214] Neutralizing antibody is present in the serum, but apparently it does not protect against development of zoster. However, reduction of neutralizing antibody titer below a certain threshold may allow reactivation of the latent virus, and a progressive decrease in titers may occur with age.[215,216]

Herpes zoster is unusual because disease may become manifest many months after the resolution of the initial illness, with no sign of activity during the interim. For reasons not yet determined, disciform keratitis, iritis, or scleritis often appears 3 to 4 months after the cutaneous eruption, sometimes with minimal early ocular involvement.

The cutaneous lesions of zoster are histopathologically identical to those of varicella. The virus replicates in the strata germinativum and spinosum. The inflammatory reaction in the stratum corneum can be severe enough to induce scarring. Lesions with typical intranuclear inclusions are found in the dorsal root ganglion of the sensory nerve supplying the affected area of skin. Pain may be caused by degeneration of small cutaneous nerve bundles and scarring of the segmental nerve and ganglion. Vasculitis is prominent, with granulomatous or diffusely lymphocytic infiltration.[217,218] Lymphocytic infiltration of nerves (particularly the long ciliary nerve), patchy necrosis of the iris and ciliary body, scleritis, and a granulomatous reaction to Descemet's membrane can also be seen.

Clinical manifestations. Zoster occurs after activation of latent VZV that has persisted after primary varicella infection. The area supplied by the trigeminal nerve is second only to the thoracic region in frequency of involvement. The first division of the fifth cranial nerve is affected 20 times more than the second and third divisions. When the disease involves the first division of the fifth nerve, it is known as herpes zoster ophthalmicus (HZO) and is of special importance because of the danger to the eye.

The first symptom of herpes zoster is pain, which is accompanied by hyperesthesia of the skin within the distribution of one or more dermatomes. At the onset, a slight elevation of temperature might occur with some evidence of meningeal irritation. A blushing of the skin develops, sometimes simultaneous with the pain, but usually 3 to 4 days later, followed by the appearance of papules that quickly become vesicles. After a few days the clear fluid within the vesicles becomes turbid and yel-

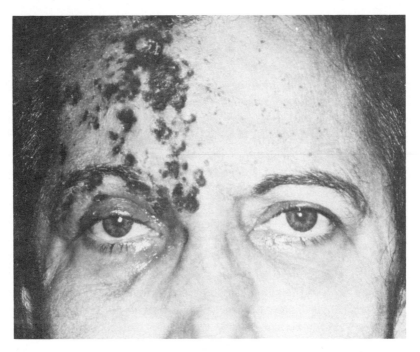

Fig. 12-27. Herpes zoster dermatitis with typical lesions along distribution of frontal nerve.

low; in a short time they burst and crusts form (Fig. 12-27). If secondary infection does not develop, the crusts disappear rapidly, often leaving white scars in the area. The entire cycle usually takes 3 to 6 weeks. Rarely, infection occurs without development of the typical skin lesions.[219-221]

The most distressing symptom is pain; occasionally it is mild, with a feeling of tingling and numbness, but usually it is throbbing and burning. The pain generally subsides with healing of the eruption, but may persist for years. Postherpetic neuralgia is absent in patients under 20 years of age, but occurs in over 50% of patients over 50 years of age. The pain may develop several months after the onset of HZO and tends to gradually diminish with time, but in approximately one fourth of cases it persists for more than a year.[222] The affected area usually is left with decreased sensation and sometimes a slight feeling of numbness and tightness. The viral infection is invariably more severe and prolonged in older patients.

In herpes zoster ophthalmicus the frontal nerve is involved most often, especially its medial branches (supratrochlear and supraorbital). The lacrimal and nasociliary branches are frequently not involved. The pain, scarring, and rash are usually more severe over the area of the skin supplied by the branches affected first. Hutchinson rule—that involvement of the eye is likely if the side of the tip of the nose is involved—is essentially true, but there are some exceptions (Fig. 12-28). Eye involvement also occurs in many patients who do not have Hutchinson's sign. A few lesions can develop outside the involved dermatome, past the midline, or even in a remote area of the body, but this usually does not indicate dissemination. The disease is rarely bilateral.[223]

Dissemination of the rash occurs most frequently in debilitated patients, particularly those with lymphomas.[224] Encephalitis and pneumonia (primary varicella pneumonia) are two of the more serious complications that can occur, but even in immunocompromised patients disseminated zoster is rarely fatal.

Ocular complications. Ocular complications occur in about 50% of cases of ophthalmic zoster, appearing at any time during the eruptive phase or weeks to months after the rash has subsided.[222,225]

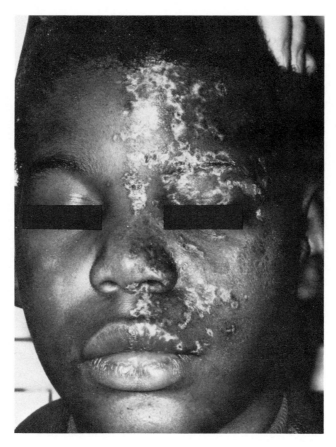

Fig. 12-28. Herpes zoster dermatitis with hemifacial involvement, including the side of the tip of the nose (Hutchinson's sign).

Upper lid. The upper lid generally is affected because of frontal nerve branch involvement. Marked edema of the upper lids with vesicle formation usually occurs. Lesions on the lid skin most often disappear with little or no scarring, but if scarring occurs lagophthalmos or entropion or ectropion of the upper lid may result. Necrosis of the lid and forehead can be seen in the most severe cases.[205] Secondary infection, usually with *Staphylococcus aureus* or streptococci, or canaliculitis, can also develop. Early in the disease ptosis is often present, usually because of mechanical edema, but paresis of the sympathetic third nerve fibers to the levator muscle and third nerve palsy can also be responsible.

Conjunctiva and sclera. The conjunctiva is injected, edematous, and may exhibit petechial hemorrhages (Fig. 12-29). Conjunctivitis is usually papillary, but a follicular or membranous form may develop. Occasionally vesicular lesions occur on the palpebral or bulbar conjunctiva and can cause scarring.

Both episcleritis and scleritis can occur. Episcleritis is common, usually develops early, and can last for months.[222] Scleritis may be seen immediately after the skin lesions have waned or 1 to 3 months later.[226] It can be nodular or diffuse and is frequently recurrent. Sclerokeratitis, with peripheral corneal edema, infiltration, and vascularization, can also be seen.

Cornea. Corneal complications occur in approximately 40% of cases of HZO and can take many forms. The most common findings are dendrites and punctate keratitis.[227] The dendritiform figures (Fig. 12-30) are not excavated, but rather are made up of swollen, heaped-up cells, and have a gray,

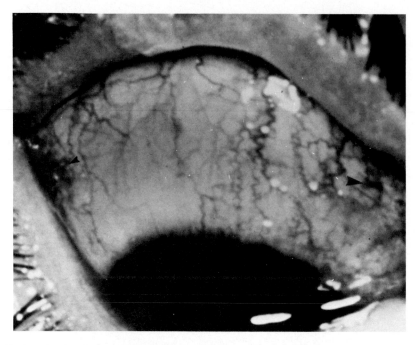

Fig. 12-29. Conjunctiva is edematous and injected. Small petechial hemorrhages are occasionally seen in ophthalmic herpes zoster *(arrows)*.

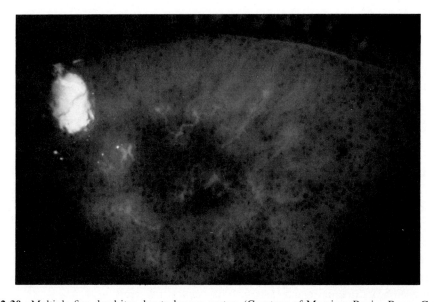

Fig. 12-30. Multiple fine dendrites due to herpes zoster. (Courtesy of Massimo Busin, Bonn, Germany)

plaquelike appearance.[228-232] In contrast to the often delicate pattern of herpes simplex dendrites, the zoster dendrite is more coarse and ropy, and is often stellate (Table 12-4). The terminal bulbs seen in simplex dendrites are not present in zoster dendrites. The dendrites of zoster stain irregularly with fluorescein but well with rose bengal. Like simplex dendrites, these figures contain live virus. The dendrites are seen most often during the acute disease (4 to 6 days) but can appear many weeks afterward, particularly in patients using topical steroids.[233] They resolve without treatment within 1 month.

Punctate keratitis is seen as multiple, peripheral, focal, raised lesions, which stain with rose bengal. These lesions probably contain live virus and may resolve or progress to dendrite formation. Both punctate and dendritic lesions can lead to anterior stromal infiltrates.[227,234] The subepithelial opacities can be nummular or irregular and can reach several millimeters in size. They usually occur 10 days after the onset of the rash and last only a few weeks. They resolve without treatment and appear to respond to topical steroids, but relapse can occur, even as late as 2 years after the onset of the disease.

Disciform keratitis, similar in appearance to that seen in varicella and herpes simplex, can occur

TABLE 12-4. Differential Points of Dendritic Lesions

PROPERTIES	HERPES ZOSTER DENDRITE	HERPES SIMPLEX DENDRITE
Appearance	Medusoid "Painted-on" appearance, like plaque heaped on cornea Coarse, swollen epithelial cells reaching in different directions, either from a central focal point or in an elongated branching figure	Delicate, fine, lacy Denuded ulcer
Terminal bulbs	None	May or may not be seen
Staining	Stains poorly with fluorescein	Edges stain with rose bengal red dye; ulcer base stains well with fluorescein, which diffuses into surrounding diseased epithelium
Response to steroid drops	Good	Made worse
Dermatologic findings and distribution	Grouped vesicles with erythematous base; may occur in crops	Grouped vesicles with erythematous base; may occur in crops May be very similar to zoster; therefore what appears to be typical shingles caused by herpes zoster may be caused by simplex virus.
	Always in dermatomal distribution	May be in dermatomal distribution but usually is not
Healing	Heals usually in 2 to 3 weeks and lasts 5 to 6 weeks	May heal in 7 to 10 days, but may persist for 3 weeks
Symptoms	Prodrome of pain and tingling paresthesias or pruritis in two thirds of cases	May have pain and paresthesias
Age incidence	Peak: over 60 years; may occur in children also	1 to 15 years and 35 to 50 years
Inflammation	Less in histologic examination	More in skin lesions in pathologic examination
Recurrence	Rare; never in same distribution	Common

after HZO (Fig. 12-31). It typically develops 3 to 4 months after the acute disease but can occur at 1 month or after years. The epithelium may not have been involved during the acute attack. Ring infiltrates and necrotizing interstitial keratitis also can occur and are clinically identical to those seen in herpes simplex keratitis. Marginal corneal ulceration can mimic Mooren's ulcer.[235] Corneal vascularization, edema, and scarring are common (Fig. 12-32). If there is stromal vascularization, lipid keratopathy can develop. The pathogenesis of stromal disease in zoster is presumed to be immunologic.

Decreased corneal sensation occurs in approximately 50% of patients, and in one third to one half of these patients it becomes permanent.[222,227] The frequency and severity of hypesthesia tend to be greater than in herpes simplex keratitis. The complications of neurotrophic keratitis are a major cause of the ocular morbidity of this disease: recurrent epithelial breakdown, persistent epithelial defects, sterile ulceration, vascularization, perforation (Fig. 12-33), and superinfection (Fig. 12-34).

Mucus plaques are commonly seen in zoster keratitis and are often confused with viral dendrites. These are gray, elevated, and linear or branching in shape, and stain well with rose bengal (Fig. 12-35).[231,236] They are usually seen 3 to 4 months after the cutaneous disease and change day to day. They lie over degenerating epithelium and stromal inflammation. Corneal sensation is usually decreased. They can be removed from the surface with gentle scraping, which can be useful in differentiating them from true dendrites.

Iris. Uveitis is frequently seen in HZO; it occurs in most eyes with corneal disease but can be seen in isolation. It usually occurs during the initial attack but also can occur months later. The uveitis is most often mild and transient; however, in a considerable number of cases, a severe anterior iridocyclitis develops, which tends to recur. Secondary glaucoma is particularly common.

Single or multiple patches of sectorial iris pigment epithelial loss and atrophy can be seen, due to an obliterative vasculitis.[237] In extreme cases, anterior segment ischemia and necrosis may develop.[238]

Other ocular complications. Herpes zoster rarely affects the retina, but retinal vasculitis,[239] hemorrhagic chorioretinitis, acute retinal necrosis, and nonrhegmatogenous detachments can be seen. Optic neuritis may appear as a retrobulbar neuritis,[224,229,240] papillitis, or neuroretinitis.[241] Pupillary abnormalities and cranial nerve palsies also can occur.[242]

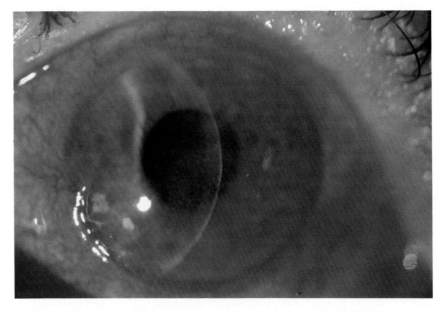

Fig. 12-31. Disciform keratitis after herpes zoster. (Courtesy of Melvin I. Roat, Pittsburgh.)

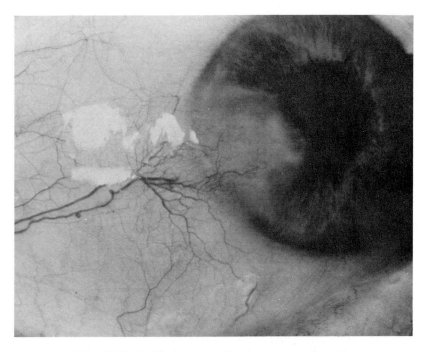

Fig. 12-32. Residual scarring after herpes zoster keratitis.

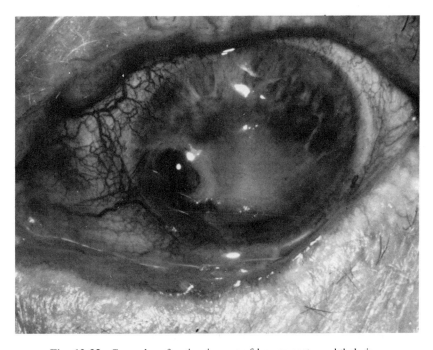

Fig. 12-33. Corneal perforation in case of herpes zoster ophthalmicus.

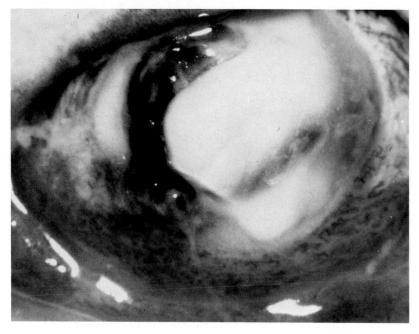

Fig. 12-34. Secondary infection by *Staphylococcus aureus* in cornea compromised by herpes zoster keratitis.

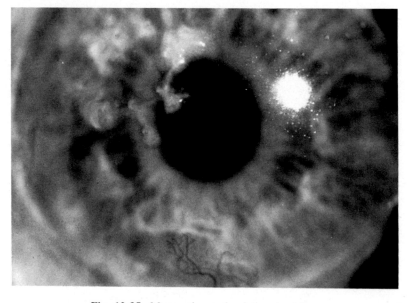

Fig. 12-35. Mucus plaque simulating dendrite.

Diagnosis

Herpes zoster usually can be diagnosed on clinical grounds, although skin lesions in some cases of herpes simplex can be similar. Confusion also can occur in those rare cases in which skin involvement is absent. Laboratory confirmation can be obtained in a number of ways: Vesicular fluid or corneal lesions can be examined with Giemsa or Papanicolaou stain, for multinucleated giant epithelial cells and intranuclear eosinophilic inclusion bodies; electron microscopy can demonstrate the virus; and immunologic tests can indicate the presence of VZV antigens.[243,244] Cultures from early ocular or cutaneous lesions can be inoculated in human tissue culture. The virus is recoverable only in the early lesions, usually during the first 48 to 72 hours.

When ocular disease becomes manifest months after the skin eruption, the diagnosis must be presumptive, based on the history, skin scarring (if present), and consistent clinical picture.

Systemic work-up for malignancy or immunodeficiency disease is generally not indicated; however, a thorough history and review of systems is worthwhile. Herpes zoster is a common presenting manifestation of AIDS, and it is important to question younger patients about their sexual preference, intravenous drug use, or possible exposure by other means and to obtain tests for HIV serum antibodies.[208] Medical evaluation is also indicated in patients with cutaneous dissemination or recurrent disease.

Treatment

General. In vitro VZV is susceptible to IDU, Ara-A, Ara-C, acyclovir, and BVDU; each has been used clinically with some success.[100,145,245-249] Of these, BVDU and acyclovir appear to be the most effective and least toxic.

High doses of oral acyclovir (600 mg five times/day for 10 days) were found to speed resolution of skin lesions, reduce viral shedding, and decrease the incidence of dendritic keratitis, stromal keratitis, and anterior uveitis.[145] In this study treatment was initiated within 7 days of disease onset; when treatment was begun within 72 hours of onset the results were even more marked. There did not appear to be any effect on the incidence or severity of postherpetic neuralgia. The drug was well tolerated. More recently this group has recommended a dose of 800 mg five times daily. Combined topical and oral BVDU also appears to be effective and well tolerated in uncontrolled studies,[246,247] but this medication is not available in the United States.

Administration of oral prednisone may reduce the incidence of postherpetic neuralgia.[250] In the most recent study, 40 mg prednisone tapered over 4 weeks reduced the incidence of postherpetic neuralgia from 65% to 15% of patients.[251] Concern has been raised that systemic steroids may cause dissemination of the infection,[252] but this possibility appears to be a significant risk only in patients with immunodeficiency.

In summary, the current recommended treatment for treatment is as follows (if begun within 7 days of disease onset): acyclovir 800 mg orally 5 times daily for 10 days; add prednisone 40 mg orally daily, gradually tapered over 4 weeks, if the patient is over 50 years of age (see box on p. 276).

Dermal eruption. When administered alone, topical idoxuridine penetrates the skin poorly, but when combined with dimethylsulfoxide (DMSO), its penetration increases. This combination has been effective in reducing symptoms[253] but is not approved for use in the United States. Application of topical acyclovir also may be beneficial, but this has not yet been adequately tested. Burrow's solution, cool compresses, and mechanical cleansing are helpful. Some recommend antibiotic ointment to decrease the risk of bacterial superinfection, but this is probably ineffective.

Punctate epithelial keratitis and dendritic keratitis. These conditions probably result from active viral replication in the epithelium, so it might be expected that antiviral agents would speed their resolution. However, no agent has clearly been demonstrated to be of benefit. Topical acyclovir alone

SUMMARY OF RECOMMENDED TREATMENT FOR ACUTE HERPES ZOSTER

General*	Acyclovir 800 mg orally five times daily for 10 days
	Prednisone 40 mg orally daily, gradually tapered over 4 weeks†
Skin	Burrows solution, cool compresses, mechanical cleansing
	Topical idoxuridine and DMSO‡
Epithelial keratitis	Debridement or none
Stromal keratitis	Topical corticosteroids
Uveitis	Topical corticosteroids
	Oral corticosteroids, ?oral acyclovir (400 mg, four times a day) in severe cases
Corneal mucus plaques	Lubricants, topical corticosteroids, acetylcysteine (10%)

*If less than 7 days after onset.
†If patient is over 50 years of age and not immunocompromised.
‡Not available in the United States.

results in faster resolution of epithelial disease than topical steroids alone or combined topical acyclovir and steroids,[254-256] but acyclovir was not compared with untreated controls. Combined topical and oral BVDU appeared to speed resolution of keratitis, but these studies were uncontrolled.[246,247]

Topical corticosteroids also appear to speed resolution of these lesions,[72,231,243] but one must be absolutely sure of the diagnosis because such treatment could be disastrous if the dendrite were actually caused by herpes simplex.[257] Debridement may be helpful.[258]

Because no treatment has been clearly demonstrated to be beneficial, and these lesions generally resolve in a few days without treatment, it seems best to withhold both antiviral medication and topical corticosteroids. Systemically administered acyclovir, given for general treatment of herpes zoster, may also treat the epithelial lesions because the drug reaches the tear film.

Stromal keratitis. Anterior stromal infiltration, disciform keratitis, interstitial keratitis, and sclerokeratitis all respond to topical corticosteroids.[206,227,250,259] The risks and benefits of treatment are identical to those for herpes simplex, except that corticosteroids do not appear to exacerbate active viral infection with herpes zoster. The minimum dose necessary to achieve the desired effect should be used. Topical corticosteroids should be used with caution in patients with neurotrophic keratitis, exposure, or epithelial defects because of the increased risk of corneal melting.

Uveitis. Corticosteroids are the mainstay of treatment. Topical treatment is usually sufficient, but in some cases oral prednisone may be necessary. Acyclovir, given systemically or topically, has been beneficial in some cases,[254-256] but concurrent corticosteroid treatment is often required.

Nonhealing epithelial defects. Most often these defects result from neurotrophic keratitis, but exposure, trichiasis, anterior stromal inflammation, and drug toxicity are also common. Lid position abnormalities should be corrected and unnecessary drugs discontinued. Lubricant drops and ointments and pressure patching are the simplest measures and are usually successful. If not, therapeutic contact lenses, lateral or total tarsorrhaphy, or a conjunctival flap may be necessary.

Corneal mucus plaques. Mucus plaques often persist for months but usually resolve without treatment. Topical corticosteroids, lubricants, and mucolytic agents can reduce their formation, but recurrences are frequent.[260]

Pain. Zoster pain can be a serious problem. Administration of levodopa (100 mg three times a day for 10 days) during the acute attack reduced the intensity of pain and appeared to reduce the frequency of postherpetic neuralgia.[261] Cimetidine (300 to 400 mg orally daily for 14 days) also has been reported to relieve pain and itching and speed resolution of vesicles,[262,263] but the most recent study did not confirm this.[264] Cimetidine, a histamine receptor (H_2) blocker, may exert its effect through modulation of lymphocyte function.[265] Topical capsaicin has been reported effective, but the number of patients tested was small.[266,267] Amitriptyline, carbamazepine, chlorprothixene, and adenosine monophosphate[268] have all been used, but do not appear to be very effective. In intractable cases stellate ganglion block can provide relief.[269]

Penetrating keratoplasty. Keratoplasty should be approached with caution. There are no large series of cases, but the success rate is generally poor if there is markedly reduced corneal sensation. However, recently two centers have reported a number of successful cases, including some with corneal anesthesia.[270,271] If surgery is contemplated, it is best to wait until at least 1 year after the disease is quiescent. Maintaining epithelial integrity is paramount and should be achieved by obtaining donor tissue with healthy epithelium, protecting this epithelium postoperatively with lubricants, and, in some cases, performing partial or total temporary tarsorrhaphy.

ADENOVIRUS

THE VIRUS

Adenoviruses contain double-stranded DNA surrounded by an icosahedral capsid composed of 252 capsomers. They are not enveloped and measure 70 to 90 nm in diameter. More than 40 immunologically distinct serotypes have been distinguished based on capsomer antigens. As with herpesviruses, viral particle assembly occurs in the nucleus. The virus is relatively easy to isolate in human cell cultures, but no animal model of infection has been developed.

EPIDEMIOLOGY

Nearly all serotypes of adenovirus have been associated with ocular infection.[272] Certain serotypes (1,2,4,5, and 6) are endemic in the population and mainly associated with respiratory and gastrointestinal infection.[273] These serotypes appear to be a common cause of mild conjunctivitis, often associated with sore throat.[274] Other serotypes (3,7,8,10,19, and 30) are seen mainly in epidemics where ocular symptoms predominate and tend to be more severe. Antibodies to these serotypes are rare in the normal population of western countries.[275] The location of the reservoir of these viruses is unclear, but they are much more common in the Orient, and chronic infections and shedding may occur in some cases.[276-278] Transmission during epidemics of ocular disease occurs by contamination of fingers, ophthalmic instruments and solutions,[279] swimming pools,[280] and possibly through sexual contact.[281] One of the most common sites of transmission is the eye clinic. The virus can persist on nonporous surfaces (for example, tonometer tips) for up to 34 days.[282] Adequate handwashing and cleansing of ophthalmic instruments are the mainstay of its control. The incubation period is 2 to 14 days, and in epidemic keratoconjunctivitis the person may remain infectious for 10 to 14 days after symptoms develop.

Two distinct clinical forms of epidemic adenoviral conjunctivitis occur, epidemic keratoconjunctivitis (EKC), and pharyngoconjunctival fever (PCF). EKC is marked by the frequent presence of corneal lesions and PCF by concurrent pharyngitis and fever and the absence of corneal lesions.

EPIDEMIC KERATOCONJUNCTIVITIS

EKC is most commonly produced by serotypes 8 and 19, but many other serotypes (2,3,4,5,7,9,10,11,14,16,21,29, and 37) can produce a similar picture.[283,284]

Clinical manifestations. Symptoms, usually rapid in onset, include watering, soreness, grittiness, and foreign body sensation.[285-290] Most cases are bilateral, with involvement of the second eye frequently occurring 3 to 7 days after the first. Symptoms and signs in the first eye are usually more severe than in the second. Follicular conjunctivitis is the earliest and most common sign. The follicles are more evident in the inferior fornix. Petechial hemorrhages are often present in the palpebral conjunctiva, and rarely, more extensive hemorrhage is seen. Pseudomembranous or membranous conjunctivitis can occur in more severe cases (Fig. 3-9 and 12-36). Lid edema is common and may be

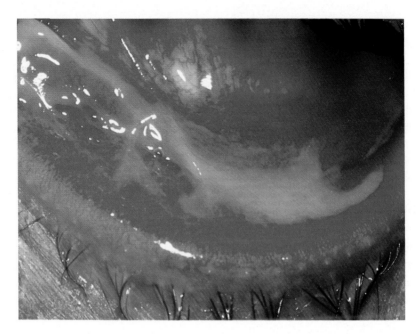

Fig. 12-36. Severe conjunctival hyperemia, follicular response, and membrane formation in EKC.

mistaken for cellulitis. Preauricular adenopathy develops in the majority of cases, usually within the first few days of symptoms. Conjunctivitis usually resolves in about 2 weeks, but corneal involvement may last much longer.

The characteristic course of the keratitis has been well documented.[291,292] Approximately 3 to 4 days after onset of symptoms, a diffuse fine epithelial keratitis appears (Fig. 12-37). Minute white dots are seen, some of which stain with fluorescein or rose bengal, and persist in the majority of cases for 2 to 3 weeks. Approximately 1 week after onset, focal epithelial keratitis develops and persists for 1 to 2 weeks (Fig. 12-38). The focal lesions are similar to those seen in other forms of viral keratitis, with central ulceration and irregular borders with gray-white dots, which may be elevated. Fluorescein stains the central portion of the lesions. Both the diffuse and focal lesions are thought to be caused by active viral infection.

Approximately 2 weeks after onset, subepithelial infiltrates can develop beneath the focal epithelial lesions (Fig. 12-39). The patient then develops increased photophobia and decreased vision. If untreated, these infiltrates gradually fade over weeks or months but can persist for more than 10 years. Histologically, they are composed of lymphocytes and can be associated with overlying defects in Bowman's membrane and epithelial basement membrane.[293] The infiltrates are most likely an immunologic response to viral antigens, which have seeped into the stroma.[294]

Rarely disciform keratitis or anterior uveitis can occur.[275] In a few cases, chronic or recurrent inflammation has occurred after typical EKC, and adenovirus was recovered again many months after the disease onset.[276-278] In some of these cases a chronic papillary conjunctivitis was the only manifestation; in others recurrent focal epithelial keratitis was noted, sometimes over stromal infiltrates. Chronic steroid use had been present in some cases but not in others.

Treatment. The most important measure is prevention of spread of the disease by the patient and physician. The patient should be informed about the length of time the disease is infectious and the types of precautions that are necessary to prevent spread.

No agent has been found to be effective against acute infection. Treatment therefore is palliative

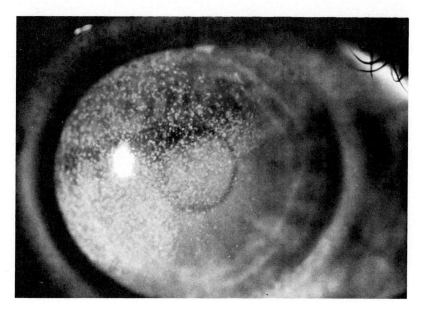

Fig. 12-37. Epithelial staining in early EKC.

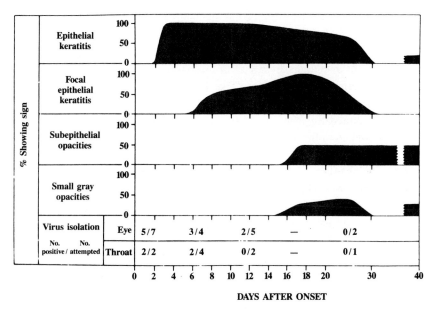

Fig. 12-38. Clinical course of keratitis and virus isolations in patients with epidemic keratoconjunctivitis. Diffuse superficial epithelial keratitis is present from the first day in most cases. Focal epithelial lesions (or coarse keratopathy) appear approximately 7 days after onset. Subepithelial opacities form at the site of some of the focal epithelial lesions from the eleventh to fifteenth day. Subepithelial involvement may persist for many months after the epithelium clears. (From Dawson C et al: Am J Ophthalmol 69:473, 1970.)

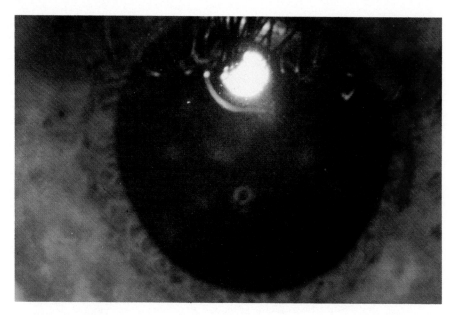

Fig. 12-39. Subepithelial corneal infiltrates seen in EKC.

and can include warm or cold compresses, lubrication, topical vasoconstrictors, and cycloplegic drops. The risk of bacterial superinfection is very low, so prophylactic antibiotic treatment is unnecessary.

If membranes form, their removal usually provides some symptomatic relief. Because membranes can result in conjunctival scarring, treatment with a mild steroid, one to two times daily, is recommended. A steroid-sulfacetamide combination drop may be used.

Topical steroids are very effective in relieving the signs and symptoms of subepithelial infiltrates; however, the end result is probably the same, and weaning patients can be very difficult. Steroids are most effective early in the course but also can be beneficial as long as 1 year after onset. In general, their use is indicated if the symptoms are severe or prolonged, if vision is markedly reduced, or if the patient is unable to perform normal activities. The risks and benefit of their use should be discussed with the patient and a mutual decision made. It is probably best to avoid their use, if possible, because they are often required for many months, may cause persistent viral infection, and often produce the common steroid complications.

Pharyngoconjunctival Fever

Pharyngoconjunctival fever (PCF) is an acute follicular conjunctivitis associated with pharyngitis and fever and seen mainly in children[295] (Fig. 12-40). It is most commonly caused by serotypes 3 and 7. PCF is highly contagious and is spread mainly via respiratory secretions, but also through contaminated swimming pools. Regional adenopathy is usually present; conjunctival hemorrhage also may occur. A mild diffuse punctate keratitis can be seen; subepithelial infiltrates are rare.

The ocular findings in PCF are similar to those of acute hemorrhagic conjunctivitis and early EKC, but patients do not have the systemic symptoms of PCF. There is no specific treatment. Resolution generally occurs in 7 to 14 days.

INFECTIOUS MONONUCLEOSIS

Infectious mononucleosis is caused by EBV, a herpesvirus. An acute conjunctivitis can occur, sometimes with follicles, hemorrhage, focal white infiltrates, or membrane development.[296,297] Con-

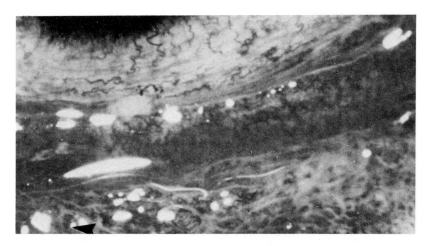

Fig. 12-40. Large follicles in lower tarsal conjunctiva in pharyngoconjunctival fever.

junctival granulomas have been seen, associated with preauricular adenopathy (see Parinaud's oculo-glandular syndrome, Chapter 6). Focal epithelial keratitis can occur during the acute disease, and, in one case, small dendritic lesions were observed from which EBV was isolated.[298] An unusual num-mular keratitis, with lamellar infiltrates at all levels of the cornea, can be seen months after the acute illness (see Chapter 11). Other ocular findings include lid edema (common), dacryoadenitis, episcleri-tis, uveitis, optic neuritis, retinal edema, and retinal hemorrhages.[192,299,300]

NEWCASTLE DISEASE

Newcastle disease is caused by a virus that produces fatal pneumonitis in fowl. Human infections occur in poultry workers and laboratory technicians and are manifested as unilateral, usually follicu-lar, conjunctivitis with scant watery discharge.[301] Preauricular adenopathy is present, and a fine epi-thelial keratitis and subepithelial infiltrates can be seen. The disease resolves spontaneously without sequelae.

ACUTE HEMORRHAGIC CONJUNCTIVITIS

Acute hemorrhagic conjunctivitis is an acute follicular conjunctivitis that occurs in epidemics. It is caused by enteroviruses, which are members of the family Picornaviridae—small, nonenveloped RNA viruses. Polioviruses, echoviruses, and coxsackieviruses are types of enteroviruses. Epidemic conjunctivitis is usually caused by enterovirus type 70 and coxsackievirus type A24.[302] After an in-cubation period of less than 24 hours, patients develop pain, foreign body sensation, tearing, and photophobia in one eye that rapidly spreads to the other.[303] A mild follicular conjunctivitis is seen, sometimes with subconjunctival hemorrhage and preauricular adenopathy[288,294,304-307] (Fig. 12-41). The frequency of these findings varies considerably in different epidemics. A fine epithelial keratitis and subepithelial infiltrates also can be seen. Nearly all cases resolve without ocular sequelae in 2 to 3 weeks, but neurologic complications, particularly radiculomyelitis, can occur.[308]

OTHER VIRAL INFECTIONS

Viral infection of the external eye can occur in mumps, rubeola, rubella, variola, and vaccinia. The ocular findings in these diseases, as well as a summary of external ocular findings in other viral diseases, are given in Table 12-5. The characteristics of epithelial cell inclusions in viral diseases and chlamydial diseases are listed in Table 4-3.

TABLE 12-5. Summary of Viral External Disease

VIRUS	LIDS	CONJUNCTIVITIS	CORNEA	ADENOPATHY	OTHER FINDINGS	COMMENTS
HERPESVIRUSES						
Herpes simplex (primary)	Vesicles, hyperemia, swelling	Follicular, membranes (50%)	FK,* dendrite	+	Canniliculitis, iritis	
Varicella	Vesicles, hyperemia, swelling	Papillary, pocks	SPK,† dendrites, phlyctenules, disciform keratitis	++	Iritis	
Zoster	Vesicles, marked edema, hyperemia	Usually papillary; can be follicles, membranes, hemorrhages	Dendrites, disciform keratitis	−	Keratouveitis, scleritis, retinitis, others	Typical skin involvement
Epstein-Barr	Mild hyperemia and swelling	Usually papillary, can be follicles, hemorrhage, membranes, infiltrate, granuloma	FK, dendrites, nummular keratitis (late)	+	Infectious mononucleosis, canniliculitis, episcleritis, uveitis, optic neuritis	Usually mild or no conjunctivitis
CMV[309]		Mild follicular		−	Mononucleosis-like illness, chorioretinitis	
ADENOVIRUSES						
EKC	Swelling, hyperemia	Follicles, hemorrhages, membranes	SPK, FK, subepithelial infiltrates	++	Iritis (rare)	Most commonly types 8, 19
PCF	Swelling, hyperemia	Follicles, hemorrhages, membranes	SPK	++	Pharyngitis, fever	Most commonly types 3, 7
ENTEROVIRUSES						
Acute hemorrhagic conjunctivitis	Mild swelling, hyperemia	Mild follicular response, hemorrhagic	SPK, subepithelial infiltrates	+ (60%)	Radiculomyelitis	Occurs in epidemics, incubation period <24 hrs

	Lids	Conjunctiva	Cornea			
PARAMYXOVIRUSES						
Newcastle disease	Mild swelling, hyperemia	Usually follicular	SPK, subepithelial infiltrates	+	Occurs in poultry workers and lab technicians	
Mumps[310-312]	Mild swelling, hyperemia	Catarrhal, occasionally follicular	SPK, disciform keratitis (Fig. 12-43)	−	Episcleritis scleritis uveitis dacryoadenitis others	
Rubeola (measles)[313-315]	Swelling of plica	Catarrhal, Koplik spots	SPK, rarely interstitial keratitis, corneal ulcers	+	Fever, rash, rarely severe systemic disease, other ocular disease	Severe corneal complications in malnourished children
POXVIRUSES						
Variola (smallpox) (Fig. 12-44)	Swelling, hyperemia	Follicular, can have hemorrhage, pus, pocks	Corneal pocks, disciform keratitis, interstitial keratitis	+	Fever, rash, can be fatal	Now rare
Vaccinia[316-320]	Marked lid swelling, "kissing lesions" (Fig. 12-45)	Catarrhal or purulent, papillary or follicular	SPK, disciform keratitis, interstitial keratitis	++	Malaise, fever	After smallpox vaccination
Molluscum contagiosum	Typical lid lesion(s)	Follicular, rarely primary lesion	SPK, pannus	−		
TOGAVIRUSES						
Rubella[321,322] (acquired)		Mild catarrhal or follicular	SPK	−	Fever, rash	Conjunctivitis 70%, keratitis 2%
PAPOVAVIRUSES						
Papilloma virus	Warts	Warts, papillae, rarely follicles	SPK	−		
ORTHOMYXOVIRUSES						
Influenza virus		Follicular	—	−	Influenza	

*Focal keratitis.
†Superficial punctate keratitis.

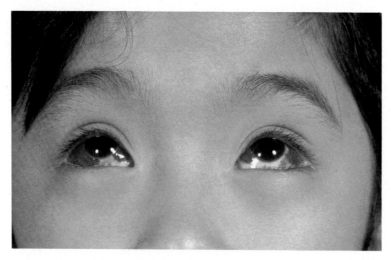

Fig. 12-41. Acute hemorrhagic conjunctivitis. (Courtesy of Eric Donnenfeld, Rockville Center, NY.)

DISEASE SUSPECTED TO BE OF VIRAL ORIGIN

DIMMER'S NUMMULAR KERATITIS

Dimmer's nummular keratitis is rare and characterized by multiple disc-shaped infiltrates in the superficial stroma. The etiology has not been demonstrated, but is suspected to be viral. Dimmer's nummular keratitis is discussed in Chapter 11.

THYGESON'S SUPERFICIAL PUNCTATE KERATITIS

Thygeson's superficial punctate keratitis (TSPK) is characterized by bilateral recurrent focal epithelial keratitis without associated conjunctival or stromal inflammation.[323-328] The etiology is unknown but is suspected to be viral. It can affect all age groups, with the greatest incidence seen in the second and third decades. Patients report photophobia, tearing, foreign body sensation, and often a mild decrease in vision. The classic corneal lesion in TSPK is a group of coarse, oval-shaped, slightly raised, white or gray dots that stain with fluorescein (Fig. 12-42). One to 50 of these lesions can be present, 20 on the average, and they tend to affect the central cornea more than the periphery. This classic picture is seen during active, symptomatic disease; during inactive stages the lesions can disappear, can be flat, gray, intraepithelial dots that do not stain, or appear stellate. The epithelium is normal between the lesions, and subepithelial opacities do not develop, unless toxic drugs, such as IDU, are used. The conjunctiva may be mildly injected; tiny, hairlike filaments may be present; and corneal sensation is normal or only slightly subnormal.

Individual attacks generally last 1 to 2 months, go into remission for 4 to 6 weeks, and then recur; the time course is variable. Usually after 2 to 4 years, the disease resolves without sequelae, but persistence as long as 20 years has been observed, particularly with steroid use.[326]

Symptoms can be relieved and signs suppressed by using soft or hard contact lenses or by applying topical steroids.[329,330] Low concentrations of steroids (for example, 0.12% prednisolone) two to three times daily, generally only for a few days to 2 weeks, are usually sufficient to bring relief. If sufficient response is not obtained or more intensive or prolonged treatment is required, bandage contact lenses can be applied. Antiviral agents do not appear to be beneficial. IDU does not speed resolution and can cause subepithelial scarring. Trifluridine has been reported to induce resolution without recurrence when used nine times/day for weeks to months[331]; however, most have not experienced success with this agent.

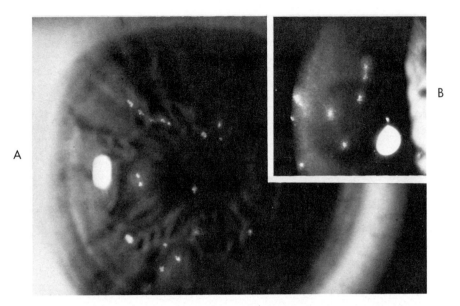

Fig. 12-42. Thygeson superficial punctate keratitis. **A,** Coarse, whitish lesions clustered in central cornea. **B,** More magnified view of lesions.

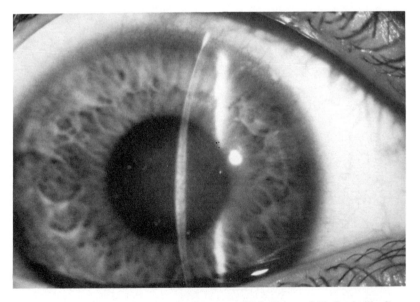

Fig. 12-43. Disciform keratitis in mumps. (Courtesy of Eric Donnenfeld, Rockville Center, NY.)

That TSPK is caused by a virus is supported by the resemblance of the epithelial lesions to those seen in measles, mumps, variola, and adenovirus infection and by electron microscopic evidence of virus particles in epithelial lesions. In two cases a virus was isolated from these lesions: In one case the virus was not identified,[332] and in the other it was identified as VZV.[333] Ostler[334] has suggested that a slow virus may be responsible.

The frequency of HLA-DR3 is significantly increased in patients with TSPK,[328] suggesting an

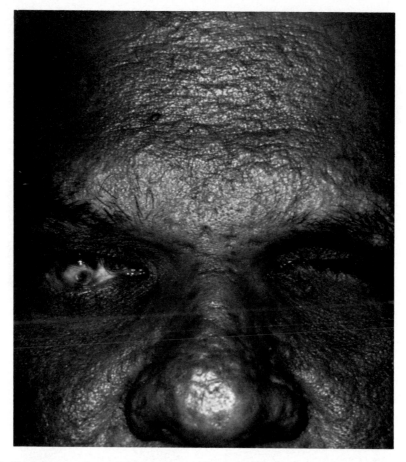

Fig. 12-44. Skin and corneal scarring in smallpox. (Courtesy of Eric Donnenfeld, Rockville Center, NY.)

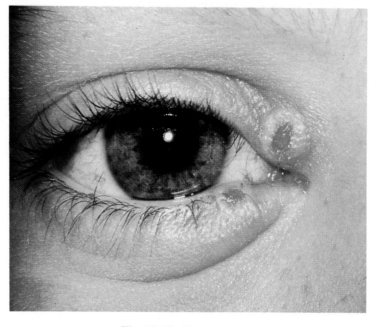

Fig. 12-45. Vaccinia of lid.

immunologic role. Further evidence for an immunologic role is the dramatic response to corticosteroids and the extended course of the disease.

REFERENCES

1. Henson D et al: Ultrastructural localization of herpes simplex virus antigens on rabbit corneal cells using sheep antihuman IgG anti-horse ferritin hybrid antibodies, Invest Ophthalmol 13:819, 1974.
2. Baringer JR and Swoveland P: Recovery of herpes simplex virus from human trigeminal ganglions, N Engl J Med 288:648, 1973.
3. Warren KG et al: Isolation of latent herpes simplex virus from the superior cervical and vagus ganglions of human beings, N Engl J Med 298:1068, 1978.
4. Rong BL et al: Detection of the herpes simplex virus genome in the human cornea, Ophthalmology 95(suppl):159, 1988.
5. Abghare SZ and Stulting RD: Recovery of herpes simplex virus from ocular tissues of latently infected inbred mice, Invest Ophthalmol Vis Sci 29:239, 1988.
6. Cook SD, Batra SK, and Brown SM: Recovery of herpes simplex virus from corneas of experimentally infected rabbits, J Gen Virol 68:2013, 1987.
7. Cook SD and Brown SM: Herpes simplex virus type 1 persistence and latency in cultured rabbit corneal epithelial cells, keratocytes, and endothelial cells, Br J Ophthalmol 70:642, 1986.
8. Claoué CMP et al: Does herpes simplex virus establish latency in the eye of the mouse? Eye 1:525, 1987.
9. Easty DL: Virus disease of the eye, Chicago, 1985, Mosby–Year Book, Inc.
10. Tullo AB et al: Spread of virus and distribution of latent infection following ocular herpes simplex in the non-immune and immune mouse, J Gen Virol 63:95, 1982.
11. Hill TJ: Ocular pathogenicity of herpes simplex virus, Curr Eye Res 6:1, 1987.
12. Gordon Y and Araullo-Cruz T: Herpesvirus inoculation of cornea, Am J Ophthalmol 97:482, 1984.
13. Chaney SMJ, Warren KG, and Subak-Sharpe JH: Variable restriction endonuclease sites of herpes simplex virus type 1 isolates form encephalic, facial and genital lesions and ganglia, J Gen Virol 64:2717, 1983.
14. Lonsdale DM et al: Variations in herpes simplex virus isolated form human ganglia and a study of clonal variation in HSV-1, Ann NY Acad Sci 354:291, 1980.
15. Gerson M: Consecutive infections with herpes simplex virus types 1 and 2 within a three-week period, J Infect Dis 149:655, 1984.
16. Lewis ME et al: Detection of multiple strains of HSV-1 within individual human hosts, Oxford, 1983, International Herpesvirus Workshop.
17. Heller M et al: Herpetic proctitis and meningitis: recovery of two strains of herpes simplex type 1 from cerebrospinal fluid, J Infect Dis 146:584, 1982.
18. Gordon YJ et al: RNA complementary to herpes simplex virus type 1 ICPO gene demonstrated in neurons of human trigeminal ganglia, J Virol 62:1832, 1988.
19. Rock DDL et al: Detection of latency-related viral RNAs in trigeminal ganglia of rabbits latently infected with herpes simplex virus type 1, J Virol 61:3820, 1987.
20. Stevens JS et al: RNA complementary to herpesvirus alpha mRNA is prominent in latently infected neurons, Science 235:1056, 1987.
21. Stevens JG et al: The herpes simplex virus latency associated transcript is prominent in trigeminal ganglia for seropositive humans, J Infect Dis 158:117, 1988.
22. Croen KD et al: Latent herpes simplex virus in human trigeminal ganglia. Detection of an immediate early gene "anti-sense" transcript by in situ hybridization, N Engl J Med 317:1427, 1987.
23. Kwon BS et al: Induction of ocular herpes simplex virus shedding by iontophoresis of epinephrine into rabbit cornea, Invest Ophthalmol Vis Sci 24:441, 1981.
24. Gordon YJ et al: The development of an improved murine iontophoresis reactivation model for the study of HSV-1 latency, Invest Ophthalmol Vis Sci 27:1230, 1986.
25. Openshaw H et al: Acute and latent infection of sensory ganglia with herpes simplex virus: immune control and virus reactivation, J Gen Virol 44:205, 1979.
26. Gerdes JC and Smith DS: Recurrence phenotypes and establishment of latency following rabbit keratitis produced by multiple herpes simplex virus strains, J Gen Virol 64:2441, 1983.
27. Wander AH, Centifanto YM, and Kaufman HE: Strain specificity of clinical isolates of herpes simplex virus, Arch Ophthalmol 98:1458, 1980.
28. Centifanto-Fitzgerald YM et al: Ocular disease pattern induced by herpes simplex virus is genetically determined by a specific region of viral DNA, J Exp Med 155:475, 1982.
29. Centifanto-Fitzgerald YM, Fenger T, and Kaufman HE: Virus proteins in herpetic keratitis, Exp Eye Res 35:425, 1982.
30. Smeraglia R et al: The role of herpes simplex virus secreted glycoproteins in herpetic keratitis, Exp Eye Res 35:443, 1982.
31. Kaufman HE et al: Effect of the herpes simplex virus genome on the response of infection to corticosteroids, Am J Ophthalmol 100:114, 1985.
32. Ahonen R, Vannas A, and Mäkitie J: Virus particles and leukocytes in herpes simplex keratitis, Cornea 3:43, 1984.
33. Gordon YJ: Herpetic stromal keratitis: a new molecular model and its clinical correlation. In Cavanagh HD, editor: The cornea: Transactions of the World Congress on the Cornea III, New York, 1988, Raven Press.
34. Pavan-Langston D: Viral diseases: herpetic infections. In Smolin G and Thoft RA, editors: The cornea: scientific foundations and clinical practice, Boston, 1983, Little, Brown & Co.
35. Zimmerman TJ et al: HLA types and recurrent corneal herpes simplex infection, Invest Ophthalmol 16:756, 1977.

36. Foster CS et al: HLA phenotypic expression in patients with recurrent and nonrecurrent herpes simplex keratitis. In Sundmacher R, editor: Herpetic eye diseases, Munich, 1981, Verlag.

37. Meyers-Elliot R et al: HLA antigens in herpes stromal keratitis, Am J Ophthalmol 89:54, 1980.

38. Smith J, Pentherer J, and MacCallum F: The incidence of herpesvirus hominis antibody in the population, J Hyg 65:396, 1967.

39. Locatcher-Khorazo D and Seegal BC: Microbiology of the eye, St Louis, 1972, Mosby–Year Book, Inc.

40. Brown DC: Ocular herpes simplex, Invest Ophthalmol 10:210, 1971.

41. Norn MS: Dendritic herpetic keratitis: 1. Incidence, seasonal variations, recurrence rate, visual impairment, therapy, Acta Ophthalmol 48:91, 1970.

42. Liesegang TJ et al: Epidemiology of ocular herpes simplex: incidence in Rochester, Minn, 1950 through 1982, Arch Ophthalmol 107:1155, 1989.

43. Liesegang TJ: Epidemiology of ocular herpes simplex: natural history in Rochester, Minn, 1950 through 1982, Arch Ophthalmol 107:1160, 1989.

44. Wilhelmus KR, Falcon MG, and Jones BR: Bilateral herpetic keratitis, Br J Ophthalmol 65:385, 1981.

45. Bell D, Holman R, and Pavan-Langston D: Epidemiological aspects of herpes simplex keratitis, Ann Ophthalmol 14:421, 1982.

46. Shuster J, Kaufman HE, and Nesburn AB: Statistical analysis of the rate of recurrence of herpesvirus ocular epithelial disease, Am J Ophthalmol 91:328, 1981.

47. Wilhelmus KR et al: Longitudinal analysis of ulcerative herpetic keratitis. In Sundmacher R, editor: Herpes eye diseases, Munich, 1981, Bergmann Verlag.

48. Norn MS: Dendritic (herpetic) keratitis: 2. Follow-up examinations of corneal opacity, Acta Ophthalmol (Kbh) 48:214, 1970.

49. Claque CMP, Menage MJ, and Easty DL: Severe herpetic keratitis. I. Prevalence of visual impairment in a clinic population, Br J Ophthalmol 72:530, 1988.

50. Change R, Fiumara NJ, and Weinstein L: Genital herpes, JAMA 229:544, 1974.

51. Tarkkanen A and Laatkainen L: Late ocular manifestations in neonatal herpes simplex infection, Br J Ophthalmol 61:608, 1977.

52. Wheeler CE Jr and Huffines WD: Primary disseminated herpes simplex of the newborn, JAMA 191:111, 1965.

53. Zaib ZM, Nahmias AJ, and Josey WE: Genital herpes infections associated with cervical dysplasia and carcinoma, Cancer 23:940, 1969.

54. Pierson RB and Kirkham TH: Neonatal keratitis due to herpesvirus: hominis type 1 infection, Can J Ophthalmol 9:429, 1974.

55. Hanna L, Ostler HB, and Keshishyan H: Observed relationship between herpetic lesions and antigenic type of *Herpesvirus hominis,* Surv Ophthalmol 21:110, 1976.

56. Oh JO and Stevens TR: Comparison of types 1 and 2 *Herpesvirus hominus* infection of rabbit eyes. I. Clinical manifestations, Arch Ophthalmol 90:473, 1973.

57. Stevens TR and Oh JO: Comparison of types 1 and 2 *Herpesvirus hominus* infection of rabbit eyes. II. His-

topathologic and virologic studies, Arch Ophthalmol 90:477, 1980.

58. Harris GJ et al: Herpetic canalicular obstruction, Arch Ophthalmol 99:383, 1981.

59. Stern GA, Zarn SZ, and Gutgesell VJ: Primary herpes simplex subepithelial dendritic keratitis, Am J Ophthalmol 91:496, 1981.

60. Egerer U and Stary A: Erosive-ulcerative herpes simplex blepharitis, Arch Ophthalmol 98:1760, 1980.

61. Darouger S et al: Acute follicular conjunctivitis and keratoconjunctivitis due to herpes simplex virus in London, Br J Ophthalmol 62:843, 1978.

62. Jones BR: Differential diagnosis of punctate keratitis, Int Ophthalmol Clin 2:291, 1962.

63. Duke-Elder S and Leigh AG: System of ophthalmology, vol VIII: Diseases of the outer eye, St Louis, 1965, Mosby–Year Book, Inc.

64. Lanier JD: Marginal herpes simplex keratitis, Ophthalmol Digest 38:15, 1976.

65. Pavan-Langston D et al: Intraocular penetration of ARA-A and IDU: therapeutic implication in clinical herpetic uveitis, Trans Am Acad Ophthalmol Otolaryngol 77:455, 1973.

66. Thygeson P: Marginal herpes simplex keratitis simulating catarrhal ulcer, Invest Ophthalmol 10:1006, 1971.

67. Lowry SF, Melnick JL, and Rawls WE: Investigation of plaque formation in chick embryo cells as a biological marker for distinguishing herpes virus type 2 from type 1, J Gen Virol 10:1, 1971.

68. Kaufman H: Epithelial erosion syndrome: metaherpetic keratitis, Am J Ophthalmol 57:984, 1964.

69. Laibson PR: Surgical approaches to the treatment of active keratitis, Int Ophthalmol Clin 13:65, 1973.

70. Kaufman HE, Konai A, and Ellison ED: Herpetic iritis: demonstration of virus in the anterior chamber by fluorescent antibody techniques and electronmicroscopy, Am J Ophthalmol 71:465, 1971.

71. Pavan-Langston D: Diagnosis and management of herpes simplex ocular infection, Int Ophthalmol Clin 15:19, 1975.

72. Pavan-Langston D and Brockhurst RJ: Herpes simplex panuveitis, Arch Ophthalmol 81:783, 1969.

73. Carrol JM et al: The recurrence of herpetic keratitis following idoxuridine therapy, Am J Ophthalmol 63:103, 1967.

74. Hendricks RL, Epstein RJ, and Tumpey T: The effect of cellular immune tolerance to HSV-1 antigens on the immunopathology of HSV-1 keratitis, Invest Ophthalmol Vis Sci 30:105, 1989.

75. Jones BR: The management of ocular herpes, Trans Ophthalmol Soc UK 79:425, 1959.

76. Oh JO: Endothelial lesions of rabbit cornea produced by herpes simplex virus, Invest Ophthalmol 9:196, 1970.

77. Collin HB and Abelson MB: Herpes simplex virus in human cornea, retrocorneal fibrous membrane, and vitreous, Arch Ophthalmol 94:1726, 1976.

78. Metcalf JF and Reichert RW: Histological and electron microscopic studies of experimental herpetic keratitis in the rabbit, Invest Ophthalmol Vis Sci 18:1123, 1979.

79. Sundmacher R and Neumann-Haefelin D: Herpes sim-

plex virus-positive and virus-negative keratouveitis. In Silverstein AM and O'Connor GR, editors: Immunology and immunopathology of the eye, New York, 1979, Masson Publishing.

80. Brightbill FS and Kaufman HE: Adenine arabinoside therapy in corneal stromal disease and iritis due to herpes simplex, Ann Ophthalmol 6:25, 1974.

81. Dawson CR, Togni B, and Moore TE Jr: Structural changes in chronic herpetic keratitis, Arch Ophthalmol 79:740, 1968.

82. Shimeld C et al: Isolation of herpes simplex virus from the cornea in chronic stromal keratitis, Br J Ophthalmol 66:643, 1982.

83. Sanitato JJ et al: Acyclovir in the treatment of herpetic stromal disease, Am J Ophthalmol 98:537, 1984.

84. Hewson GE: Iritis due to herpes virus, Ir J Med Sci 372, 1957.

85. Witmer R and Iwamoto T: Electron microscope observation of herpes-like particles in the iris, Arch Ophthalmol 79:331, 1968.

86. Robin JB, Steigner JB, and Kaufman HE: Progressive herpetic corneal endotheliitis, Am J Ophthalmol 100:336, 1985.

87. Vannas A and Ahonen R: Herpetic endothelial keratitis: a case report, Acta Ophthalmol 59:296, 1981.

88. Plotkin J, Reynaud A, and Olumoto M: Cytologic study of herpetic keratitis, Arch Ophthalmol 85:597, 1971.

89. Smith TF: Clinical uses of the diagnostic virology laboratory, Med Clin North Am 67:935, 1983.

90. Roat MI et al: Antiviral effects of rose bengal and fluorescein, Arch Ophthalmol 105:1415, 1987.

91. Kaufman HE: The diagnosis of corneal herpes simplex infection by fluorescent antibody staining, Arch Ophthalmol 64:382, 1960.

92. Dunkel EC et al: Rapid detection of herpes simplex virus (HSV) antigen in human ocular infections, Curr Eye Res 7:661, 1988.

93. Cleveland PH and Richman DD: Enzyme immunofiltration staining assay for the immediate diagnosis of herpes simplex virus and varicella zoster virus directly from clinical specimens, J Clin Microbiol 25:416, 1987.

94. Kowalski RP and Gordon YJ: Evaluation of immunologic tests for the detection of ocular herpes simplex virus, Ophthalmology 96:1583, 1989.

95. Gebhardt BM, Reidy J, and Kaufman HE: An affinity membrane test for superficial corneal herpes, Am J Ophthalmol 105:686, 1988.

96. Kohne D: Application of DNA probe tests to the diagnosis of infectious disease, Am Clin Prod Rev 5:20, 1986.

97. Mulcahy L: DNA probes: an overview, Am Clin Prod Rev 5:14, 1986.

98. Rao NA: A laboratory approach to rapid diagnosis of ocular infections and prospects for the future, Am J Ophthalmol 107:283, 1988.

99. Oh JO: Infectious agents: viruses. In Smolin G and Thoft RA, editors: The cornea: scientific foundations and clinical practice, Boston, 1983, Little, Brown & Co.

100. Kaufman HE, Nesburn AB, and Maloney ED: IDU therapy of herpes simplex, Arch Ophthalmol 64:382, 1960.

101. Kaufman HE: Clinical cure of herpes simplex keratitis by 5-iodo-2'-deoxyuridine, Proc Soc Exp Biol Med 109:251, 1962.

102. Gasset AR and Katzin D: Antiviral drugs and corneal wound healing, Invest Ophthalmol 14:628, 1975.

103. Langston RHS, Pavan-Langston D, and Dohlman CH: Antiviral medication and corneal wound healing, Arch Ophthalmol 92:490, 1974.

104. Polack FM and Rose J: The effect of 5-iodo-2-deoxyuridine (IDU) in corneal healing, Arch Ophthalmol 71:520, 1964.

105. Kaufman HE, Martola EL, and Dohlman CH: Use of 5-iodo-2'-deoxyuridine (IDU) in treating herpes simplex keratitis, Arch Ophthalmol 68:235, 1962.

106. Laibson PR and Leopold IH: An evaluation of double blind IDU therapy in 100 cases of herpetic keratitis, Trans Am Acad Ophthalmol Otolaryngol 68:21, 1964.

107. Patterson A et al: Controlled studies of IDU in the treatment of herpetic keratitis, Trans Ophthalmol Soc UK 83:583, 1963.

108. Hart DRL et al: Treatment of human herpes simplex keratitis with idoxuridine, Arch Ophthalmol 73:623, 1965.

109. Jones BR: Rational regimen of administration of antivirals, Trans Am Acad Ophthalmol Otolaryngol 79:104, 1975.

110. Laibson PR: Current therapy of herpes simplex virus infection of the cornea, Int Ophthalmol Clin 13:39, 1973.

111. Laibson PR et al: ARA-A and IDU therapy of human superficial herpetic keratitis, Invest Ophthalmol 14:762, 1975.

112. Falcon MG et al: Adverse reactions in the eye from topical therapy with idoxuridine, adenine arabinoside and trifluorothymidine. In Sundmacher R, editor: Herpetic eye diseases, Munich, 1981, Verlag.

113. Itoi M et al: Teratogenicities of ophthalmic drugs. I. Antiviral ophthalmic drugs, Arch Ophthalmol 93:46, 1975.

114. Payrau P and Dohlman CH: IDU in corneal wound healing, Am J Ophthalmol 57:999, 1964.

115. Pavan-Langston D: New developments in the therapy of ocular herpes simplex, Int Ophthalmol Clin 13:53, 1973.

116. Pavan-Langston D, Langston RHS, and Geary PA: Prophylaxis and therapy of experimental ocular herpes simplex. Comparison of idoxuridine adenine arabinoside and hypoxanthine arabinoside, Arch Ophthalmol 92:417, 1974.

117. Pavan-Langston D et al: Intravenous and possibly subconjunctival injection of soluble antiviral ARA AMP may be useful in treatment of deep ocular herpetic disease, Arch Ophthalmol 94:1585, 1976.

118. Pavan-Langston D: New developments in the therapy of ocular herpes simplex, Int Ophthalmol Clin 13:53, 1973.

119. Markham RHC et al: Double blind clinical trial of adenine arabinoside and idoxuridine in herpetic corneal ulcers, Trans Ophthalmol Soc UK 97:33, 1977.

120. Coster DL et al: Clinical evaluation of adenine arabi-

noside and trifluorothymidine in the treatment of corneal ulcers caused by herpes simplex virus, J Infect Dis 133(suppl A):173, 1976.

121. Pavan-Langston D and Buchanan RA: Vidarabine therapy of herpetic keratitis, Trans Am Acad Ophthalmol Otolaryngol 81:813, 1976.

122. Whitley RJ et al: Adenine arabinoside therapy of biopsy-proved herpes simplex encephalitis, N Engl J Med 297:289, 1977.

123. Gasset AR and Akaboshi T: Teratogenicity of adenine arabinoside (Ara-A), Invest Ophthalmol 15:556, 1976.

124. McGill J, Fraunfelder FT, and Jones BR: Current and proposed management of ocular herpes simplex, Surv Ophthalmol 20:358, 1976.

125. McGill J et al: Some aspects of the clinical use of trifluorothymidine in the treatment of herpetic ulceration of the cornea, Trans Ophthalmol Soc UK 94:342, 1974.

126. Pavan-Langston D and Foster CS: Trifluorothymidine and idoxuridine therapy of ocular herpes, Am J Ophthalmol 84:818, 1977.

127. Wellings PC et al: Clinical evaluation of trifluorothymidine in the treatment of herpes simplex corneal ulcer, Am J Ophthalmol 73:932, 1972.

128. Laibson PR et al: Double controlled comparison of IDU and trifluorothymidine in 33 patients with superficial herpetic keratitis, Trans Am Ophthalmol Soc 75:316, 1977.

129. Van Bijsterveld OP and Post HJ: Trifluorothymidine and adenine arabinoside in the treatment of dendritic keratitis. In Sundmacher R, editor: Herpetic eye diseases, Munich, 1981, Verlag.

130. McKinnon JR, McGill JI, and Jones BR: A coded clinical evaluation of adenine arabinoside and trifluorothymidine in the treatment of ulcerative herpetic keratitis. In Pavan-Langston D, Buchanan RA, and Alford CA, editors: Adenine arabinoside: an antiviral agent, New York, 1975, Raven Press.

131. Hyndiuk RA et al: Trifluridine in resistant human herpetic keratitis, Arch Ophthalmol 96:1839, 1978.

132. Pavan-Langston D and Nelson DJ: Intraocular penetration of trifluridine, Am J Ophthalmol 87:814, 1979.

133. Langston RHS and Pavan-Langston D: Penetrating keratoplasty for herpetic keratitis: decision making and management, Int Ophthalmol Clin 15:125, 1975.

134. Wellings PC et al: Clinical evaluation of trifluorothymidine in the treatment of herpes simplex corneal ulcers, Am J Ophthalmol 73:932, 1972.

135. Poirier RH et al: Intraocular antiviral penetration, Arch Ophthalmol 100:1964, 1982.

136. Yeakley WR et al: A double-controlled evaluation of acyclovir and vidarabine for the treatment of herpes simplex epithelial keratitis, Trans Am Ophthalmol Soc 79:168, 1981.

137. LaLau C et al: Multicenter trial of acyclovir and trifluorothymidine in herpetic keratitis (acyclovir symposium), Am J Med 79:305, 1985.

138. Collum L, Benedict-Smith A, and Hillary I: Randomized double-blind trial of acyclovir and idoxuridine in dendritic corneal ulceration, Br J Ophthalmol 64:766, 1980.

139. Coster DJ et al: A comparison of acyclovir and idoxuridine as treatment for ulcerative herpetic keratitis, Br J Ophthalmol 64:763, 1980.

140. Pavan-Langston D et al: Acyclovir and vidarabine in therapy of ulcerative herpes simplex keratitis: a comparative masked clinical trial, Am J Ophthalmol 92:829, 1981.

141. Collum LM et al: Randomized double-blind trial of acyclovir (Zovirax) and adenine arabinoside in herpes simplex amoeboid corneal ulceration, Br J Ophthalmol 69:847, 1985.

142. Lass JH, Pavan-Langston D, and Park N: Acyclovir and corneal wound healing, Am J Ophthalmol 88:102, 1979.

143. Kaufman HE and Rayfield MA: Viral conjunctivitis and keratitis. In Kaufman HE et al, editors: The cornea, New York, 1988, Churchill Livingstone.

144. Nilsen AE et al: Efficacy of oral acyclovir in the treatment of initial and recurrent genital herpes, Lancet 2:571, 1982.

145. Cobo LM et al: Oral acyclovir in the treatment of acute herpes zoster ophthalmicus, Ophthalmology 93:763, 1986.

146. Bialasiewicz AA and Jahn GJ: Systemic acyclovir therapy in recurrent keratouveitis caused by herpes simplex virus, Klin Monatsbl Augenheilkd 185:539, 1984.

147. Schwab I: Oral acyclovir in the management of herpes simplex ocular infections, Ophthalmology 95:423, 1988.

148. Colion J et al: Combination therapy for dendritic keratitis with acyclovir and vidarabine, J Ocular Pharmacol 3:39, 1987.

149. Hung SO et al: Oral acyclovir in the management of dendritic herpetic corneal ulceration, Br J Ophthalmol 68:398, 1984.

150. Collum LMT, Akhtar J, and McGettrick P: Oral acyclovir in herpetic keratitis, Trans Ophthalmol Soc UK 104:629, 1985.

151. Sanitato JJ et al: Acyclovir in the treatment of herpetic stromal disease, Am J Ophthalmol 98:537, 1984.

152. Mindel A et al: Prophylactic oral acyclovir in recurrent genital herpes, Lancet 2:57, 1984.

153. Straus SE et al: Suppression of frequently recurring genital herpes: a placebo-controlled double-blind trial of oral acyclovir, N Engl J Med 310:1543, 1984.

154. Douglas JM et al: A double-blind study of oral acyclovir for suppression of recurrences of genital herpes simplex virus infection, N Engl J Med 310:1551, 1984.

155. Meyrick Thomas RH et al: Oral acyclovir in the suppression of recurrent non-genital herpes simplex virus infection, Br J Dermatol 113:731, 1985.

156. Kaufman HE et al: Oral antiviral drugs in experimental herpes simplex keratitis, Antimicrob Agents Chemother 24:888, 1983.

157. Nesburn AB, Willey DE, and Trousdale MD: Effect of intensive acyclovir therapy during artificial reactivation of latent herpes simplex virus (41563), Proc Soc Exp Biol Med 172:316, 1983.

158. Beyer CF et al: Oral acyclovir reduces the incidence of recurrent herpes simplex keratitis in rabbits after penetrating keratoplasty, Arch Ophthalmol 107:1200, 1989.

159. Jones BR et al: Topical therapy of ulcerative herpetic keratitis with human interferon, Lancet 2:128, 1976.

160. Sundmacher R, Neumann-Haefelin D, and Cantell K: Successful treatment of dendritic keratitis with human leukocyte interferon, Graefes Arch Clin Exp Ophthalmol 201:39, 1976.

161. Kaufman HE et al: Human leukocyte interferon for the prevention of recurrences of herpetic keratitis, J Infect Dis 133:A165, 1976.

162. Shuster JJ, Kaufman HE, and Nesburn AB: Statistical analysis of the rate of recurrence of herpesvirus ocular epithelial disease, Am J Ophthalmol 91:328, 1981.

163. Sundmacher R, Cantell K, and Neumann-Haefelin D: Combination therapy of dendritic keratitis with trifluorothymidine and interferon, Lancet 2:687, 1978.

164. de Koning EWJ, van Bijsterveld OP, and Cantell K: Combination therapy for dendritic keratitis with human leukocyte interferon and trifluorothymidine and interferon, Br J Ophthalmol 66:509, 1982.

165. Colin J et al: Combination therapy for dendritic keratitis with human leukocyte interferon and acyclovir, Am J Ophthalmol 95:346, 1983.

166. de Koning EWJ, van Bijsterveld OP, and Cantell L: Combination therapy for dendritic keratitis with acyclovir and alpha-interferon, Arch Ophthalmol 101:1866, 1983.

167. Maudgal P, De Clercq E, and Missotten L: Efficacy of bromovinyl-deoxyuridine in the treatment of herpes simplex virus and varicella zoster eye infections, Antiviral Res 4:281, 1984.

168. Kibrick S, Takahashi GH, and Liebowitz HM: Local corticosteroid therapy and reactivation of herpetic keratitis, Arch Ophthalmol 86:694, 1971.

169. Coster DJ, Jones BR, and Falson MG: Role of debridement in the treatment of herpetic keratitis, Trans Ophthalmol Soc UK 97:314, 1977.

170. Wittpenn JR and Pepose JS: Impression debridement of herpes simplex dendritic keratitis, Cornea 5:245, 1986.

171. Jawetz E et al: Studies on herpes simplex. XI. The antivirus dynamics of 5-iodo-2-deoxyuridine in vivo, J Immunol 95:635, 1965.

172. Hyndiuk RA and Kaufman HE: Newer compounds in therapy of herpes simplex keratitis, Arch Ophthalmol 78:600, 1967.

173. Laibson PR: Current therapy of herpes simplex virus infection of the cornea, Int Ophthalmol Clin 13:39, 1973.

174. Rice NSC and Jones BR: Problems of corneal grafting in herpetic keratitis. In Corneal graft failure, Ciba Foundation Symposium 15, Amsterdam, 1973, Elsevirer.

175. Witmer R: Results of keratoplasty in metaherpetic keratitis. In Sundmacher R, editor: Herpetic eye diseases, Munich, 1981, Verlag.

176. Langston R, Pavan-Langston D, and Dohlman CH: Penetrating keratoplasty for herpetic keratitis, Trans Am Acad Ophthalmol Otolaryngol 79:577, 1975.

177. Foster CS and Duncan J: Penetrating keratoplasty for herpes simplex keratitis, Am J Ophthalmol 92:336, 1981.

178. Polack FM and Kaufman HE: Penetrating keratoplasty in herpetic keratitis, Am J Ophthalmol 73:908, 1972.

179. Ficker LA et al: Long-term prognosis for corneal grafting in herpes simplex keratitis, Eye 2:400, 1988.

180. Cohen E, Laibson P, and Arentsen J: Corneal transplantation for herpes simplex keratitis, Am J Ophthalmol 95:645, 1983.

181. Kaufman HE and Rayfield MA: Viral conjunctivitis and keratitis. In Kaufman HE et al, editors: The cornea, New York, 1988, Churchill Livingstone.

182. Patten JT, Cavanagh HD, and Pavan-Langston D: Penetrating keratoplasty in acute herpetic corneal perforations, Ann Ophthalmol 8:287, 1976.

183. Pfister RR, Richards JS, and Dohlman CH: Recurrence of herpetic keratitis in corneal grafts, Am J Ophthalmol 73:192, 1972.

184. Cobo LM et al: Prognosis and management of corneal transplantation for herpetic keratitis, Arch Ophthalmol 98:1755, 1980.

185. Fine M and Cignetti F: Penetrating keratoplasty in herpes simplex keratitis, Arch Ophthalmol 95:613, 1977.

186. Beyer CF et al: Oral acyclovir reduces the incidence of recurrent herpes simplex keratitis in rabbits after penetrating keratoplasty, Arch Ophthalmol 107:1200, 1989.

187. Irvine JA, Dunkel EC, and Langston DP: Varicella zoster virus (VZV) induced ocular pathology in guinea pig, Invest Ophthalmol Vis Sci 29(suppl):41, 1988.

188. Weller TH and Whitton HM: The etiologic agents of varicella and herpes zoster: isolation, propagation, and cultural characterization in vitro, J Exp Med 108:843, 1958.

189. Croen KD et al: Patterns of gene expression and sites of latency in human nerve ganglia are different for varicella-zoster and herpes simplex virus, Proc Natl Acad Sci USA 85:9773, 1988.

190. Charles NC, Bennett TW, and Margolis S: Ocular pathology of the congenital varicella syndrome, Arch Ophthalmol 95:2034, 1977.

191. De Luise VP and Wilson FM II: Varicella and herpes zoster ophthalmicus. In Duane T and Jaeger E, editors: Clinical ophthalmology, vol 5, Philadelphia, 1988, Harper & Row.

192. Ostler HB and Thygeson P: The ocular manifestations of herpes zoster, varicella, infectious mononucleosis and cytomegalovirus disease, Surv Ophthalmol 21:148, 1976.

193. Duke-Elder S and Leigh AG: System of ophthalmology, vol VIII: Diseases of the outer eye, St Louis, 1965, Mosby–Year Book, Inc.

194. Falls HF and Beall JG: Ocular varicella, Arch Ophthalmol 43:411, 1945.

195. Nesburn AB et al: Varicella dendritic keratitis, Invest Ophthalmol 13:764, 1974.

196. Uchida Y, Kaneko M, and Hayashi K: Varicella dendritic keratitis, Am J Ophthalmol 89:259, 1980.

197. Pickard R: Varicella of the cornea, Br J Ophthalmol 20:15, 1936.

198. Awan KJ: Corneal complications of varicella, Pak J Ophthalmol 1:147, 1985.

199. Kielar RA, Cunningham GC, and Gerson KC: Occurrence of herpes zoster ophthalmicus in a child with absent immunoglobulin A and deficiency of delayed hypersensitivity, Am J Ophthalmol 72:555, 1971.

200. David TJ and Williams ML: Herpes zoster in infancy, Scand J Infect Dis 11:185, 1979.
201. Dworsky M, Whitley R, and Alford C: Herpes zoster in early infancy, Am J Dis Child 134:618, 1980.
202. Baba K et al: Increased incidence of herpes zoster in normal children infected with varicella zoster virus during infancy: community-based follow-up study, J Pediatr 108:372, 1986.
203. Brunell PA, Miller LH, and Lovejoy F: Zoster in infancy: failure to maintain virus latency following intrauterine infection, J Pediatr 98:71, 1981.
204. Blodi F: Ophthalmic zoster in malignant disease, Am J Ophthalmol 65:686, 1968.
205. Goodman ML and Maher E: Four uncommon infections in Hodgkin's disease, JAMA 198:1129, 1966.
206. Scheie HG: Herpes zoster ophthalmicus, Trans Ophthalmol Soc UK 90:899, 1970.
207. Sandor EV et al: Herpes zoster ophthalmicus in patients at risk for AIDS, N Engl J Med 310:1118, 1984.
208. Sandor EV et al: Herpes zoster ophthalmicus in patients at risk for the acquired immune deficiency syndrome (AIDS), Am J Ophthalmol 101:153, 1986.
209. Dolin R et al: Herpes zoster varicella infections in immunosuppressed patients, Ann Intern Med 89:375, 1978.
210. Whitley RJ et al: Early vidarabine therapy to control the complications of herpes zoster of immunosuppressed patients, N Engl J Med 307:971, 1982.
211. Lightman S, Marach RJ, and Powell D: Herpes zoster ophthalmicus: a medical review, Br J Ophthalmol 65:539, 1981.
212. Ragossino MW et al: Population-based study of herpes zoster and its sequelae, Medicine 61:310, 1982.
213. Guess HA et al: Epidemiology of herpes zoster in children and adolescents: a population-based study, Pediatrics 76:512, 1985.
214. Weller TH: Varicella and herpes zoster, N Engl J Med 309:1362, 1983.
215. Weller TH: Varicella-herpes zoster virus. In Evans AS, editor: Viral infections of humans: epidemiology and control, New York, 1976, Plenum.
216. Friedlander MH: Allergy and immunology of the eye, Hagerstown, MD, 1979, Harper & Row.
217. Hedges TR and Albert DM: The progression of the ocular abnormalities of herpes zoster. Histopathologic observations of nine cases, Ophthalmology 89:165, 1982.
218. Naumann G, Gass JDM, and Font RL: Histopathology of herpes zoster ophthalmicus, Am J Ophthalmol 65:533, 1968.
219. Lewis G: Zoster sine herpete, Br Med J 2:418, 1958.
220. Uchida Y, Kaneko M, and Onishi Y: Ophthalmic herpes zoster without eruption. In Henkind P, editor: Acta XXIV International Congress of Ophthalmology, vol 2, Philadelphia, 1983, JB Lippincott.
221. Ross JVM: Herpes zoster sine eruptione, Arch Ophthalmol 42:808, 1949.
222. Cobo M et al: Observations on the natural history of herpes zoster ophthalmicus, Curr Eye Res 6:195, 1987.
223. Edgarton AE: Herpes zoster ophthalmicus: report of cases and review of literature, Arch Ophthalmol 34:40, 114, 1945.
224. Pemberton JW: Optic atrophy in herpes zoster ophthalmicus, Am J Ophthalmol 58:852, 1964.
225. Duke-Elder S and Leigh AG: System of ophthalmology, vol VIII: Diseases of the outer eye, St Louis, 1965, Mosby–Year Book, Inc.
226. Dugmore W: Intercalary staphyloma in a case of herpes zoster ophthalmicus, Br J Ophthalmol 51:350, 1967.
227. Liesegang TJ: Corneal complications of herpes zoster ophthalmicus, Ophthalmology 92:316, 1985.
228. Acers TE and Vaille V: Co-existent herpes zoster and herpes simplex, Am J Ophthalmol 63:992, 1967.
229. Ahmad M, Bowen SF Jr, and Burke R: Optic atrophy following herpes zoster ophthalmicus in a child, Can J Ophthalmol 4:387, 1969.
230. Marsh RJ et al: Herpetic epithelial disease, Arch Ophthalmol 94:1899, 1976.
231. Piebenga LW and Laibson PR: Dendritic lesions in herpes zoster ophthalmicus, Arch Ophthalmol 90:268, 1973.
232. Sugar HS: Herpetic keratouveitis: clinical experiences, Ann Ophthalmol 3:355, 1971.
233. Jones DB: Herpes zoster ophthalmicus. In Golden B, editor: Ocular inflammatory disease, Springfield, Ill, 1974, Charles C Thomas.
234. Marsh RJ: Herpes zoster keratitis, Trans Ophthalmol Soc UK 93:181, 1973.
235. Mondino BJ, Brown SI, and Mondzelewski JP: Peripheral corneal ulcers with herpes zoster ophthalmicus, Am J Ophthalmol 86:611, 1978.
236. Marsh RJ, Fraunfelder FT, and McGill JI: Herpetic corneal epithelial disease, Arch Ophthalmol 94:1899, 1976.
237. Marsh RJ, Easty DL, and Jones BR: Iritis and iris atrophy in herpes zoster ophthalmicus, Am J Ophthalmol 78:2, 1974.
238. Crock G: Clinical syndromes of anterior segment ischemia, Trans Ophthalmol Soc UK 87:513, 1967.
239. Hesse RJ: Herpes zoster ophthalmicus associated with delayed retinal thrombophlebitis, Am J Ophthalmol 84:329, 1977.
240. Harrison EQ: Complications of herpes zoster ophthalmicus, Am J Ophthalmol 60:1111, 1965.
241. Bartlett RE, Mumma CS, and Irvine AR: Herpes zoster ophthalmicus with bilateral hemorrhagic retinopathy, Am J Ophthalmol 34:45, 1951.
242. Goldsmith MO: Herpes zoster ophthalmicus with sixth nerve palsy, Can J Ophthalmol 3:279, 1968.
243. Hayashi K, Uchida Y, and Oshima M: Fluorescent antibody study of herpes zoster keratitis, Am J Ophthalmol 75:795, 1973.
244. Pavan-Langston D and McCulley JP: Herpes zoster dendritic keratitis, Arch Ophthalmol 89:25, 1973.
245. Valtuch G and Sachs F: Herpes zoster in a patient with Hodgkin's disease, Arch Intern Med 121:458, 1971.
246. De Clercq E: Oral (E)-5-(2-Bromovinyl)-2-deoxyuridine in severe herpes zoster, Br Med J 281:1, 1980.
247. Maudgal P, De Clercq E, and Missotten L: Efficacy of bromovinyl-deoxyuridine in the treatment of herpes simplex virus and varicella zoster eye infections, Antiviral Res 4:281, 1984.
248. Balfour H et al: Acyclovir halts progression of herpes zoster in immunocompromised patients, N Engl J Med 308:1448, 1983.

249. Bean B, Braum C, and Balfour H: Acyclovir therapy for acute herpes zoster, Lancet 2:118, 1982.

250. Scheie HG and McLellan TG Jr: Treatment of herpes zoster ophthalmicus with corticotropin and corticosteroids, Arch Ophthalmol 62:579, 1959.

251. Keckes L and Basheer A: Do corticosteroids prevent postherpetic neuralgia? Br J Dermatol 102:551, 1980.

252. Merselis JG Jr, Kaye D, and Hook EW: Disseminated herpes zoster: a report of 17 cases, Arch Intern Med 113:679, 1964.

253. Juel-Jensen BE et al: Treatment of zoster with idoxuridine in dimethyl sulfoxide: results of two double-blind controlled trials, Br Med J 4:776, 1970.

254. McGill J and Chapman C: A comparison of topical acyclovir with steroids in the treatment of herpes zoster keratouveitis, Br J Ophthalmol 67:746, 1983.

255. McGill J et al: A review of acyclovir treatment of ocular herpes zoster and skin infections, J Antimicrob Chemother 12(Suppl B):45, 1983.

256. McGill J, Chapman C, and Mahakasingam M: Acyclovir therapy in herpes zoster infection: a practical guide, Trans Ophthalmol Soc UK 103:111, 1983.

257. Forrest WM and Kaufman HE: Zosteriform herpes simplex, Am J Ophthalmol 81:86, 1976.

258. Wilson FM II: Varicella and herpes zoster ophthalmicus. In Tabbara KF and Hyndiuk RA, editors: Infections of the eye, Boston, 1986, Little, Brown & Co.

259. Berghaust G and Westerby R: Zoster ophthalmicus: local treatment with cortisone, Acta Ophthalmol 45:787, 1967.

260. March RJ: Current management of ophthalmic herpes zoster, Trans Ophthalmol Soc UK 96:334, 1976.

261. Kernbaum S and Hauchecome J: Administration of levodopa for relief of herpes zoster pain, JAMA 246:132, 1981.

262. van der Spuy S, Levy DW, and Levin W: Cimetidine in the treatment of herpes virus infections, S Afr Med J 58:112, 1980.

263. Mavligit GM and Talpaz M: Cimetidine for herpes zoster, N Engl J Med 310:318, 1984.

264. Levy DW, Banerje AK, and Glenny HP: Cimetidine in the treatment of herpes zoster, J Coll Physicians Lond 19:96, 1985.

265. Barr W: Cimetidine, an immunomodulating drug, Mayo Clin Proc 56:580, 1981.

266. Bernstein JE et al: Treatment of chronic postherpetic neuralgia with topical capsaicin, Am Acad Dermatol 17:93, 1987.

267. Bucci FA, Gabriels CF, and Krohel GB: Successful treatment of postherpetic neuralgia with capsaicin, Am J Ophthalmol 106:758, 1988.

268. Sklar SH et al: Herpes zoster: the treatment and prevention of neuralgia with adenosine monophosphate, JAMA 253:1427, 1985.

269. Olson ER and Ivy HB: Stellate block for trigeminal zoster, J Clin Neuro Ophthalmol 1:53, 1981.

270. Reed JW, Joyner SJ, and Knauer WJ: Penetrating keratoplasty for herpes zoster keratopathy, Am J Ophthalmol 107:257, 1989.

271. Marsh RJ and Cooper M: Ocular surgery in ophthalmic zoster, Eye 3:313, 1989.

272. Adenovirus keratoconjunctivitis, Br J Ophthalmol 61:73, 1977 (editorial).

273. Fox JP, Hall CE, and Cooney MK: Observations of adenovirus infections, The Seattle Virus Watch VII 105:362, 1977.

274. Gigliotti F et al: Etiology of acute conjunctivitis in children, J Pediatr 98:531, 1981.

275. Tullo AB and Higgins PG: An outbreak of adenoviral conjunctivitis in Bristol, Br J Ophthalmol 63:621, 1979.

276. Petit TH and Holland GN: Chronic keratoconjunctivitis associated with ocular adenovirus infection, Am J Ophthalmol 61:73, 1979.

277. Boniuk M, Phillips CA, and Friedman JB: Chronic adenovirus type 2 keratitis in man, N Engl J Med 273:924, 1965.

278. Darougar S et al: Epidemic keratoconjunctivitis and chronic papillary conjunctivitis in London due to adenovirus type 19, Br J Ophthalmol 61:76, 1977.

279. Sprague JB et al: Epidemic keratoconjunctivitis: a severe industrial outbreak due to adenovirus type 8, N Engl J Med 289:1341, 1973.

280. D'Angelo LJ et al: Pharyngoconjunctival fever caused by adenovirus type 4: report of a swimming pool-related outbreak with recovery of virus from pool water, J Infect Dis 140:42, 1979.

281. Harnett GB and Newnhamm WA: Isolation of adenovirus type 19 from the male and female genital tracts, Br J Vener Dis 57:55, 1981.

282. Nauheim R et al: Survival of adenovirus on various surfaces, Invest Ophthalmol Vis Sci 30(suppl):362, 1989.

283. Tullo A: The adenoviruses. In Easty DL: Virus diseases of the eye, Chicago, 1985, Mosby–Year Book, Inc.

284. Centers for Disease Control: Keratoconjunctivitis due to adenovirus type 19-Canada, MMWR 23:185, 1974.

285. Jawetz E et al: The etiology of epidemic keratoconjunctivitis, Am J Ophthalmol 43:79, 1957.

286. Laibson PR, Ortolan G, and Dupre-Strachan S: Community and hospital outbreak of epidemic keratoconjunctivitis, Arch Ophthalmol 80:467, 1968.

287. Dawson CR, Hanna L, and Tagni B: Adenovirus type 8 infections in the United States: ten observations on the pathogenesis of lesions in severe eye disease, Arch Ophthalmol 87:258, 1972.

288. Hart JCD et al: Epidemic keratoconjunctivitis: a virological and clinical study. Trans Ophthalmol Soc UK 92:795, 1972.

289. Hierholzer JC et al: Adenovirus type 19 keratoconjunctivitis, N Engl J Med 290:1436, 1974.

290. O'Day DM et al: Clinical and laboratory evaluation of epidemic keratoconjunctivitis due to adenovirus types 8 and 19, Am J Ophthalmol 81:207, 1976.

291. Dawson CR et al: Adenovirus type 8 keratoconjunctivitis in the United States, Am J Ophthalmol 69:473, 1970.

292. Jones BR: The clinical features of viral keratitis and a concept of their pathogenesis, Proc R Soc Med 51:13, 1958.

293. Lund OE and Stefani JF: Corneal histology after epidemic keratoconjunctivitis, Arch Ophthalmol 96:2085, 1978.

294. Jones BR: Epidemic hemorrhagic conjunctivitis in London, 1971, Trans Ophthalmol Soc UK 92:625, 1972.

295. Kimura SJ et al: Sporadic cases of pharyngoconjunctival fever in northern California, Am J Ophthalmol 43:14, 1957.

296. Bernstein A: Infectious mononucleosis, Medicine 19:85, 1940.

297. Librach IM: Ocular symptoms in glandular fever, Br J Ophthalmol 40:619, 1956.

298. Wilhelmus KR: Ocular involvement in infectious mononucleosis, Am J Ophthalmol 91:117, 1981.

299. Piel JJ, Thelander HE, and Shur EB: Infectious mononucleosis of the central nervous system with bilateral papilledema, J Pediatr 37:661, 1950.

300. Tanner OR: Ocular manifestations infectious mononucleosis, Arch Ophthalmol 51:229, 1954.

301. Hales RH and Ostler BH: Newcastle disease conjunctivitis with subepithelial infiltrates, Br J Ophthalmol 57:694, 1973.

302. Higgins PG: Acute hemorrhagic conjunctivitis. In Easty DL: Virus disease of the eye, Chicago, 1985, Mosby–Year Book, Inc.

303. Yang YF et al: Epidemic hemorrhagic keratoconjunctivitis, Am J Ophthalmol 80:192, 1975.

304. Kono R et al: Neurologic complications associated with acute hemorrhagic conjunctivitis virus infection and its serologic complication, J Infect Dis 129:590, 1974.

305. Whitcher JP et al: Acute hemorrhagic conjunctivitis in Tunisia, Arch Ophthalmol 94:51, 1976.

306. Wolken SH: Acute hemorrhagic conjunctivitis, Surv Ophthalmol 19:71, 1974.

307. Sklar VEF et al: Clinical findings and results of treatment in an outbreak of acute hemorrhagic conjunctivitis in southern Florida, Am J Ophthalmol 95:45, 1983.

308. Hung PT and Sung SM: Neurologic complications with elevated antibody titer after subacute hemorrhagic conjunctivitis, Am J Ophthalmol 80:832, 1975.

309. Garau J et al: Spontaneous cytomegalovirus mononucleosis with conjunctivitis, Arch Intern Med 137:1977.

310. Danielson RW and Long JC: Keratitis due to mumps, Arch Ophthalmol 24:655, 1941.

311. Riffenburgh RS: Ocular manifestations of mumps, Arch Ophthalmol 66:739, 1961.

312. Mickatavage R and Amadur J: A case report of mumps keratitis, Arch Ophthalmol 69:758, 1963.

313. Sandford-Smith JH and Whittle H: Corneal ulceration following measles in Nigerian children, Br J Ophthalmol 63:720, 1983.

314. Foster A and Sommer A: Childhood blindness from corneal ulceration in Africa: causes, presentation and treatment, Bull World Health Organ 64:619, 1986.

315. Dekkers NWHM: The cornea in measles, The Hague, 1981, Dr W Junk Publishers.

316. Ellis P and Winograd LA: Ocular vaccinia: a specific treatment, Arch Ophthalmol 68:600, 1962.

317. Petit TH: The poxviruses: vaccinia and variola, Int Ophthalmol Clin 15:203, 1975.

318. Jones BR and Al-Hussaine MD: Therapeutic considerations in ocular vaccinia, Trans Ophthalmol Soc UK 83:613, 1963.

319. Kaufman H, Nesburn AB and Maloney ED: Cure of vaccinia infection by 5-iodo-2-deoxyuridine, Virology 18:567, 1962.

320. Ruben FL and Lane MJ: Ocular vaccinia: an epidemiologic analysis of 348 cases, Arch Ophthalmol 84:45, 1970.

321. Boger WP, Peterson RA, and Robb RM: Keratoconus and acute hydrops in mentally retarded patients with congenital rubella syndrome, Am J Ophthalmol 91:231, 1981.

322. Hara J et al: Ocular manifestations of the 1976 rubella epidemic in Japan, Am J Ophthalmol 87:642, 1979.

323. Thygeson P: Superficial punctate keratitis, JAMA 144:1544, 1950.

324. Thygeson P: Further observations on superficial punctate keratitis, Arch Ophthalmol 66:158, 1962.

325. Thygeson P: Clinical and laboratory observation on superficial punctate keratitis, Am J Ophthalmol 61:1344, 1966.

326. Tabbara KF et al: Thygeson's superficial punctate keratitis, Ophthalmology 88:75, 1981.

327. Abbott RL and Forster RK: Superficial punctate keratitis of Thygeson associated with scarring and Salzmann's nodular degeneration, Am J Ophthalmol 87:296, 1979.

328. Darrell RW: Thygeson's superficial punctate keratitis: natural history and association with HLA DR3, Trans Am Ophthalmol Soc 79:486, 1981.

329. Forstot SL and Bender PS: Treatment of Thygeson's superficial punctate keratopathy with soft contact lenses, Am J Ophthalmol 88:186, 1979.

330. Goldberg DB, Schanzlin DJ, and Brown SI: Management of Thygeson's superficial punctate keratitis, Am J Ophthalmol 89:22, 1980.

331. Nesburn AB et al: Effect of topical trifluridine on Thygeson's superficial punctate keratitis, Ophthalmology 91:1188, 1984.

332. Braley AEK and Alexander RC: Superficial punctate keratitis: isolation of a virus, Arch Ophthalmol 50:147, 1953.

333. Lemp MA, Chambers RW, and Lurdy J: Viral isolation in superficial punctate keratitis, Arch Ophthalmol 91:8, 1974.

334. Ostler HB: Suspected infectious etiology. In Smolin G and Thoft RA, editors: The cornea: scientific foundations and clinical practice, Boston, 1983, Little, Brown & Co.

BLEPHARITIS

The term "blepharitis" encompasses a common yet not well-understood group of diseases. Clinically these diseases have been divided into those that affect mainly the base of the lashes (anterior blepharitis), and those that affect primarily the meibomian glands (posterior blepharitis) (Table 13-1). This division is somewhat artificial in that signs of both types frequently are present, and the nature of their interrelation is obscure.

ANTERIOR LID MARGIN

Anterior blepharitis is a very common disease and often a difficult problem for both the physician and the patient. It is characterized by the accumulation of material around the base of the lashes and erythema of the anterior lid margin. The most common types of anterior blepharitis are the staphylococcal and seborrheic varieties. These are defined clinically; their relationship to staphylococcal infection and seborrhea (overaction of sebaceous glands) is inconsistent.

STAPHYLOCOCCAL BLEPHARITIS

Clinical manifestations. Patients with staphylococcal blepharitis may be asymptomatic or may report burning, itching, and irritation, which frequently is worse in the morning.[1-3] Hard, brittle, fibrinous scales commonly are seen at the base of the lashes. Scales that encircle the lash are known as *collarettes*. These collarettes are thought to formed by fibrin exudation from the ulcerated skin at the base of the cilium. As the lash grows, it carries the fibrin out from the lid margin. Less commonly, matted, hard crusts surround the individual cilium (Fig. 13-1). When these crusts are removed, small

TABLE 13-1. Common Types of Blepharitis

FEATURE	STAPHYLOCOCCAL	SEBORRHEIC	MEIBOMITIS	*MORAXELLA*
Scales	Hard, brittle tenacious	Greasy, easily removed	Greasy	Macerated epithelium, minimal scaling
Meibomian glands	—	Meibomian abnormalities common	Inspissated plugs, pouting orifices	—
Associated forms of blepharitis	Seborrheic common	Staphylococcal and meibomitis	Seborrheic common	—
Associated skin disease	Seborrheic dermatitis (10%)	Seborrheic dermatitis (100%)	Acne rosacea (two thirds), seborrheic dermatitis (one third)	Occasionally
Bilateral or unilateral	May be unilateral, especially early	Bilateral	Bilateral	Often unilateral
Ulceration	Yes	No	No	No
Keratitis	SPK (most); marginal infiltrates, phlyctenules	SPK (occasional)	SPK (common), rapid tear breakup time	Marginal infiltrates, occasionally ulcers
Keratitis sicca	50%	33%	33%	—
Hordeola	Frequent	Rare	Common	No
Lash abnormalities	Madarosis, poliosis	No	No	No
Conjunctivitis (injection, papillary response)	Common	Occasional	Common	Always, may be follicular
Treatment	Lid hygiene, topical antibiotics	Lid hygiene, treat dermatitis	Lid hygiene, expression, systemic antibiotics	Topical antibiotics

SPK, Superficial punctate keratopathy.

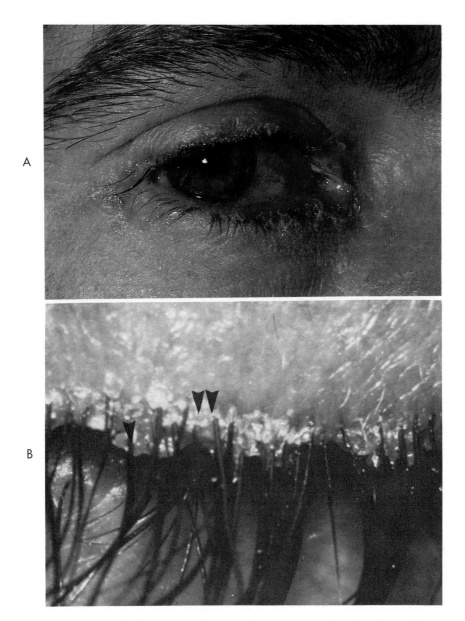

Fig. 13-1. A, Ulcerative blepharitis with conspicuous crusting of the lid margin. **B,** When the crust was removed, a bleeding area was visible *(double arrow)*. Collarette formation *(single arrow)* is noted around a cilium.

ulcers of the hair follicles can be seen, and bleeding may occur. Blood vessels on the lid margins may be dilated, and there may be thinning or loss of the lashes *(madarosis)* (Fig. 13-2), white lashes *(po-liosis)*, misdirected lashes *(trichiasis)*, broken lashes, or irregularity of the lid margin *(tylosis)*.

Seborrheic blepharitis, described later, often is present, but meibomian gland dysfunction usually is not seen. A chronic papillary conjunctivitis also is often present, and this may be accompanied by mucopurulent (predominantly polymorphonuclear) exudate. The conjunctivitis is typically worse in the morning. Hordeola, both external and internal, can accompany the blepharitis. Corneal complications are common, including punctate keratopathy, catarrhal infiltrates, phlyctenules, ulceration, and pannus formation. The punctate keratopathy predominantly affects the inferior third of the cornea and

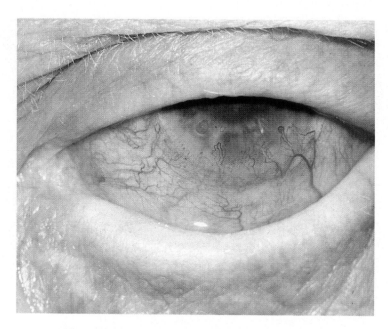

Fig. 13-2. Loss of cilia after staphylococcal blepharitis.

consists of fine, flat lesions that are regular in shape and may stain with fluorescein or rose bengal. Catarrhal infiltrates and phlyctenules are discussed in Chapter 19.

Pathogenesis. The relationship between staphylococcal blepharitis and *Staphylococcus aureus* infection is unclear. Staphylococci are common on unaffected lids; *S. epidermidis* can be isolated from 90% to 95% of normal lids, and *S. aureus* from 10% to 35%.[4-6] In patients with signs of staphylococcal blepharitis, *S. aureus* is isolated from the lid margin significantly more often, but still only about half of the time. *S. epidermidis* and *Propionibacterium acnes* are isolated in nearly all cases, and many other bacteria are found occasionally.[4,7] *S. epidermidis,* or other nonaureus species, may be able to produce the same clinical disease as *S. aureus.* Some researchers have attempted to differentiate the *S. epidermidis* strains found on the lids of patients with blepharitis from those strains found on unaffected lids, but the results have not been very illuminating.[8,9]

The role of staphylococci is suggested by several findings: In 1937 both Allen[10] and Thygeson[11] demonstrated that topical application of a filtrate prepared from a culture of *S. aureus* produced a toxic type of conjunctivitis and keratitis in human volunteers. Later, a filtrate prepared from *S. epidermidis* also was found capable of producing toxic conjunctivitis.[12] Staphylococci produce many enzymes and toxins that may injure the ocular surface. Alpha-toxin, also known as dermonecrotic factor, was suggested by Thygeson to be the one most responsible for such injury. Alpha-toxin appears to increase cell membrane permeability, and it probably is responsible for the inferior punctate keratitis seen in affected eyes. However, other toxins such as beta-toxin (beta-hemolysin), gamma-toxin, delta-toxin, exfoliative toxin (responsible for signs of toxic epidermal necrolysis), and toxic shock syndrome toxin-1 are elaborated by some staphylococcal strains, and these may play a role in blepharoconjunctivitis.[13] Also, enzymes such as lysozyme, lipase, fatty wax esterase, and cholesterol esterase can be produced by both *S. aureus* and *S. epidermidis;* these enzymes may alter the ocular flora and meibomian secretions.

In the past *Pityrosporum ovale* and *Demodex folliculorum* were thought to play a role in staphylococcal blepharitis, but this seems not to be true. *D. folliculorum* is a microscopic, eight-legged, transparent mite (Fig. 13-3) that commonly infests humans and lives in sebaceous follicles. It covers the base of the lash with a tubular sleeve (Fig. 13-4), and waxy debris forms cuffs around the lashes. Since bacteria are found on *D. folliculorum* bodies, it is possible that the mite serves as a vector for staphylococcal infection.[14-16] The diagnosis of *D. folliculorum* infection can be made by extracting the lash and suspending it in viscous fluid; examination of the base will reveal the mite clinging to the lash. McCulley and Dougherty[7] examined lashes from patients in this manner and found *Demodex* in approximately equal frequency in controls and in patients with blepharitis.

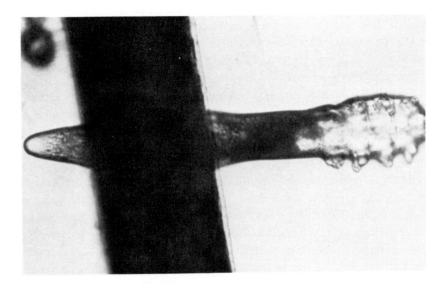

Fig. 13-3. *Demodex folliculorum.*

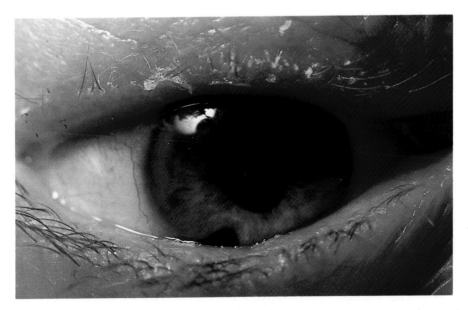

Fig. 13-4. Cuffing of the base of a cilium, as seen in an infection of the lid margin caused by *Demodex folliculorum.*

Differential diagnosis. One of the complications of chronic blepharitis is poliosis, a sign also seen in Vogt-Koyanagi-Harada, Waardenburg's, and Behçet's syndromes. Loss of lashes is also seen in trichotillomania (a compulsion to pull out one's own hair).

Staphylococcal blepharitis must be differentiated from dry eyes, although the two conditions frequently occur in the same eye. The corneal staining in staphylococcal blepharitis usually involves the lower third of the cornea, but keratitis sicca is associated with diffuse stain in the interpalpebral zone. Filaments usually are not seen in staphylococcal blepharitis, but they may be seen in dry eye. If the diagnosis is uncertain, Schirmer testing should be performed.

Treatment. Blepharitis can be very difficult to eradicate; often the disease persists throughout the patient's life. The patient's understanding of the chronic nature of the disease is crucial to its management. However, blepharitis usually can be controlled with a combination of lid hygiene and antibiotic application. The lids can be washed with diluted baby shampoo (one half or one third strength) for approximately 1 minute, using a cotton swab, cotton ball, washcloth, or the tip of the finger. Recently, commercially prepared kits (EV Care and EV Lid Cleanser II, Eagle Vision, Memphis; OCuSOFT Lid Scrub, OCuSOFT, Richmond, Texas), have become available for this purpose, and they may be superior. Initially the routine is performed twice daily; after 1 month the frequency is decreased to once daily and continued indefinitely.

Antibiotic ointments also seem to be helpful and can be applied up to four times daily. Erythromycin and bacitracin are the most commonly used antibiotics, but gentamicin also can be used. (Approximately 50% of *S. aureus* isolated from the lids of patients with staphylococcal blepharitis are resistant to sulfonamides, so those drugs should not be used unless sensitivity testing has been performed.) Infection of the meibomian, sweat, and sebaceous glands of the cilia follicles may play a role in the resistance to therapy, since it is difficult or impossible to obtain a therapeutic concentration of any antibiotic in these structures. In resistant cases or cases associated with catarrhal infiltrates or phlyctenulosis, cultures of the lid margin should be performed to direct antibiotic treatment and monitor staphylococcal colonization. I usually instruct patients to apply the antibiotic ointment twice daily, after scrubbing, for 1 month; then to decrease applications to once daily for another month. In most cases this is sufficient. If exacerbations occur, repeat cultures might be advisable to detect colonization by new bacteria.

If lid and conjunctival redness or keratitis persist despite these measures, topical steroids can be used. These can relieve the signs and symptoms of inflammation but should be used cautiously. Usually applying the ointment to the lids twice daily for 1 to 2 weeks is sufficient.

When treating pediculi, the nits should be removed manually and the adult organism should be dealt with (suffocated) by applying petroleum jelly.

The treatment of catarrhal ulcers and phlyctenules is discussed in Chapter 19.

It is important to realize the difficulties in treating staphylococcal blepharokeratoconjunctivitis. Treatment may have to be continued for a long period, and the patient must understand the chronic nature of the disease. Also, the physician must recognize the atypical forms of the disease, the different types of corneal involvement, and how tear dysfunction and immunologic complications influence the disease.

SEBORRHEIC BLEPHARITIS

Patients with seborrheic blepharitis complain mainly of burning and itching in the eye. They tend to be older than patients with staphylococcal blepharitis and often have had symptoms for many years.

Large, yellow, greasy scales are seen loosely attached to the side of the cilia (Fig. 13-5). Crusting is present on the lashes and lids *(scurf),* and the lid margins often are red. Staphylococcal blepharitis, meibomian seborrhea, or meibomitis also may be present.[7] Approximately 15% of patients also have

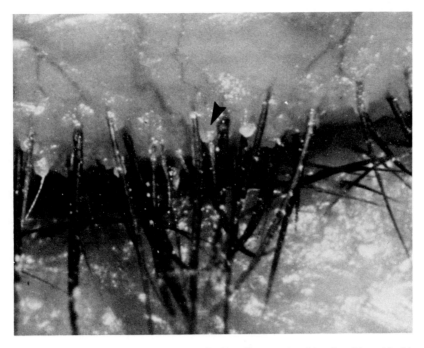

Fig. 13-5. Sebaceous blepharitis *(single arrow).* Scales adhere to the side of a cilium *(double arrow).*

corneal involvement, a punctate keratopathy that is found either in the interpalpebral space or over the lower third of the cornea.

Nearly all patients have seborrheic dermatitis, but it usually is mild and is easily overlooked.[5,17] Seborrheic dermatitis is seen as greasy scales over an erythematous patch of skin. The scalp, eyebrows, eyelids, nasolabial folds, and retroauricular or sternal skin may be involved.

Dysfunction of the sebaceous glands is thought to be the cause of seborrheic blepharitis, but the pathogenesis of the clinical findings is unclear. *Pityrosporum ovale,* a yeast, frequently is seen on scrapings, but its significance is unknown.

This disease also tends to be chronic and incurable, and it is important for the patient to understand this. Treatment consists mainly of lid hygiene, as described for staphylococcal blepharitis. If meibomitis is present, warm compresses, expression of meibomian glands, and oral antibiotics may be helpful. Associated dermatologic abnormalities should be recognized and treated in conjunction with a dermatologist.

Usually symptoms improve over 1 to 2 months, and they then can be controlled with daily scrubs. However, prolonged use of hot compresses, lid massage, and oral antibiotics may be necessary.

POSTERIOR LID MARGIN

The role of meibomian gland dysfunction in blepharitis and blepharoconjunctivitis was not sufficiently appreciated in the past. McCulley, who helped draw attention to meibomian gland dysfunction, has divided the disorder into several types: meibomian seborrhea, primary meibomitis, and secondary meibomitis associated with seborrheic blepharitis.[7,17]

CLINICAL MANIFESTATIONS

Meibomian seborrhea is excessive meibomian secretion in the absence of inflammatory signs. The symptoms, mainly a burning feeling in the eye, tend to be more prominent than the signs. The mei-

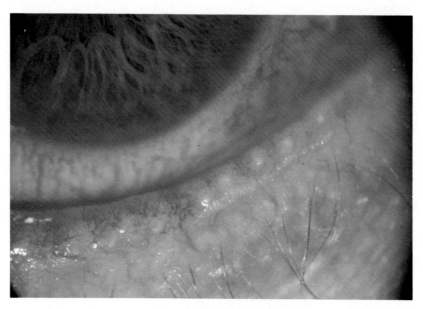

Fig. 13-6. Meibomitis, with erythema of the lid margin and inspissation of secretions in the gland orifices.

bomian glands are dilated and are easily expressed, releasing large amounts of clear fluid. Excessive foam often is present in the tear film. The orifices are not plugged with inspissated secretions. Meibomian seborrhea usually is seen in conjunction with mild seborrheic blepharitis.

Primary meibomitis is characterized by inflammation around the meibomian gland orifices, pouting of the gland orifices, and solidification of meibomian secretions (Fig. 13-6). The symptoms include burning, tearing, itching, dryness, irritation, and photophobia. The most prominent feature is stagnation of the meibomian gland secretions. This is manifest as dilation of the glands and inspissation of the secretions. The dilated glands can be seen through the tarsal conjunctiva with the aid of a slit-lamp microscope, and the inspissated secretions are oily and often semisolid or yellow. Expression of the secretions is more difficult and often preceded by extrusion of an inspissated plug.

Hyperemia, thickening, and an irregularity of contour (tylosis) may affect the posterior lid margin. Chalazia, tarsitis, or nodules may be seen on the posterior lid; occasionally, the Zeis glands become inflamed. Foamy tears can accumulate in the canthi, or a thick greasy film may be noted. The tear breakup time is reduced. Papillary conjunctivitis and interpalpebral superficial punctate keratopathy often are present.

In the secondary form, associated with seborrheic blepharitis, the meibomitis is spotty, with scattered glands or clusters of glands affected. Otherwise the findings are similar.

Virtually all patients with meibomian gland dysfunction have evidence of sebaceous gland dysfunction elsewhere, but it is often subtle. When seborrheic blepharitis is more prominent, seborrheic dermatitis is nearly always present, but when meibomitis is dominant, approximately two thirds of patients have acne rosacea and only one third have seborrheic dermatitis. Acne rosacea may give rise to erythema, telangiectasia, papules, follicular pustules, and hypertrophic sebaceous glands. These signs are found on the forehead, nose, and cheeks (see also Chapter 25).

PATHOGENESIS

Meibomitis does not appear to be related to bacterial infection. No bacteria have been isolated with greater than normal frequency. The superficial punctate keratopathy looks like that seen in conditions with an unstable tear film, not like that described as secondary to staphylococcus toxin[11] or with anterior blepharitis.[10] An unstable tear film in patients with meibomian keratoconjunctivitis can account for the keratopathy without necessitating the presence of a bacterial exotoxin; however, this may be only one of several pathways involved.

The stagnation of the meibomian glands, which produce the lipid layer of the tear film, may account for the tear film instability. In accordance with this, stabilization of the tear film occurs when fresh secretions from deep within the glands are added by expressing them into the tear film.[18] The observed instability does not appear to be caused by a quantitative decrease in the tear lipid layer, but there may be a qualitative abnormality. Strains of *S. epidermidis* isolated from patients with meibomian gland dysfunction have significantly greater lipase activity than strains from normal eyes,[19] and increased breakdown of lipids into free fatty acids could destabilize the tear film. However, experiments to date have not found a biochemical abnormality in secretions from these patients.[20-22]

The consistent finding of more generalized sebaceous gland dysfunction (the meibomian gland is a specialized sebaceous gland) suggests that these patients have a systemic predisposition to disease in these glands.

TREATMENT

Like anterior blepharitis, meibomitis is a chronic disease that can be controlled but not cured. Helpful measures include hot compresses, lid massage, lid scrubs, and systemic antibiotics. Hot compresses are applied to the lids for 5 to 10 minutes up to four times daily. Massaging the lids helps express meibomian secretions, relieving stagnation. Systemic tetracycline usually is very effective, both for the meibomitis and for acne rosacea, if it is present. The initial dose is 250 mg by mouth four times daily. The drug should be taken on an empty stomach and should not be given to pregnant women or to children under 8 years of age. The mechanism of the beneficial effect is unknown, but it has been proposed that tetracycline stabilizes the lipid secretions by inhibiting bacterial enzymes.[22] In sensitive patients, doxycycline, erythromycin, or trimethoprim-sulfamethoxazole can be used.

The value of topical antibiotics is not as clear, but erythromycin, tetracycline, or bacitracin can be used. Topical steroids probably have no benefit.

HORDEOLA

A hordeolum, commonly known as a sty, is an acute, suppurative, nodular inflammation of the lid margin. Hordeola may affect primarily the internal (posterior) portion of the lid, when they arise from the meibomian glands, or the external portion (anterior), when they arise from the Zeis glands, sweat glands, or hair follicles (Fig. 13-7). Hordeola often are infectious, most commonly staphylococcal, but they may be sterile acute inflammations in obstructed glands. They often are associated with blepharitis.

Hordeola can rupture spontaneously or resolve slowly. They are treated with hot compresses and topical antibiotics. If these measures do not succeed, incision and drainage can be performed. Associated blepharitis should also be treated.

CHALAZIA

A chalazion is a sterile, chronic nodular inflammation of a Zeis or meibomian gland (Fig. 13-8). It is a granulomatous reaction to sebaceous material that has been extruded from a plugged gland into the surrounding tissue. It may be insidious in onset or develop acutely and be indistinguishable from a hordeolum. Recently chronic chalazia were found to be associated with hypercholesterolemia in some patients, and lowering serum cholesterol decreased their occurrence.[23]

Hot compresses may be of benefit. The chalazia can be incised and curetted or left alone. Injection of corticosteroid (approximately 0.1 ml triamcinolone 5 mg/ml) may be of benefit.[24,25]

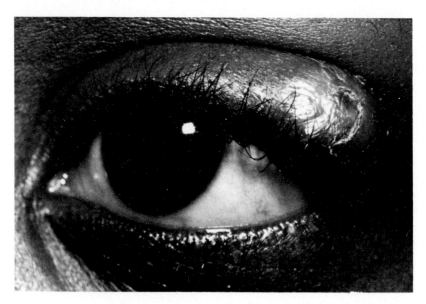

Fig. 13-7. External hordeolum (stye).

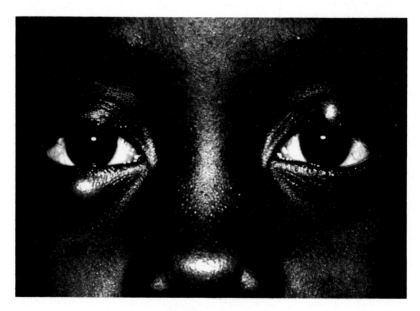

Fig. 13-8. Chalazia.

OTHER CAUSES OF MARGINAL LID INFLAMMATION

Marginal lid ulcers may be caused by vaccinia virus and other poxviruses, as well as by herpes virus. If these viruses are suspected, one should look for other skin lesions and perform scrapings and cultures of the lid lesions.

Herpes simplex can cause a marginal vesicular and ulcerative blepharitis, most commonly in the primary infection. Also, grouped lesions can occur on the anterior surface of the lids, either in primary or recurrent infection. The lesions begin as clear vesicles on an erythematous base and then open, ulcerate, crust over, and heal without scarring, over 7 to 14 days (see Fig. 12-3). Scrapings of the base of a lesion may demonstrate multinucleated giant cells or intranuclear inclusions. If there is no associated keratitis, no treatment is necessary, but I commonly prescribe prophylactic antiviral medication (idoxuridine or vidarabine ointment). Topical acyclovir may speed healing, but it is available only as a dermatologic preparation, and its safety around the eye is unknown. Systemic acyclovir can be considered in severe cases.

Angular blepharitis often is associated with a *Moraxella* infection. The lateral lid margins are wet, macerated, and may be ulcerated (see Fig. 6-8). The gram-negative diplobacillus can be identified on smears. *Moraxella* are sensitive to most antibiotics, and the infection responds rapidly to lid scrubs and antibiotic ointment.

Phthiriasis palpebrum is an uncommon cause of blepharitis and conjunctivitis and can easily be overlooked.[26] Pubic lice *(Phthirus pubis)* have a predilection for lashes as well pubic hairs because of the appropriate spacing of the cilia (Fig. 13-9). With phthiriasis palpebrum a severe blepharoconjunctivitis can be seen, particularly in children. Symptoms include itching, irritation and redness of the lid margins, and conjunctiva. A high index of suspicion and careful examination of the patient's lid margins and eyelashes lead to the proper diagnosis. Nits (louse eggs) usually are seen as small ovoid bodies stuck to the lashes (Fig. 13-10). The adult louse is transparent and can be difficult to see unless it contains blood or other ingested material. The feces of the louse are toxic and cause a follicular conjunctivitis and mild epithelial keratitis.

The condition is best treated by carefully removing the lice and nits from the patient's lashes. Local application of a pediculicide such as yellow mercuric oxide 1% ophthalmic ointment (twice daily for 7 days) or physostigmine ointment (twice daily for 10 days) should be considered when total mechanical removal is impossible. An application of 20% fluorescein also has been found effective.[27] Body hair should be examined for infestation with lice, and family members and contacts also should be examined and treated if infected.

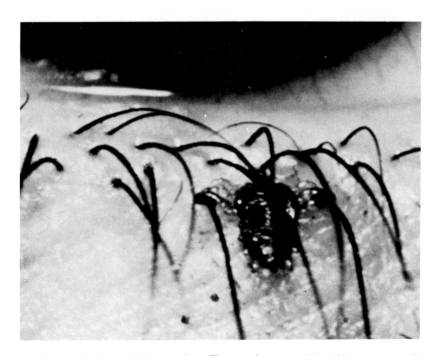

Fig. 13-9. Pediculosis *(Phthirus pubis)*. The parasite suspends itself between two cilia.

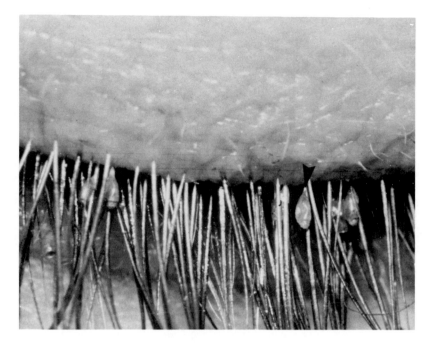

Fig. 13-10. Nits *(arrow)*.

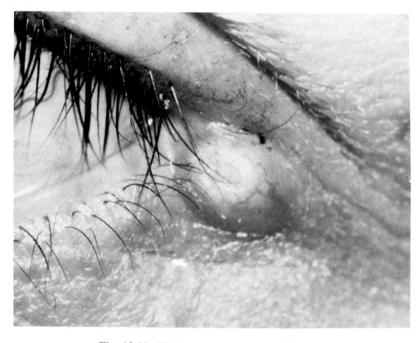

Fig. 13-11. Molluscum contagiosum lid lesion.

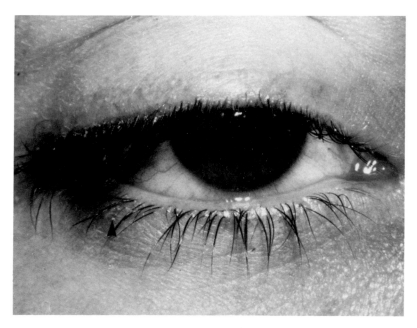

Fig. 13-12. Inconspicuous molluscum contagiosum lesion, hidden by cilia *(arrow),* which causes persistent injection of the eye with follicular conjunctivitis.

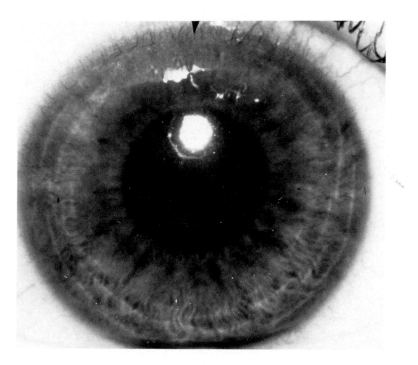

Fig. 13-13. Left untreated, a molluscum contagiosum infection can cause pannus *(arrow).*

Molluscum contagiosum is a poxvirus that commonly infects the lid margins. It occurs most often in adolescents and young adults and is spread by close contact, including sexual contact. The molluscum nodule is a pearly white, raised, round, noninflamed lesion with a craterous center. It may be obvious (Fig. 13-11) or subtle (Fig. 13-12). Conjunctival lesions also can occur and are seen as a small, white pimples containing caseous material on an erythematous base. Chronic follicular conjunctivitis can occur. In long-standing cases superior micropannus and fine epithelial keratitis can affect the superior cornea, simulating trachoma (Fig. 13-13). A scraping of the conjunctiva reveals mononuclear cells. Molluscum bodies are seen in microscopic section of the lesion (Figs. 13-14 and 13-15). Treatment is by surgical excision.

Verrucae are pedunculated or sessile multilobular lesions caused by papovavirus. When located on the lid margin or conjunctiva, they can cause a mild papillary conjunctivitis or fine epithelial keratitis. A mononuclear response is seen in conjunctival scrapings.

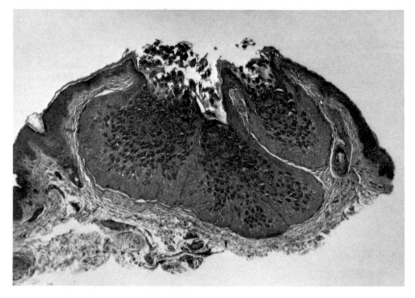

Fig. 13-14. A skin lesion caused by molluscum contagiosum with typical cytoplasmic inclusions. (H & E ×100) (Courtesy of Bruce L Johnson, Pittsburgh, Pa.)

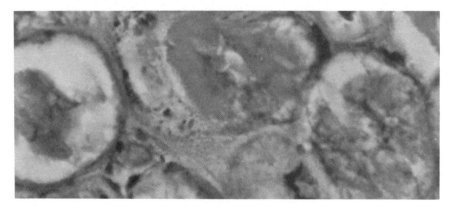

Fig. 13-15. Higher magnification of molluscum bodies.

Blepharoconjunctivitis can develop as a side effect of oral 13-cis-retinoic acid, which is used to treat basal cell carcinoma, keratinizing dermatoses, and cystic acne.[28]

Other causes of blepharitis include syphilis, tuberculosis, psoriasis, yaws, pinta, and atopic dermatitis.[6] Patients with atopic disease also have a tendency to develop staphylococcal blepharitis.

REFERENCES

1. Smolin G and Okumoto M: Staphylococcal blepharitis, Arch Ophthalmol 95:812, 1977.
2. Thygeson P: The etiology and treatment of blepharitis: study in military personnel, Milit Surg 98:191, 1946.
3. Thygeson P: Complications of staphylococcal blepharitis, Am J Ophthalmol 68:446, 1969.
4. Dougherty JM and McCulley JP: Comparative bacteriology of chronic blepharitis, Br J Ophthalmol 68:524, 1984.
5. McCulley JP and Sciallis GF: Meibomian keratoconjunctivitis: oculodermal correlates, CLAO J 9:130, 1983.
6. Smolin G, Tabbara K, and Whitcher J: Infectious diseases of the eye, Baltimore, 1984, Williams & Wilkins.
7. McCulley JP, Dougherty JM, and Deneau DG: Classification of chronic blepharitis, Ophthalmology 89:1173, 1982.
8. Dougherty JM and McCulley JP: Bacterial lipases and chronic conjunctivitis, Invest Ophthalmol Vis Sci 27:486, 1986.
9. Bowers R et al: Non-*aureus* staphylococcus in corneal disease, Invest Ophthalmol Vis Sci 30(suppl):380, 1989.
10. Allen JH: Staphylococcic conjunctivitis, Am J Ophthalmol 20:1025, 1937.
11. Thygeson P: Bacterial factors in chronic catarrhal conjunctivitis: role of toxin-forming staphylococci, Arch Ophthalmol 18:373, 1937.
12. Valenton M and Okumoto M: Toxin producing strains of *Staphylococcus epidermidis,* Arch Ophthalmol 89:186, 1973.
13. Okumoto M: Infectious agents: bacteria. In Smolin G and Thoft RA, editors: The cornea: scientific foundations and clinical practice, Boston, 1983, Little, Brown & Co, Inc.
14. Coston TO: *Demodex folliculorum* blepharitis, Trans Am Ophthalmol Soc 65:361, 1967.
15. English FP et al: The vector potential of *Demodex folliculorum,* Arch Ophthalmol 84:83, 1970.
16. Jeffery MP: Ocular diseases caused by nematodes, Am J Ophthalmol 40:411, 1955.
17. McCulley JP and Dougherty JM: Blepharitis associated with acne rosacea and seborrheic dermatitis, Int Ophthalmol Clin 25:159, 1985.
18. McCulley JP and Sciallis GF: Meibomian keratoconjunctivitis, Am J Ophthalmol 84:788, 1977.
19. Dougherty JM and McCulley JP: Bacterial lipases and chronic blepharitis, Invest Ophthalmol Vis Sci 27:486, 1986.
20. Keith CG: Seborrheic blepharo-kerato-conjunctivitis, Trans Ophthalmol Soc UK 87:85, 1967.
21. Cory CC et al: Meibomian gland secretions in the red eyes of rosacea, Br J Dermatol 88:25, 1973.
22. McCulley JP: Meibomitis. In Kaufman HE et al, editors: The cornea, New York, 1988, Churchill Livingstone, Inc.
23. Gottsch JD and Greenberg KA: An association of elevated serum cholesterol and multiple recurrent chalazia, Invest Ophthalmol Vis Sci 30(suppl):502, 1989.
24. Pizzarello LD et al: Intralesional corticosteroid therapy of chalazia, Am J Ophthalmol 85:818, 1978.
25. Sloas HA et al: Treatment of chalazia with injectable triamcinolone, Ann Ophthalmol 15:78, 1983.
26. Couch JM et al: Diagnosing and treating *Phthirus pubis* palpebrarum, Surv Ophthalmol 26:219, 1982.
27. Matthew M, D'Souza P, and Mehta DK: A new treatment of phthiriasis palpebrarum, Ann Ophthalmol 14:439, 1982.
28. Blackman HJ et al: Blepharoconjunctivitis: a side effect of 13-cisretinoic acid therapy for dermatologic diseases, Ophthalmology 86:753, 1980.

Tear Film Abnormalities

Tear film abnormalities are common and a great source of irritation, both for the patient and the physician. Yet despite the prevalence of these disorders, our understanding of the cause is poor, diagnostic tests are limited and relatively insensitive, and treatment is inadequate. Classification of tear abnormalities is limited by this lack of knowledge, but generally the conditions can be divided into those involving an abnormality in the composition of the tear film, and those in which the spreading or "surfacing" of the tear film is abnormal. By far the most common abnormality of composition is aqueous tear deficiency, but abnormalities in other tear components such as lipid and mucin also can occur. Impaired lid function, such as lagophthalmos, or seventh nerve paresis, proptosis, or localized conjunctival elevations are examples of conditions that interfere with tear surfacing.

ABNORMALITIES OF TEAR FILM COMPOSITION

AQUEOUS

Aqueous deficiency most frequently occurs idiopathically in women in their forties and fifties; however, it can develop at any age, can affect men, and can be associated with many local and systemic conditions (see box on p. 311).

Sjögren's syndrome. The classic triad of Sjögren's syndrome consists of dry eyes, dry mouth (xerostomia), and a connective tissue disease, most commonly rheumatoid arthritis.[1,2] However, the syndrome often is incomplete, and its definition has varied in the past. The term should not be used to

CONDITIONS ASSOCIATED WITH AQUEOUS TEAR DEFICIENCY

CONGENITAL CONDITIONS

Riley-Day syndrome
Cri-du-chat syndrome
Multiple endocrine neoplasia
Lacrimal gland hypoplasia
Anhidrotic ectodermal dysplasia
Holmes-Adie syndrome
Paralytic hyposecretion

LOCAL CONDITIONS

Dacryoadenitis (viral or bacterial)
Irradiation
Trauma
Benign lymphoepithelial lesion
    (Mikulicz's disease)
Seventh nerve palsy
Blepharitis

AUTOIMMUNE DISEASES

Rheumatoid arthritis
Lupus erythematosus
Polyarteritis nodosa
Hashimoto's thyroiditis
Polymyositis
Others

HEMATOPOIETIC DISEASES

Lymphoma
Thrombocytopenic purpura
Hypergammaglobulinemia
Waldenström's macroglobulinemia

OTHER SYSTEMIC CONDITIONS

Celiac disease
Sarcoidosis
Graft versus host disease
Pulmonary fibrosis
Chronic hepatobiliary disease
Amyloidosis

MEDICATIONS

Anticholinergic drugs
Antihistamines
Tricyclic antidepressants
Monoamine oxidase inhibitors
Beta-blockers
Hydrochlorothiazide
Oral contraceptives?
Antidiarrheals
Decongestants
Thiabendazole
Anti-parkinsonian agents
Antineoplastic agents
Retinoids (etretinate, isotretinoin)
Many others[4]

refer to cases of isolated dry eyes. The syndrome currently is divided into two forms: primary dry eyes and dry mouth, and secondary dry eyes and/or dry mouth in association with systemic autoimmune disease.[3] Associated autoimmune diseases include all of those listed in the box above.

Sjögren's syndrome usually develops between 30 and 60 years of age, and women are affected nine times more frequently than men.[5] Besides the lacrimal and salivary glands, the mucus-secreting glands, respiratory mucosa, and vagina also may be involved. Xerostomia (Fig. 14-1) may cause difficulty in swallowing and chewing, and ulcers may develop on the tongue and buccal mucous membrane.[2] Other sites of extraglandular involvement include the joints, skin, lungs, kidneys, peripheral and central nervous systems, blood, and muscles. Autoimmune thyroiditis is relatively common, and some patients require thyroid supplementation. Lymphocyte function is impaired, and lymphoreticular neoplasms also occur.[3,6] Surprisingly, these manifestations are more common in the primary form of the syndrome than in the secondary type. Central nervous system complications occur in more than 20% of patients with primary Sjögren's syndrome,[7] and there is a strong association of central nervous system disease with peripheral vasculitis.[8]

Tear and salivary deficiencies are caused by infiltration of the lacrimal and salivary glands with lymphocytes and plasma cells.[9] Areas of mononuclear cell infiltration are associated with focal degeneration of the glandular acini. Cellular infiltration and glandular atrophy increase, and proliferating ductal epithelial cells form myoepithelial islands. The gland tissue eventually is replaced with connective tissue. Biopsy of the more accessible minor glands of the lip and palate demonstrate changes similar to those noted in the lacrimal gland and can facilitate diagnosis.[5]

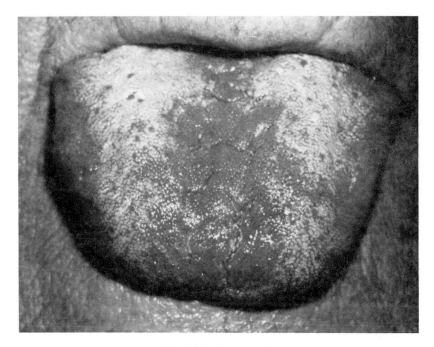

Fig. 14-1. Xerostomia.

Patients with Sjögren's syndrome have a number of immunologic abnormalities, some of which are helpful in diagnosis. Approximately half of these patients have hypergammaglobulinemia, which usually involves all immunoglobulin classes. Monoclonal gammopathies also can occur, and immune complexes and autoantibodies are common.[10] Rheumatoid factor, antinuclear factor, and antibodies to ribonucleoprotein La (SS-B) are seen in most patients. SS-B is relatively specific for Sjögren's syndrome, although it can also be seen in systemic lupus erythematosus. Another antibody to ribonucleoprotein, SS-A, appears to be present in most of the patients with the more serious systemic complications of Sjögren's syndrome.[11] In addition, infants born to women with SS-A antibodies have a greater risk of having cardiac conduction defects.[12]

The pathogenesis of Sjögren's syndrome is unknown. There is a high incidence of HLA-Dw3, and anti-salivary duct antibodies have been found in a high percentage of patients.[13] Some researchers have suggested that Epstein-Barr or cytomegalovirus infection plays a role in the development of Sjögren's syndrome.[14-16] Antibodies against Epstein-Barr virus nuclear antigen are more often found in patients with Sjögren's syndrome.[15,16]

MUCIN

The relationship of mucin abnormalities to clinical disease is unclear. It has been proposed that mucin is important in stabilizing the tear film, by increasing the wettability of the epithelial surface.[17-20] Clinically wettability is measured by tear film breakup time, and some symptomatic patients are found to have normal tear volume but rapid tear film breakup. Theoretically, any disease that causes conjunctival scarring will reduce the number of goblet cells and lead to decreased tear mucin. Therefore relatively severe mucin deficiency would be expected in cicatricial pemphigoid, erythema multiforme major, vitamin A deficiency, and chemical burns. However, the relationship of mucin deficiency to the changes seen in these conditions has not been well demonstrated.

The correlation between goblet cell density and tear mucin content is poor,[21] and even in cases with severe goblet cell loss, tear mucin content is only moderately reduced.[22] It is possible that a qualitative change in tear mucin occurs, but to date this has not been demonstrated.

Excessive mucin often is noted as mucous strands or plaques. The condition may be caused by increased production or by relative overabundance in aqueous deficiency. Ocular infection, allergies, foreign bodies, and trauma all can stimulate increased production.

LIPID

The only cause of true lipid deficiency is congenital absence of the meibomian glands, a condition that can occur in ectodermal dysplasia. The lack of tear lipids causes increased evaporation of tears, which can lead to corneal thinning.[23] Increased lipid production and abnormal lipid composition may be present in meibomitis, but their role in tear and corneal surface disease remains unclear (see Chapter 13).

CLINICAL MANIFESTATIONS

The patient complains of burning and irritation, usually in both eyes. Occasionally a foreign body sensation or mucous discharge also is present. The symptoms are exacerbated by reading, watching television, or other tasks involving concentration, drafts or winds, hot, dry environments, and smoke or other particulate matter in the air. The symptoms may be most marked in the morning, on awakening, or in the evening.

Examining the eye with the slit-lamp microscope reveals an increased amount of debris in the tear film, resulting from the poor tear flow. The tear meniscus, or marginal tear strip, may be reduced. Normal meniscus height is 0.2 to 0.3 mm,[24] and if it is lower than this, keratoconjunctivitis sicca is likely to be present. Viscous mucous threads may be present in the inferior cul-de-sac. Corneal findings include decreased luster, punctate keratopathy (Fig. 14-2), filaments (Fig. 14-3), mucous plaques, keratinization, band keratopathy,[25] and ulceration.

Dry eyes are prone to infections such as conjunctivitis, blepharitis, and keratitis. Sterile corneal

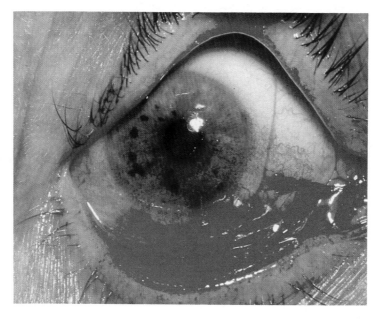

Fig. 14-2. Rose bengal red staining of the cornea and conjunctiva in keratoconjunctivitis sicca. Note the extensive amount of stained mucoid material.

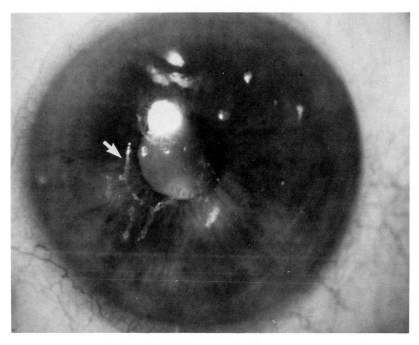

Fig. 14-3. Filamentary keratitis *(arrow)* in a patient with Sjögren's syndrome.

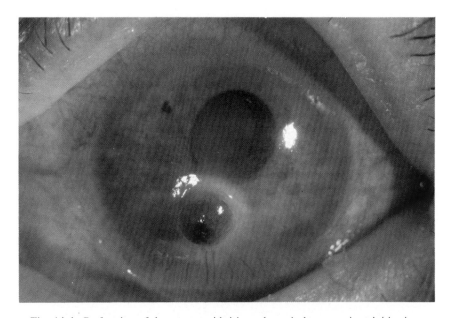

Fig. 14-4. Perforation of the cornea with iris prolapse in keratoconjunctivitis sicca.

ulceration also is relatively common in patients with dry eyes. Typically the ulcer is round or horizontally oval, noninfiltrated, and located in the interpalpebral cornea. The ulcers tend to progress rapidly, forming deep, steep-walled craters that often perforate (Fig. 14-4). The ulceration usually can be halted with a bandage contact lens or by sealing with cyanoacrylate adhesive, but healing is slow. Penetrating keratoplasty may be required.

DIAGNOSTIC TESTS

There is no reliable, sensitive test to diagnose dry eyes. If the condition is relatively severe, the diagnosis can easily be made by clinical examination and Schirmer testing. However, in milder cases establishing the diagnosis often is difficult or impossible. The three simplest and most common tests are rose bengal staining, the Schirmer test, and tear breakup time.

Rose bengal stain is quite valuable in the diagnosis of keratoconjunctivitis sicca. It stains devitalized epithelial cells and mucus. It is the pattern of epithelial injury that suggests dry eyes: interpalpebral cornea and conjunctiva (see Fig. 14-2). In milder cases the staining is limited to the conjunctiva, and in the severest cases most of the cornea also stains. Mucous filaments may be present on the interpalpebral corneal surface.

The *Schirmer test* is a means of estimating tear production (see box below). A Schirmer I (unanesthetized) value less than 5 mm after 5 minutes is considered significant.[26] Test values are reduced in normals after anesthesia, and therefore a reading of 3 mm or less is recommended for this test.[27] Tear production is greatest during the first 1 to 2 minutes after placement of the strip and then slows to a nearly constant rate after 5 minutes.[28] The lower steady rate may be more diagnostic, but this hypothesis has not been tested.

Tear breakup time is the amount of time it takes for a dry spot to appear in the tear film. The test

---

TEAR FUNCTION TESTS

The Schirmer tests of tear quantity are a measurement of the aqueous layer only. The tests are performed with 5 × 30 mm strips of Whatman filter paper (available commercially from Smith Miller & Patch Laboratories). The paper is folded so that 5 mm of the strip will lie within the lower conjunctival sac, and the remaining 25 mm will project over the lower eyelid. The amount of moistening of the exposed paper is recorded at the end of 5 minutes. It is paramount to remember that these tests are rough measurements only. They are clinically useful as gross indicators of tear function.

SCHIRMER TEST I (measures total reflex and basic tear secretion)

To minimize reflex tearing, avoid a brightly lit room and instillation of ocular medications before testing. The patient may keep his or her eyes open or closed. If the paper is wetted completely before 5 minutes, note this time; if not, note the amount of wetting at the end of 5 minutes.

Results: Normals will wet approximately 10 to 30 mm at the end of 5 minutes. This amount decreases with age but probably should not be less than 10 mm. If wetting is greater than 30 mm, reflex tearing is intact but not controlled or tear drainage is insufficient. Tear secretion between 5 and 30 mm may be normal, or basal secretion may be low and compensated for by reflex stimulation. A value of less than 5 mm indicates hyposecretion.

BASIC SECRETION TEST (measures basic tear secretion)

Instill topical anesthetic and wait until anesthesia is achieved. The cul-de-sac should be dried before inserting strips. Only basic secretion is being measured. The difference between this test and the Schirmer test I is the amount of reflex secretion. Basic secretion of 3 mm or less after 5 minutes is abnormal.

SCHIRMER TEST II (measures reflex tear secretion)

Instill topical ocular anesthetic and irritate unanesthetized nasal mucosa by rubbing it with a cotton swab. Measure wetting after 2 minutes. Less than 15 mm wetting represents failure of reflex secretion. This test is seldom employed, since reflex tearing usually is intact.

is performed as follows: Fluorescein is instilled in the eye, and the patient is asked to blink several times to distribute the dye. The patient is then asked to look straight ahead (the lids should not be held open), and the examiner observes the tear film with cobalt blue light for development of a black island within the green film. The tear breakup time is the time between the last blink and the appearance of the dry spot. An abnormal tear breakup time is less than 10 seconds. This test is useful in diagnosing tear abnormalities without significant aqueous deficiency. It is not useful if the corneal surface is irregular or if large particles are present in the tear film.

A number of laboratory tests have been used to detect dry eyes. However, none of these have proved sufficiently sensitive or easy to perform to warrant widespread use.

Tear osmolality appears to be a relatively sensitive laboratory test for dry eyes, but it requires special laboratory equipment to perform.[29] Tear film osmolality presumedly is increased because of decreased aqueous flow and increased tear evaporation. This is determined by collecting a tear sample in a glass micropipette and measuring the freezing point in a nanoliter osmometer. An osmolality of more than 312 mOsm/L is considered indicative of dry eyes and in one study was found to have a sensitivity of 76% and specificity of 84%.[30]

Tear lysozyme is decreased in dry eyes. The most common means of measuring this in the laboratory is by an agar diffusion test. Wetted Schirmer strips are placed on agarose gel containing a suspension of *Micrococcus lysodeikticus,* a bacteria whose cell wall is destroyed by lysozyme (Fig. 14-5). The greater the tear lysozyme concentration, the larger the zone of bacterial lysis.[5,26] (The plates are available from the Kallestad Co., Austin, Texas.)

In one comparative study tear lysozyme was found to be more accurate than rose bengal staining or Schirmer testing.[12] However, decreased tear lysozyme is not specific for dry eyes; it is also found in herpes simplex infection, bacterial conjunctivitis, smog irritation, and malnutrition.[28] Also, concentrations vary with age and time of the day.[31]

Tear lactoferrin is also reduced in dry eyes. This can be measured using a commercially available antibody assay kit (Lactoplate, Mackeen Consultants, Bethesda, Md.). Both basal and reflex tears are

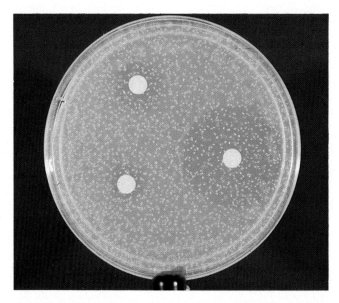

Fig. 14-5. Lysozyme activity assay. Note the zone of lysis of the agar medium inoculated with a suspension of *Micrococcus lysodeikticus.*

measured, and the percent increase in lactoferrin from basal to reflex tears is determined. This test was found to be 96% sensitive in one study[30] but only 35% sensitive and 70% specific in a more recent comparison with tear osmolarity.[32]

TREATMENT

Once the diagnosis of dry eyes is made, it is important to consider the possibility of an association with a systemic disease. The patient should be questioned about dryness of the mouth or other mucous membranes, arthritis, and other symptoms of autoimmune disease. Laboratory testing (for example, erythrocyte sedimentation rate, ANA, rheumatoid factor, complete blood count) is indicated if the dryness is severe, if dryness of the mouth or other mucous membranes is present, if the patient is male or under 30 years of age, or if a review of systems suggests systemic disease.

If Sjögren's syndrome is present, thyroid function tests probably are worthwhile. Immunosuppression with corticosteroid or cyclophosphamide is indicated in the treatment of systemic complications such as glomerulonephritis and pneumonitis. Tabbara[13] also has recommended a short course of prednisone in patients with early Sjögren's syndrome, in whom the diagnosis has been confirmed histologically. He has observed rapid clinical improvement in some patients.

Medications that decrease tear production should be discontinued whenever possible. Using a humidifier in the home often is helpful.

Artificial tear solutions. The mainstay of the treatment of dry eyes is artificial tears. Many types of artificial tear solutions are commercially available, and no particular type has been demonstrated to be superior. Most have a polymeric agent such as polyvinyl alcohol, methylcellulose, or dextran to increase viscosity. The solutions with polymeric agents seem to be retained for longer periods, but inspissated material tends to form on the lid margin and in the fornix.[33] Hypotonic solutions have been developed, based on the assumption that reducing the hyperosmolality of the tears in dry eyes will provide more symptomatic relief. Although the effect on osmolality appears to be short-lived,[34] many patients do prefer these drops.

The preservatives in artificial tear solutions, particularly thimerosal and benzalkonium chloride, can elicit contact sensitivity reactions or cause toxicity to the surface epithelium. Nonpreserved solutions are available (Unisol, CooperVision, San German, Puerto Rico; Refresh, Allergan, Irvine, Calif.) and can be very useful, particularly in patients with severe dryness, who must use the drops frequently. However, these drops are less convenient and must be discarded 24 to 48 hours after opening.

The use of viscoelastic materials, hyaluronic acid and chondroitin sulfate, in artificial tear solutions has been recommended,[35-37] but one double-blind study found no difference in patient preference between these and an artificial tear solution with polyvinyl alcohol.[38]

Autologous serum has been reported to be an effective artificial tear solution,[39] but this has not been tested in a controlled manner. All-trans retinoic acid ointment initially was reported to be very effective,[40] but a subsequent controlled study did not find it to be more effective than a standard artificial tear ointment.[41]

Ointments. Petrolatum-based ointments relieve the symptoms, primarily through lubrication. However, they tend to interfere with vision, so most patients use them only at bedtime. Ointments without preservatives are available and are preferable.

Artificial tear inserts. A unique product, Lacrisert (Merck, Sharp & Dome, West Point, Pa.) is a small pellet of polymer (hydroxypropyl cellulose) that is placed in the inferior fornix. In the presence of tears it slowly dissolves, releasing the polymer into the tear film and retarding its evaporation.[42-45] It generally is used once or twice daily. Lacriserts can be very helpful in some patients with dry eyes, but several problems limit their use. Since many of these patients do not produce enough tears to melt the insert, artificial tear drops must also be used. Some patients have difficulty inserting the pellets in the fornix. Other problems are blurred vision, particularly when looking through the enlarged tear meniscus, and irritation from the presence of the pellet.

Mucolytic agents. In some patients with marked mucous strands, globs, or filaments, a mucolytic agent will increase comfort. N-acetylcysteine (10% to 20%) can be effective in dissolving excess mucus when given two to four times daily. The Food and Drug Administration has not approved this use of the drug, but it is available and can be formulated by most pharmacists. It burns upon instillation and has a distasteful odor. In many patients a course of 3 to 4 weeks of treatment provides prolonged relief; others require chronic treatment.

Punctal occlusion. Occlusion of the lacrimal puncta can be performed to aid retention of naturally produced and artificial tears.[46,47] The ability of punctal occlusion to improve objective clinical findings has not been well documented, but the procedure often is helpful in patients whose symptoms are not relieved by frequent use of artificial tears.

The main complication of punctal occlusion is epiphora, which can be prevented by (1) limiting the procedure to patients whose Schirmer test values are consistently less than 3 mm and (2) testing with temporary occlusion. Temporary occlusion can be achieved with collagen plugs (Lacrimedics, San Marino, Calif.), silicone plugs (Fig. 14-6) (Eagle Vision, Memphis), cyanoacrylate adhesive, by suturing the punctum with 10-0 nylon, or by placing a heated spatula on the punctum for 1 second. If symptoms are improved or the frequency of drop use can be reduced and epiphora does not occur, permanent occlusion may be performed. This is most easily accomplished with cautery, using an electrocautery device (Hyfrecator, Birtcher, Los Angeles), or a hand-held cautery. Recanalization can occur, and if several attempts are unsuccessful, the punctum or a portion of the canaliculus can be extirpated.

Moisture chambers. Evaporation can be retarded by surrounding the eye with a moisture-retaining chamber. Many different types of moisture chambers can be fashioned, including swimming goggles, clear plastic wrap, silicone breast implants, or moist chamber spectacles. These are most useful for comatose patients and those with nocturnal lagophthalmos, but they also can aid many severely affected patients. The main drawbacks are their cosmetic unacceptability and their tendency to fog, blurring vision.

Bandage contact lenses. Bandage contact lenses are most useful in treating filamentary keratitis. The lens is placed after the filaments are removed from the cornea; the patient experiences immediate

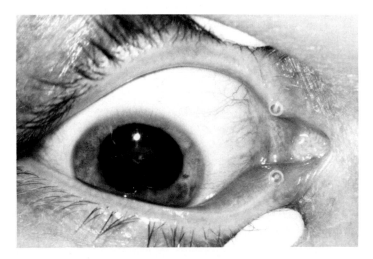

Fig. 14-6. Silicone punctal plugs.

symptomatic relief and the filaments usually do not reappear as long as the lens is in place. Bandage lenses are also helpful in cases of recurrent epithelial breakdown or delayed healing, in eyes that are mucin deficient but have relatively good aqueous flow, and in some cases of exposure keratitis. The lenses can provide some symptomatic relief in patients with marked drying, but other means of treatment should be exhausted first[48] because of the relatively high risk of complications such as infection, vascularization, and chemical reactions.[49] Thicker lenses with a lower water content are preferred to thinner, higher water content lenses. The former tend not to dehydrate as much, but concomitant artificial tear use is recommended.

Other treatments. Symptomatic improvement and increased tear lysozyme with oral bromhexine has been reported.[24,50] Lateral tarsorrhaphy may be necessary in some patients to help prevent surface breakdown and ulceration. Parotid duct transposition was explored in the past but has been largely abandoned.[51-53] The surgery is tedious, and the secretion usually is excessive and increases during eating.

Penetrating keratoplasty can be performed for scarring or ulceration caused by dry eyes, but the results usually are poor. Keratoprosthesis can be performed as a last resort.

Psychologic aspects. The physician's task does not end with prescribing artificial tears. Patients with dry eyes in particular require attention to other, psychologic needs. Dry eye conditions are chronic, annoying, and sometimes debilitating diseases. Patients must come to realize the limitations of treatment but also that good vision nearly always is maintained. Many patients require reassurance, attention, and compassion from the physician. They also need time to adapt to their condition and to adjust their life-style, and this usually occurs over several visits. Informational pamphlets, videotaped presentations, and discussions with auxiliary personnel can be very useful. In many communities support groups have been established to help people with dry eyes deal with their condition, and I have found this to be one of the most effective forms of treatment.

ABNORMALITIES OF TEAR SURFACING

The term "tear surfacing" was introduced by Lemp[54] to refer to the spreading of tears across the corneal and conjunctival surfaces. The lids are primarily responsible for this spreading, and it requires an intact lid margin, contact of the lid with the globe, and complete closure of the lid during blinking. Interference with any of these properties can result in drying of the surface areas affected. Lid surfacing abnormalities include the following:

Lid position	*Lid movement (blinking)*	*Localized surface elevations*
Entropion	Seventh nerve palsy	Pterygium
Ectropion	Symblepharon	Limbal tumor
Tumors	Severe proptosis	Postsurgical edema
Colobomas and other lid defects	Parkinsonism	Subconjunctival hemorrhage
Ptosis surgery	Bilateral fifth nerve palsy	Filtering bleb
Floppy eyelid syndrome	Coma	Many others
	Graves syndrome	

Dellen (*delle* is the singular form) are localized thinnings of the cornea (Fig. 14-7) or sclera (Fig. 14-8) that form adjacent to corneal or conjunctival elevations. They represent localized dehydration caused by lack of wetting by the lid.

CLINICAL MANIFESTATIONS

Dellen are differentiated from ulceration by their rapid onset, lack of infiltration, location adjacent to elevations, and coverage by intact epithelium. Their nature can be confirmed by taping the eyelids shut; most will improve in 1 to 2 hours and disappear in 24 to 48 hours.

In most types of tear surfacing abnormalities, the diagnosis is obvious. However, infrequent or incomplete blinking and lagophthalmos may be difficult to appreciate unless the physician specifically

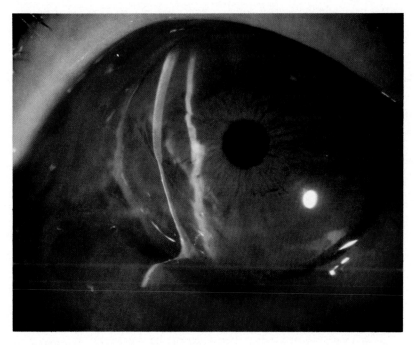

Fig. 14-7. Corneal delle adjacent to the area of conjunctival elevation.

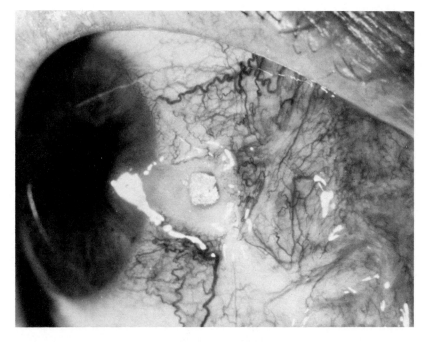

Fig. 14-8. Scleral delle.

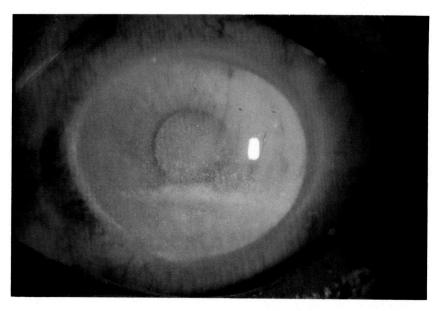

Fig. 14-9. Corneal staining in lagophthalmos.

looks for them. The pattern of staining may suggest their presence (see Fig. 3-12); chronic punctate keratopathy of the central or lower cornea usually occurs. Occasionally, the entire lower half of the cornea is involved, or more frequently a horizontal band of keratopathy is seen across the cornea (Fig. 14-9). There usually is a lack of corneal luster, as well as diffuse haziness and desiccation of the involved area.

Lagophthalmos sometimes is present only during sleep. The physician should check specifically for this common condition (Fig. 14-10), because otherwise it may be missed. The diagnosis can be

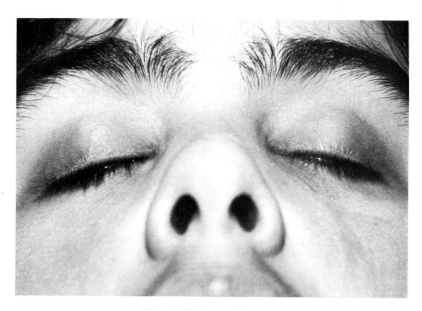

Fig. 14-10. Lagophthalmos.

definitely made only by the response to nocturnal taping of the lids, since mild surface changes may be present in the morning and then heal later in the day. However, in chronic disease the exposed cornea can develop map-dot-fingerprint lines, spheroidal degeneration, nodules similar to small deposits of Salzmann's nodular dystrophy, and, the most common sign, a horizontal brown line of iron deposition, which indicates chronic epithelial damage and irritation.[55]

TREATMENT

If possible the primary cause of exposure should be addressed. Abnormalities of lid position usually can be corrected surgically. Most other conditions usually can be adequately treated with artificial tear solutions or ointment. Taping the lids, swimming goggles, or other forms of moisture chambers often are necessary at night. Occasionally, punctal occlusion can be performed to increase the height of lacrimal lake; in some cases epiphora is preferable to severe drying. If these measures do not provide comfort or maintain epithelial integrity, lateral tarsorrhaphy can be performed. In the most severe cases a total tarsorrhaphy or conjunctival flap can provide comfort and prevent ulceration or perforation.

Corneal dellen and other forms of localized surface drying usually occur adjacent to acute elevations, and tear drops or ointments are sufficient until the elevation subsides. Pterygia and other limbal masses may require surgical excision, and subconjunctival hemorrhages may require drainage.

REFERENCES

1. Bloch KJ et al: Sjögren's syndrome: a clinical, pathological and serological study of sixty-two cases, Medicine (Baltimore) 44:187, 1965.
2. Sjögren H and Bloch KJ: Keratoconjunctivitis sicca and the Sjögren syndrome, Surv Ophthalmol 16:145, 1971.
3. Moustsopoulos HM et al: Sjögren's syndrome (sicca syndrome): current issues, Ann Intern Med 92:212, 1980.
4. Fraunfelder FT: Drug-induced ocular side effects and drug interactions, ed 3, Philadelphia, 1989, Lea & Febiger.
5. Tabbara KF et al: Sjögren's syndrome: a correlation between ocular findings and labial salivary gland histology, Trans Am Acad Ophthalmol Otolaryngol 78:467, 1974.
6. Anderson LG and Talal N: The spectrum of benign to malignant lymphoproliferation in Sjögren's syndrome, Clin Exp Immunol 9:199, 1971.
7. Alexander EL et al: Neurologic complications of primary Sjögren's syndrome, Medicine 61:247, 1982.
8. Molina R, Provost TT, and Alexander EL: Peripheral inflammatory vascular disease in Sjögren's syndrome: association with nervous system complications, Arthritis Rheum 28:1341, 1985.
9. Williamson J: Keratoconjunctivitis sicca, histology of lacrimal gland, Br J Ophthalmol 57:852, 1973.
10. Talal N: Sjögren's syndrome. In Samter M, editor: Immunologic diseases, ed 4, Boston, 1988, Little, Brown & Co, Inc.
11. Land HC and Fauci AS: Sjögren's syndrome. In E Braunwald et al, editors: Harrison's principles of internal medicine, ed 11, New York, 1987, McGraw-Hill, Inc.
12. Franco HL et al: Autoantibodies directed against sicca syndrome antigens in the neonatal lupus syndrome, Am Acad Dermatol 4:67, 1981.
13. Tabbara KF: Sjögren's syndrome. In Smolin G and Thoft RA, editors: The cornea: scientific foundations and clinical practice, Boston, 1983, Little, Brown & Co, Inc.
14. Venables P: Sjögren's syndrome: differential diagnosis, immunopathology and genetics. In Scott T et al, editors: Topical reviews, reports of rheumatic diseases, London, 1988, ARC Publications.
15. Fox RI, Pearson G, and Vaughan JH: Detection of Epstein-Barr virus-associated antigens and DNA in salivary biopsies from patients with Sjögren's syndrome, J Immunol 137:3162, 1986.
16. Pflugfelder SC et al: Epstein-Barr virus infection and immunologic dysfunction in patients with aqueous tear deficiency, Ophthalmology 97:313, 1990.
17. Holly FJ: Formation and rupture of the tear film, Exp Eye Res 15:515, 1973.
18. Lemp MA, Dohlman CH, and Holly FJ: Corneal desiccation despite normal tear volume, Ann Ophthalmol 2:258, 1970.
19. Lemp MA et al: Dry eye secondary to mucus deficiency, Trans Am Acad Ophthalmol Otolaryngol 75:1223, 1971.
20. Holly FJ and Lemp MA: Wettability and wetting of corneal epithelium, Exp Eye Res 11:239, 1971.
21. Friend J, Kiorpes T, and Thoft RA: Conjunctival goblet cell frequency after alkali injury is not accurately reflected by aqueous tear mucin content, Invest Ophthalmol Vis Sci 24:612, 1983.
22. Kinoshita S et al: Goblet cell density in ocular surface disease: a better indicator than tear mucin, Arch Ophthalmol 101:1284, 1983.
23. Mishima S and Maurice DM: Oily layer of tear film and evaporation from corneal surface, Exp Eye Res 1:39, 1961.
24. Scharf JM et al: Influence of bromhexine on tear lysozyme level in keratoconjunctivitis sicca, Am J Ophthalmol 92:21, 1981.

25. Lemp MA and Ralph RA: Rapid development of band keratopathy in dry eyes, Am J Ophthalmol 83:657, 1977.

26. van Bijsterveld OP: Diagnostic tests in the sicca syndrome, Arch Ophthalmol 82:10, 1969.

27. Lamberts DW, Foster CS, and Perry HD: Schirmer test after topical anesthesia and the tear meniscus height in normal eyes, Arch Ophthalmol 97:1082, 1979.

28. Lamberts DW: Keratoconjunctivitis sicca. In Smolin G and Thoft RA, editors: The cornea: scientific foundations and clinical practice, Boston, 1983, Little, Brown & Co, Inc.

29. Gilbard JP, Farris RL, and Santamaria J: Osmolarity of tear microvolumes in keratoconjunctivitis sicca, Arch Ophthalmol 96:677, 1978.

30. Farris RL et al: Diagnostic tests in keratoconjunctivitis sicca, CLAO J 9:23, 1983.

31. Sen DK and Sarin GS: Biological variations of lysozyme concentration in the tear fluids of healthy persons, Br J Ophthalmol 70:246, 1986.

32. Luce A, Farris RL, and Nunez JN: A comparison of two diagnostic tests for keratoconjunctivitis sicca: lactoplate and tear osmolarity, Invest Ophthalmol Vis Sci 30(suppl):523, 1989.

33. Swanson A, Jeter D, and Tucker P: Ophthalmic vehicles. II. Comparison of ointment and polyvinyl alcohol 1.4%, Ophthalmologica 160:265, 1970.

34. Holly FJ and Lamberts DW: Effect of nonisotonic solutions on tear film osmolality, Invest Ophthalmol Vis Sci 20:236, 1981.

35. DeLuise VP and Peterson WS: The use of topical Healon tears in the management of refractory dry-eye syndrome, Ann Ophthalmol 16:823, 1984.

36. Polack FM and McNiece MT: The treatment of dry eyes with Na hyaluronate (Healon), Cornea 1:133, 1982.

37. Hammer ME and Burch TG: Viscous corneal protection by sodium hyaluronate, chondroitin sulfate, and methylcellulose, Invest Ophthalmol Vis Sci 25:1329, 1984.

38. Limberg MB et al: Topical application of hyaluronic acid and chondroitin sulfate in the treatment of dry eyes, Am J Ophthalmol 103:194, 1987.

39. Fox RI et al: Beneficial effect of artificial tears made with autologous serum in patients with keratoconjunctivitis sicca, Arthritis Rheum 27:459, 1984.

40. Tseng SCG et al: Topical retinoid treatment for various dry-eye disorders, Ophthalmology 92:717, 1985.

41. Soong HK et al: Topical retinoid therapy for squamous metaplasia of various ocular surface disorders, Ophthalmology 95:1442, 1988.

42. Bloomfield SE et al: Soluble artificial tear inserts, Arch Ophthalmol 95:247, 1977.

43. Werblin TP, Rheinstrom SD, and Kaufman HE: The use of slow-release artificial tears in the long-term management of keratitis sicca, Ophthalmology 88:78, 1981.

44. Guatheron PD, Lotli VJ, and LeDouarec JC: Tear film breakup time prolonged with unmedicated cellulose polymer inserts, Arch Ophthalmol 97:1944, 1979.

45. Hill JC: Slow-release artificial tear inserts in the treatment of dry eyes in patients with rheumatoid arthritis, Br J Ophthalmol 73:151, 1989.

46. Tuberville AW, Frederick WR, and Wood TO: Punctal occlusion in tear deficiency syndromes, Ophthalmology 89:1170, 1982.

47. Freeman JM: The punctum plug: evaluation of a new treatment for the dry eye, Trans Am Acad Ophthalmol Otolaryngol 79:874, 1975.

48. Gassett AR and Kaufman HE: Hydrophilic lens therapy of severe keratoconjunctivitis sicca and conjunctival scarring, Am J Ophthalmol 71:1185, 1971.

49. Dohlman CH, Boruchoff SA, and Mobilia E: Complications in use of soft contact lenses in corneal disease, Arch Ophthalmol 90:367, 1973.

50. Frost-Larsen K et al: Sjögren's syndrome, Arch Ophthalmol 98:836, 1980.

51. Katsuelson AB and Zhak EM: Surgical therapy of xerophthalmia by transplantation of parotid duct into conjunctival sac, Vestn Oftalmol 30:3, 1951.

52. Bennett JE: The management of total xerophthalmia, Arch Ophthalmol 81:667, 1969.

53. Soll DB: Vein grafting in nasolacrimal system reconstruction, Ophthalmic Surg 14:696, 1983.

54. Lemp MA et al: The precorneal tear film. I. Factors in spreading and maintaining a continuous tear film over the corneal surface, Arch Ophthalmol 3:39, 1970.

55. Katz J and Kaufman HE: Corneal exposure during sleep (nocturnal lagophthalmos), Arch Ophthalmol 95:499, 1977.

EPITHELIAL DISEASES

NORMAL EPITHELIAL HEALING

Normal epithelial wound healing is a process of cell migration, mitosis, and adhesion. Small defects are covered by migration of adjacent epithelial cells, and this is followed by cell division until the thickness of the epithelium returns to normal.[1,2] With larger defects both migration and mitosis are involved in covering the defect, and more time is required. If the basement membrane is intact, the epithelial cells attach rapidly, forming hemidesmosomes over remaining anchoring fibrils (within 24 hours).[3] Healing after injuries that destroy the basement membrane is more complex and can take much longer.

After epithelial wounding, a temporary layer of fibrin and fibronectin forms on the denuded surface and facilitates epithelial migration and attachment.[4-10] The process of cell sliding involves detachment from underlying fibronectin through activation of plasmin, a proteolytic enzyme, and advancement to adjacent fibronectin.[11] The epithelial cells are stimulated by fibrin and fibronectin to release plasminogen activator. Plasminogen activator then causes the conversion of plasminogen into plasmin. The active plasmin decreases epithelial adhesion to the fibrin and fibronectin, allowing advancement of the cell.

Once epithelial integrity is restored, the temporary matrix of fibrin and fibronectin is resorbed.

After the epithelial layer is intact, basement membrane and anchoring fibrils are formed. If stroma has been removed, collagen is laid down beneath the epithelium and new anchoring fibrils may constantly be reformed until normal stromal thickness is achieved.[12]

NEUROTROPHIC KERATITIS

The sensory innervation of the cornea can be impaired by many conditions (see box below). Whenever corneal sensation is decreased, epithelial dysfunction occurs. The pathogenesis of the epithelial disease is unclear, but it is believed that the corneal nerves normally provide some type of trophic influence on the epithelium. The nerves may release substances from their sensory endings that are necessary for epithelial cell function. In the absence of innervation, cell metabolism is reduced, permeability is increased,[19] acetylcholine and choline acetyltransferase concentrations are reduced,[20,21] and the mitotic rate decreases.[22,23] The epithelial cell vitality is decreased, and defects, vascularization, and opacification can occur, even in the absence of injury.[24] However, these eyes are also prone to infection and trauma, and their ability to heal is markedly reduced.[25] Stromal ulceration often occurs, usually in the presence of persistent epithelial defects.

CORNEAL MANIFESTATIONS

Early signs of corneal involvement are the development of a corneal haze and injection of the conjunctiva. These changes may be apparent within 24 hours after section of the trigeminal nerve. Damage and focal loss of epithelial cells lead to punctate keratopathy and decreased corneal luster (Fig. 15-1). In many cases larger erosions develop, and eventually so do broad epithelial defects, most commonly in the interpalpebral cornea. These defects usually are slow to heal, even with treatment. Iritis often accompanies a persistent epithelial defect, and a sterile hypopyon can be seen, usually after placement of a bandage contact lens. Ulceration (Fig. 15-2), perforation, and vascularization often develop.

CAUSES OF DECREASED CORNEAL SENSATION

FIFTH NERVE PALSY
Surgical
Tumors
Aneurysms
Others

CONGENITAL CAUSES
Familial dysautonomia (Riley-Day syndrome)
Goldenhar's syndrome
Möbius syndrome
Parry-Romberg syndrome
Bassen-Kornzweig syndrome
Isolated congenital trigeminal anesthesia

CORNEAL DYSTROPHIES
Lattice
Granular (rare)

IATROGENIC
Contact lens wear[13]
Trauma to ciliary nerves by laser, cryotherapy, scleral buckling, or diathermy
Corneal incisions: cataract, keratoplasty, epikeratophakia

INFECTION
Herpes simplex
Herpes zoster
Leprosy

SYSTEMIC DISEASE
Diabetes[14,15]

MEDICATIONS
Topical anesthetic abuse
Atropine[16]
Timolol (usually temporary)[17]
Sulfacetamide 30%[18]

TOXIC CAUSES
Chemical burns
Carbon disulfide exposure
Hydrogen sulfide exposure

FUNCTIONAL CAUSES
Hysteria

MISCELLANEOUS CAUSES
Any condition involving chronic epithelial injury or stromal inflammation

---

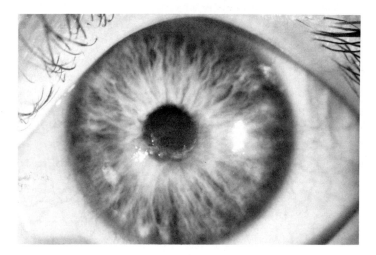

Fig. 15-1. Anesthetic cornea with loss of epithelial luster and irregular thickening of central epithelium.

The course of neurotrophic keratitis varies considerably. In many patients with congenital or acquired corneal hypesthesia, the cornea can appear normal or exhibit only mild punctate staining for years. Then, spontaneously or after minor trauma, an epithelial defect develops; it heals poorly, and infection or sterile ulceration often follow.

TREATMENT

The only form of treatment available is protecting the corneal surface with lubricants, tarsorrhaphy, and bandage contact lenses. Punctate staining and corneal haziness are treated with artificial tear

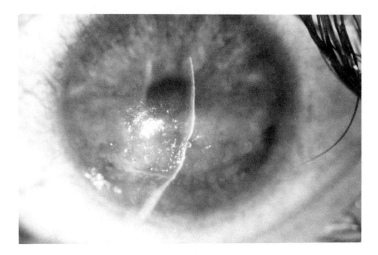

Fig. 15-2. Anesthetic cornea with ulceration.

solutions during the day and ointment at bedtime. If defects develop, patching may result in healing, but often a bandage contact lens or tarsorrhaphy is required. Using bandage contact lenses is more likely to cause complications in these patients. A sterile hypopyon often develops, usually within 1 or 2 days of lens application. For unknown reasons, of a cycloplegic agent usually prevents this complication. Both sterile and infectious infiltrates also are common.

A complete tarsorrhaphy usually results in healing of the epithelium and prevents further ulceration. Once the epithelium is intact, the tarsorrhaphy can gradually be opened. Partial closure may be required permanently, and occasionally total closure must be performed repeatedly or a conjunctival flap must be placed.

RECURRENT EROSIONS

Recurrent erosions are a common problem. Most cases are related to corneal injury, most commonly from fingernails or paper.[26] These erosions also may be seen in diabetes,[27] corneal dystrophies,[28] other forms of anterior stromal injury, exposure, and Cockayne's syndrome.[29] Causes of recurrent corneal erosions are presented in the box below.

The erosions reflect an abnormality of the epithelial attachment complex, which comprises the basement membrane, hemidesmosomes, anchoring fibrils, and anterior stroma.[30-32] After trauma, discontinuities and duplications of attachment complexes are seen for 8 to 12 weeks, and during this period the epithelium is easily removed.[32,33] Damage to Bowman's layer and anterior stroma or active inflammation in these layers also can prevent adhesion. Primary abnormalities in the attachment complex are seen in map-dot-fingerprint dystrophy (see Chapter 17) and diabetes. Thickening of the

---

CAUSES OF RECURRENT CORNEAL EROSIONS

TRAUMA
Fingernail or paper cuts
Alkali burns
Thermal injury

CORNEAL DYSTROPHIES
Meesmann's
Fuchs'
Reis-Bücklers'
Grayson-Wilbrandt
Epithelial basement membrane
Lattice
Macular
Granular

CORNEAL ANESTHESIA
Herpes simplex
Herpes zoster
Alkali burns
Others

OTHER CORNEAL CONDITIONS
Nontraumatic anterior stromal injury (for example, infection)
Corneal edema

SYSTEMIC DISEASE
Diabetes
Cockayne's syndrome
Epidermolysis bullosa

---

basement membrane, with reduced penetration of the anchoring fibrils into the stroma, and duplications of anchoring fibrils are seen in the corneas of patients with diabetes.[34] In lattice dystrophy, amyloid deposition occurs between the epithelium and Bowman's layer, disrupting the epithelial attachment complex.[35]

CLINICAL MANIFESTATIONS

With recurrent erosions the patient experiences pain, photophobia, tearing, and foreign body sensation.[36] The onset usually is sudden, most often on awakening, but can occur anytime. The symptoms vary in severity and duration with the size of the erosion; they can last for minutes to days. The frequency of attacks also varies considerably, and as many as four or five brief attacks may occur each day.

During an acute attack one may see epithelial loss, epithelial microcysts, bullae, loose sheets of epithelium, or epithelial filaments. Visual acuity can be markedly reduced if the visual axis is affected. Between attacks epithelial cysts, surface irregularity, or subepithelial scarring often can be detected.[37,38] The healed epithelial area may even resemble a dendritic figure and may be misdiagnosed as herpetic keratitis. As with any epithelial defect, bacterial infection can develop.

The physician should look for evidence of abnormal epithelial adhesion in other portions of the cornea and the fellow eye to detect epithelial basement membrane dystrophy. It has been stated that approximately half of patients with recurrent erosions have evidence of epithelial basement membrane dystrophy.[29]

TREATMENT

The treatment of recurrent corneal erosion is directed toward reestablishing tight adhesion of the epithelium by a normal epithelial attachment complex. The first goal is healing of the erosion, which usually is accomplished with patching. Removal of loose epithelium and a bandage contact lens can aid healing.

In many cases little or no treatment is required; the attacks are relatively infrequent and short-lived. Erosions usually abate spontaneously after 1 to 3 years. The simplest method of reducing recurrences is by lubrication, and hypertonic drops and ointments appear to be superior. A 5% sodium chloride drop is instilled four or five times daily, and the ointment form is given at bedtime. Treatment should be continued for at least 3 months.

If further treatment is necessary, several options are available, including anterior stromal puncture, debridement, superficial keratectomy, and bandage contact lens wear. Anterior stromal puncture was introduced by McLean, MaCrea, and Rich[39] to treat recurrent erosions occurring consistently in the same portion of the extraaxial cornea. A 25- or 27-gauge needle is used to create several shallow (one fourth to one third depth) punctures in the anterior stroma of the affected area. The needle tip can be bent at 90 degrees to ensure that only the desired depth is achieved. The mechanism of action is unclear, but in rabbits epithelial plugs persist in the wounds for at least 5 months after surgery.[40] I have found this technique to be very effective, but it can be used in only a limited number of patients, since the erosions must consistently occur in the same area and the visual axis should be avoided.

Scraping of the epithelium and basement membrane can improve adhesion after healing. If the recurrences consistently affect the same portion of the cornea, the epithelium can be removed and the base gently scraped with a blunt instrument, such as a Kimura spatula. If epithelial basement membrane dystrophy is present, some have recommended more aggressive debridement of the entire corneal surface[41] or superficial keratectomy.[42,43] Of course, these procedures carry a theoretic risk of scarring and infection.

A bandage contact lens can provide comfort and lessen or eliminate erosions. It usually must be worn for at least 3 months and should not be removed until the epithelium appears normal in the affected area.

I perform anterior stromal puncture if recurrences affect only a localized extraaxial area. Localized axial lesions are gently scraped at the slit-lamp microscope, using a Paton or Kimura spatula. When basement membrane disease is more generalized or when patients are reluctant to undergo the above procedures, a bandage contact lens is placed. If this is not possible or sufficient, a near total epithelial debridement is performed.

PERSISTENT EPITHELIAL DEFECTS

Nonhealing epithelial defects (Fig. 15-3) are relatively common problems, but a systematic approach to diagnosis and treatment can nearly always lead to resolution.

The most common conditions associated with delayed epithelial healing are listed in the box on p. 330). A thorough search for these conditions should be performed in any patient with a persistent defect; often a number of conditions are present.

Stromal Ulceration

If epithelial healing is delayed, stromal substance can be lost. This has been hypothesized to result from several mechanisms. With a chronic epithelial defect, polymorphonuclear leukocytes (PMNs) invade the stroma, and excess amounts of the enzymes plasmin and collagenase may be produced. Collagenase can split collagen, making it more vulnerable to destruction by other proteases. Collagenase has been isolated from ulcerating corneas and is thought to be produced by epithelial cells, PMNs, and keratocytes.[44]

Plasmin also can be secreted by epithelial cells, PMNs, and keratocytes. Plasmin degrades fibrin, fibronectin, and basement membrane components and activates collagenase.[45] Theoretically, excess plasmin production could prevent the formation of an adequate fibrin-fibronectin layer for epithelial attachment and resurfacing. Plasmin also stimulates keratocyte secretion of latent collagenase, converts latent collagenase to active collagenase, and cleaves complement component C3 to produce fragments chemotactic for PMNs. In addition to the experimental support for the role of plasmin, elevated tear levels of plasmin have been found in some patients with persistent epithelial defects.[46]

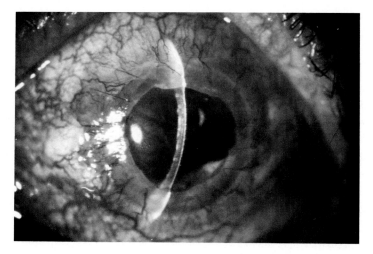

Fig. 15-3. Persistent epithelial defect after penetrating keratoplasty. (Courtesy of Stuart I. Brown, La Jolla, Calif.)

COMMON CAUSES OF DELAYED EPITHELIAL HEALING

ABNORMAL LID FUNCTION

Entropion
Ectropion
Lagophthalmos
Trichiasis

MEDICATIONS

Topical antibiotics
Topical antivirals
Preservatives
Anesthetic abuse

SYSTEMIC DISEASE

Diabetes mellitus
Severe malnutrition
Vitamin A deficiency

PRIMARY EPITHELIAL DISEASE

Cicatricial pemphigoid
Erythema multiforme major (Stevens-Johnson syndrome)
Atopic keratoconjunctivitis
Other dermatologic conditions

LOCAL CONDITIONS

Corneal anesthesia
Stromal injury: viral (see Fig. 12-10), traumatic, chemical
Keratoconjunctivitis sicca
Active stromal inflammation or infection
Occult foreign body

TREATMENT

If possible, any conditions that impair epithelial healing should be corrected. Dry eyes are treated with lubricants and punctal occlusion, lid position abnormalities are corrected surgically, and unnecessary toxic medications are discontinued.

Progressive measures are then taken, in a stepwise manner, from the least complicated or invasive measure to the most, to obtain healing. Pressure patching, bandage contact lens, or total tarsorrhaphy can be used. If some healing is not obtained within 2 or 3 days, the next measure is taken. Since contact lens wear for 1 to 3 weeks usually is required, hydrophilic polymer contact lenses are preferred to short-lived collagen lenses. It is best to have several types of bandage lenses available because no one type fits all patients. In eyes with marked conjunctival inflammation or elevation, smaller-diameter lenses can be helpful. Pediatric aphakic lenses can be used for this purpose, since they are approximately 12 mm in diameter and are relatively stiff. Larger lenses can be trephined to the correct size. Tarsorrhaphy should be total, or near total, with only a small medial opening for instillation of medications. The tarsorrhaphy should be left in place for at least 10 days. One of the sutures can be tied with a bow knot, over bolsters, allowing loosening for examination and reclosure if healing is incomplete.

Epithelial transplantation. Transplantation of conjunctival epithelium or limbal corneal epithelium can be used for eyes with recalcitrant epithelial defects.[47-51] The procedure has been used chiefly after chemical or thermal burns but also can be performed in other conditions, such as after penetrating keratoplasty or in cases of herpes simplex keratitis. Transplantation often is successful in those cases not amenable to other forms of treatment.

Experimental treatments. Various topical medications have been proposed for enhancing epithelial healing.

Fibronectin and epidermal growth factor. Considerable interest has developed in the use of fibronectin and epidermal growth factor (EGF). As mentioned previously, fibronectin appears to play an important role in epithelial cell migration over a defect. Epidermal growth factor promotes epithelial cell proliferation, another important process in epithelial healing.[10,52,53] Both topical fibronectin[54-56] and EGF[10,52,53,57-59] promote epithelial healing after various types of injury in rabbits. However, in experimental animals the epithelial defects recur, even with continued fibronectin or EGF treatment. The incidence of secondary epithelial breakdown was reduced by combined use of EGF and fibronectin[60] or by adding topical steroid treatment to EGF or fibronectin treatment.[61]

In uncontrolled patient trials, autologous fibronectin drops appeared to aid closure of persistent epithelial defects,[62,63] and epidermal growth factor was reported to promote epithelial healing in patients with corneal disease.[64] However, in a controlled study, EGF did not promote epithelial healing in patients undergoing penetrating keratoplasty.[65] Controlled clinical trials currently are under way to better evaluate the efficacy of these medications. However, I suspect that they will not prove very valuable clinically, except possibly in the most severe cases.

Plasmin inhibitors. In view of the elevated tear levels of plasmin found in some patients with persistent epithelial defects and the possible role of plasmin in persistence of epithelial defects and the associated stromal ulceration, the use of inhibitors of plasmin also has been investigated recently. Treatment with topical aprotinin, a proteinase inhibitor, appeared to promote epithelial healing.[46] Further studies are needed, and aprotinin currently is not commercially available.

Collagenase inhibitors. The identification of collagenase in ulcerating corneas caused a great deal of excitement about the possible therapeutic role of collagenase inhibitors. EDTA (ethylenediaminetetraacetic acid), cysteine, acetylcysteine (Mucomyst), and alpha$_2$-macroglobulin have anticollagenase activity and have been tried. As yet none has been convincingly demonstrated to be of clinical benefit in preventing stromal ulceration.[66]

Once the epithelial defect is closed, the surface should be protected to facilitate thickening and attachment of the epithelial layer. Lubricants can be continued, a bandage contact lens can be left in place for several weeks, or the tarsorrhaphy can gradually be taken down.

REFERENCES

1. Kuwabara T, Perkins DG, and Cogan DG: Sliding of the epithelium in experimental corneal wounds, Invest Ophthalmol 15:4, 1976.
2. Pfister RR: The healing of corneal epithelial abrasions in the rabbit: a scanning electron microscopic study, Invest Ophthalmol 14:468, 1975.
3. Gipson IK et al: Hemidesmosomal formation in vitro, J Cell Biol 97:849, 1983.
4. Fujikawa LS et al: Fibronectin in healing rabbit corneal wounds, Lab Invest 45:120, 1981.
5. Suda T et al: Fibronectin appears at the site of corneal stromal wound in rabbits, Curr Eye Res 1:553, 1981.
6. Ohashi Y et al: Appearance of fibronectin in rabbit cornea after thermal burn, Jpn J Ophthalmol 27:547, 1983.
7. Fujikawa LS et al: Basement membrane components in healing rabbit corneal epithelial wounds: immunofluorescence and ultrastructural studies, J Cell Biol 98:128, 1984.
8. Nishida T et al: Fibronectin promotes epithelial migration of cultured rabbit cornea in situ, J Cell Biol 97:1653, 1983.
9. Berman M et al: Ulceration is correlated with degradation of fibrin and fibronectin at the corneal surface, Invest Ophthalmol Vis Sci 24:1358, 1983.
10. Watanabe K, Nakagawa S, and Nishida T: Stimulatory effects of fibronectin and EGF on migration of corneal epithelial cells, Invest Ophthalmol Vis Sci 28:205, 1987.
11. Berman M et al: The pathogenesis of epithelial defects and stromal ulceration. In Cavanagh HD, editor: The cornea: transactions of the World Congress on the Cornea III, New York, 1988, Raven Press.
12. Goodman WM et al: Unique parameters in the healing of linear partial thickness penetrating corneal incisions in rabbit: immunohistochemical evaluation, Curr Eye Res 8:305, 1989.
13. Millodot M: Effect of long-term wear of hard contact lenses on corneal sensitivity, Arch Ophthalmol 96:1255, 1978.
14. Schwartz DE: Corneal sensitivity in diabetics, Arch Ophthalmol 91:174, 1974.
15. Schultz RO et al: Diabetic keratopathy as a manifestation of peripheral neuropathy, Am J Ophthalmol 96:368, 1983.
16. Von Oer S: Ueber die Beziehung des Acetylcholine des Hornhautepithels zur Erregungsu: Bertragung von Diesem auf die Sensiblen Nervenenden, Pflugers Arch 273:325, 1961.
17. Van Buskirk EM: Corneal anesthesia after timolol maleate therapy, Am J Ophthalmol 88:739, 1979.
18. Chang FW, Reinhart S, and Fraser NM: Effect of 30% sulfacetamide on corneal sensitivity, Am J Optom Physiol Opt 61:318, 1984.
19. Simone S: de Ricerche sul contenuto in acqua totale ed in azoto totale della cornea di coniglio in condizione di cheratite neuroparalytica sperimentale, Arch Ottalmol 62:151, 1958.
20. Mittag TW, Mindel JS, and Green JP: Trophic functions of the neuron. V. Familial dysautonomia: choline acetyltransferase in familial dysautonomia, Ann NY Acad Sci 228:301, 1974.
21. Hallerman W: Zur lakalbehandlung des Auges mit Acetycholin, Klin Monatsbl Augenheilkd 121:397, 1952.
22. Sigelman S and Friedenwald JS: Mitotic and wound healing activities of the corneal epithelium: effect of sensory denervation, Arch Ophthalmol 52:46, 1954.
23. Mishima S: The effects of the denervation and the stimulation of the sympathetic and the trigeminal nerve on the mitotic rate of the corneal epithelium in the rabbit, Jpn J Ophthalmol 1:56, 1957.
24. Alper MG: The anesthetic eye: an investigation of

changes in the anterior ocular segment of the monkey caused by interrupting the trigeminal nerve at various levels along its course, Trans Am Ophthalmol Soc 72:323, 1976.

25. Schimmelpfennig B and Beuerman R: Sensory deprivation of the rabbit cornea affects epithelial properties, Exp Neurol 69:169, 1980.

26. Cavanaugh DW et al: Pathogenesis and treatment of persistent epithelial defects, Trans Am Acad Ophthalmol Otolaryngol 81:754, 1976.

27. Mandelcorn MS, Blankenship G, and Machemer R: Pars plana vitrectomy for management of severe diabetic retinopathy, Am J Ophthalmol 81:561, 1976.

28. Akiya S and Brown SI: The ultrastructure of Reis-Bücklers' dystrophy, Am J Ophthalmol 72:549, 1971.

29. Brown NA and Bron AJ: Recurrent erosion of the cornea, Br J Ophthalmol 60:84, 1976.

30. Goldman JM, Dohlman CH, and Kravit BA: The basement membrane of the human cornea in recurrent epithelial erosion syndrome, Trans Am Acad Ophthalmol Otolaryngol 73:471, 1969.

31. Kenyon K: The synthesis of basement membrane by epithelium in bullous keratopathy, Invest Ophthalmol 8:156, 1969.

32. Khodadoust AA et al: Adhesion of regenerating corneal epithelium: the role of the basement membrane, Am J Ophthalmol 65:339, 1968.

33. Kenyon KR et al: Regeneration of corneal epithelial basement membrane following thermal cauterization, Invest Ophthalmol Vis Sci 16:292, 1977.

34. Kenyon KR: Recurrent corneal erosion: pathogenesis and therapy, Int Ophthalmol Clin 19:169, 1979.

35. Fogle JA et al: Defective epithelial adhesion in anterior corneal dystrophies, Am J Ophthalmol 79:925, 1975.

36. Chandler PA: Recurrent erosions of the cornea, Am J Ophthalmol 28:355, 1945.

37. Tripathi RG and Bron AJ: Cystic disorders of the corneal epithelium. II. Ultrastructural study of nontraumatic recurrent erosion, Br J Ophthalmol 56:73, 1972.

38. Wales HJ: A family history of corneal erosions, Trans Ophthalmol Soc NZ 8:77, 1955.

39. McClean EN, MaCrea SM, and Rich LF: Recurrent erosion: treatment by anterior stromal puncture, Ophthalmology 93:784, 1986.

40. Judge D et al: Anterior stromal micropuncture: electron microscopic changes in the rabbit cornea, Cornea 9:152, 1990.

41. Wood TO and Griffith ME: Surgery for corneal epithelial basement membrane dystrophy, Ophthalmic Surg 19:20, 1988.

42. Buxton JN and Constad WH: Superficial epithelial keratectomy in the treatment of epithelial basement membrane dystrophy, Cornea 6:292, 1987.

43. Buxton JN and Constad WH: Superficial epithelial keratectomy in the treatment of epithelial basement membrane dystrophy, Ann Ophthalmol 19:92, 1987.

44. Pfister RR et al: Collagenase activity of intact corneal epithelium in peripheral alkaline burns, Arch Ophthalmol 86:308, 1971.

45. Berman M et al: Plasmin regulates corneal collagenase secretion by degrading fibroblast cell surface/matrix fibronectin, Invest Ophthalmol Vis Sci 25(suppl):6, 1984.

46. Salonen EM et al: Plasmin in tear fluid of patients with corneal ulcers: basis for new therapy, Acta Ophthalmol (Copenh) 65:3, 1987.

47. Thoft RA: Conjunctival transplantation, Arch Ophthalmol 95:1425, 1977.

48. Thoft RA: Conjunctival transplantation as an alternative to keratoplasty, Ophthalmology 86:1084, 1979.

49. Thoft RA: Indications for conjunctival transplantation, Ophthalmology 89:335, 1982.

50. Thoft RA: Keratoepithelioplasty, Am J Ophthalmol 97:1, 1983.

51. Kenyon KR and Tseng SCG: Limbal autograft transplantation for ocular surface disorders, Ophthalmology 96:709, 1989.

52. Frati L et al: Selective binding of the epidermal growth factor and its specific effects on the epithelial cells of the cornea, Exp Eye Res 14:135, 1972.

53. Savage CR and Cohen S: Proliferation of corneal epithelium induced by epidermal growth factor, Exp Eye Res 15:361, 1973.

54. Nishida T et al: Fibronectin enhancement of corneal epithelial wound healing of rabbits in vivo, Arch Ophthalmol 102:455, 1984.

55. Caron LA et al: Topical fibronectin in a rabbit alkali burn model of corneal ulceration, Invest Ophthalmol Vis Sci 26(suppl):176, 1985.

56. Tenn PF et al: Fibronectin in alkali burned rabbit cornea: enhancement of epithelial wound healing, Invest Ophthalmol Vis Sci 26(suppl):92, 1985.

57. Singh G and Foster CS: Epidermal growth factor in alkali-burned corneal epithelial wound healing, Am J Ophthalmol 103:802, 1987.

58. Chung JH and Fagerholm P: Treatment of rabbit corneal alkali wounds with human epidermal growth factor, Cornea 8:122, 1989.

59. Reim M et al: Effect of epidermal growth factor in severe experimental alkali burns, Ophthalmic Res 20:327, 1988.

60. Singh G and Foster CS: Treatment of nonhealing corneal ulcers and recurrent corneal erosions. In Cavanagh HD, editor: The cornea: transactions of the World Congress on the Cornea III, New York, 1988, Raven Press.

61. Singh G and Foster CS: Growth factors in treatment of nonhealing corneal ulcers and recurrent erosions, Cornea 8:45, 1989.

62. Phan TM et al: Topical fibronectin in the treatment of persistent corneal epithelial defects and trophic ulcers, Am J Ophthalmol 104:494, 1987.

63. Nishida T: Role of fibronectin in corneal epithelial wound healing. In Cavanagh HD, editor: The cornea: transactions of the World Congress on the Cornea III, New York, 1988, Raven Press.

64. Daniele S et al: The effect of the epidermal growth factor (EGF) on the corneal epithelium in humans, Graefes Arch Clin Exp Ophthalmol 210:159, 1979.

65. Kandarakis AS, Page CS, and Kaufman HE: The effect of epidermal growth factor on epithelial healing after penetrating keratoplasty in human eyes, Am J Ophthalmol 98:411, 1984.

66. Berman MB: Collagenase and corneal ulceration. In Wolley DR and Evanson JA, editors: Collagenase in normal and pathological connective tissues, New York, 1980, John Wiley & Sons, Inc.

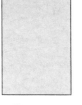

DEGENERATIONS

Involutional changes
- Morphologic changes
- Pinguecula
- Limbal girdle (white limbal girdle of Vogt)
- Corneal arcus (arcus corneae, gerontoxon, arcus senilis)
- Cornea farinata
- Descemet striae (glass striae)
- Hassall-Henle bodies
- Mosaic (crocodile) shagreen
- Furrow degeneration
- Other involutional changes

Noninvolutional degenerations
- Pterygium
- Amyloid degeneration
- Band-shaped keratopathy
   Treatment
- Spheroid degeneration
- Salzmann's degeneration
- Terrien's marginal degeneration
- Coats' white ring
- Pellucid marginal degeneration
- Lipid degeneration
- Dellen (Fuchs dimples)

The term "degeneration" is used to describe changes in tissues that cause deterioration and sometimes impair function. Degeneration can occur as a relatively normal aging process or may be related to a specific disease. It may be unilateral or bilateral; if bilateral it is often asymmetric. With rare exceptions there is no family history of or genetic predisposition to the condition. Degeneration commonly affects the peripheral cornea, can be accompanied by vascularization, and generally begins in middle age or older.

In contrast, the term "dystrophy" refers to a hereditary, symmetric, bilateral disease that usually affects the central cornea, is avascular, begins early in life, and is unrelated to other systemic or local diseases (Table 16-1).

For instructive purposes degeneration can be divided into two types: those that are common and appear to be primarily related to age (involutional) and those that are less common and usually related to specific local and systemic conditions.

INVOLUTIONAL CHANGES
MORPHOLOGIC CHANGES

Advancing age frequently brings about minor changes in the gross morphologic characteristics of the cornea, including flattening of the vertical meridian, generalized thinning that is most prominent

TABLE 16-1. Differentiation of Degeneration and Dystrophy

FEATURE	DEGENERATION	DYSTROPHY
Onset	Middle age or older	Usually first decade
Laterality	Often unilateral or asymmetric	Bilateral and symmetric
Family history	Uncommon	Common
Vascularization	Common	No
Corneal location	Peripheral	Central

peripherally, increased stromal relucency, and decreased transparency and luster. Also, the cornea's refractive index increases slightly, and in some individuals the corneal nerves become more visible. Histopathologically, the epithelial basement membrane and Descemet's membrane show irregular thickening, there is nonspecific degeneration of stromal ground substance and collagen, corneal guttae develop, and endothelial cell density decreases. Usually these changes are of little or no clinical importance, except that the vertical flattening of the cornea may alter the refractive error, requiring relatively more plus cylinder at the 180-degree axis. Of course, in some cases the decrease in endothelial cell density can lead to corneal edema (Fuchs' dystrophy).

The aging conjunctiva undergoes changes similar to those of the cornea. It becomes thinner, less transparent, and more relucent, mainly because of atrophy of the subepithelial layers. Laxity develops as a result of the loss of elastic tissue, occasionally producing frank redundancy, known as *conjunctivochalasis*. The conjunctival vessels become more prominent, particularly in the interpalpebral area, and tortuosities, varicosities, and small telangiectases may appear.

PINGUECULA

A pinguecula is a triangular or polygonal, gray-white to yellowish, slightly elevated conjunctival nodule adjacent to the limbus in the horizontal meridian (Fig. 16-1). Pingueculae are most commonly seen on the nasal side and usually occur bilaterally. More densely opacified material often can be seen within the nodule, obscuring the underlying vessels.

Histopathologically, a pinguecula consists of a mass of abnormal subepithelial collagen. The connective tissue is hyalinized, with increased basophilia and curling of the collagen fibrils. The abnormal collagen takes on the staining characteristics of elastic tissue (elastotic degeneration) but is not elastin, as it is resistant to digestion by elastase. The overlying epithelium usually is normal or slightly thinned, but it may be thickened or even mildly dysplastic.

Pingueculae are thought to be caused by the combined effects of age and exposure to sunlight, perhaps with further contribution by exposure to dust and wind or repeated trauma from lid closure.[1-3] The predilection of pingueculae for the nasal aspect of the interpalpebral conjunctiva probably is related to the fact that this area of the conjunctiva receives the greatest amount of ultraviolet exposure through reflection of sunlight from the side of the nose. Rather than a degeneration of existing collagen, the abnormal material may be abnormal elastic fibers produced by damaged fibroblasts.[4]

Pingueculae have little clinical significance and generally do not require treatment. They can grow in width and height and can extend onto the cornea, at which point they are called pterygia. Occasionally, for unknown reasons, they become inflamed and symptomatic (pingueculitis).[5] Pingueculitis can be treated by observation only, with topical steroids, or by excision.

In rare cases pingueculae have been mistaken for epithelial tumors. The two should be differentiated easily by the subepithelial location of the pingueculae, by their lack of staining with rose bengal, and by their fluorescence in ultraviolet light. Conjunctival scrapings from pingueculae show es-

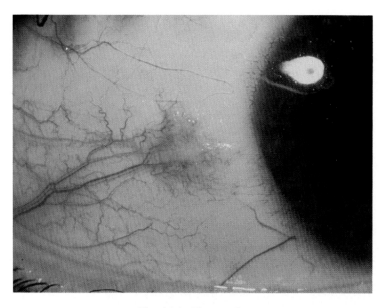

Fig. 16-1. Pinguecula.

sentially normal epithelial cells, whereas scrapings from epithelial tumors usually contain cells with neoplastic characteristics. Brown, pinguecula-like lesions also have been noted in patients with Gaucher's disease.[6]

LIMBAL GIRDLE (WHITE LIMBAL GIRDLE OF VOGT)

Vogt's girdle is a narrow, crescentic, yellow-white line running along the nasal and temporal limbal areas of the cornea in the interpalpebral zone (Fig. 16-2). It is composed of small, irregular, chalklike flecks and opacities lying immediately beneath the epithelium and usually is more prominent nasally. As described by Vogt, type I is separated from the limbus by a narrow lucid interval, and type II extends to the limbus without an intervening clear zone.[7]

Limbal Girdles of Vogt

TYPE I (EARLY CALCIFIC BAND KERATOPATHY)	TYPE II (TRUE VOGT'S GIRDLE)
Lucid interval	No lucid interval
Fine crystals	Chalklike flecks
"Swiss cheese holes"	No "holes"
Slightly more superficial	Slightly deeper
Rather smooth central edge	Thornlike extensions from central edge
Calcium	Elastosis
Calcium adjacent conjunctiva	Pinguecula adjacent conjunctiva

Type II appears to represent elastotic degeneration of subepithelial collagen, such as that found in pingueculae, and is considered the characteristic and true Vogt's girdle; type I actually is thought to represent early calcific band keratopathy.[8] The lucid interval of type I can be explained by the fact that calcium deposition ends at the termination of Bowman's membrane, still some distance from the opaque sclerolimbal junction. The elastosis of type II occurs between the end of Bowman's membrane and the sclerolimbal junction so that no lucid interval is seen.

Vogt's girdle (type II) can be found in about 60% of patients over 40 years of age and in all

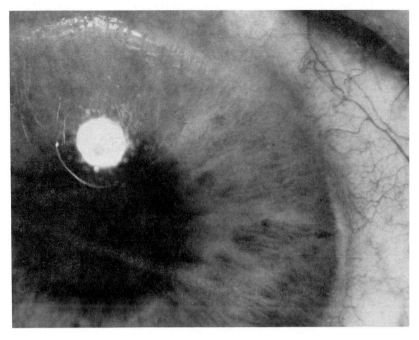

Fig. 16-2. Vogt's limbal girdle, type II. No lucid interval is seen; chalklike flecks are noted in opacity *(arrow)*.

patients over 80 years of age, if searched for carefully by indirect lateral illumination.[8] Its occurrence probably depends largely on exposure to sunlight, as is true of pingueculae.

Vogt's girdle has no clinical significance except that it must be distinguished from minimal calcific band keratopathy. Perhaps the severity of the girdle can provide some insight into the degree of actinic radiation to which a patient has been exposed.

CORNEAL ARCUS (ARCUS CORNEAE, GERONTOXON, ARCUS SENILIS)

Corneal arcus is a bilateral hazy ring of yellow-white deposits in the peripheral cornea (Fig. 16-3). The deposits appear first in the inferior cornea and then in the superior cornea, eventually encircling the cornea. Deposition occurs first in the posterior cornea, near Descemet's membrane, then near Bowman's layer. With progression, an anvil- or hourglass-shaped distribution is seen. On slit-lamp examination one can see numerous crisscrossing lines of relative clarity throughout the arcus, and in very early cases the posterior corneal haze and lucent lines may simulate a posterior crocodile shagreen.

A lucid interval is present between the peripheral border of the arcus and the limbus. This area is not entirely free of lipid, however, since the deposits extend across the limbus into the adjacent sclera at the level of Descemet's membrane. The central edge of the lucid interval is located at the termination of Bowman's layer, but it is unclear whether the lucid interval is related to the lack of Bowman's layer or to the proximity to the limbal vasculature, since the arcus and its lucid interval can be seen to be displaced centrally in an area of abnormal corneal vascularization. At times the arcus can be rather extensive and extend axially without corneal vascularization, at which time it probably should be classified as a lipid keratopathy (Fig. 16-4).

The incidence of corneal arcus is directly related to age; it is present in 60% of people between 40 and 60 years of age and in nearly everyone over 80.[9] However, arcus is rarely seen in certain populations, such as Canadian Eskimos. It tends to occur earlier in men than in women, and earlier in blacks than in whites.

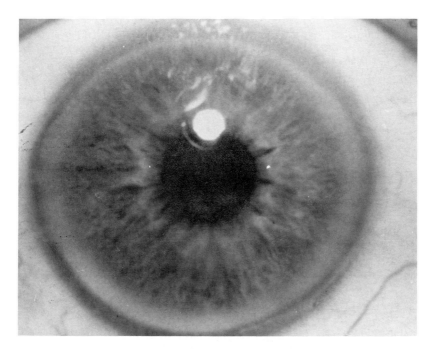

Fig. 16-3. Corneal arcus.

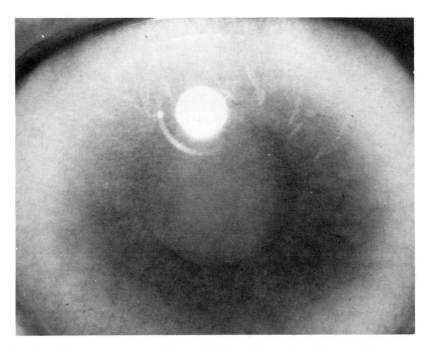

Fig. 16-4. Extensive arcus, resulting in lipid deposition in the axial area of the cornea.

The arcus is composed of cholesterol esters, cholesterol, and neutral glycerides in the extracellular corneal stroma.[10,11] The development of arcus is related to increasing age, elevation of cholesterol and low-density lipoproteins, and increased vascular permeability.[12-17] Corneal arcus generally carries no implication of systemic disease, but some cases are related to hyperlipoproteinemia, particularly types II and III.[13] The presence of arcus in a person under 50 years of age is a significant risk factor for coronary heart disease,[18] and therefore a serum lipid profile should be obtained in these patients. The presence of a unilateral arcus suggests vascular occlusion on the side without arcus.[19] Arcus is rarely a congenital finding (see Chapter 5) and can occur prematurely in lethicin cholesterol acyltransferase (LCAT) deficiency[20] and phytosterolemia.[21]

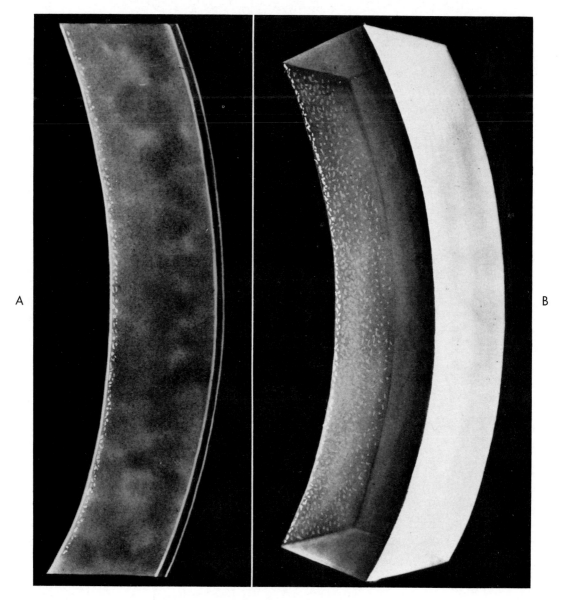

Fig. 16-5. A, Cornea farinata consists of punctate opacities in deep stroma, as seen in parallelepiped section. These are best seen by retroillumination. **B,** Same lesion and location in optical section.

CORNEA FARINATA

Cornea farinata is an age-related corneal change comprising innumerable tiny, dustlike gray dots and flecks in the deep corneal stroma (Figs. 16-5 and 16-6). The name "farinata" refers to the farinaceous, or flourlike, appearance of the deposits, which classically are more prominent centrally and best seen with retroillumination. The condition usually is bilateral, but unilateral cases have been reported. The deposits do not interfere with vision. Cornea farinata sometimes occurs as a familial trait.[22] The histopathologic characteristics of cornea farinata are unknown, but the deposits probably are composed of lipofuscin,[23] a degenerative pigment that accumulates in aged cells. Lipofuscin has been found in pre-Descemet dystrophy, a condition that bears a close clinical resemblance to cornea farinata (see Chapter 17). Cornea farinata sometimes is mistaken for cornea guttata. Careful examination of the posterior surface of the cornea by specular reflection reveals the normal endothelial mosaic pattern underlying the opacities of cornea farinata, which are smaller and more gray-white than those of cornea guttata.

DESCEMET'S STRIAE (GLASS STRIAE)

Small, linear striations in Descemet's membrane often are seen in otherwise normal corneas, perhaps more commonly in older patients.[24] The striae are finer and more subtle than those of striate keratopathy and are not large enough to cause gross irregularities of Descemet's membrane or of the posterior corneal surface. Descemet's striae generally are oriented vertically, but they may tilt slightly away from the vertical in either the nasal or temporal direction. They have a double-walled (pipestem) configuration. They have no clinical significance, except that some ophthalmologists think that they are slightly more common in patients with diabetes (Fig. 16-7).

HASSALL-HENLE BODIES

Descemet's membrane normally has a uniform thickness except in the corneal periphery, where localized thickenings are common, particularly with advancing age. These nodular thickenings are called Hassall-Henle bodies, or Descemet's "warts." They project toward the anterior chamber and

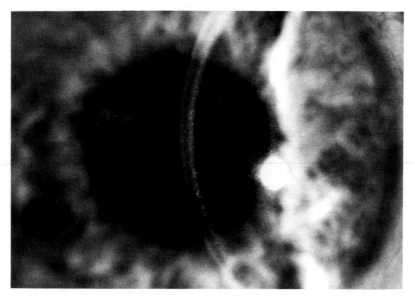

Fig. 16-6. Cornea farinata.

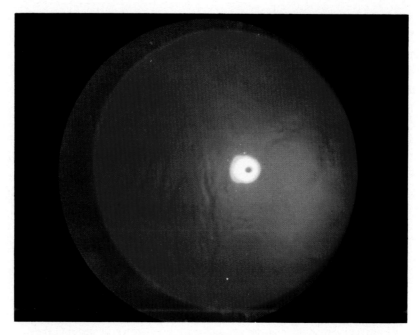

Fig. 16-7. Glassy striae, or Descemet's striae, are vertically oriented.

can be seen in the area of specular reflection as small, circular, dark areas within the normal endothelial mosaic.

Hassall-Henle bodies are histopathologically the same as the excrescences that occur in cornea guttata but are peripheral and do not indicate corneal disease.

MOSAIC (CROCODILE) SHAGREEN

Mosaic shagreen of Vogt consists of grayish white, polygonal opacities separated by relatively clear spaces, creating an appearance likened to crocodile leather (Fig. 16-8).[7] This pattern may be seen in either the anterior or posterior corneal layers, usually is bilateral, and is most prominent centrally. Vascularization does not occur, and only rarely are the opacities dense enough to reduce vision.

Most cases of mosaic shagreen are involutional in origin, but anterior mosaic shagreen has been seen after trauma, in association with band keratopathy, or in a dominantly inherited juvenile form.

The cause of both forms is unknown, but Bron[25] and Tripathi[26] have proposed that anterior mosaic shagreen results from relaxation of the normal tension on Bowman's layer. The collagen lamellae insert obliquely into Bowman's layer and, according to the researchers' theory, when tension on Bowman's layer is released, the lamellae support the layer in ridges, which are noted as the clear spaces of the mosaic. A similar pattern can be seen in the fluorescein-stained cornea after applying pressure to the cornea through the lid. It also can be seen in hypotony, or when a hard contact lens flattens a cornea with keratoconus.[27]

In one case of posterior crocodile shagreen, an irregular saw-toothed configuration of the collagen lamellae was noted on electron microscopy,[28] but the significance of this finding is unclear.

FURROW DEGENERATION

In rare cases thinning can develop in the lucid interval between an arcus and the limbus in the elderly (Fig. 16-9). This is noninflammatory and asymptomatic. The epithelium is intact, and vascu-

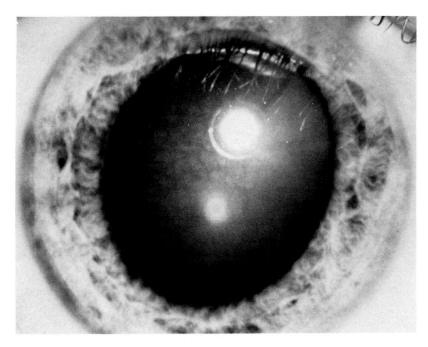

Fig. 16-8. Posterior mosaic shagreen. Gray polygonal patches are noted in deep stroma and Descemet's membrane area.

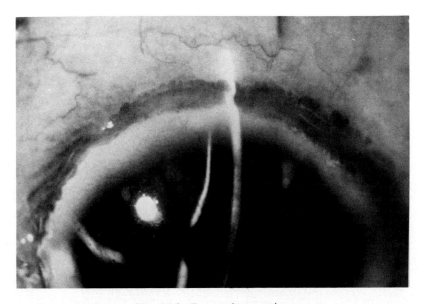

Fig. 16-9. Furrow degeneration.

larization and perforation do not occur. More commonly, the false appearance of a furrow can be created by the pattern of lipid deposition, with relative lucency of the anterior lamellae.

OTHER INVOLUTIONAL CHANGES

On occasion the nerves in an aging cornea may become more visible. A Hudson-Stähli line also can be seen as an involutional change (see Chapter 27).

NONINVOLUTIONAL DEGENERATIONS
PTERYGIUM

Pterygia are fibrovascular overgrowths of the bulbar conjunctiva onto the cornea (Fig. 16-10). They usually are triangular and horizontally oriented, with the base peripheral and the apex central over the cornea. They are located in the palpebral fissure, most commonly on the nasal side, but can occur on the temporal side as well. A grayish, flat, avascular zone usually lies at the apex. An iron line, called Stocker's line, may be seen in advance of the pterygium head. Just within the avascular cap fine anastomosing and budding vessels are present, particularly in actively growing pterygia. The body of the pterygium varies in thickness and injection, these being most prominent during active growth. The vessels are straight and appear to be under tension. Although the head is firmly attached to the cornea, the body usually can be lifted from the globe.

Pseudopterygia must be distinguished from true pterygia. In pseudopterygia the conjunctiva becomes attached to the cornea during peripheral inflammatory disease. A probe can be passed between the conjunctival mass and the globe (Fig. 16-11), which is not possible with true pterygia.

Pterygia most likely are related to ultraviolet radiation and other environmental factors such as heat, wind, dust, and dry atmosphere.[29,30] The prevalence of pterygia in a population is directly related to proximity to the equator. In the Western hemisphere the highest prevalence is seen in Central America and the Caribbean; in the United States the highest rates are seen in the South.[31] Pterygia are more common in men, in people who work outdoors, and in people who do not wear spectacles.[31] However, the mechanism of development of the conjunctival lesion and the reason for its growth onto

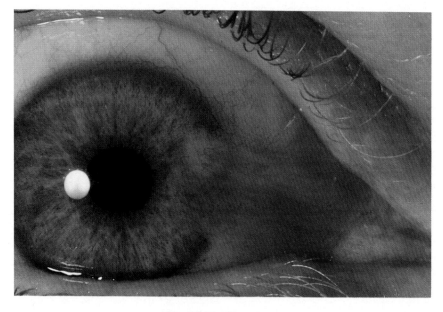

Fig. 16-10. Pterygium.

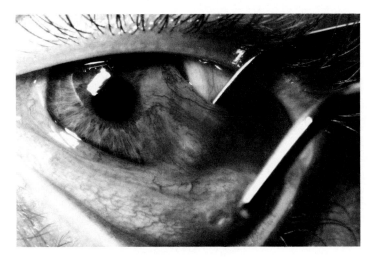

Fig. 16-11. Pseudopterygium.

the cornea are unknown. Barraquer[32] has proposed that the limbal elevation produced by the conjunctival lesion causes peripheral corneal drying and microulceration, which induces vascular invasion. However, this is not consistently noted in active pterygia.

Histologically, the conjunctival changes in pterygia are identical to those in pingueculae, with thickening and elastotic degeneration of the subepithelial connective tissue (Fig. 16-12).[3,33] Vascularity is increased, and the overlying epithelium may be mildly dysplastic. In primary cases the abnormal material does not extend beneath Tenon's layer and therefore does not become adherent to the sclera. Fibroblasts are present at the head of the pterygium, advancing between Bowman's layer and the epithelial basement membrane. Vessels and connective tissue invade this zone, fragmenting and detaching Bowman's layer.

The peak incidence of pterygia is between 20 and 40 years of age. The natural course of pterygia varies considerably. Most commonly they arise from long-standing pingueculae and grow rapidly, over several months, to the limbus.[34] They then progress slowly over the cornea and can take several years to reach the pupil. Growth can stop at any time, and this is indicated by decreased injection, shrinkage of the cap, and regression of the most central vessels. With further involution the head and body flatten and the number of larger vessels decreases.

Pterygia usually are asymptomatic, but they can cause photophobia, tearing, and foreign body sensation. They also can decrease vision by inducing with the rule and irregular astigmatism (Fig. 16-13) or by growing across the visual axis. Limited rotation, causing diplopia in peripheral gaze, can be a consequence, usually in recurrent pterygia.

Pterygia usually are removed because of the cosmetic blemish, astigmatism, or the risk of involvement of the visual axis. Unfortunately, the recurrence rate is high, averaging approximately 40% in various studies.[31,35-37] Recurrences generally occur rapidly, within 2 to 3 months of surgery, arising from the cut conjunctival edge and progressing across the bed of the resection and onto the cornea. The highest rates of recurrence are after surgery on active pterygia; less risk is attached to operating on inactive or atrophic pterygia. The high recurrence rate prompts a conservative approach to pterygia. They should be removed only when necessary because vision has been decreased or because documented recent progression threatens vision.

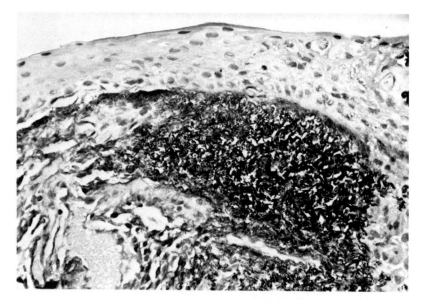

Fig. 16-12. Pterygium. Subepithelial curled and fragmented fibers that pick up elastic stain. (Elastic stain ×500) (Courtesy of Bruce L. Johnson, Pittsburgh.)

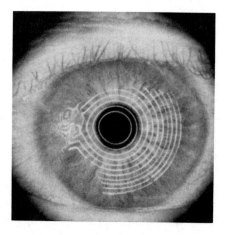

Fig. 16-13. Induction of with-the-rule irregular astigmatism by pterygium can be seen with photokeratoscopy.

A number of excision techniques have been described, but none has been clearly demonstrated to be superior. Beta-irradiation,[31,38-42] conjunctival grafts,[43] and lamellar corneal grafts[44-46] appear to reduce the recurrence rate, but most practitioners reserve these to treat recurrent cases. After surgery, thiotepa (0.5 mg/ml, one drop every 3 hours while awake for 6 to 8 weeks) may also be beneficial,[47-49] but it also can cause skin and lash depigmentation, conjunctivitis, and scleral ulceration.[49] Mitomycin appears to be effective in reducing recurrences, but experience with it has been limited.[50,51] The dose has varied from 0.2 mg/ml, one drop twice daily for 5 days to 0.4 mg/ml, one drop every 6 hours for 14 days. Townsend[34] presents a more extensive discussion of these techniques.

For primary pterygia, I perform a simple excision, leaving bare sclera. The corneal surface should be smoothed as much as possible (a diamond corneal burr can be used for this purpose). If the pterygium recurs, excision is combined with a conjunctival flap, free or sliding. If it recurs despite these measures, resection is combined with both a conjunctival flap and a peripheral lamellar corneal graft.

AMYLOID DEGENERATION

Corneal deposits of amyloid may be seen in primary or secondary localized amyloidosis and primary systemic disease. The most common form is secondary localized amyloidosis, which is seen in the cornea (or conjunctiva) after trauma or chronic ocular disease (Figs. 16-14 and 16-15). Some of the problems that cause secondary localized amyloidosis are trachoma, sarcoidosis, lipid proteinosis (Urbach-Wiethe disease), retrolental fibroplasia, phlyctenular disease, interstitial keratitis, uveitis, glaucoma, leprosy, and keratoconus.

The amyloid may appear as a small, salmon pink to yellow-white, fleshy, waxy, sometimes nodular mass or masses on the cornea or conjunctiva; as grayish perivascular deposits; as lamellar deposits; or as a subepithelial pannus. The diagnosis usually is made histologically; its only clinical significance is that it can contribute to decreased vision.

Primary localized amyloidosis occurs as lattice dystrophy, gelatinous droplike dystrophy, or polymorphic stromal dystrophy. (The last is most likely a degeneration.) These conditions are discussed in Chapter 17. The cornea does not become involved in secondary systemic amyloidosis. In primary systemic amyloidosis, purpuric and papillary lesions of the eyelids and conjunctiva may be seen (see Fig. 24-10). Ophthalmoplegias and ptosis also can occur, and in the familial form veil-like vitreous opacities or glaucoma are seen.[52] In rare cases families have been reported that exhibit both lattice dystrophy and signs of primary systemic amyloidosis (see Chapter 17).[53,54] Skin changes, cranial nerve palsies, and visceral symptoms have been present. The visual loss usually is milder or delayed, since central deposits are decreased, but in contrast to typical lattice dystrophy, the deposits extend to the limbus.

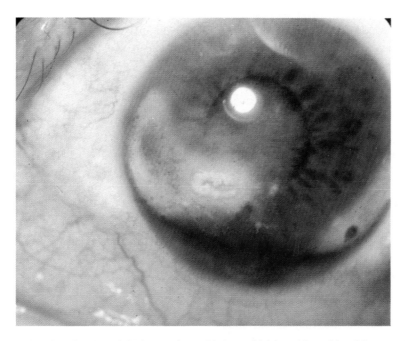

Fig. 16-14. Secondary localized amyloid in a patient with interstitial keratitis and band keratopathy. (Courtesy F. Wilson II, Indianapolis.)

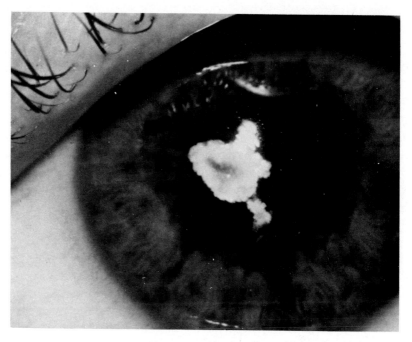

Fig. 16-15. Secondary localized amyloidosis of the cornea.

BAND-SHAPED KERATOPATHY

Band keratopathy of calcific origin usually occurs from drugs, localized ocular inflammatory disease, or systemic disease that causes hypercalcemia. Most commonly it develops in eyes with chronic ocular inflammatory disease, particularly uveitis. Children with juvenile rheumatoid arthritis and uveitis are especially prone to development of band keratopathy. Chronic exposure of the ocular surface to mercury, in eye drops or fumes, can induce calcium deposition. Old interstitial keratitis, corneal edema, glaucoma, trauma, and phthisis also can be associated with band keratopathy.

Following are some of the conditions that result in band keratopathy:

1. Hypercalcemia
    a. Sarcoidosis and other granulomatous disease
    b. Renal failure
    c. Hyperparathyroidism
    d. Hematologic malignancies (for example, multiple myeloma, lymphoma, leukemia)
    e. Acute osteoporosis (including Paget's disease)
    f. Idiopathic hypercalcemia of infancy
    g. Excess vitamin D intake
    h. Bone metastases
    i. Lithium therapy
    j. Milk-alkali syndrome
    k. Thiazides
2. Gout (urate)
3. Ocular disease
    a. Chronic nongranulomatous uveitis (juvenile rheumatoid arthritis)
    b. Prolonged glaucoma
    c. Long-standing corneal edema

    d. Phthisis

    e. Spheroid degeneration (can occur in band form)

    f. Norrie's disease

    g. Interstitial keratitis

4. Idiopathic origin

5. Mercury

    a. Mercury fumes[55]

    b. Eye drops containing mercury[56]

6. Chronic irritants (for example, calomel, calcium bichromate vapor)

7. Discoid lupus erythematosus

8. Tuberous sclerosis

9. Ichthyosis

10. Rothmund-Thomson syndrome

11. Progressive facial hemiatrophy (Parry-Romberg syndrome)

12. Intracameral Viscoat[57-60]

In rare cases band keratopathy can occur in a hereditary form. Calcareous degeneration of the cornea is a similar process that involves all layers of the cornea. This type of degeneration is seen in phthisis bulbi, necrotic intraocular neoplasm, extensive trauma, and other conditions in which "bone" is formed in other parts of the eye. In rare cases it occurs unaccompanied by ocular disease or systemic hypercalcemia.[61] In hyperuricemia, urate crystals can be deposited in the cornea in a band form. In this instance the band keratopathy takes on a brownish color instead of the gray-white opacity seen in calcific band keratopathy. Keratopathy in band form also can occur in extensive spheroid degeneration of the cornea.

Band keratopathy is most often seen in the interpalpebral area. It begins in the periphery (Fig. 16-16) and can extend to involve the visual axis (Fig. 16-17). A lucid interval is seen between the calcific band and the limbus. Small holes in the calcific opacity are noted throughout the band keratopathy, representing areas in which corneal nerves penetrate Bowman's layer. These small holes give

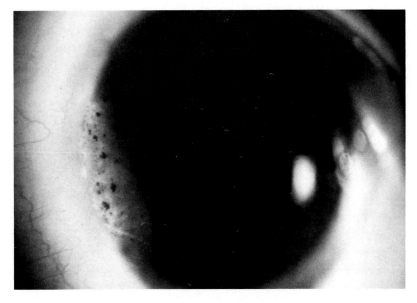

Fig. 16-16. Early band keratopathy in a patient with juvenile rheumatoid arthritis. (Courtesy of Richard A. Thoft, Pittsburgh.)

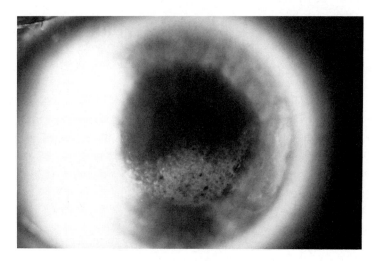

Fig. 16-17. More advanced band keratopathy.

a "Swiss cheese" appearance to the layer on slit-lamp examination. The deposits initially are grayish and flat, but with progression they become white and elevate the overlying epithelium. The band usually develops slowly, over years, but can develop rapidly, particularly in dry eyes.[62]

Histologically, the earliest changes consist of a basophilic staining of the basement membrane of the epithelium. Later, calcium deposits are seen in Bowman's layer (Fig. 16-18) and sometimes in the anterior stroma, and fragmentation and destruction of Bowman's layer occurs.[63,64] The deposition of the calcium in Bowman's layer accounts for the lucid interval, since Bowman's layer does not extend to the absolute limbus. The calcium is deposited extracellularly in local disease, whereas in systemic hypercalcemia the deposits are intracellular.

The mechanism of calcium deposition has not been determined.[63,64] In other tissues calcium and phosphate concentrations are very close to those that favor precipitation. Mild elevation of either calcium or phosphate levels, elevation of the pH, or concentration by evaporation can lead to precipitation. Uveitis may alter corneal metabolism, resulting in a rise in tissue pH and thus favoring precipitation of calcium salts.[65] However, in experimental animals combined ocular inflammation and hypercalcemia did not cause band keratopathy unless the lids were open.[66] Evaporation of tears may favor calcium precipitation by making the pH more alkaline. Carbon dioxide is lost from the tears in the palpebral fissure, and this may locally elevate pH. The lack of blood vessels in the cornea may prevent the normal buffering ability of blood serum to inhibit variations in tissue pH.[63]

Treatment. Band keratopathy can be treated if vision is reduced, if the deposits cause mechanical irritation of the lids, or if the epithelium breaks down over the deposits. The easiest means is by use of ethylenediaminetetraacetic acid (EDTA).*

To apply EDTA, 4% cocaine drops or other topical anesthetic must first be instilled into the cul-de-sac. Cocaine will facilitate removal of the epithelium, which is necessary for the EDTA to act. I have found the following to be the most effective method: A 3 ml plastic syringe is cut approximately 1.5 cm from the handled end; this is inverted and placed firmly against the cornea. The EDTA is

---

*The solution is prepared using Endrate (Abbott Laboratories) in a 20 ml ampule containing 150 mg/ml. The ampule is diluted with water to 175 ml. A 0.05 M, 1.7% solution of neutral disodium EDTA is obtained.

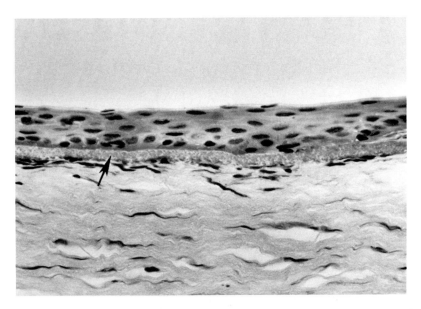

Fig. 16-18. Early band keratopathy. Deposition of calcium salts gives Bowman's layer a stippled appearance *(arrow)*(hematoxylin and eosin,   ×800). (Courtesy of Bruce L. Johnson, Pittsburgh.)

dropped into the well thus created and allowed to react for approximately 1 minute. The liquid then is absorbed with a cellulose sponge, and the cornea is gently scraped with a Kimura spatula or scalpel blade. The process is repeated until the band is removed. Alternatively, the EDTA can be placed on a small strip of cellulose sponge that is resting on the cornea; the cellulose strip is kept moist by dropping the solution onto the sponge continuously. If necessary, a diamond burr can be used to polish the cornea. Patching, cycloplegics, and mild antibiotics are employed until reepithelialization has occurred.

If no EDTA is available, anesthetic drops can be instilled, and the cornea can be scraped with a scalpel blade (for example, no. 15 Bard-Parker).[67] The scraping is continued until all gritty-feeling material is removed.

SPHEROID DEGENERATION

Spheroid degeneration is one of many names applied to spherical, golden brown, translucent, droplike deposits that may be seen in the subepithelial layers of the cornea and conjunctiva.[67-73] These deposits begin peripherally, most often at the 3 o'clock and 9 o'clock positions, and advance centrally. They may progressively darken, opacify, and coalesce. Extensive spheroid degeneration, such as that seen in tropical and climatic types, can extend in plaquelike fashion across the central cornea, reducing vision (noncalcific, spheroid band keratopathy, Fig. 16-19). In severe cases the deposits become nodular, elevating the epithelium. Clinically (and histopathologically) they brightly fluoresce in ultraviolet light.

Fraunfelder, Hanna, and Parker[68,74,75] divide spheroid degeneration into three types: the primary corneal type, the secondary corneal type, and the conjunctival type, which can occur with the primary or secondary corneal types. Primary corneal spheroid degeneration is unrelated to the coexistence of any other ocular disease but is related to advancing age and usually is bilateral. In rare cases primary band-shaped spheroidal degeneration can develop in childhood. These cases are associated with photophobia, intermittent pain, and slow deterioration in vision.[76] Familial cases have been reported.[77]

The secondary corneal type is a degenerative change that can occur after various long-standing

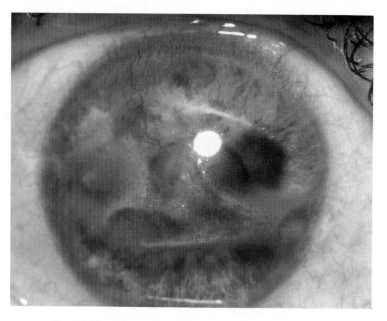

Fig. 16-19. Spheroid degeneration in bandlike distribution.

ocular diseases (Fig. 16-20), including glaucoma, herpetic infection, and dystrophies, especially Fuchs' endothelial dystrophy and lattice dystrophy (Fig. 16-21). This type can be unilateral or bilateral, central or peripheral, depending on the location of the predisposing disease. The secondary corneal form also may be caused by chronic climatic insults. These cases usually are bilateral, can occur in young people, and often are referred to as tropical or climatic corneal degeneration.

The conjunctival form can occur alone or with either of the corneal types. It is more common in older age-groups and may be associated with pinguecula or pterygium.

This classification of spheroid degeneration is somewhat arbitrary in that the primary corneal type is probably largely climatic in origin as well, and local corneal inflammation may enhance production of the abnormal material in each type.

Spheroid degeneration occurs almost exclusively in the interpalpebral zones of the cornea and conjunctiva, suggesting that actinic exposure plays a role in its development. It is more common in parts of the world with greater amounts of sunlight, with increasing age, and in those with outdoor occupations.[30,71] There is a strong association between conjunctival spheroidal degeneration and pingueculae, and both probably are related to exposure to ultraviolet light.[3,78,79] Chronic mild trauma from wind, sand, or ice, low humidity, and possibly extremes of temperature also may be responsible.

The spheroid material is acidophilic and amorphous by light microscopy (Fig. 16-22), finely granular by electron microscopy, extracellular, and proteinaceous.* The spheroids are located mainly in the superficial stroma but occasionally may be seen in the deep stroma or within the epithelium.

The composition of spheroid degeneration long has been unclear and to some extent controversial. Different researchers have described the material variously as being colloid, high-tyrosine protein, lipid, keratin-like, a secretory product of abnormal fibrocytes, and elastotic degeneration of collagen. Garner, Morgan, and Tripathi[81] initially believed that the material was a form of keratin and

---

*References 33, 70, 71, 74, 75, 80, 81.

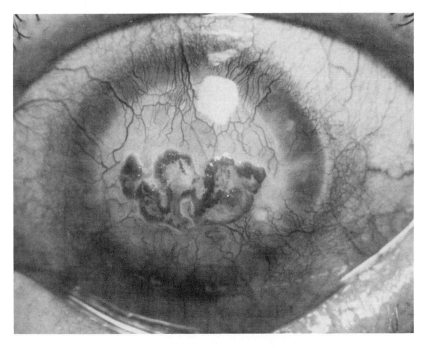

Fig. 16-20. Spheroid degeneration occurring secondarily in failed corneal graft.

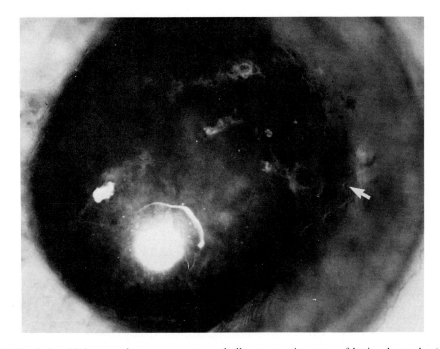

Fig. 16-21. Spheroid degeneration can occur secondarily, as seen in a case of lattice dystrophy *(arrow)*.

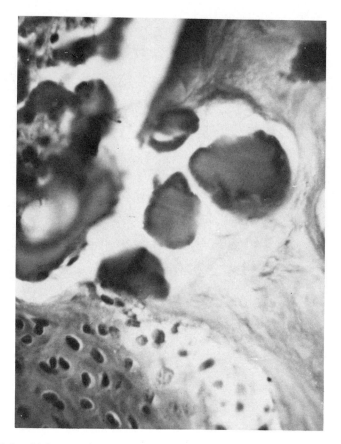

Fig. 16-22. Spheroid degeneration. Acidophilic amorphous material as seen by light microscopy.

thus originated from the epithelium; however, Garner and colleagues[71] later concluded that it was more likely collagenous. Hanna and Fraunfelder[75] thought that the substance was of stromal origin, consisting of a fibrocyte-derived granular protein deposited on adjacent collagen fibrils. The composition is not lipid, despite the "oil droplet" clinical appearance. Most researchers now think that the process is basically a stromal one and that epithelial involvement occurs only secondarily after destruction of Bowman's membrane.[3,33,75,80,81] Most likely spheroid degeneration is a type of elastotic degeneration of collagen. The clinically descriptive term of spheroid degeneration will be used until the histopathologic nature of the disorder finally is determined.

In most cases the lesions are asymptomatic and require no treatment. If vision is reduced by central involvement, lamellar keratectomy or keratoplasty is indicated. Recurrence is common after conjunctival resection, but the number of lesions is much smaller.[82]

SALZMANN'S DEGENERATION

Salzmann's degeneration is a noninflammatory condition comprising elevated, bluish white and sometimes yellow-white subepithelial corneal nodules usually arranged in a circular fashion around the pupillary area (Figs. 16-23 and 16-24). These nodules often appear within or adjacent to an area of previous scarring or at the edge of a long-standing pannus, but they can occur in any area of the cornea. They usually develop slowly and are asymptomatic unless they occur in the visual axis, where they can decrease vision. Occasionally the epithelium can break down over the surface, causing irritation. Salzmann's degeneration occurs in adults of any age and is most commonly bilateral. A

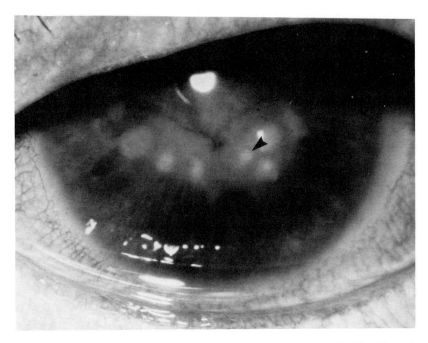

Fig. 16-23. Salzmann's degeneration is characterized by small, elevated, round, bluish white lesions *(arrow)* in the cornea.

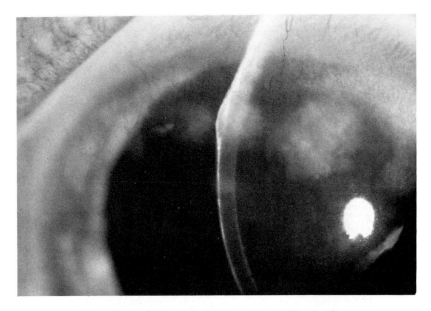

Fig. 16-24. Salzmann's degeneration, slit illumination.

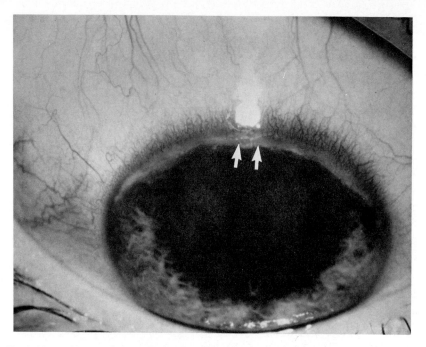

Fig. 16-25. Terrien's marginal thinning in the superior aspect of the cornea. A thin lipid line occurs at the central edge of the thinned area *(double arrow)*.

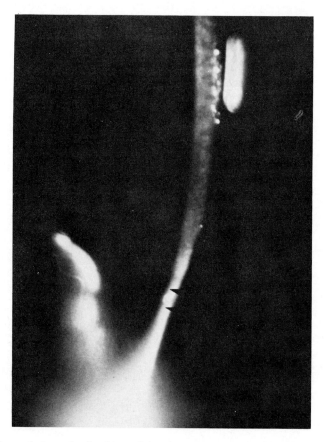

Fig. 16-26. Slit-lamp photograph of a thin peripheral cornea in Terrien's degeneration *(double arrow)*.

history of previous corneal inflammation is common, particularly of phlyctenular and trachomatous disease.[83,84]

The raised areas consist of hyaline plaques located between the epithelium and Bowman's layer, replacing Bowman's layer in most areas. The nature of the hyaline material is not known, but it does not stain for elastin, amyloid, or reticulin.[84] The epithelium varies in thickness but usually is thinned over the nodules, and the amount of subepithelial basement membrane material is markedly increased.

Treatment usually is not necessary, but surgery may be required if visual acuity is reduced because of involvement of the pupillary area. Simple excision of the nodules may be sufficient, but sometimes lamellar or penetrating keratoplasty is required.

TERRIEN'S MARGINAL DEGENERATION

Terrien's marginal degeneration is an uncommon marginal thinning of the cornea. It occurs more often in males than females, is commonly bilateral, and can occur at any age. It may develop gradually over many years and may be unilateral at first. It usually is asymptomatic, unless astigmatism develops.

Marginal thinning with opacification and superficial vascularization are the dominant features. The degeneration generally begins superonasally, as punctate stromal opacities separated by a lucid zone from the limbus. With time these coalesce, superficial vessels extend over them from the limbus, and the stroma thins. The thinning is in an arcuate shape, without a steep edge, and remains covered by epithelium. A yellow-white line, which appears to be lipid deposition, is seen at the central edge of the thinned area (Figs. 16-25 and 16-26).

The thinning can progress circumferentially and in rare cases centrally (Fig. 16-27). Marked thinning can lead to severe astigmatism because of the tilting forward of the central cornea. Perforation is uncommon but can occur spontaneously or after minor trauma. Occasionally the thinning is associated with recurrent inflammation, episcleritis, or scleritis.[85] Breaks in Descemet's membrane can occur, but in contrast to keratoconus, intracorneal pockets of aqueous result, not corneal edema.[86,87]

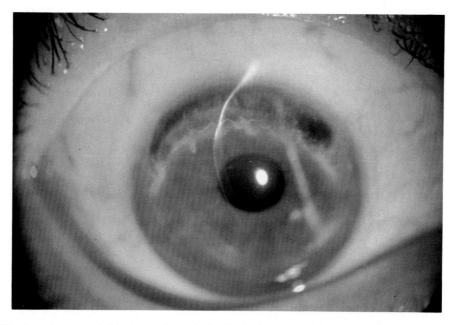

Fig. 16-27. Superior corneal thinning and ectasia in Terrien's marginal degeneration. (Courtesy of Bartly J. Mondino, Los Angeles.)

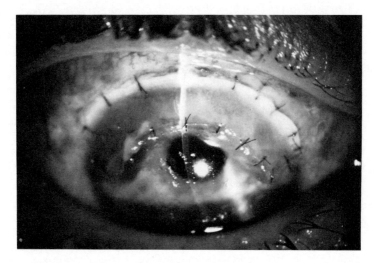

Fig. 16-28. Crescentic lamellar graft for Terrien's marginal degeneration. (Courtesy of Frank Cignetti, Pittsburgh.)

The cause of Terrien's marginal degeneration is unknown. Histologically, the stromal thinning, vascularization, and lipid deposition is evident, as well as local absence of Bowman's membrane, and in some cases healed breaks in Descemet's membrane. Fibrillar degeneration of collagen also is seen.[88,89] An electron microscopic study demonstrated phagocytosis of collagen by histiocytic cells with a high degree of lysosomal activity.[90]

If the thinning becomes so extreme that perforation is threatened or if astigmatism severely reduces vision, a reconstructive full-thickness or lamellar corneoscleral graft can alleviate the problem.[91,92] These grafts must be hand-fashioned to fit the defect (Fig. 16-28).

Terrien's marginal degeneration may be confused with Mooren's ulcer. The differences between these two conditions are as follows:

MOOREN'S ULCER	TERRIEN'S MARGINAL DEGENERATION
Unilateral or bilateral	Usually symmetrical and bilateral; can be unilateral
Pain and inflammation	Usually painless and not inflamed
Epithelial breakdown at central edge of active ulcers, stains with fluorescein	Epithelium intact, no fluorescein staining
Spreads centrally and circumferentially; slow or rapid progression	Spreads circumferentially; slow progression
Overhanging central edge; can become vascularized with healing; no lipid	Gradual central edge; vascularized base; lipid deposits
Can cause severe corneal melting; destructive	Usually main problem is astigmatism caused by corneal ectasia
Perforation occurs in severe cases	Perforation occurs in 15% of cases as a result of minor trauma

COATS' WHITE RING

Coats' white ring is a small corneal opacity that is the residue of previous injury by a metallic foreign body. On slit-lamp examination the ring is seen as a small, anterior, granular, white, oval ring (Fig. 16-29). Iron deposition is found in Bowman's layer or the anterior stroma.

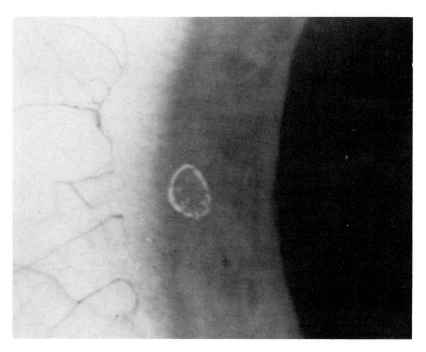

Fig. 16-29. Coats' white ring.

PELLUCID MARGINAL DEGENERATION

Pellucid marginal degeneration is an uncommon form of corneal thinning and ectasia. A narrow, arcuate band of corneal thinning is seen in the inferior cornea, usually between 4 o'clock and 8 o'clock (Fig. 16-30). The stroma is clear, epithelialized, and nonvascularized. The thinned area usually is 1 to 2 mm in width and is separated from the limbus by 1 to 2 mm of clear cornea. The cornea central to the thinning is of normal thickness and protrudes forward, creating against-the-rule astigmatism (Figs. 16-31 and 16-32). In contrast to keratoconus, no Fleischer ring, Vogt striae, or conical shape are seen.

Pellucid marginal degeneration usually appears between 20 and 40 years of age; There is no sexual predilection or family history. However, increased amounts of astigmatism have been reported in family members.[93] The condition may progress, usually gradually over several years. Hydrops and corneal scarring can develop, and rupture can occur with trauma.[94-97]

On histologic examination, stromal thinning with localized loss of Bowman's layer has been noted.[95,98-100] Collagen with 110 nm banding also has been found.

Pellucid marginal degeneration has features similar to those seen in keratoconus: progressive thinning and ectasia, hydrops, and scarring. It differs, however, in the more peripheral location of the thinning; the lack of a Fleischer ring, Vogt striae, or a conical shape; and the slightly older age of affected patients. Some feel that keratoconus and pellucid marginal degeneration are different presentations of the same disease, but this can be determined only by further study of the biochemical processes underlying the diseases.

The major problem for patients with pellucid marginal degeneration is astigmatism caused by protrusion of the central cornea. Usually correction with eyeglasses is inadequate, and contact lens correction often is difficult. When the astigmatism cannot be corrected with either eyeglasses or hard contact lenses, any of several surgical approaches can be tried. Large, inferiorly eccentric penetrating grafts can be performed, but these are prone to vascularization, rejection, and high postoperative

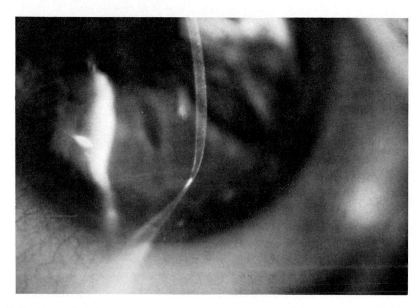

Fig. 16-30. Pellucid marginal degeneration. Inferior corneal thinning without vascularization or lipid deposition.

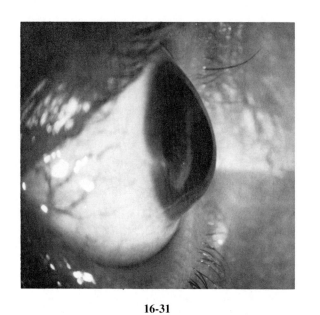

16-31

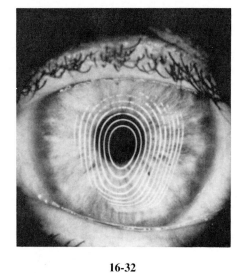

16-32

Fig. 16-31. Inferior corneal ectasia in pellucid marginal degeneration.

Fig. 16-32. Pellucid marginal degeneration. Photokeratoscopy demonstrates marked central corneal flattening and inferior peripheral steepening in the vertical meridian.

astigmatism.[94,101] Resection of the thinned cornea,[101,102] central lamellar keratoplasty, and crescentic peripheral lamellar keratoplasty[103] also have been performed. Crescentic peripheral lamellar keratoplasty appears to be the best option at this time.

LIPID DEGENERATION

Lipid degeneration of the cornea occurs in primary and secondary forms. Secondary lipid deposition is much more common and usually is related to corneal vascularization. It is most commonly associated with trauma, ulceration, hydrops,[104] interstitial keratitis, or herpes zoster keratitis (Fig. 16-33). The pathogenesis of the deposition of lipids is unclear, but it may involve increased vascular permeability, excess production of lipids, or inability to metabolize lipids.

The lipid is seen as a dense, yellow-white opacity that may fan out with feathery edges from blood vessels (Fig. 16-34).[105] Multicolored crystals (cholesterol) also may be seen at the edge of the opacity, where it is not so dense. The opacity usually develops rapidly, in an area with long-standing vascularization. Histologically, the material consists of neutral fats, phospholipids, and cholesterol, as in corneal arcus.[11,106,107]

Much less frequently, lipid deposits develop in a cornea with no previous history of disease or vascularization.[9,107,108-111] Serum lipids usually are within normal limits. In one case histologic examination indicated vascularization, chronic nongranulomatous inflammation, and extracellular lipids, with the same composition as in secondary lipid keratopathy.[111] Therefore some cases may be secondary, with the original corneal inflammatory disease undiagnosed. Penetrating keratoplasty may be required to preserve vision, but deposits can occur in the graft.[109]

In primary lipid degeneration the practitioner should consider some rare causes of serum lipoprotein abnormalities, such as Tangier disease and lecithin cholesterol acyltransferase (LCAT) deficiency (see Chapter 21). In Tangier disease visual acuity is good, and hazy stromal infiltrates consisting of fine dots are seen throughout the cornea, densest posteriorly and in the horizontal meridian. A lipid arcus is not present, and vision is not affected. The serum cholesterol is low, high-density lipopro-

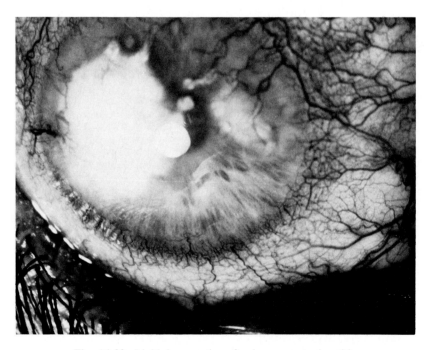

Fig. 16-33. Lipid degeneration after herpes zoster keratitis.

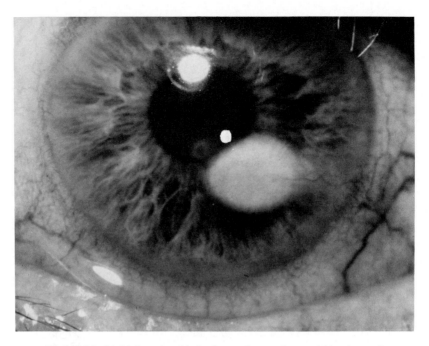

Fig. 16-34. Lipid deposit with feathery edges and central blood vessel.

teins (HDL) usually are markedly deficient, low-density lipoproteins (LDL) are low, and very–low density lipoproteins (VLDL) are increased. In LCAT deficiency, granular stromal clouding also is seen, but with a peripheral arcus and an outer lucid interval. Vision usually is not affected. LDL is decreased, and lipoproteins of abnormal structure are seen in the plasma as well as in other tissues of the body, including the cornea.[112] Fish-eye disease is an inherited disorder in which marked corneal clouding can occur, with elevated LDL and VLDL and reduced HDL.[113]

Argon laser treatment can reduce the extent or density of the lipid opacities and improve vision in some cases.[114] However, several treatments, with thousands of burns, are required, and rapid corneal thinning, leading to keratoplasty, can occur.

DELLEN (FUCHS' DIMPLES)

Dellen are areas of localized thinning of the cornea or sclera caused by tear film instability and dryness. The thinning is caused by reversible water loss from the corneal stroma or sclera. Dellen usually are seen in the peripheral cornea adjacent to acute elevations of the conjunctiva (for example, after surgery or with marked chemosis). Dellen are discussed more fully in Chapter 14 but are mentioned here because they may occur idiopathically in elderly people.

REFERENCES

1. Hogan MJ and Alvarado J: Pterygium and pinguecula: electron microscopic study, Arch Ophthalmol 78:74, 1967.
2. Sugar S and Kobernick S: The pinguecula, Am J Ophthalmol 47:341, 1959.
3. Klintworth GK: Chronic actinic keratopathy: a condition associated with conjunctival elastosis (pingueculae) and typified by characteristic extracellular concretions, Am J Pathol 67:327, 1972.
4. Austin P, Jakobiec HA, and Iwamoto T: Elastodysplasia and elastodystrophy as pathologic bases of ocular pterygium and pinguecula, Ophthalmology 90:96, 1983.
5. Sugar S and Kobernick S: Localized irritative lesions involving pingueculae, Am J Ophthalmol 57:94, 1964.
6. Petrohelos M et al: Ocular manifestations of Gaucher's disease, Am J Ophthalmol 80:1006, 1975.
7. Vogt A: Corneal degenerations of various etiology. In Blodi FC, editor: Textbook and atlas of slit lamp microscopy of the living eye, Bonn, 1981, Wayenbargh Editions.
8. Sugar SH and Kobernick S: The white limbal girdle of Vogt, Am J Ophthalmol 50:101, 1960.

9. Duke-Elder S and Leigh AG: System of ophthalmology, vol 8, diseases of the outer eye, St Louis, 1965, Mosby–Year Book, Inc.

10. Cogan DG and Kuwabara T: Arcus senilis, its pathology and histochemistry, Arch Ophthalmol 61:353, 1959.

11. Andrews JS: The lipids of arcus senilis, Arch Ophthalmol 68:264, 1962.

12. Walton KW: Studies on the pathogenesis of corneal arcus formation, J Pathol 111:263, 1973.

13. Vinger PF and Sachs BA: Ocular manifestations of hyperlipoproteinaemia. Am J Ophthalmol 70:563, 1970.

14. Rifkind BM: Corneal arcus and hyperlipoproteinaemia, Surv Ophthalmol 16:295, 1972.

15. Walton KW and Dunkerley DJ: Studies on the pathogenesis of corneal arcus formation. II. Immunofluorescent studies on lipid deposition in the eye of the lipid-fed rabbit, J Pathol 114:217, 1974.

16. Winder AF: Factors influencing the variable expression of xanthelasmata and corneal arcus in familial hypercholesterolemia, Birth Defects 18:449, 1982.

17. Pe'er J et al: Association between corneal arcus and some of the risk factors for coronary artery disease, Br J Ophthalmol 67:795, 1983.

18. Rosenman RH et al: Relation of corneal arcus to cardiovascular risk factors and incidence of coronary disease, N Engl J Med 291:1322, 1974.

19. Smith JL and Susac JO: Unilateral arcus senilis: sign of occlusive disease of the carotid artery, JAMA 225:676, 1973.

20. Horven I, Effe K, and Gjone E: Corneal and fundus changes in familial LCAT deficiency, Acta Ophthalmol (Copenh) 52:201, 1974.

21. Björkhem I and Skrede S: Familial diseases with storage of sterols other than cholesterol: cerebrotendinous xanthomatosis and phytosterolemia. In Scriver CR et al, editors: The metabolic basis of inherited disease, ed 6, New York, 1989, McGraw-Hill, Inc.

22. Paufique L and Etienne R: La cornea farinata, Bull Soc Ophtalmol Fr 50:522, 1950.

23. Curran RE, Kenyon KR, and Green WR: Pre-Descemet's membrane corneal dystrophy, Am J Ophthalmol 77:711, 1974.

24. Sturrock G: Glassy corneal striae, Graefes Arch Klin Ophthalmol 188:245, 1973.

25. Bron AJ and Tripathi RC: Anterior corneal mosaic: further observations, Br J Ophthalmol 53:760, 1969.

26. Tripathi RC and Bron AJ: Secondary anterior crocodile shagreen of Vogt, Br J Ophthalmol 59:59, 1975.

27. Dangel ME, Kracher GP, and Stark WJ: Anterior corneal mosaic in eye with keratoconus wearing hard contact lenses, Arch Ophthalmol 102:888, 1984.

28. Krachmer JH et al: Corneal posterior crocodile shagreen and polymorphic amyloid degeneration, Arch Ophthalmol 101:54, 1983.

29. Moran DJ and Hollows FC: Pterygium and ultraviolet radiation: a positive correlation, Br J Ophthalmol 68:343, 1984.

30. Taylor HR et al: Corneal changes associated with chronic UV irradiation, Arch Ophthalmol 107:1481, 1989.

31. Cameron ME: Pterygium throughout the world, Springfield, Ill, 1965, Charles C Thomas.

32. Barraquer JI: Etiologia y patogenia del pterigiom y de las excavaciones de la cornea de Fuchs, Arch Soc Am Oftalmol Optom 5:45, 1964.

33. Rodrigues MM, Laibson PR, and Weinreb S: Corneal elastosis: appearance of band-like keratopathy and spheroidal degeneration, Arch Ophthalmol 93:111, 1975.

34. Townsend WM: Pterygium. In Kaufman HE et al, editors: The cornea, New York, 1988, Churchill Livingstone, Inc.

35. Pearlman G et al: Recurrent pterygium and treatment with lamellar keratoplasty with presentation of a technique to limit recurrences, Ann Ophthalmol 2:763, 1970.

36. Zauberman H: Pterygium and its recurrence, Am J Ophthalmol 63:1780, 1967.

37. Youngson RM: Recurrence of pterygium after excision, Br J Ophthalmol 56:120, 1972.

38. Alaniz-Cancino F: The use of postoperative beta irradiation in the treatment of pterygium, Ophthalmic Surg 13:1022, 1982.

39. Cooper JS and Lerch IA: Postoperative irradiation of pterygia, Radiology 135:743, 1980.

40. Hilgers JH: Pterygium, Am J Ophthalmol 50:635, 1960.

41. Pico G: Pterygium: current concept of etiology and management. In King JH and McTigue JW, editors: The cornea: World Congress, Washington, 1965, Butterworth Publishers.

42. Bahrassa F and Datta R: Postoperative beta radiation treatment of pterygium, Int J Radiat Oncol Biol Phys 9:679, 1983.

43. Kenyon KR, Wagoner MD, and Hettinger ME: Conjunctival autograft transplantation for advanced and recurrent pterygium, Ophthalmology 92:1461, 1985.

44. Poirier RH and Fish JR: Lamellar keratoplasty for recurrent pterygium, Ophthalmic Surg 7:38, 1976.

45. Laughrea PA and Arentsen JJ: Lamellar keratoplasty in the management of recurrent pterygium, Ophthalmic Surg 17:106, 1986.

46. Busin M et al: Precarved lyophilized tissue for lamellar keratoplasty in recurrent pterygium, Am J Ophthalmol 102:222, 1986.

47. Meacham CT: Triethylene thiophosphoramide in prevention of pterygium recurrence, Am J Ophthalmol 54:751, 1962.

48. Harrison M, Kelly A, and Ohlrich J: Pterygium: thiotepa versus beta radiation, a double-blind trial, Tr Aust Coll Ophthalmol 1:64, 1969.

49. Asregadoo ER: Surgery, thio-tepa, and corticosteroid in the treatment of pterygium, Am J Ophthalmol 74:960, 1972.

50. Singh G, Wilson MR, and Foster CS: Mitomycin eye drops as treatment for pterygium, Ophthalmolology 95:813, 1988.

51. Hayasaka S et al: Postoperative instillation of low-dose mitomycin C in the treatment of primary pterygium, Am J Ophthalmol 106:715, 1988.

52. Kaufman HE and Thomas IB: Vitreous opacities diagnostic of familial primary amyloidosis, N Engl J Med 261:1267, 1959.

53. Kirk HQ et al: Primary familial amyloidosis of the cor-

nea, Trans Am Acad Ophthalmol Otolaryngol 77:411, 1973.

54. Meretoja J: Comparative histopathological and clinical findings in eyes with lattice corneal dystrophy of two different types, Ophthalmologica 165:15, 1972.

55. Kennedy RE, Roca PD, and Platt DS: Further observations on atypical band keratopathy in glaucomatous patients, Trans Am Ophthalmol Soc 72:107, 1974.

56. Kennedy RE, Roca PD, and Landers PH: Atypical band keratopathy in glaucomatous patients, Am J Ophthalmol 72:917, 1971.

57. Binder PS, Deg JK, and Kohl FS: Calcific band keratopathy after intraocular chondroitin sulfate, Arch Ophthalmol 105:1243, 1987.

58. Coffman MR and Mann PM: Corneal subepithelial deposits after use of sodium chondroitin, Am J Ophthalmol 102:279, 1986.

59. Ullman S, Lichtenstein SB, and Heerlein K: Corneal opacities secondary to Viscoat, J Cataract Refract Surg 12:489, 1986.

60. Nevyas AS et al: Acute band keratopathy following intracameral Viscoat, Arch Ophthalmol 105:958, 1987.

61. Henriksen E: Primary calcareous corneal dystrophy, Acta Ophthalmol (Copenh) 60:759, 1982.

62. Lemp MA and Ralph RA: Rapid development of band keratopathy in dry eyes, Am J Ophthalmol 83:657, 1977.

63. O'Connor GR: Calcific band keratopathy, Trans Am Ophthalmol Soc 70:58, 1972.

64. Pouliquen Y: Ultrastructure of band keratopathy, Arch Ophtalmol 27:149, 1967.

65. Doughman DJ et al: Experimental band keratopathy, Arch Ophthalmol 81:264, 1969.

66. Economon JW, Silverstein AM, and Zimmerman LE: Band keratopathy in a rabbit colony, Invest Ophthalmol 2:361, 1963.

67. Young JDH and Finlay RD: Primary spheroidal degenerations of the cornea in Labrador and northern Newfoundland, Am J Ophthalmol 79:129, 1975.

68. Fraunfelder F and Hanna C: Spheroid degeneration of the cornea and conjunctiva. III. Incidences, classification and etiology, Am J Ophthalmol 76:41, 1973.

69. Freedman A: Climatic droplet keratopathy. I. Clinical aspects, Arch Ophthalmol 89:193, 1973.

70. Johnson GJ and Ghosh M: Labrador keratopathy: clinical and pathological findings, Can J Ophthalmol 10:119, 1975.

71. Garner A et al: Spheroidal degeneration of cornea and conjunctiva, Br J Ophthalmol 60:473, 1976.

72. Ahmad A et al: Climatic droplet keratopathy in a 16-year-old boy, Arch Ophthalmol 95:149, 1977.

73. Anderson J and Fuglsang H: Droplet degeneration of the cornea in North Cameroon: prevalence and clinical appearance, Br J Ophthalmol 60:256, 1976.

74. Fraunfelder FT, Hanna C, and Parker JM: Spheroid degeneration of the cornea and conjunctiva. I. Clinical course and characteristics, Am J Ophthalmol 74:821, 1972.

75. Hanna C and Fraunfelder FT: Spheroid degeneration of the cornea and conjunctiva. II. Pathology, Am J Ophthalmol 74:829, 1972.

76. Hida T et al: Primary band-shaped spheroidal degener-

ation of the cornea: three cases from two consanguineous families, Br J Ophthalmol 70:347, 1986.

77. Hida T et al: Familial band-shaped spheroid degeneration of the cornea, Am J Ophthalmol 97:651, 1984.

78. Norn MS: Prevalence of pinguecula in Greenland and Copenhagen, Acta Ophthalmol (Copenh) 57:96, 1979.

79. Norn MS: Spheroid degeneration, pinguecula, and pterygium among Arabs in the Red Sea territory, Jordan, Acta Ophthalmol (Copenh) 60:949, 1982.

80. Brownstein S et al: The elastotic nature of hyaline corneal deposits: a histochemical, fluorescent, and electron microscopic examination, Am J Ophthalmol 75:799, 1973.

81. Garner A, Morgan G, and Tripathi RC: Climatic droplet keratopathy. II. Pathologic findings, Arch Ophthalmol 89:198, 1973.

82. Norn MS: Conjunctival spheroid degeneration: recurrence after excision, Acta Ophthalmol (Copenh) 60:434, 1982.

83. Katz D: Salzmann's nodular corneal dystrophy, Acta Ophthalmol (Copenh) 31:377, 1953.

84. Vannas A, Hogan MJ, and Wood I: Salzmann's nodular degeneration of the cornea, Am J Ophthalmol 79:211, 1975.

85. Austin P and Brown SI: Inflammatory Terrien's marginal corneal disease, Am J Ophthalmol 98:189, 1981.

86. Soong HK et al: Corneal hydrops in Terrien's marginal degeneration, Ophthalmology 93:340, 1986.

87. Ashenhurst M and Slomovic A: Corneal hydrops in Terrien's marginal degeneration: an unusual complication, Can J Ophthalmol 22:328, 1987.

88. Süveges MD, Levai G, and Alberth B: Pathology of Terrien's disease, Am J Ophthalmol 74:1191, 1972.

89. Guyer DR et al: Terrien's marginal degeneration: clinicopathologic case reports, Graefes Arch Clin Exp Ophthalmol 225:19, 1987.

90. Iwamoto T, DeVoe AG, and Farris RL: Electron microscopy in cases of marginal degeneration of the cornea, Invest Ophthalmol 11:241, 1972.

91. Brown AC, Rao GN, and Aquavella JV: Peripheral corneal grafts in Terrien's marginal degeneration, Ophthalmic Surg 14:931, 1983.

92. Caldwell DR et al: Primary surgical repair of several peripheral marginal ectasias in Terrien's marginal degeneration, Am J Ophthalmol 97:332, 1984.

93. Nagy M and Vigvary L: Beitrage zur atiologie der degeneratio marginalis pellucida corneae, Klin Monatsbl Augenheilkd 161:604, 1972.

94. Krachmer J: Pellucid marginal corneal degeneration, Arch Ophthalmol 96:1217, 1978.

95. Pouliquen Y et al: Acute corneal edema in pellucid marginal degeneration or acute marginal keratoconus, Cornea 6:169, 1987.

96. Golubovíc S and Parunovíc A: Acute pellucid marginal corneal degeneration, Cornea 7:290, 1988.

97. Carter JB, Jones DB, and Wilhelmus KR: Acute hydrops in pellucid marginal corneal degeneration, Am J Ophthalmol 107:167, 1989.

98. Francois J, Hassens M, and Stockman L: Degenerescence marginale pellucide de la corneé, Ophthalmolgica 155:337, 1968.

99. Pouliquen Y et al: Degenerescence pellucide marginale

de la corneé ou keratocone marginale, J Fr Ophtalmol 3:109, 1980.

100. Rodrigues MM et al: Pellucid marginal corneal degeneration: a clinicopathologic study of two cases, Exp Eye Res 33:277, 1981.

101. Barraquer JI: Results of the crescent resection in keratotorus, Dev Ophthalmol 5:49, 1981.

102. Dubroff S: Pellucid marginal corneal degeneration: report on corrective surgery, J Cataract Refract Surg 15:89, 1989.

103. Schanzlin DJ, Samo EM, and Robin JB: Crescentic lamellar keratoplasty in pellucid marginal corneal degeneration, Am J Ophthalmol 96:253, 1983.

104. Shapiro LA and Farkas TG: Lipid keratopathy following corneal hydrops, Arch Ophthalmol 95:456, 1977.

105. Jack RL and Lase SA: Lipid keratopathy, an electron microscopic study, Arch Ophthalmol 83:678, 1970.

106. Ciccarelli EC and Kuwabara T: Experimental aberrant lipogenesis, Arch Ophthalmol 62:125, 1959.

107. Baum JL: Cholesterol keratopathy, Am J Ophthalmol 67:372, 1969.

108. Fine BS, Townsend WM, and Zimmerman LE: Primary lipoidal degeneration of the cornea, Am J Ophthalmol 78:12, 1974.

109. Friedlander MH et al: Bilateral central lipid infiltrates of the cornea, Am J Ophthalmol 84:78, 1977.

110. Savino DF, Fine BS, and Alldredge OC: Primary lipidic degeneration of the cornea, Cornea 5:191, 1986.

111. Alfonso E et al: Idiopathic bilateral lipid keratopathy, Br J Ophthalmol 72:338, 1988.

112. Gjone E and Bergaust B: Corneal opacity in familial plasma cholesterol ester deficiency, Acta Ophthalmol (Copenh) 47:222, 1969.

113. Bron AJ: Corneal changes in the dyslipoproteinemias, Cornea 8:135, 1989.

114. Marsh RJ: Argon laser treatment of lipid keratopathy, Br J Ophthalmol 72:900, 1988.

DYSTROPHIES OF THE EPITHELIUM, BOWMAN'S LAYER, AND STROMA

Although a dystrophy may be apparent at birth, it usually is initially seen later in the first decade or in the second decade of life. Dystrophies show a hereditary pattern (usually autosomal dominant), are bilateral, symmetric, and may be progressive. They tend to affect the central cornea more than the periphery and to be avascular, and they usually are unrelated to any other local or systemic disease. Of course, there are exceptions to each of these generalizations.

Corneal dystrophies are most easily classified anatomically, since they usually affect only one corneal layer. A pathogenic classification would be preferable, but as yet understanding of the pathogenesis of corneal dystrophies is limited. Some conditions that traditionally have been classified as dystrophies usually do not show a hereditary pattern and probably are forms of degeneration. Pre-Descemet's dystrophy, epithelial basement membrane dystrophy, and possibly Fuchs' dystrophy are such conditions.

DYSTROPHIES OF THE EPITHELIUM AND BASEMENT MEMBRANE

Anterior corneal dystrophies affect the epithelium, basement membrane, and Bowman's layer (Table 17-1). Primary involvement of any one of these layers frequently leads to or is accompanied by changes in the other two layers, so exact classification as to level of involvement often is difficult and arbitrary. However, the following dystrophies affect primarily the epithelium and basement membrane:

1. Meesmann's dystrophy (juvenile epithelial corneal dystrophy)
2. Epithelial basement membrane dystrophy (Cogan's map-dot-fingerprint dystrophy, bleblike dystrophy, dystrophic recurrent erosions)

MEESMANN'S DYSTROPHY

Meesmann's dystrophy is a rare, bilateral, symmetric, familial corneal disease that begins early in life.[1-6] The major finding is epithelial vesicles, which may be seen as early as 6 months of age and tend to increase in number with age. Meesmann's dystrophy is inherited as an autosomal dominant trait with incomplete penetrance.

This epithelial dystrophy usually is asymptomatic until early adulthood or middle age, when symptoms of lacrimation, photophobia, and irritation may develop. The discomfort is caused by microcysts that rupture onto the epithelial surface. In most instances visual acuity remains good, but irregularity in the corneal surface and mild opacification, which occur in older patients, can impair vision. Different families vary widely in the degree of progression with time and visual impairment.[7]

The bleblike lesions in the epithelium appear in direct focal illumination as small, white-gray, punctate opacities that are diffusely distributed over the corneal surface but are more pronounced in the interpalpebral zone (Fig. 17-1). On retroillumination the opacities appear as clear, spherical vesicles that are regular in size and shape (Fig. 17-2). The cysts can coalesce into refractile lines or clusters. In rare cases other forms are seen, such as a whorl-like pattern at the level of Bowman's layer, peripheral limbal lesions, or focal wedge-shaped lesions.[3,8] The intervening epithelium is clear. Some of the opacities stain with fluorescein and rose bengal, presumably those that have rup-

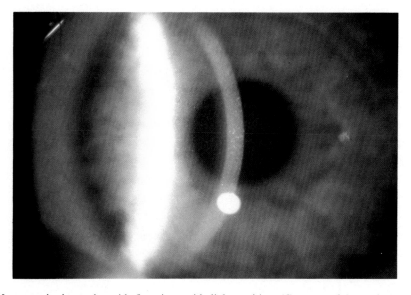

Fig. 17-1. Meesmann's dystrophy with fine, intraepithelial opacities. (Courtesy of Stuart I. Brown, La Jolla, Calif.)

TABLE 17-1. Epithelial and Bowman's Layer Dystrophies

DYSTROPHY	VISION	INHERITANCE	AGE AT MANIFESTATION	PATHOLOGIC FEATURES
Meesman's	Not usually affected but may decrease	Autosomal dominant	Childhood	Intraepithelial cysts that contain cellular debris PAS-positive material within epithelial cells and in basement membrane zone
Epithelial basement membrane (map-dot-fingerprint)	Normal or reduced	Usually none; in rare cases autosomal dominant	Adulthood	Debris containing intraepithelial cysts Insinuation of basement membrane and collagen intraepithelially, accounting for fingerprint and map appearance Recurrent epithelial erosions
Reis-Bücklers'	Reduced	Autosomal dominant	Childhood	?Primary epithelial abnormality Replacement of Bowman's layer with abnormal collagen fibers
Grayson-Wilbrandt	Reduced	Autosomal dominant	Adolescence	PAS-positive material in abnormal amounts in basement membrane zone; extends in undulating fashion into epithelium Infrequent epithelial erosions May be variant of Reis-Bücklers' dystrophy
Honeycomb	Reduced	Autosomal dominant	Childhood	May be variant of Reis-Bücklers' dystrophy
Inherited band keratopathy	Can be reduced	?Autosomal dominant	Adulthood	Calcium deposition in epithelial basement membrane and Bowman's layer
Anterior crocodile shagreen	Not affected	None	Adulthood	Anterior polygonal opacities seen as an involutional change
Local mucopolysaccharide accumulation	May be reduced	None	Infants	Bilateral diffuse clouding caused by acid mucopolysaccharide in Bowman's layer

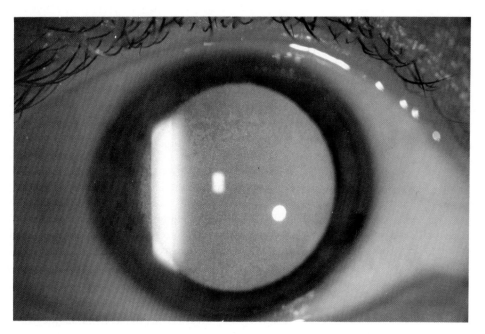

Fig. 17-2. Meesmann's dystrophy. On retroillumination small, clear, vesicles are seen.

tured onto the corneal surface. Central corneal thickness is reduced, particularly in younger patients, and increases with increasing epitheliopathy.[7] The corneal sensation may be reduced.

Similar epithelial cysts can be seen in contact lens wearers, map-dot-fingerprint dystrophy, and toxicity from local anesthetics, but the uniform size, diffuse distribution, and bilaterality distinguish Meesmann's dystrophy. This condition also can be confused with diffuse marked punctate keratopathy, such as that caused by vernal conjunctivitis, meibomitis, or dry eyes.[9] It is helpful therefore to establish the familial nature of the disease.

Histopathologically, the epithelial layer usually is thickened, but it may be thinned. There is disorganization, with poor maturation from the basal layer to the surface. Small debris-containing cysts are found throughout the epithelium; these are the vesicles seen with retroillumination on slit-lamp examination. The cysts are most numerous in the anterior third of the epithelium, and some may open to the corneal surface. The amorphous material within the cysts stains with alcian blue and colloidal iron, indicating the presence of glycosaminoglycans, and with PAS. Increased glycogen is seen in the superficial epithelium in some cases and most likely is related to the rapid turnover of cells.[10] The epithelial basement membrane may be abnormally thick and multilaminar and may show fingerlike projections extending into the basal epithelium.[11] Bowman's layer, stroma, endothelium, and Descemet's membrane appear normal.

Electron microscopy reveals an unusual, characteristic material called *peculiar substance* in the epithelial cell cytoplasm.[4-13] This substance is described as a mass of fibrillogranular material intermixed with cytoplasmic filaments. It is seen most prominently in the basal cells and may be the result of degeneration of cytoplasmic filaments.[4] In some cases electron-dense bodies that appear similar to lysosomes have been seen in the basal epithelial cells.[14] The cysts appear to contain degenerated cellular material, such as organelles, and a vacuolated homogenous substance. The walls of the intraepithelial cysts are formed by the cell membranes of adjacent epithelial cells.

There appears to be a primary epithelial cell abnormality, which probably is manifested by the development of peculiar substance. This abnormality leads to poor maturation of the epithelial cells and early cell death. The cysts appear to represent pockets of degenerated cells. The other changes, such as increased cell turnover and thickening of the basement membrane, are secondary to the epithelial disease.

Treatment is often unnecessary. However, wearing soft contact lenses has been reported to reduce greatly the number of cysts and the severity of symptoms.[15] The epithelial disease recurs after epithelial debridement and lamellar and penetrating keratoplasty, but it may be delayed or less severe.[5,12] Therefore, if vision is reduced by subepithelial scarring or irregular astigmatism, one of these procedures may be worthwhile. It has been asserted that superficial keratectomy results in reepithelialization without recurrence of epithelial disease.[10]

EPITHELIAL BASEMENT MEMBRANE DYSTROPHY

Epithelial basement membrane dystrophy (also called Cogan's microcystic epithelial dystrophy or map-dot-fingerprint dystrophy) is a common, bilateral, epithelial dystrophy.[10,16-19] Usually there is no hereditary pattern, but some cases show autosomal dominant inheritance.[20-22] The condition occurs mainly in adults, usually between 40 and 70 years of age, and is slightly more common in women. In familial cases the onset is between 4 and 8 years of age, and the frequency of attacks gradually decreases with age, being rare after 50.

Clinical manifestations. The pattern of epithelial and basement membrane abnormalities varies considerably among patients. It may be seen as dots, maps, fingerprints, blebs, nets, or any combination

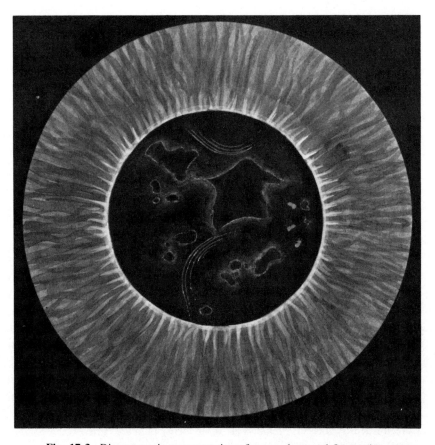

Fig. 17-3. Diagrammatic representation of maps, dots, and fingerprints.

of these patterns (Fig. 17-3). All types tend to come and go spontaneously and move to affect different portions of the cornea.

Dots are gray-white intraepithelial opacities that vary in size and may be round, oblong, or comma shaped (Fig. 17-4). With focal illumination larger dot opacities look like putty. Smaller dots may be closely clustered and clear, and these are best seen on retroillumination. Fluorescein may stain the superficial microcysts or may show negative staining where the epithelium is elevated over cysts.

Fingerprints are clusters of concentric, contoured lines that can occur in any area of the cornea. On direct illumination they usually are seen as white lines, but they are best appreciated by retroillumination, in which they appear refractile (Fig. 17-5). Some lines branch or have club-shaped terminations. Leashes of long, thick lines, described as "mares' tails," can be seen. Fingerprint-like lines can also be seen in Fuchs' dystrophy.[9]

Maps are irregular, geographic-shaped, circumscribed areas that are commonly seen, usually alone or combined with dots (Fig. 17-6). These areas vary in size and have a ground-glass appearance, often with clear lacunae. Maps may be surrounded by gray-white borders or may blend gradually into the normal cornea. They are best seen with broad, oblique illumination.

Blebs are fine, clear, round, and bubblelike and are seen best in retroillumination (Fig. 17-7). They are uniform in size and shape and can be numerous. In the past, cases with only blebs have been called *bleblike dystrophy. Nets* are refractile lines or rows of blebs that follow the normal anterior corneal mosaic.[23,24] Nets and blebs do not result in erosions, but they may be associated with maps and fingerprints, which do.

Most patients with anterior basement membrane dystrophy are asymptomatic; however, in many cases epithelial erosions occur or vision is decreased because of surface irregularity.[9,10,24] After an erosion occurs, the patient experiences foreign body sensation, pain, photophobia, or tearing. These most commonly develop upon awakening but can occur at any time of the day, and they vary consid-

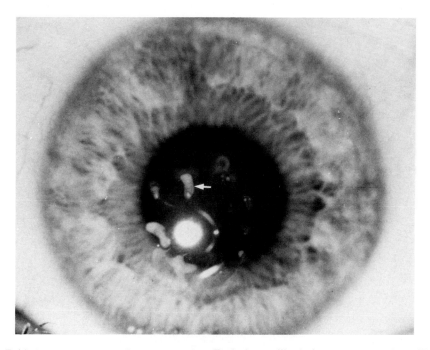

Fig. 17-4. Epithelial basement membrane dystrophy. Typical puttylike lesions *(arrow)* and maplike lines are noted in epithelium.

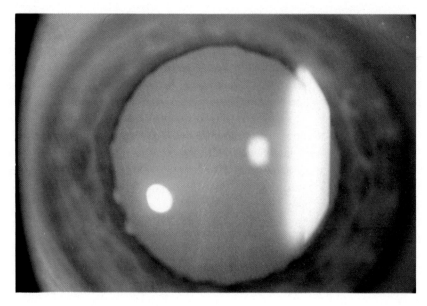

Fig. 17-5. Epithelial basement membrane dystrophy. Fingerprint lines often are best appreciated with retroillumination.

erably in severity and duration. Patients with nonfamilial disease tend to suffer recurrent erosions for no more than a few years, with spontaneous improvement and no significant residual visual loss.[25] A large percentage of patients with recurrent erosions have evidence of epithelial basement membrane dystrophy.[26] Similar changes can be seen after corneal trauma, particularly that caused by fingernails or paper cuts, but they are localized to the traumatized area. These changes also have been noted in patients who have undergone radial keratotomy.[25,27]

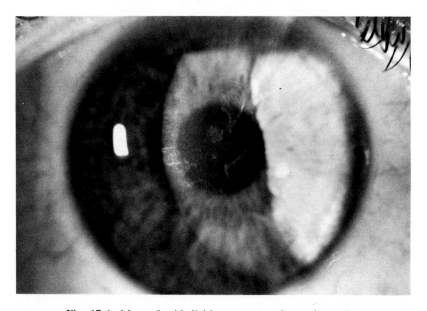

Fig. 17-6. Maps of epithelial basement membrane dystrophy.

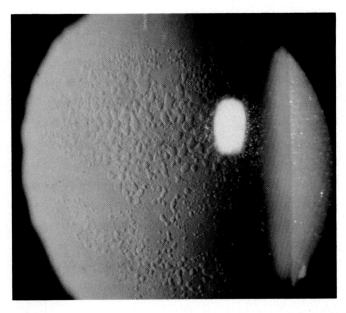

Fig. 17-7. Bleb form of epithelial basement membrane dystrophy. (Courtesy of Y. Jerold Gordon, Pittsburgh.)

Histopathology. In each of these patterns of abnormality, the epithelial basement membrane is abnormal and shows intraepithelial extensions. The maplike changes are related to multilaminar thickening of the basement membrane, with extension of the aberrant membrane into the overlying epithelium (Fig. 17-8). The extensions contain fine fibrillogranular material and are 2 to 6 μm in thickness. Epithelial cells anterior to the abnormal basement membrane do not form hemidesmosomal connections to the membrane, and this probably accounts for their tendency to erode.

The gray-white dot opacities correspond to intraepithelial microcysts (pseudocysts), which contain nuclear debris, cytoplasmic debris, and lipid (Fig. 17-9). There is no visible lining, and the cyst's wall is created by the normal border of the neighboring cell. The cysts form posterior to an intraepithelial extension of aberrant epithelial basement membrane. Epithelial cells beneath the aberrant membrane become vacuolated and liquified, forming the cyst. The cysts may discharge spontaneously onto the corneal surface and thus disappear,[28] producing an erosion in the process.

Fingerprint lines are linear projections of fibrillogranular material into the epithelial layer. The material is covered by a basement membrane, which may be thickened.[29] Blebs are localized mounds of fibrillogranular protein between Bowman's layer and the epithelial basement membrane, indenting the basal epithelium.[30]

Treatment. The treatment of recurrent erosions is discussed in Chapter 15. Photokeratoscopy (Fig. 17-10) and trial of a hard contact lens can document whether a reduction in acuity is related to epithelial irregularity. For these patients, wearing a contact lens improves vision and usually reduces the severity of the basement membrane changes.

DYSTROPHIES OF BOWMAN'S LAYER

Dystrophies that primarily affect Bowman's layer include the following:
1. Reis-Bücklers' dystrophy
2. Grayson-Wilbrandt dystrophy
3. Anterior crocodile shagreen
4. Hereditary calcific band keratopathy

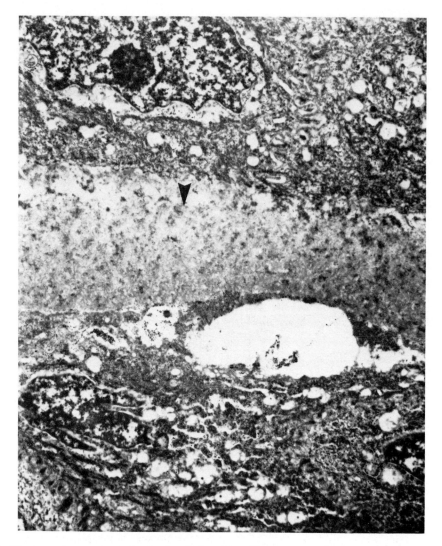

Fig. 17-8. Electron microscopic study showing insinuation of basement membrane substance *(arrow)* between epithelial cells in a case of epithelial basement membrane dystrophy.

REIS-BÜCKLERS' DYSTROPHY

Reis-Bücklers' dystrophy is transmitted as an autosomal dominant trait with strong penetrance.[31-34] It is bilateral and symmetric. The corneal disease is discernible in early childhood; symptoms usually begin about 5 years of age. Recurring attacks of erosion produce photophobia, foreign body sensation, injection, and pain, which last for several weeks. The erosions recur approximately three to four times a year and gradually decrease in frequency over 5 to 20 years. Vision usually begins to deteriorate in the twenties.

The earliest finding is a fine reticular opacification at the level of Bowman's layer. With time the cornea becomes progressively more clouded by superficial, gray-white opacities.[35] The opacities may be linear, geographic, honeycombed, or ringlike[31,34] and remain localized to Bowman's layer, except for peaklike projections into the epithelial layer (Figs. 17-11 and 17-12). The opacities are most dense in the central or midperipheral cornea, and the extreme periphery remains transparent. The corneal surface becomes rough and irregularly thickened, producing irregular astigmatism. Corneal sen-

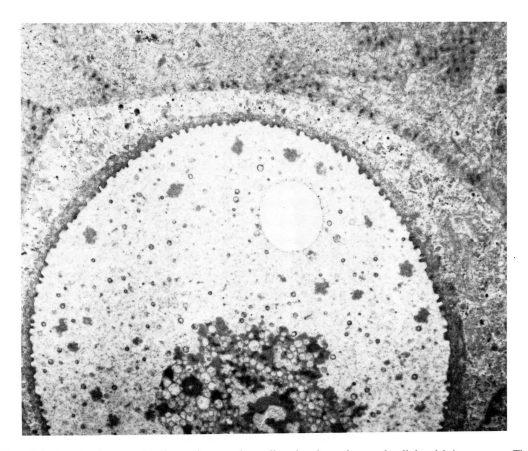

Fig. 17-9. Pseudomicrocyst showing a degenerating cell; pyknotic nucleus and cellular debris are seen. The cyst's wall is created by a normal border of neighboring cell.

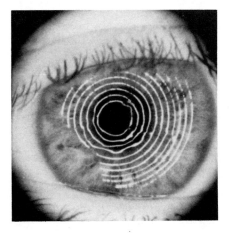

Fig. 17-10. Photokeratoscopy demonstrates surface irregularity in epithelial basement membrane dystrophy.

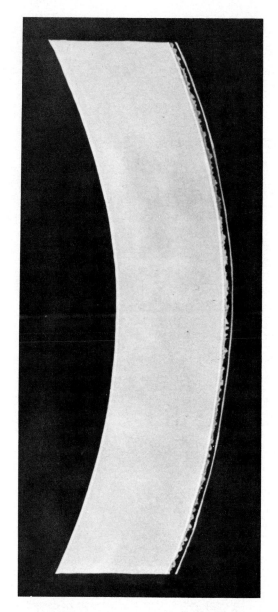

Fig. 17-11. Reis-Bücklers' dystrophy. Peaklike projections from the area of Bowman's layer extend into the epithelium.

sation decreases with increasing epithelial thickness.[36-38] Hudson-Stähli lines and prominent corneal nerves are often present; vascularization is unusual.[34]

Bowman's layer is absent in many areas and is replaced by fibrocellular connective tissue, which extends into the epithelium in projections (Fig. 17-13).[33-43] The fibrocellular material consists of a mixture of larger collagen fibrils with a diameter of 250 to 400 Å and short, dense, curly fibrils 80 to 120 Å in diameter. In areas where Bowman's layer remains intact, the fibrocellular material accumulates between Bowman's layer and the epithelium. Degenerative changes occur in the basal epithelial cells, and the basement membrane is irregular or absent. The posterior surface of the epithelial layer

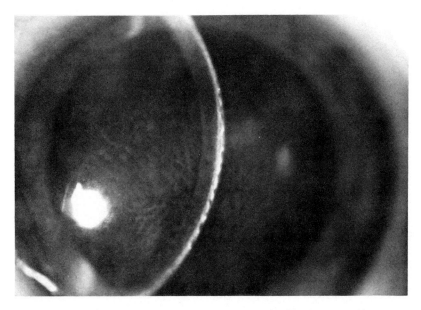

Fig. 17-12. Opacities of Reis-Bücklers' dystrophy are interwoven ringlike figures making up a geographic pattern. (Courtesy of Stuart I. Brown, La Jolla, Calif.)

has a saw-toothed configuration. The posterior stroma, Descemet's membrane, and endothelium do not exhibit disease.

The nature and location of the primary abnormality in Reis-Bücklers' dystrophy is unclear. Some have proposed that the superficial keratocytes produce abnormal collagen fibrils, damaging Bowman's layer, with secondary epithelial injury.[39,40] Others feel that a primary epithelial cell abnormality leads to the recurrent epithelial erosions, with secondary activation of stromal cells, leading to deposition of the fibrocellular material and absorption of Bowman's layer.[40]

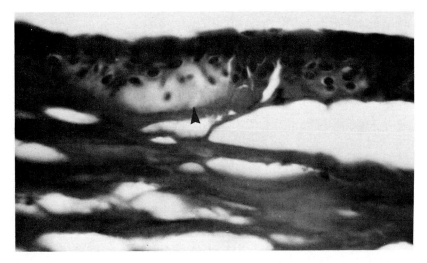

Fig. 17-13. In Reis-Bücklers' dystrophy Bowman's layer is absent in some areas and replaced by fibrocellular connective tissue *(arrow)*. (From Grayson M: Degeneration, dystrophies, and edema of the cornea. In Duane TD, editor: Clinical ophthalmology, vol 4, Hagerstown, Md, 1978, Harper & Row, Publishers, Inc.)

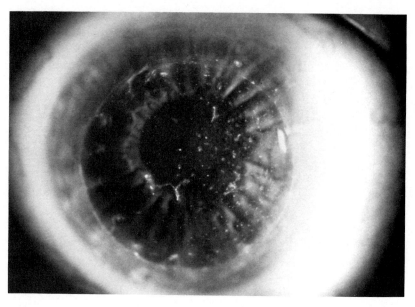

Fig. 17-14. Recurrent Reis-Bücklers' dystrophy in a graft. (Courtesy of Stuart I. Brown, La Jolla, Calif.)

Treatment. The erosions are treated in the same way as erosions of other causes, described in Chapter 15. Surgery is indicated in cases with debilitating recurrent erosions or severe impairment of vision. Lamellar and penetrating keratoplasty have been successful,[33,34,36,39] but the disease can recur in the graft (Fig. 17-14).[44,45] Superficial keratectomy appears to be equally effective and may eliminate the necessity for a penetrating graft,[39,41,46-48] but the disease can recur after this procedure also.[49]

ANTERIOR MEMBRANE DYSTROPHY OF GRAYSON-WILBRANDT

A dystrophy with a clinical appearance similar to Reis-Bücklers' dystrophy was described by Grayson and Wilbrandt.[50] Two generations of a single family were affected, and the inheritance appeared to be autosomal dominant. The onset of the disease did not occur until 10 or 11 years of age, and erosions were infrequent. Vision was variably affected, with some retaining 20/20 and others reduced to 20/200, mainly by epithelial irregularity.

On examination moundlike opacities with a gray-white, macular appearance were seen in central Bowman's layer, extending into the epithelium. The lesions varied in size, and the intervening cornea was clear. Corneal sensation was normal.

On light microscopy the epithelium varied in thickness and in some places was reduced to several layers. The epithelial cells were irregular in size and shape. PAS-staining material was present between Bowman's layer and the epithelium. The material was irregular in thickness and appeared to correspond to the clinical opacity. Bowman's layer was absent in some locations.

It is possible that this disorder is an attenuated form of Reis-Bücklers dystrophy. However, it differs from most cases of Reis-Bücklers' dystrophy in the later onset, infrequency of erosions, variable effect on vision, and the normal corneal sensation.

HONEYCOMB DYSTROPHY OF THIEL AND BEHNKE

Honeycomb dystrophy is a bilateral, subepithelial dystrophy that was described in a single family, transmitted as an autosomal dominant trait.[51] It begins in childhood and runs a progressive course of recurrent erosions and decrease in vision. The vision varies from 20/25 in younger patients to 20/100 in patients 40 to 60 years of age. Corneal erosions cease between the thirties and fifties. A characteristic honeycomb-like opacity is seen at the level of Bowman's layer, with projections into the epithelium. The corneal surface remains smooth, and sensation is not affected.

The results of histopathologic examination were reported in one case with the clinical appearance of honeycomb dystrophy but a family history of Reis-Bücklers' dystrophy.[52] The authors observed a thickened, split, or duplicated epithelial basement membrane and a fibrillogranular subepithelial layer with nodular projections into the epithelium.

Honeycomb dystrophy probably is another variant of Reis-Bücklers' dystrophy, especially in view of its occurrence in a pedigree with the Reis-Bücklers' disorder.

INHERITED BAND KERATOPATHY

Although band-shaped keratopathy usually is seen as a degeneration in local ocular disease or systemic disease, it can occur as an inherited trait. Onset has been described in late adulthood, puberty, and at birth.[53-55] In most cases it has been described in siblings of a single generation, but in one report a father and son were affected.[54] Whether this was truly a dystrophy or resulted from undiagnosed ocular or systemic disease is unclear.

Meisler et al.[56] described a family with early onset of yellow-amber–colored anterior stromal globules in a band-shaped distribution.

ANTERIOR CROCODILE (MOSAIC) SHAGREEN

Anterior crocodile shagreen is discussed in Chapter 16.

LOCAL ANTERIOR MUCOPOLYSACCHARIDE ACCUMULATION

Bilateral diffuse corneal clouding with increased acid mucopolysaccharide accumulation in Bowman's layer occurred in two infants without evidence of systemic mucopolysacccharidosis.[57] Bowman's layer was diffusely thickened with abnormal acid mucopolysaccharide (Fig. 17-15). The epithelium, stroma, Descemet's membrane, and endothelium were normal. There were no intracellular vacuoles containing fibrillogranular inclusions or extracellular granular material, which are seen in macular dystrophy.

STROMAL DYSTROPHIES

Stromal dystrophies are hereditary disorders of the cornea. They are typified by the development of noninflammatory, nonvascularized stromal opacifications of various sizes and shapes. The opaci-

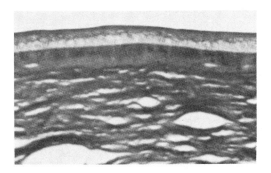

Fig. 17-15. Corneal clouding caused by accumulation of acid mucopolysaccharide in Bowman's layer. (From Rodrigues MM, Calhoun J, and Harley RD: Am J Ophthalmol 79:916, 1975.)

TABLE 17-2. Stromal Corneal Dystrophies: Histopathologic Features

DYSTROPHY	MASSON TRICHROME STAIN	PAS STAIN	ALCIAN BLUE	COLLOID IRON	CONGO RED	OIL RED 0	THIOFLAVINE T	BIREFRINGENCE*	DICHROISM†
Granular (Groenouw type I)	+ (red)	± (weak)	–	–	–	–	–	–	–
Macular (Groenouw type II)	–	+ (pink)	+ (blue)	+	–	–	–	–	–
Lattice	+ (red)	+ (pink)	–	–	– (orange)	–	+	+	+ (red/green)
Schnyder's crystalline	–	–	–	–	–	+ (red)	–	–	–
Fleck (speckled or mouchetée)	–	–	+ keratocytes (blue)	+	–	+ (red)	–	–	–
Pre-Descemet's	–	–	–	–	–	+ (red)	–	–	–

*Birefringence (The linear molecules of the Congo red dye arrange themselves along the axis of the amyloid fibrils; thus dichroism and birefringence can be demonstrated.)

1. Place a polarizing filter in front of the eyepiece lens.
2. Place a polarizing filter between the microscope light and slide.
3. Normally, when perpendicular to each other, no light is seen. However, when the amyloid fibrils stained with Congo red lie in a parallel direction, polarization of the light results. Thus some of the light passing through the first polarizing filter is rotated by the amyloid and passes through the second filter as yellow-green color against a black background.

†Dichroism

1. Place a green filter in front of the microscope light.
2. Place a polarizing filter between the green light and the slide.
3. The parallel-stained Congo red amyloid fibrils absorb green light.
4. If the polarizing is parallel to the fibril axis, the green light is absorbed.
5. If the polarizing plane is at right angles to the fibril, it is not absorbed; thus rotating the polarizing filter will produce red and green colors.

TABLE 17-3. Abnormal Substances of Stromal Dystrophies

DYSTROPHY	ABNORMAL SUBSTANCE
Granular	Amino acids and phospholipid
Lattice	Amyloid
Gelatinous droplike	Amyloid
Macular	Glycosaminoglycan (abnormal keratan sulfate?)
Central crystalline	Cholesterol
Fleck	Intracellular glycosaminoglycan
Pre-Descemet's	Intracellular lipids
Parenchymatous	Amyloid?

ties are bilateral and show specific physical characteristics on biomicroscopic examination. The histologic (Table 17-2) and histochemical (Table 17-3) nature of most of these stromal dystrophies have now been identified. There is no treatment, other than penetrating keratoplasty when vision is reduced. Table 17-4 summarizes the features of the stromal dystrophies.

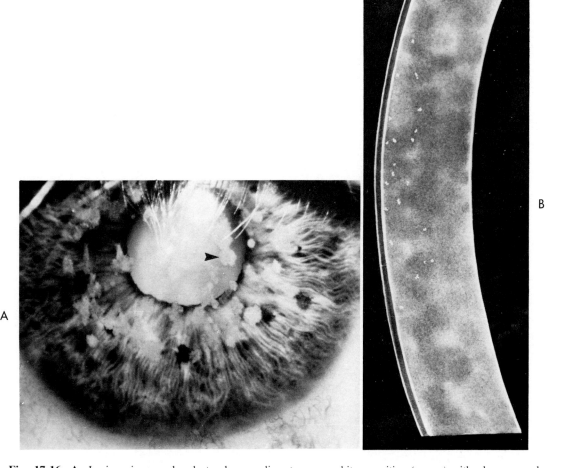

Fig. 17-16. A, Lesions in granular dystrophy are discrete, gray-white opacities *(arrow)* with clear corneal stroma between opacities. **B,** Optical section showing distribution of lesions throughout stroma.

TABLE 17-4. Stromal Corneal Dystrophies

DYSTROPHY	CHARACTER OF OPACITY	CLINICAL FEATURES	VISION	ELECTRON-MICROSCOPIC FEATURES	INHERITANCE	EROSION SYMPTOMS
Granular (Groenouw type I)	Discrete, gray-white opacities with sharp borders; Clear cornea between opacities	Axial region; All depths of stroma; No involvement of epithelium or Descemet's membrane	Usually good until age 40	Electron-dense, rhomboid-shaped rods; Endothelium not affected	Autosomal dominant; In rare cases sporadic	−
Lattice	Gray lines resembling pipestemlike threads that are translucent by retroillumination; dot and stromal opacities between these give ground-glass appearance; threadlike opacities may show bulbous areas and dichotomous branching	Scattered latticelike network with bifurcating pipestemlike threads, mainly limited to zone between center of cornea and periphery; seen throughout the stroma and may involve epithelium	Reduced early in life (usually late adolescence)	Nonbranching fibrils (8 to 10 mm) characteristic of amyloid; Endothelium not affected	Autosomal dominant	+
Gelatinous droplike	Raised multinodular subepithelial mounds	White on direct illumination, transparent on retroillumination; Central	Reduced in first decade	Amyloid in and beneath basal epithelium	?Autosomal recessive	+
Macular (Groenouw type II)	Poorly demarcated, gray-white opacities; Diffusely cloudy cornea between large, irregular opaque areas	Entire cornea may be involved, but more dense in axial region; Some spots extend to limbus; Deep epithelium and endothelium are affected	Affected in late teens	Membrane-bound vacuoles with fibrillogranular material; Keratocytes and endothelium affected	Autosomal recessive	+
Schnyder's crystalline	Crystalline deposits, usually	Mostly located in axial area of cornea; Hyperlipidemia often present; Chondrodystrophy and gene valgum in some families	Usually not markedly disturbed; may be decreased	Notched rectangular crystals	Autosomal dominant	−

Dystrophy	Clinical appearance	Location	Vision	Histology	Inheritance	
Fleck (speckled or mouchetée)	Well-demarcated, small, round, doughnutlike opacities	Opacities are located in all levels of stroma	Vision usually is not affected; however, photophobia may be marked	Keratocytes contain cytoplasmic, membrane-bound vacuoles with fibrillogranular material	Autosomal dominant	—
Marginal crystalline (Bietti)	Crystals in cornea	Superficial stromal deposition in paralimbal area	Vision is not affected by crystals Fundus albipunctatus	No studies available	Not definitely established	—
Central cloudy (François)	Diffuse posterior opacity in pupillary zone broken up into segmental areas Seen best via sclerotic scatter In direct illumination opacities are multiple, small, fuzzy-outlined gray areas, polygonal in shape and separated by clearer areas	Opacity densest posteriorly but extends to level of Bowman's layer Does not involve Descemet's membrane May be same as posterior crocodile shagreen	No decrease in vision	No studies available	Autosomal dominant	—
Parenchymatous (Pillat)	Central punctate and filamentous opacities Peripheral ones are also seen but are finer Central opacities affect posterior stroma	Most opacities are larger than those seen in pre-Descemet's dystrophy Appear gray on focal illumination and clear on retroillumination Noted in seventh decade	No decrease in vision	No studies available	?	—
Posterior amorphous	Gray sheets of indistinct corneal opacities	Opacities are at various levels but mostly deep stroma and may involve Descemet's membrane	Vision may be reduced to 20/40	No studies available	Autosomal dominant	—
Pre-Descemet's	Small opacities of varied shapes and sizes: round, comma, dots, dendritic, or linear	Best seen in retroillumination All opacities are in deep stroma	Vision is not affected	Posterior keratocytes contain membrane-bound vacuoles with fibrillogranular material	Autosomal dominant	—

GRANULAR DYSTROPHY

Granular dystrophy is transmitted as an autosomal dominant trait. The corneal opacities usually are apparent in the first decade as small, discrete, sharply demarcated, grayish white opacities in the anterior axial stroma (Fig. 17-16). At this stage the vision is not impaired, and the patient feels no discomfort. As the condition advances, the lesions become larger, increase in number, coalesce, and extend into the deeper stroma. The opacities can vary in shape; they can be round with solid (Fig. 17-16) or relatively clear centers; they can take the form of a "Christmas tree" (Fig. 17-17); they can resemble snowflakes; or they may look like sinuous, interlacing tracks or like a sponge imprint (Fig. 17-18). The stroma between the discrete opacities is clear until relatively late in the disease. The opacities can extend toward the periphery of the cornea but never reach the limbus. Corneal sensation usually is normal. In some families recurrent erosions can be common, but in most they are unusual.

Atypical, more severe forms have been described. Diffuse subepithelial opacification, developing as early as 6 years of age, has been reported in some cases.[58-60] In one type snowflakelike opacities are seen in the superficial stroma, sometimes extending into the periphery and developing into a diffuse superficial haze by the teens. In another form the lesions are small and flecklike, and normal vision is maintained throughout life.[61]

The histopathology of granular dystrophy is characteristic. Eosinophilic, hyaline deposits are seen in the stroma and beneath the epithelium. These deposits stain an intense red with Masson's trichrome (Fig. 17-19)[62] and sometimes stain weakly positive with PAS.[63] The peripheral portions of the deposits may stain with Congo red.[64,65] Electron microscopy shows electron-dense trapezoid- or rod-shaped extracellular deposits (Fig. 17-20). These deposits are 100 to 500 μm wide, and their inner structure can display a homogenous, filamentous, or moth-eaten pattern.[25,62,65-67] The stromal keratocytes in some instances show degenerative changes, with dilation of the endoplasmic reticulum and Golgi apparatus and vacuolization of the cytoplasm.[66] Histochemical studies indicate that the de-

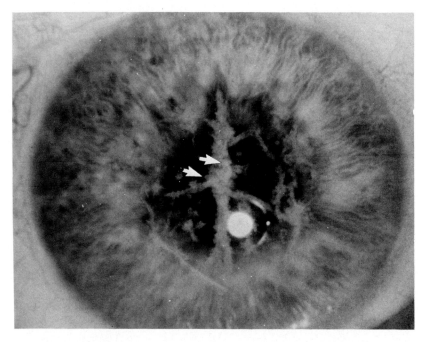

Fig. 17-17. Christmas tree opacity *(arrows)* in a case of granular dystrophy. (From Grayson M: Degeneration, dystrophies, and edema of the cornea. In Duane TD, editor: Clinical ophthalmology, vol 4, Hagerstown, Md, 1978, Harper & Row, Publishers, Inc.)

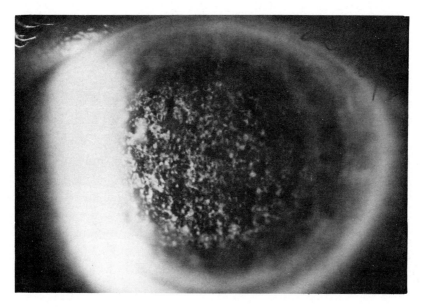

Fig. 17-18. Sponge-imprint type of opacities in granular dystrophy.

posits contain tyrosine, tryptophan, and sulfur-containing amino acids, and some contain arginine as well.[68,69] Microfibrillar protein and phospholipid also were demonstrated.[69]

The exact nature and source of the deposits is not known. Protein and phospholipids, which make up the deposits, are the principal components of cell membranes. It is unclear whether the deposits are produced by epithelium, stromal keratocytes, or both. The characteristic rod-shaped structures have been seen within both epithelial cells and keratocytes.[67] In some recurrences the disease appears to be confined to the epithelium.[70]

Treatment. Most patients with granular dystrophy do not require treatment. Some patients have recurrent erosions, and the treatment of these is discussed in Chapter 15. If vision is markedly reduced,

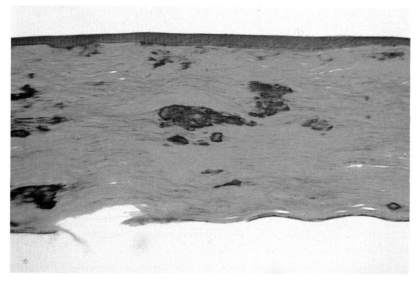

Fig. 17-19. Positive Masson's trichrome stain seen in granular dystrophy.

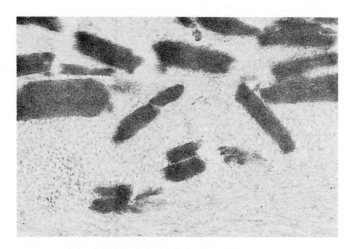

Fig. 17-20. Dense, homogeneous, rod-shaped structures characteristic of granular dystrophy as noted with transmission electron microscopy (X36,000). (From Haddad R, Font RL, and Fine BS: Am J Ophthalmol 83:213, 1977.)

surgery can be performed. If the opacities are largely superficial, epithelial scraping or superficial keratectomy may be sufficient.[71] For deeper opacities penetrating keratoplasty can be performed. Granular dystrophy can recur in the grafts and can appear as early as 1 year after surgery (Fig. 17-21).[72-77] Clinically, it usually is noted as a diffuse, subepithelial haze in the peripheral graft or as typical granular lesions in the stroma. The former type represents avascular fibrous tissue between the epithelium and Bowman's layer; it can be removed by a superficial keratectomy to restore good vision.[78] The typical electron-dense trapezoid- and rod-shaped deposits can be seen in the stroma and epithelium.[70,73,79]

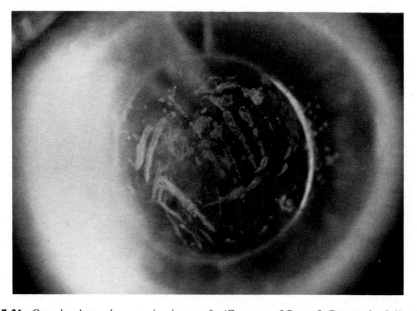

Fig. 17-21. Granular dystrophy recurring in a graft. (Courtesy of Stuart I. Brown, La Jolla, Calif.)

LATTICE DYSTROPHY

Lattice dystrophy is inherited as an autosomal dominant trait and varies in penetrance and expression.[80] Most cases are bilateral, but unilateral cases have been reported.[81-83] Clinical evidence of corneal disease appears early, usually by 2 to 7 years of age. Visual impairment gradually increases and usually requires keratoplasty by the twenties or thirties. Recurrent erosions are fairly common.

The early corneal lesions typically appear as fine, irregular lines and dots, mainly in the axial cornea and involving anterior stroma and Bowman's layer.[84] In other cases it appears as discrete round or ovoid nonrefractile subepithelial opacities or as diffuse axial anterior stromal haze.[85] With progression the lesions can appear as small nodules, dots, threadlike spicules (Fig. 17-22), or thicker, radially oriented branching lines. The lines are typically refractile with a double contour and a clear core on retroillumination. With time the lattice lines can extend into the deep stroma and epithelium, and they tend to become opacified. Between the lines refractile dots or small irregular opacities usually are present, but the stroma between these opacities initially is clear. With time the opacities coalesce, and a diffuse ground-glass haze can involve the anterior and midstroma (Fig. 17-23). Anterior involvement leads to recurrent erosions and surface irregularity.

Once the anterior cornea becomes opacified, the appearance can resemble that seen in the later stages of macular and granular dystrophies. However, the typical branching lattice lines usually can be seen. Also, refractile opacities usually can be found in lattice dystrophy but not in macular or granular dystrophies.

Histopathology. On histologic examination the epithelial layer is irregular, with areas of thickening and thinning.[63,86,87] The basal epithelial cells degenerate, and the basement membrane is thickened and discontinuous, without normal hemidesmosomes.[88,89] Bowman's layer may be absent, thick, or thin in different areas. Deposits of eosinophilic material are seen between the epithelium and Bowman's layer and throughout the stroma (Fig. 17-24). These deposits stain with Congo red (Fig. 17-25), PAS, Masson's trichrome, and thioflavin T; manifest green birefringence when viewed with a polarizing microscope (Fig. 17-26); and exhibit dichroism when viewed with polarization and a green

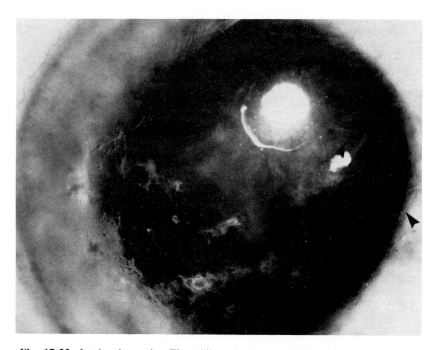

Fig. 17-22. Lattice dystrophy. Threadlike spicules branch dichotomously *(arrows)*.

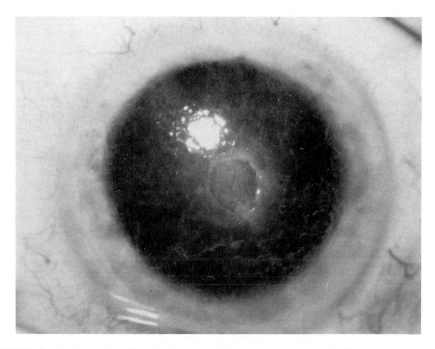

Fig. 17-23. Lattice dystrophy. Opacity has ground-glass appearance on biomicroscopic examination.

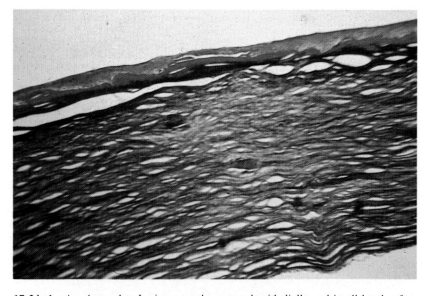

Fig. 17-24. Lattice dystrophy. Lesions may be seen subepithelially and in all levels of stroma.

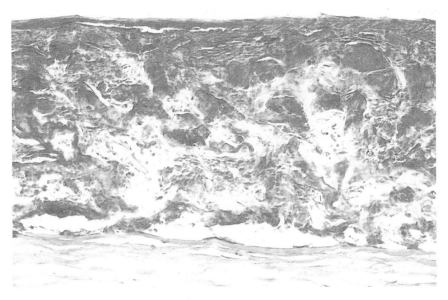

Fig. 17-25. Congo red stain of corneal amyloid. (Courtesy F. Wilson II, Indianapolis.)

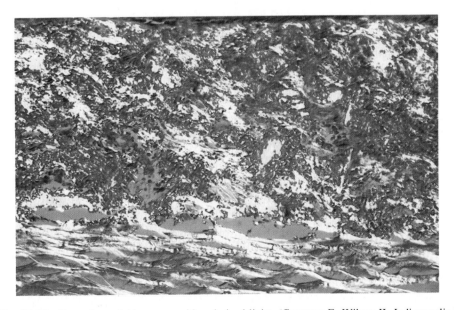

Fig. 17-26. Corneal amyloid as seen with polarized light. (Courtesy F. Wilson II, Indianapolis.)

TABLE 17-5. Comparison of Different Types of Lattice Corneal Dystrophy

CHARACTERISTIC	TYPE I	TYPE II (MERETOJA)	TYPE III	POLYMORPHIC AMYLOID DEGENERATION
Inheritance	Autosomal dominant	Autosomal dominant	Autosomal recessive?	None
Onset	Under age 10	20 to 35 years	Over age 40	Over age 40
Visual acuity	Poor after age 40	Good until age 65	Impaired after age 60	Unaffected
Erosions	Frequent	Infrequent	None	None
Cornea	Numerous, delicate lines; many amorphous deposits; periphery clear	Few thick lines; extend to periphery; few amorphous deposits	Thick lines	Polymorphic punctate opacities, filaments; central, peripheral, or annular distribution
Systemic involvement	None	Amyloidosis involving skin, nerves, arteries, and other organs	None	None
Face	Normal	Facial paresis and blepharochalasis after age 40	Normal	Normal

filter.[90-92] These findings are consistent with amyloid, and the amyloid nature has been confirmed by immunofluorescence studies using antisera to human amyloid.[93] In long-standing cases a degenerative pannus can be seen.[93] Descemet's membrane and the endothelium are essentially normal, although amyloid deposits have rarely been seen in the former.

An electron microscope shows the deposits to be composed of fine, electron-dense, nonbranching fibrils of 8 to 10 nm in diameter without periodicity.[94-96] Most of the fibrils are highly aligned, which explains the phenomena of dichroism and birefringence. Keratocytes in the involved areas are decreased in number; some of them appear quite active, but others appear degenerated.[80,90,91,96]

Amyloid is a noncollagenous, fibrous protein containing 2% to 5% carbohydrate. The structure of the amyloid deposits varies in the different forms of amyloidosis. In immunoglobulin primary systemic amyloidosis, the amyloid contains fragments of immunoglobulin light chains. In hereditary systemic amyloidosis, the most frequent protein accumulated is transthyretin, plasma prealbumin. The major component of amyloid deposits associated with secondary systemic amyloidosis is a protein (protein AA) that appears to be a degradation product of a serum acute phase reactant (serum AA) unrelated to immunoglobulins. Both primary and secondary amyloid deposits are associated with a structural protein (protein AP), which is also present in normal serum. In lattice corneal dystrophy, protein AP is present but not immunoglobulin light chains or protein AA.[97,98]

Other forms of lattice corneal dystrophy. Other forms of latticelike dystrophy have been described (Table 17-5). In rare cases a similar corneal picture can be seen in association with systemic amyloidosis. This condition originally was described by Meretoja[99-102] and has been called type II lattice dystrophy and familial amyloid polyneuropathy type IV. The latticelike corneal changes usually become manifest between 20 and 35 years of age; in later decades the skin, peripheral nerves, and cranial nerves become involved. In contrast to lattice type I, the corneal disease in type II is milder and later in onset. Vision is good until the seventh decade, and erosive symptoms are less frequent. In lattice dystrophy type II, fewer lattice lines (8 to 20) are present; they are radially oriented, coarser, and extend to the limbus. Also, there are fewer amorphous dots.

Histologic examination of corneas with lattice dystrophy type II showed a uniform thin layer of amyloid deposits posterior to Bowman's layer.[100] The lattice lines also were composed of amyloid, and they appeared to have replaced corneal nerves. Amyloid was also found beneath the basement membrane of the conjunctival epithelium and in sclera, arteries, skin, peripheral nerves, and other tissues. The amyloid protein in Meretoja's syndrome has not been identified, but it is related to transthyretin.[103]

Another type of latticelike corneal dystrophy (type III) recently was reported in two families in Japan.[104,105] These patients had thick, translucent lattice lines and few amorphous dots. Vision was good until after 40 years of age, and recurrent erosions did not develop. There was no evidence of systemic amyloidosis.

Punctate and filiform stromal amyloid deposits, which are transparent on retroillumination, can be seen in patients over 40 years of age (Fig. 17-27).[106] The deposits are bilateral and found at all levels, but mostly in the middle and deep stroma. There is no progression, vision is not affected, and the cornea remains lustrous. No hereditary pattern has been demonstrated. The amyloid nature of the deposits has been confirmed histologically.[106] This condition most likely is a degenerative disease rather than a dystrophy and should be called *polymorphic amyloid degeneration*. It probably is the same condition as parenchymatous dystrophy of Pillat (see below).

Treatment. If visual acuity is impaired, penetrating keratoplasty can be performed (Fig. 17-28). The likelihood of obtaining a clear graft is high, but the dystrophy can appear in the graft in as little as 3 years.[73,107,108] Lattice dystrophy recurs more frequently than granular or macular dystrophy: In one study 48% of patients had evidence of recurrence, from 2 to 26 years after grafting, and 15% required

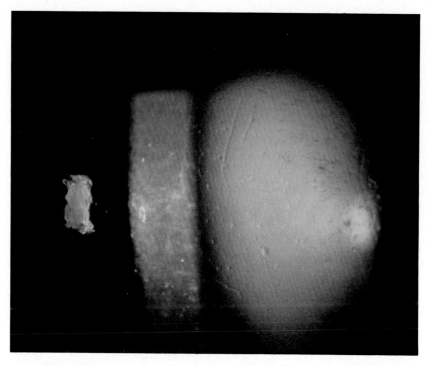

Fig. 17-27. Deep stromal punctate and filamentous opacities in polymorphic amyloid degeneration. The opacities appear gray-white on direct illumination and clear on retroillumination. (Courtesy of Robert W. Weisenthal, Syracuse, NY.)

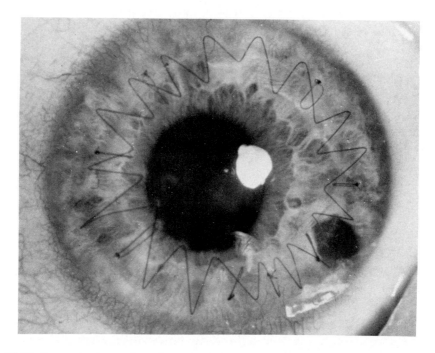

Fig. 17-28. Penetrating keratoplasty is used to obtain good vision in patients with lattice dystrophy.

regrafting.[109] Recurrence of lattice lines is unusual; more commonly, dotlike, diffuse, or filamentous subepithelial opacities or diffuse anterior stromal haze are seen.

GELATINOUS DROPLIKE DYSTROPHY

Gelatinous droplike dystrophy is a rare form of primary familial amyloidosis of the cornea.[110-116] It has been seen in Europe and the United States but is much more common in Japan.[117] The pattern of inheritance is unclear, but most likely autosomal recessive.[112] The disorder usually appears in the first decade with photophobia, lacrimation, and decreased visual acuity. Bilateral, central, raised, multinodular, subepithelial mounds of amyloid are seen (Fig. 17-29). These are white on direct illumination and transparent on retroillumination but can become yellow and milky with time. Flat subepithelial opacities can be seen surrounding the mounds. Early in the dystrophy the deposits are fairly flat and can resemble band-shaped keratopathy.[118] In the late stages the cornea can have a diffuse, mulberry-like appearance, and neovascularization can occur.

The amyloid nature of these deposits has been demonstrated histologically.[111-115,119] Bowman's layer usually is absent, and amyloid is deposited in the basal epithelial cells, beneath the epithelium, and occasionally in the stroma. The deposits contain protein AP but not protein AA or immunoglobulins.

Recurrence is seen after penetrating keratoplasty.[114,119]

MACULAR DYSTROPHY

Clinical findings. Macular dystrophy is transmitted as an autosomal recessive trait. Of the three classic stromal dystrophies, macular dystrophy is the most severe. The patient has progressive loss of vision and attacks of irritation and photophobia. In most cases vision is severely impaired by the twenties or thirties. Recurrent erosions are seen, but they are less frequent than in lattice dystrophy. Heterozygous carriers do not manifest any corneal abnormalities.

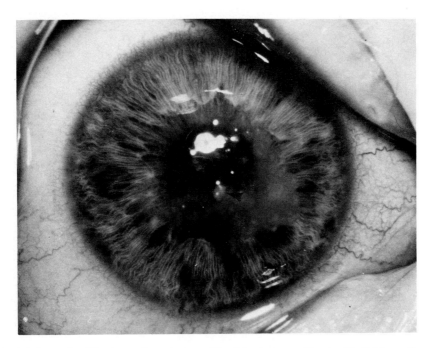

Fig. 17-29. Gelatinous droplike dystrophy; raised, multinodular lesions with subepithelial formations of amyloid *(arrow).*

The corneal changes usually are first noted between 3 and 9 years of age, when a diffuse clouding is seen in the central superficial stroma. With time the clouding extends peripherally and into the deeper stroma. By the teens the opacification involves the entire thickness of the cornea and may extend out to the limbus. As the condition progresses, the cornea becomes increasingly cloudy. Within this sea of haziness are gray-white, denser opacities with indistinct borders (Fig. 17-30). These denser, macular opacities can protrude anteriorly, resulting in irregularity of the epithelial surface (Fig. 17-31), or posteriorly, causing irregularity, grayness, and guttate appearance of Descemet's membrane (Fig. 17-32). They can enlarge with time and coalesce. The stroma is thinner than normal.[120,121]

Pathology. Histologically, macular dystrophy is characterized by the accumulation of glycosaminoglycans (acid mucopolysaccharide) between the stromal lamellae, underneath the epithelium, within stromal keratocytes, and within the endothelial cells.[63,64,122-124] The glycosaminoglycans stain with alcian blue, colloidal iron, and PAS (Figs. 17-31 and 17-32). Degeneration of the basal epithelial cells and focal epithelial thinning is seen over the accumulated material. Bowman's layer is thinned or absent in some areas.

Electron microscopy shows accumulation of mucopolysaccharide within stromal keratocytes.[64,90,124-126] The keratocytes are distended by numerous intracytoplasmic vacuoles, which appear to be the dilated cisternae of the rough endoplasmic reticulum. Some of these vacuoles are clear, but many contain fibrillar or granular material, and occasionally membranous lamellar material. The endothelium contains material similar to that found in the keratocyte. The posterior, nonbanded portion of Descemet's membrane is infiltrated by vesicular and granular material deposited by the abnormal endothelium.

The accumulated material appears to be abnormal keratan sulfate.[127] In culture the keratocytes produce only glycoprotein precursors of keratan sulfate.[128-130] The accumulated material varies; its staining by different anti−keratan sulfate antibodies differs between patients (Fig. 17-33).[131,132] In

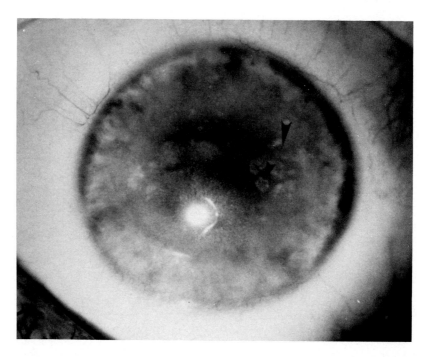

Fig. 17-30. Macular dystrophy shows diffuse corneal haze with gray-white dense opacities in the area of haze *(arrows)*.

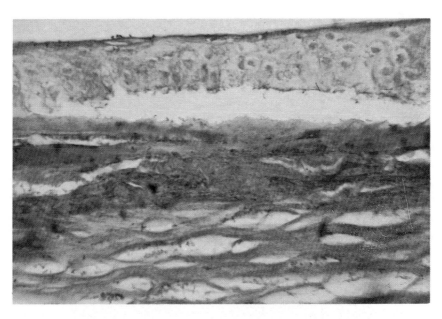

Fig. 17-31. Macular dystrophy. Colloidal iron stain indicates accumulation of acid mucopolysaccharide under epithelium.

some patients normal keratan sulfate is also absent from the serum and cartilage.[131,133] In another study the deposits were found to contain an antigen associated with intermediate-type filament.[134]

The corneal pathology of macular corneal dystrophy differs from that of the systemic mucopolysaccharidoses in several respects. There appears to be an abnormality in the synthesis of mucopolysaccharide in macular dystrophy, and an abnormality in the breakdown of mucopolysaccharide in the systemic mucopolysaccharidoses. In the systemic mucopolysaccharidoses, the abnormal material accumulates in lysosomal vacuoles, whereas in macular dystrophy it accumulates in endoplasmic re-

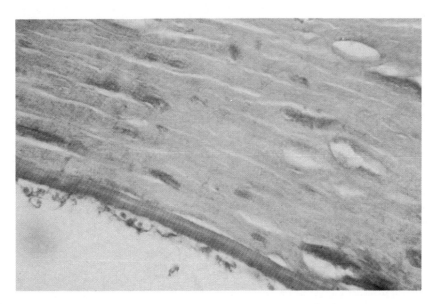

Fig. 17-32. Macular dystrophy. Colloidal iron stain shows accumulation of acid mucopolysaccharide in endothelium.

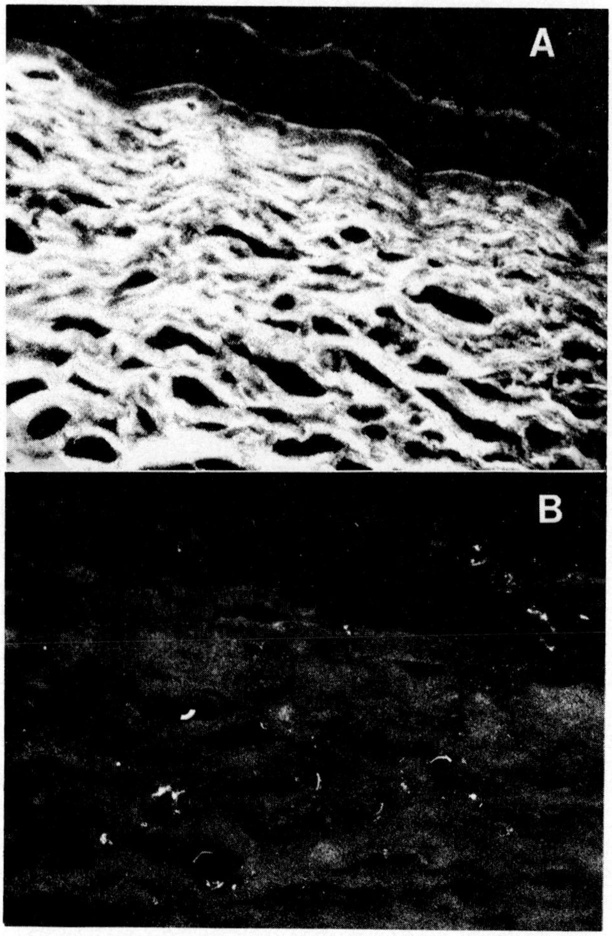

Fig. 17-33. Distribution of keratan sulfate in normal cornea, *(A)* and cornea from patients with macular corneal dystrophy *(B)*. Cryostat sections of the cornea were reacted with a monoclonal antibody against keratan sulfate using an indirect immunofluorescence technique. Note the strong staining of keratan sulfate in the normal cornea *(A)* but the absence of staining in the cornea from the patient with macular corneal dystrophy *(B)*. (Courtesy of Nirmala Sundar-Raj, PhD, Pittsburgh.)

ticulum. In the systemic mucopolysaccharidoses, epithelial involvement is prominent, and Descemet's membrane usually is not affected.

Treatment. Good results are obtained from penetrating keratoplasty for macular dystrophy (Fig. 17-34). Recurrences can be seen in both lamellar and penetrating grafts, but they usually are delayed for many years.[135,136] Host keratocytes invade the graft and produce abnormal glycosaminoglycan. The periphery of the graft is most affected, particularly the superficial and deep layers. Surprisingly, the endothelium and Descemet's membrane also are affected.

FLECK DYSTROPHY

Fleck dystrophy is a rare dystrophy that also has been called speckled dystrophy or mouchetée dystrophy. It is transmitted as an autosomal dominant trait.[137-143] The condition usually is noted during a routine examination; it is stationary with no loss of visual acuity. Some degree of photophobia may be present.[140] The lesions appear during the first decade of life and usually are bilateral, al-

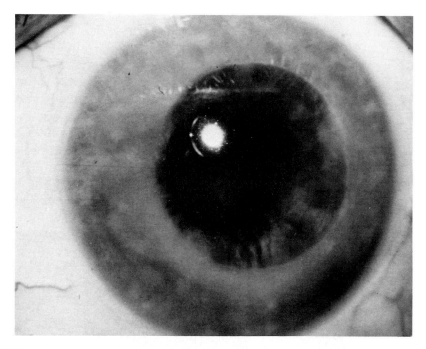

Fig. 17-34. Good visual results can be obtained with penetrating keratoplasty in macular dystrophy.

though they can be asymmetric or unilateral. Small opacities are present in all layers of the corneal stroma except Bowman's layer, and they involve the peripheral as well as the central stroma (Fig. 17-35 and 17-36). The lesions are semiopaque, flattened opacities that may be oval, round, comma-shaped, granular, or stellate. Many have a doughnutlike appearance with a relatively clear center. These small opacities are well demarcated, and the intervening stroma is clear. The best way to demonstrate them is on retroillumination. Corneal sensation is normal in most cases, but in some families sensation is decreased.[138]

Fleck dystrophy has been noted in association with a variety of disorders such as keratoconus,[138] limbal dermoids,[138] central cloudy dystrophy,[137,144,145] angioid streaks,[137] papillitis,[137] and punctate cortical lens opacities.[146] It is unclear whether the relationship is more than coincidental.

Histopathologic studies reveal abnormal, distended keratocytes throughout the stroma. Bowman's layer, epithelium, Descemet's membrane, and endothelium are normal. The keratocytes stain with oil red O and Sudan black B, indicating the presence of lipid, and alcian blue and colloidal iron, indicating the presence of mucopolysaccharide.[147,148] On electron microscopy the keratocytes are seen to contain varying numbers of membrane-limited intracytoplasmic vacuoles containing a fibrillogranular material.[146,147] Some of these vacuoles also contain membranous inclusions or pleomorphic, electron-dense deposits. The vacuoles appear to arise from the Golgi apparatus and therefore would be lysosomal vacuoles. Because of this fleck dystrophy seems to be a storage disorder of glycosaminoglycans and complex lipids that is limited to the cornea.

CENTRAL CRYSTALLINE DYSTROPHY OF SCHNYDER

Central crystalline dystrophy is transmitted as an autosomal dominant trait. It is absent at birth but may be seen as early as 18 months of age. Visual acuity usually is not affected, but occasionally it is moderately reduced. The chief characteristic of the dystrophy is the presence of bilateral, ring-shaped or disciform opacities in the central cornea.[149-154] The opacities usually appear to consist of fine,

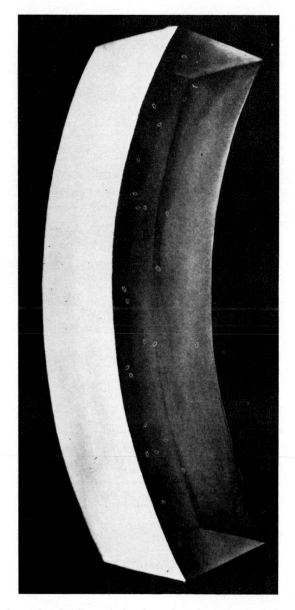

Fig. 17-35. Fleck dystrophy. Small, oval, doughnut-shaped, gray-white lesions are seen in stroma.

polychromatic, needle-shaped crystals (Fig. 17-37), but in some cases a disciform opacity is present without evident crystals.[155] The opacity primarily involves the anterior stroma but may extend into the deeper layers. The intervening stroma usually is clear, but punctate white opacities can be scattered in the stroma or the stroma can exhibit a milky opalescence.[150,152] Corneal arcus and Vogt's limbal girdle frequently are present, even at an early age.[154] Corneal sensation is normal.

The opacities progress slowly and usually stabilize in later life. Progression is more frequent in patients with diffuse opacities than in those with crystalline deposits, and there is no relation to the serum lipoprotein levels.[156]

A significant number of patients have hyperlipidemia, but the type and severity of the hyperlipi-

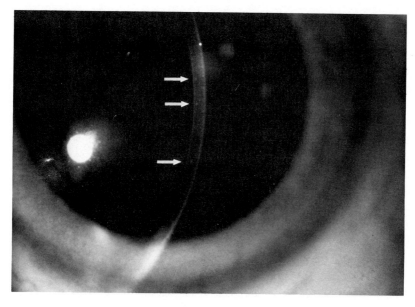

Fig. 17-36. Fleck dystrophy.

demia vary.[150,152] Within a single family some individuals have only crystalline dystrophy, others have hyperlipidemia and crystalline dystrophy, and others have only hyperlipidemia. Chondrodystrophy and genu valgum also are present in some families.[150,152,154,157]

The main histopathologic feature of Schnyder's dystrophy is the presence of cholesterol crystals, noncrystalline cholesterol, cholesterol esters, and neutral fats in the stroma.[149,152,158,159] The deposits are most numerous in the anterior stroma, but they can extend posteriorly to Descemet's mem-

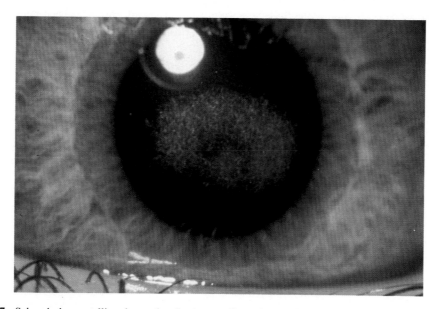

Fig. 17-37. Schnyder's crystalline dystrophy. Lesion consists of fine, polychromatic needle-like crystals in area of Bowman's layer and anterior stroma.

brane.[160] Frozen sections must be performed to avoid dissolution of the crystals during fixation. Destruction of Bowman's layer and superficial stroma with disorganization of collagen have often been observed. Some keratocytes contain cholesterol crystals, and occasionally similar deposits have been noted in basal epithelial cells.[161]

Schnyder's dystrophy is most likely a localized disorder of cholesterol metabolism, and it may be exacerbated by systemic hyperlipoproteinemia. Burns, Connor, and Gipson[162] administered radiolabeled cholesterol intravenously to a patient with crystalline dystrophy 2 weeks before keratoplasty. The radioactivity in the cornea was higher than in the blood, suggesting active deposition of cholesterol in the cornea.

In most cases of crystalline dystrophy the corneal disease requires no treatment. Serum lipid profiles should be obtained. Penetrating or lamellar keratoplasty can be performed for visual rehabilitation, but the dystrophy can recur.[62,154] It is important to consider other causes of corneal crystals. (These are discussed in Chapter 3.)

MARGINAL CRYSTALLINE DYSTROPHY OF BIETTI

Marginal crystalline dystrophy was described in two brothers who had crystalline material in the superficial stroma of the paralimbal cornea; their vision was not affected[163] (Fig. 17-38). Both brothers also had fundus albipunctatus. A few similar cases have been described, and in one case a pathologic examination was performed.[164,165] Cholesterol or cholesterol ester and complex lipid inclusions were seen in corneal fibroblasts and circulating lymphocytes.

CENTRAL CLOUDY DYSTROPHY OF FRANÇOIS

Central cloudy dystrophy is transmitted as an autosomal dominant trait, with early onset and no progression with age.[166,167] Vision is not affected, and there are no other symptoms, so the diagnosis often is not made until late in life.

A diffuse clouding is present in the axial cornea; it is densest posteriorly and fades anteriorly and peripherally (Figs. 17-39 and 17-40). The cloud is broken into segments by an interlacing network of clear lines, creating a mosaic pattern. Sometimes the opacification extends to or in rare cases involves Bowman's layer; in this location the opacities are smaller and less numerous.

Most likely this condition is the same as posterior mosaic shagreen. It has been noted in association with fleck dystrophy,[168] fleck dystrophy and pseudoxanthoma elasticum,[169] and pre-Descemet's dystrophy.[138]

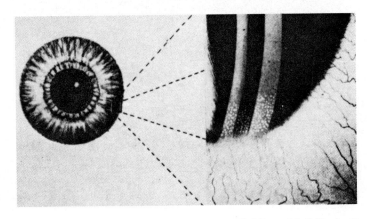

Fig. 17-38. Marginal crystalline changes in cornea. (From Bagolini B and Ioli-Spada G: Am J Ophthalmol 65:53, 1968.)

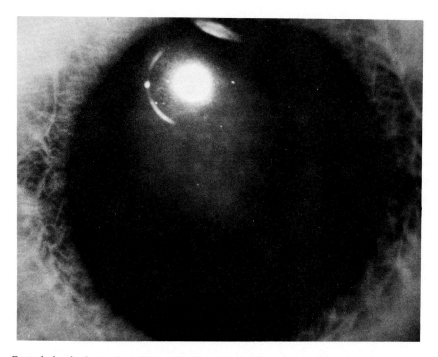

Fig. 17-39. Central cloudy dystrophy of François. General clouding of cornea is broken up into segmental areas of opacity by intervening clear tissue.

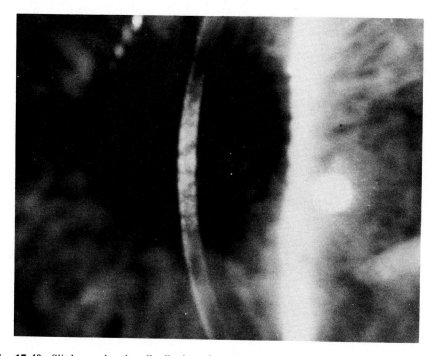

Fig. 17-40. Slit-beam showing distribution of opacity in central cloudy dystrophy of François.

Parenchymatous Dystrophy of Pillat

Parenchymatous dystrophy of the cornea is rare; only a few cases have been reported.[170,171] Thomsitt and Bron[172] called it polymorphic stromal dystrophy. Most likely this is a degenerative change and is the same as polymorphic amyloid degeneration.[106]

Deep stromal opacities are seen, which are gray-white on focal illumination and clear on retroillumination (see Fig. 17-27). The deposits are punctate and filamentous and can be central, peripheral, or annular in distribution. The punctate opacities are polymorphic flecklike, stellate, linear, or guttate. The filaments are identical to those seen in lattice dystrophy; they can have beading, striations, or dichotomous branching.

The deposits usually are noted in patients in the sixth decade, and progression has not been demonstrated. Vision and corneal sensation are not affected. Although the condition has been noted in two siblings, no heritability has been demonstrated.

Posterior Amorphous Dystrophy

Posterior amorphous dystrophy, an autosomal dystrophy, has been described in only two families.[173,174] Changes have been noted as early as 16 weeks of age and thus may be present at birth. Progression has not been documented, and visual acuity has not been worse than 20/40.

Gray, sheetlike opacities can involve any portion of the stroma but are most prominent posteriorly. They can affect the central or peripheral portions of the cornea or both. Descemet's membrane may show posterior bowing and distortion of the endothelial mosaic. Central corneal thinning, flattened keratometry, and hyperopia may be present. Various iris and angle abnormalities have been noted, including a prominent Schwalbe ring with numerous fine iris processes, pupillary remnants, corectopia, iridocorneal adhesions, and anterior stromal tags.

It is important to differentiate this type of dystrophy from interstitial keratitis, since both can show posterior corneal opacification. However, no vascularization or inflammation is seen in posterior amorphous dystrophy. In view of the early onset, lack of progression, and association with iris abnormalities, this condition may be a dysgenesis rather than a dystrophy.[173]

PRE-DESCEMET'S DYSTROPHIES

A variety of fine posterior stromal opacities have been described in patients in the fourth decade or older. Most likely these are degenerative diseases rather than dystrophies.[25] However, some of these conditions have been reported in a number of family members, over two to four generations.[169,175-177] In one family the mother had typical cornea farinata, whereas her daughter had pre-Descemet's dystrophy.

Cornea farinata is sometimes classified with pre-Descemet's dystrophies, but it is more often considered an age-related degeneration. Cornea farinata consists of tiny, punctate, gray opacities in the deep stroma immediately anterior to Descemet's membrane. It is discussed in Chapter 16.

The opacities in pre-Descemet's dystrophy resemble those in cornea farinata, but they are larger and more polymorphous. Grayson and Wilbrandt[178] described primary pre-Descemet's dystrophies that consisted of mixtures of six types of tiny, deep, stromal opacities: (1) dendritic or stellate, (2) boomerang, (3) circular or dot, (4) comma, (5) linear, and (6) filiform (Fig. 17-41). The deposits could be axial, peripheral, or diffuse. The type and location of the opacities showed no correlation with age or with the presence or absence of coexisting ocular or systemic disease. More recently a pedigree was described with more uniform, polychromatic filaments in a diffuse pattern extending to the limbus.[176] Four generations were affected, and the inheritance appeared to be autosomal dominant.

Histopathologic examination of one case of pre-Descemet's dystrophy demonstrated that the pathologic condition was limited to the keratocytes of the posterior stroma.[179] Within the keratocytes

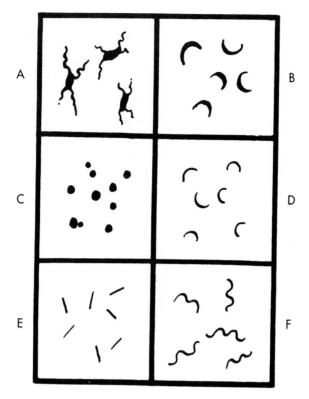

Fig. 17-41. Patterns of opacities in the pre-Descemet's dystrophies. **A,** Dendritic. **B,** Boomerang. **C,** Circular. **D,** Comma. **E,** Linear. **F,** Filiform.

were cytoplasmic vacuoles (secondary lysosomes) that contained lipidlike material, which on electron microscopy consisted of fibrillogranular and electron-dense lamellar inclusions. These findings suggest that the accumulated material most likely was lipofuscin, a degenerative "wear and tear" lipoprotein associated with aging.

Similar opacities have been noted in association with other ocular or systemic abnormalities, and these have been called secondary pre-Descemet's dystrophies. Pre-Descemet's dystrophy has been reported in association with keratoconus and has been called deep filiform dystrophy of Maeder and Danis.[180] It also has been reported in patients with epithelial basement membrane dystrophy,[177] posterior polymorphous dystrophy,[177] ichthyosis (deep punctate dystrophy of Franceschetti and Maeder),[181,182] central cloudy corneal dystrophy,[169] pseudoxanthoma elasticum,[169] and in female carriers of sex-linked ichthyosis.[183]

ECTATIC DYSTROPHIES

ANTERIOR KERATOCONUS

Anterior keratoconus has also been called conical cornea (Fig. 17-42). It may be congenital but usually appears at puberty or soon thereafter. It has a tendency to progress for about 7 to 8 years and then remain stable, but this varies considerably. Progression can be rapid, gradual, or intermittent. In general it is more likely to occur between 10 and 30 years of age than after age 30.

The condition usually is bilateral but may be unilateral or highly asymmetric. Most cases have no familial history of keratoconus, but pedigrees with autosomal dominant and recessive inheritance have been described.[184-188] Photokeratoscopy has shown that apparently unaffected family members

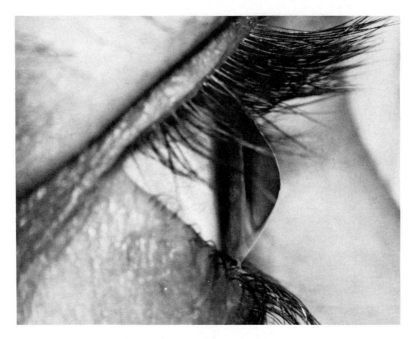

Fig. 17-42. Keratoconus.

have increased central steepening and astigmatism.[189] In familial keratoconus approximately two thirds of affected members have other evidence of connective tissue abnormalities such as syndactyly, Raynaud's phenomenon, and brachydactyly.[190] Keratoscopy is the most sensitive means of diagnosis, since the characteristic pattern is present even in early keratoconus (Fig. 17-43).[191-193] Typically the central mires are oval, pointing inferonasally, with decreased separation (steepening) of the inferonasal mires and increased separation (flattening) of the superotemporal mires. This is usually associated with myopic astigmatism. With progression the keratoscopic findings become more marked (Fig. 17-44), and the position, size, and shape of the cone can vary. Most commonly the cone is relatively round and only slightly displaced inferonasally. However, cones can be oval, sagging, small nipple-like, large, or more peripheral (usually inferior). The conical deformation of the cornea results in a convexity of the lower lid on down gaze, called *Munson's sign*. A *Fleischer ring* is iron deposition in the epithelium around a portion or the entire circumference of the base of the cone. It is most easily appreciated with oblique cobalt blue illumination (Fig. 17-45). The ring can be useful in determining the size and position of the cone. The cone also can be visualized by retroillumination with the slit-lamp microscope or retinoscope.

The apex of the cornea thins in proportion to the progression of the disease. However, perforation is rare. Vertical stress lines appear deep in the corneal stroma *(Vogt's striae)* (Fig. 17-46). These lines disappear with gentle pressure on the apex of the cone. Increased visibility of the corneal nerves, posterior crocodile shagreen, and guttae also may be present. Interruptions in Bowman's layer can be seen as clear spaces in the anterior stroma of the thinned cornea, usually with a vertical orientation.[194] Corneal sensation is reduced, particularly in the inferior cornea.[195] A scissors reflex often is present on retinoscopy. Keratometry mires are irregular, and corneal curvature can exceed 70 diopters.

Fine anterior stromal scars can be seen near the cone apex, caused by ruptures of Bowman's layer. Acute tears in Descemet's membrane can occur in advanced cases, leading to stromal edema in

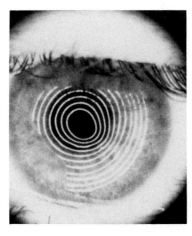

17-43

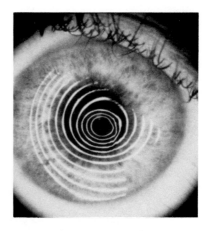

17-44

Fig. 17-43. Photokeratoscopy in moderate keratoconus demonstrates ovaling of central mires, with superonasal flattening and inferotemporal steepening.

Fig. 17-44. Central steep nipplelike cone.

the cone *(corneal hydrops)* (Fig. 17-47). This appears to occur more often in patients with Down's syndrome.[196-199] The edema can thicken the cornea twofold to threefold but usually resolves in 2 to 3 months, leaving an apical scar (Fig. 17-48). Sometimes the vision is improved or contact lens wear is facilitated by the scarring, as a result of the flattening of the cone.

Associated conditions. Keratoconus can be associated with the following ophthalmic conditions:

Retinitis pigmentosa	Congenital cataract	Retinopathy of prematurity[298]
Leber's congenital amaurosis	Aniridia	Blue sclera
Ectopia lentis	Microcornea	Vernal keratoconjunctivitis

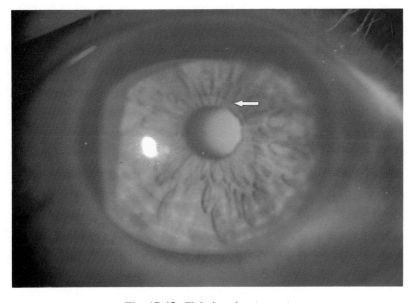

Fig. 17-45. Fleischer ring *(arrow).*

Atopic dermatitis

Other atopic diseases

Down's syndrome

Mitral valve prolapse[211]

False chordae tendinaea[299]

Marfan's syndrome[300,301]

Ehlers-Danlos syndrome[302,303]

Osteogenesis imperfecta[304]

Apert's syndrome

Noonan's syndrome[305]

Crouzon's syndrome[306]

Little's disease[303]

Duane's syndrome[307]

Addison's disease

Xeroderma pigmentosa[308]

Laurence-Moon-Bardet-Biedel syndrome[303]

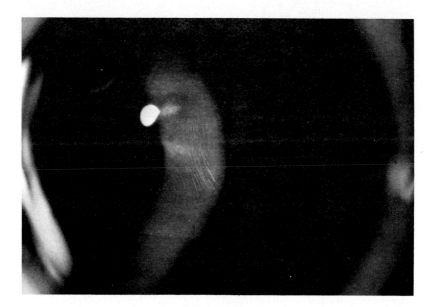

Fig. 17-46. Vogt's striae.

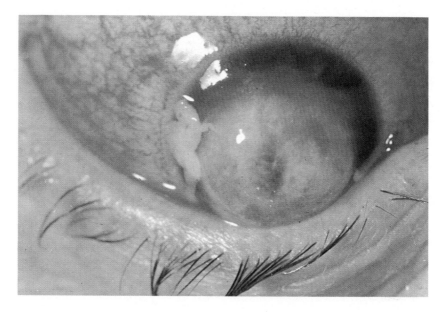

Fig. 17-47. Acute corneal hydrops.

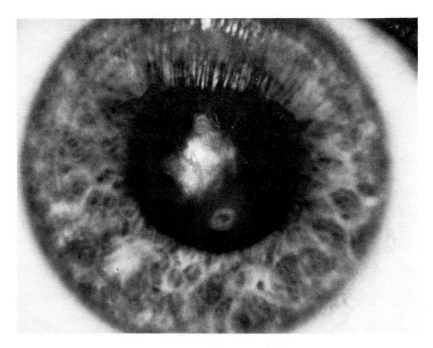

Fig. 17-48. Residual scarring from hydrops of the cornea secondary to keratoconus.

The association of keratoconus with vernal keratoconjunctivitis,[200-202] atopic dermatitis,[200,203,204] and other atopic diseases[205-207] is well documented. The relationship is unclear, but the frequency of their coexistence appears to be significantly greater than expected by chance.[208,209] Individuals with Down's syndrome are significantly more likely to have keratoconus.[195-198,210] Patients with mitral valve prolapse also appear to have a higher incidence of keratoconus.[211]

Histopathology. Fragmentation and fibrillation of Bowman's layer and the epithelial basement membrane are noted in the area of the cone (Fig. 17-49).[212-214] Interruptions of Bowman's layer are common, and scar tissue and activated keratocytes are noted in these areas.[215] Electron-dense, PAS-positive material is seen in the stroma and adjacent to the activated keratocytes.[213,214,216-218] It is presumed to be an abnormal proteoglycan.

The corneal epithelium may be irregular and thinned over the cone. Fleischer ring is seen as the accumulation of ferritin particles within and between the basal epithelial cells at the base of the cone.[212,219,220] Corneal hydrops is seen as tears in Descemet's membrane, with extension of adjacent endothelium over the exposed stroma and deposition of new Descemet's material.[221,222]

As the stroma thins, the number of corneal lamellae decreases.[214,223] The diameter of the collagen fibrils increases, as does the interfibrillary distance.[222] However, the hexagonal arrangement of the fibrils is not changed, and the distance does not increase to the point that clarity is lost. The content and distribution of the different collagen types appear to be normal.[224-226]

Biochemical studies. A variety of biochemical abnormalities have been reported in keratoconus corneas. Unfortunately, many of these have not been confirmed or have been contradicted by other studies. Increased reducible collagen cross-linking was found in one study,[227] but this was not confirmed in others.[228,229] In tissue culture some of the keratocytes were found to have defects in RNA translation, leading to reduced protein synthesis.[230] Collagenolytic activity has been consistently reported to be higher than normal.[223,231,232] Several studies have suggested that an abnormality in proteoglycans is present. Keratocyte proteoglycan metabolism was found to be abnormal,[233,234] and abnormalities were found in the glycoproteins on the surface of the keratocytes.[235] Total proteoglycan content was

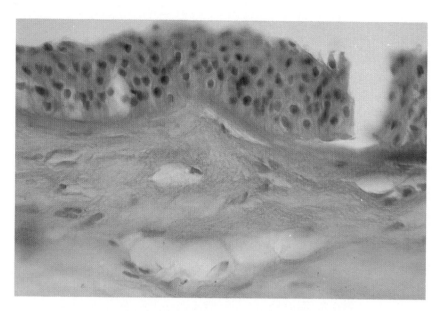

Fig. 17-49. Fragmentation and fibrillation of Bowman's layer and basement membrane in keratoconus. (From Grayson M: Degeneration, dystrophies, and edema of the cornea. In Duane TD, editor: Clinical ophthalmology, vol 4, Hagerstown, Md, 1978, Harper & Row, Publishers, Inc.)

found to be increased,[236] and an abnormal noncollagenous component of the stroma was reported.[228] Proteoglycan location, in relation to collagen fibrils, was found to be abnormal by electron histochemistry and x-ray diffraction.[237] The interaction between the collagen fibrils and proteoglycans may be important in maintaining normal corneal strength. Therefore, these abnormalities could result in stretching and thinning of the stroma.[238]

Pathogenesis. In view of the diversity of biochemical findings in keratoconus, it has been proposed that keratoconus can be caused by more than one mechanism.[237,239] Collagen may be defective in some patients; for instance, in Ehlers-Danlos type VI, in which keratoconus can occur, collagen cross-linking is deficient. Supporting this mechanism are studies that show abnormal collagen synthesis by keratocytes, abnormal cross-linking, and increased collagenolytic activity. Other studies have suggested that proteoglycan abnormalities are responsible in some patients.

The wearing of hard contact lenses also has been proposed as a cause for keratoconus. Many patients wearing hard contact lenses have developed keratoconus,[240-244] and a relatively high percentage of patients diagnosed as having keratoconus wore hard contact lenses in the past.[245,246] Certainly wearing hard contact lenses, particularly PMMA lenses, can alter the corneal surface, increasing or decreasing curvature and producing regular and irregular astigmatism (corneal warping).[247,248] Most of the time these changes disappear when the patient stops wearing contact lenses, but in some cases they are permanent.[249] Such corneal warping can appear similar to early keratoconus; however, they usually can be differentiated. Patients with corneal warping do not have corneal thinning, Descemet's striae, Fleischer rings, or other changes typical of keratoconus. Also, keratoscopy demonstrates the irregular astigmatism but not the characteristic egg-shaped mires pointing inferotemporally. Whether the full-blown clinical picture of keratoconus can be induced by wearing contact lenses remains to be determined, but it seems unlikely.

Rubbing the eyes also has been suggested as a cause of keratoconus. The evidence in favor of this is limited; many patients with atopy and Down's syndrome, which often are associated with keratoconus, rub their eyes excessively. Also, in one case an initially normal cornea developed keratoconus after intensive daily massage.[250]

Treatment. When eyeglasses are no longer sufficient to correct vision, contact lenses are indicated. Most patients with keratoconus can be fitted successfully with lenses, although it often entails a great deal of time, patience, and trial and error.[251-254] A number of authors have described fitting techniques.[255-257] In some cases this requires use of double posterior curve lenses (Soper),[256] combined soft and hard (piggyback) lenses,[258] or a hard lens with a soft peripheral skirt (for example, Softperm lens, Sola/Barnes-Hind, Sunnyvale, Calif.).

If scarring prevents adequate vision or if the patient cannot wear contact lenses, keratoplasty can be performed. Overall there is a 10% to 20% probability of a patient with keratoconus eventually requiring keratoplasty.[251,259] The prognosis for a clear graft and visual acuity of 20/40 or better is very good (greater than 80%).[260-265] The average astigmatism after surgery is greater than in other keratoplasty patients (approximately 4 to 5 diopters), and one fourth to one fifth of patients will have greater than 6 diopters of astigmatism.[259-262] Approximately 60% of patients will require contact lens fitting after keratoplasty, for correction of myopia or astigmatism or both.[253] Unfortunately, contact lens wear is associated with endothelial cell injury[266] and probably an increased risk of infection and rejection. Recurrence of keratoconus in the graft has been reported but is rare.[267,268]

Permanent mydriasis can occur after keratoplasty (Urrets-Zavalia syndrome).[269] The mechanism is unknown, but use of strong mydriatics[268] and iris ischemia caused by pressure of the corneal wound against the iris[270] have been implicated.

Lamellar keratoplasty also can be of value, but it is more difficult and the visual results are not quite as good.[271-274] Still, it may be useful, particularly in patients who cannot cooperate well with postoperative care (for example, in cases involving Down's syndrome or very large or peripheral cones).

Epikeratophakia for keratoconus is a form of onlay lamellar keratoplasty. A lamellar graft lathed to a uniform thickness of 0.3 mm is sutured on top of the cornea, to flatten the cone.[275,276] Only patients without central corneal scarring are candidates. An average of 9 diopters of corneal flattening is obtained, and approximately 80% of patients obtain 20/40 vision or better.[277,278] The rate of visual recovery varies widely but appears to be similar to that after penetrating keratoplasty. If necessary, penetrating keratoplasty can be performed after epikeratophakia, and the results appear similar to those in virgin eyes.[279] The main advantages of epikeratophakia are that it is an extraocular procedure, there is no risk of rejection, and it is technically simpler than lamellar keratoplasty. In general the reported results have been good, and my own experience is similar, but the procedure must be evaluated further to determine its value compared to keratoplasty.

Thermokeratoplasty has been used with limited success. Heat is applied to the corneal stroma, shrinking the collagen and flattening the cone.[280-282] The visual results were disappointing, and many complications occurred, including persistent epithelial defects, stromal scarring, instability of the corneal curvature, and aseptic corneal necrosis.[279,283,284]

Acute hydrops should be treated conservatively, and the patient should be assured that the condition nearly always improves. Some scarring usually remains, but in some cases the cornea is flattened, and contact lens wear is facilitated. Cycloplegia and hypertonic solutions or ointment may provide some symptomatic relief. The condition usually resolves in 8 to 10 weeks, but some cases take 6 months or more, and others never clear. If the condition is not improving after 3 months, keratoplasty is indicated.

KERATOGLOBUS

Keratoglobus is a rare, bilateral, globular corneal ectasia. The stroma is diffusely thinned to one third to one fifth normal thickness and is often thinnest in the periphery (Figs. 17-50 and 17-51). The cornea is transparent, and its diameter is normal. The intraocular pressure is normal. The corneal ectasia can lead to high myopia and astigmatism (Fig. 17-52). Acute hydrops can occur,[285] and perforation after minimal trauma has occurred in most reported cases.[286-289] Pathologic examination has

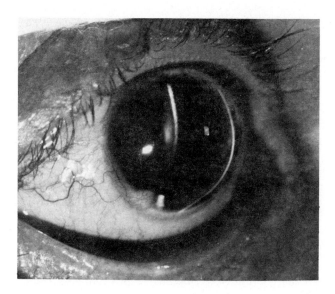

Fig. 17-50. Diffusely thin and ectatic cornea in keratoglobus.

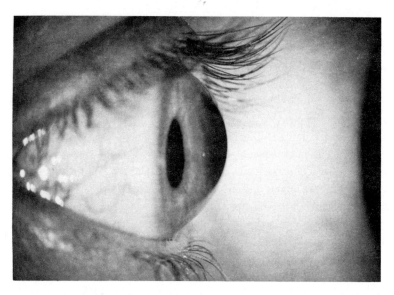

Fig. 17-51. Globular cornea in keratoglobus.

demonstrated focal breaks in or absence of Bowman's layer and stromal thinning to one third to one fifth normal thickness.[288,290]

Keratoglobus can be associated with Leber's congenital amaurosis,[291,292] blue sclera, hyperextensibility of the joints of the hand and ankles, sensorineural hearing defects, and mottling of the teeth (Fig. 17-53).[285,287,288] Keratoconus and keratoglobus have been observed in different members of the same family; in one family the father had keratoglobus and a son had keratoconus,[293] and in another family a brother had keratoglobus and a sister had keratoconus.[294] Treatment options are limited and not very successful. Contact lens wear is not recommended because of the risk of perforation, but it

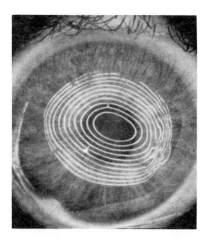

Fig. 17-52. Marked astigmatism in keratoglobus.

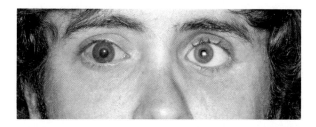

Fig. 17-53. Individual with keratoglobus, blue sclera (right eye), and hyperextensible joints. Left eye was enucleated as a result of rupture after minor trauma.

usually is not possible anyway. Total keratoplasty can be performed, but the sclera often is thin as well, making closure difficult. If surgery is necessary, onlay lamellar keratoplasty (that is, epikeratophakia) may be preferable. A penetrating graft can be performed later into the thickened bed.

Differential diagnosis. It is important to differentiate among keratoglobus, keratectasia, and congenital anterior staphyloma. In keratectasia the cornea is bulging, protruding through the lids, and is opaque, with variable thinning and scarring of the stroma. It usually occurs unilaterally. If the ectatic cornea also contains uveal tissue, the condition is called congenital anterior staphyloma. Megalocornea may appear similar to keratoglobus, but the corneal diameter is normal in keratoglobus. The normal diameter and normal intraocular pressure differentiate keratoglobus from congenital glaucoma.

POSTERIOR KERATOCONUS

Posterior keratoconus is a rare condition characterized by a focal or generalized increase in the curvature of the posterior corneal surface, with normal curvature of the anterior surface.[295-297] It is more commonly unilateral then bilateral. The condition usually is present at birth and is nonprogressive. It most likely is a form of dysgenesis and thus is discussed in Chapter 5.

REFERENCES

1. Pameijer JK: Ueber eine Fremdartige Familiäre Oberflächliche Hornhautveränderung, Klin Monatsbl Augenheilkd 95:516, 1935.

2. Meesmann A: Ueber eine Bisher Nicht Beschriebene Dominant Vererbte Dystrophia Epithelialis Corneae, Ber Dtsch Ophthalmol Ges 52:154, 1938.

3. Meesmann A and Wilke F: Klinische und Anatomische

Untersuchungen Über eine Bisher Unbekannte, Dominant Vererbte Epitheldystrophie der Hornhaut, Klin Monatsbl Augenheilkd 103:361, 1939.

4. Kuwabara R and Ciccarelli EC: Meesmann's corneal dystrophy, Arch Ophthalmol 71:676, 1964.

5. Stocker FW and Holt LB: Rare form of hereditary epithelial dystrophy, Arch Ophthalmol 53:536, 1955.

6. Snyder WB: Hereditary epithelial corneal dystrophy, Am J Ophthalmol 55:56, 1963.

7. Wittebol-Post D, van Bijsterveld OP, and Delleman JW: Meesmann's epithelial dystrophy of the cornea: biometrics and a hypothesis, Ophthalmologica 194:44, 1987.

8. Tripathi RG and Bron AJ: Cystic disorders of the corneal epithelium. II. Pathogenesis, Br J Ophthalmol 57:375, 1973.

9. Bron AJ and Brown NA: Some superficial corneal disorders, Trans Ophthalmol Soc UK 91:13, 1971.

10. Cogan DG et al: Microcystic dystrophy of the corneal epithelium, Trans Am Ophthalmol Soc 62:213, 1964.

11. Fine BS et al: Meesmann's epithelial dystrophy of the cornea, Am J Ophthalmol 83:633, 1977.

12. Burns RP: Meesmann's corneal dystrophy, Trans Am Ophthalmol Soc 66:531, 1968.

13. Tremblay M and Dubé I: Meesmann's corneal dystrophy: ultrastructural features, Can J Ophthalmol 17:24, 1982.

14. Nakaniski I and Brown SI: Ultrastructure of epithelial dystrophy of Meesmann, Arch Ophthalmol 93:259, 1975.

15. Bourne WM: Soft contact lens wear decreases epithelial microcysts in Meesmann's corneal dystrophy, Trans Am Ophthalmol Soc 84:170, 1986.

16. Cogan DG et al: Microcystic dystrophy of the cornea, Arch Ophthalmol 92:470, 1974.

17. King RG Jr and Geeraets R: Cogan-Guerry microcystic corneal epithelial dystrophy, Med Coll Va Q 8:241, 1972.

18. Trobe JD and Laibson PR: Dystrophic changes in the anterior cornea, Arch Ophthalmol 87:378, 1972.

19. Wolter JR and Fralick FB: Microcystic dystrophy of the corneal epithelium, Arch Ophthalmol 75:380, 1966.

20. Laibson PR and Krachmer JH: Familial occurrence of dot, map, and fingerprint dystrophy of the cornea, Invest Ophthalmol 14:397, 1975.

21. Franceschetti A: Hereditäre Rezidivierende Erosion der Hornhaut, Z Augenheilkd 66:309, 1928.

22. Bron AJ and Burgess SEP: Inherited recurrent corneal erosion, Trans Ophthalmol Soc UK 101:239, 1981.

23. Bron AJ and Tripathi RC: Anterior corneal mosaic: further observations, Br J Ophthalmol 53:760, 1969.

24. Bron AJ and Tripathi RC: Cystic disorders of the corneal epithelium. I. Clinical aspects, Br J Ophthalmol 53:760, 1969.

25. Waring GO, Rodriquez MM, and Laibson PR: Corneal dystrophies. I. Dystrophies of the epithelium, Bowman's layer, and stroma, Surv Ophthalmol 23:71, 1978.

26. Brown NA and Bron AJ: Recurrent erosion of the cornea, Br J Ophthalmol 60:84 1976.

27. Nelson JD et al: Map-dot-fingerprint changes in the corneal epithelial basement membrane following radial keratotomy, Ophthalmology 92:199, 1985.

28. Polack FM: Contributions of electron microscopy to the study of corneal pathology, Surv Ophthalmol 20:375, 1976.

29. Broderick JD, Dark AJ, and Peace GW: Fingerprint dystrophy of the cornea, Arch Ophthalmol 92:483, 1974.

30. Dark AJ: Bleb dystrophy of the cornea: histochemistry and ultrastructure, Br J Ophthalmol 61:65, 1977.

31. Reis W: Familiäre, Fleckige Hornhautentartung, Dtsch Med Wochenschr 43:575, 1917.

32. Bücklers M: Ueber eine Weitere Familiäre Hornhautdystrophie (Reis), Klin Monatsbl Augenheilkd 114:386, 1949.

33. Rice NSC et al: Reis-Bücklers' dystrophy, Br J Ophthalmol 52:577, 1968.

34. Jones ST and Stauffer LH: Reis-Bücklers' corneal dystrophy, Trans Am Acad Ophthalmol Otolaryngol 74:417, 1970.

35. Paufique L and Bonnet M: La dystrophie cornéenne hérédo-familiale de Reis-Bücklers, Ann Oculist 199:14, 1966.

36. Hall P: Reis-Bücklers' dystrophy, Arch Ophthalmol 91:170, 1974.

37. Kaufman HG and Clowe FW: Irregularities of Bowman's membrane, Am J Ophthalmol 62:227, 1966.

38. Wittebol-Post D, van Bijsterveld OP, and Delleman JM: The honeycomb type of Reis-Bücklers' dystrophy of the cornea: biometrics and interpretation, Ophthalmologica 194:65, 1987.

39. Griffith DG and Fine BS: Light and electron microscopic observations in a superficial corneal dystrophy, Am J Ophthalmol 63:1659, 1967.

40. Hogan M and Wood I: Reis-Bücklers' corneal dystrophy, Trans Ophthalmol Soc UK 91:41, 1971.

41. Kanai A, Kaufman HE, and Polack FM: Electron microscopic study of Reis-Bücklers' dystrophy, Ann Ophthalmol 5:953, 1973.

42. Perry HD, Fine BS, and Caldwell CR: Reis-Bücklers' dystrophy, Arch Ophthalmol 97:664, 1979.

43. Yamaguchi T, Polack F, and Valenti J: Reis-Bücklers' corneal dystrophy, Am J Ophthalmol 90:95, 1980.

44. Olson RJ and Kaufman HE: Recurrence of Reis-Bücklers' corneal dystrophy in a graft, Am J Ophthalmol 85:349, 1978.

45. Caldwell DR: Postoperative recurrence of Reis-Bücklers' corneal dystrophy, Am J Ophthalmol 85:567, 1978.

46. Wood TO et al: Treatment of Reis-Bücklers' corneal dystrophy by removal of subepithelial fibrous tissue, Am J Ophthalmol 85:360, 1978.

47. Wagoner MD and Kenyon KR: Stripping of subepithelial fibrous tissue for treatment of anterior corneal dystrophies, Ophthalmology 91(suppl):122, 1984.

48. Schwartz MF and Taylor HR: Surgical management of Reis-Bücklers' corneal dystrophy, Cornea 4:100, 1985.

49. Yamaguchi T, Polack FM, and Valenti J: Electron microscopic study of recurrent Reis-Bčklers' corneal dystrophy, Am J Ophthalmol 90:95, 1980.

50. Grayson M and Wilbrandt H: Dystrophy of the anterior

limiting membrane of the cornea (Reis-Bücklers' type), Am J Ophthalmol 63:345, 1966.

51. Thiel HJ and Behnke H: Eine Bisher Unbekannte Subepitheliale Hereditäre Hornhautdystrophie, Klin Monatsbl Augenheilkd 150:862, 1967.

52. Yamaguchi T, Polack FM, Rowsey JJ: Honeycomb-shaped corneal dystrophy: a variation of Reis-Bücklers' dystrophy, Cornea 1:71, 1982.

53. Streiff EB and Zwahlen P: Une famille avec dégénérescence en bandelette de la cornée, Ophthalmologica (Paris) 111:129, 1947.

54. Glees M: Ueber Familiaeres Auftreten der Primaeren, Bandfoermigen Hornhoatdegeneration, Klin Monatsbl Augenheilkd 116:185, 1950.

55. Duke-Elder S and Leigh AG: System of ophthalmology, vol 8, Diseases of the outer eye, St Louis, 1965, Mosby–Year Book, Inc.

56. Meisler DM et al: Familial band-shaped nodular keratopathy, Ophthalmology 92:217, 1985.

57. Rodrigues MM, Calhoun J, and Harley RD: Corneal clouding with increased acid mucopolysaccharide accumulation in Bowman's membrane, Am J Ophthalmol 79:916, 1975.

58. Waardenburg PJ and Jonkers GH: A specific type of dominant progressive dystrophy of the cornea, developing after birth, Acta Ophthalmol (Copenh) 39:919, 1961.

59. Haddad R, Font RL, and Fine BS: Unusual superficial variant of granular dystrophy of the cornea, Am J Ophthalmol 83:213, 1977.

60. Rodrigues MM, Gaster RN, and Pratt MV: Unusual superficial confluent form of granular corneal dystrophy, Ophthalmology 90:1507, 1983.

61. Forsius H et al: Granular corneal dystrophy with late manifestation, Acta Ophthalmol (Copenh) 61:514, 1983.

62. Garner A and Tripathi RD: Hereditary crystalline stromal dystrophy of Schnyder. II. Histopathology and ultrastructure, Br J Ophthalmol 56:400, 1972.

63. Jones ST and Zimmerman LE: Histopathologic differentiation of granular, macular, and lattice dystrophies of the cornea, Am J Ophthalmol 51:394, 1961.

64. Garner A: Histochemistry of corneal macular dystrophy, Invest Ophthalmol 8:473, 1969.

65. Iwamoto T et al: Ultrastructural variations in granular dystrophy of the cornea, Graefes Arch Clin Exp Ophthalmol 194:1, 1975.

66. Sornson E: Granular dystrophy of the cornea: an electron microscopic study, Am J Ophthalmol 59:1001, 1965.

67. Wittebol-Post D, van der Want JJ, and van Bijsterveld OP: Granular dystrophy of the cornea (Groenouw type I): is the keratocyte the primary source after all? Ophthalmologica 195:169, 1987.

68. Garner A: Histochemistry of corneal granular dystrophy, Br J Ophthalmol 53:799, 1969.

69. Rodrigues MM et al: Microfibrillar protein and phospholipid in granular corneal dystrophy, Arch Ophthalmol 101:802, 1983.

70. Johnson BL, Brown SI, and Zaidman GW: A light and electron microscopic study of recurrent granular dystrophy of the cornea, Am J Ophthalmol 92:49, 1981.

71. Moller HU and Ehlers N: Early treatment of granular dystrophy (Groenouw type I), Acta Ophthalmol (Copenh) 63:597, 1985.

72. Brownstein S et al: Granular dystrophy of the cornea: electron microscopic confirmation of recurrence in a graft, Am J Ophthalmol 77:701, 1974.

73. Herman SJ and Hughes WF: Recurrence of hereditary corneal dystrophy following keratoplasty, Am J Ophthalmol 75:689, 1973.

74. Pouliquen Y et al: Ophthalmol Clinic, Hotel-Dieu, Place de Parvis, Notre-Dame, Paris, Exp Eye Res 18:163, 1974.

75. Rodrigues MM and McGavic JS: Recurrent corneal granular dystrophy: a clinicopathologic study, Trans Am Ophthalmol Soc 73:306, 1975.

76. Stuart JC and Mund ML: Recurrent granular corneal dystrophy, Am J Ophthalmol 79:18, 1975.

77. Tripathi R and Garner A: Corneal granular dystrophy: a light and electron microscope study of its recurrence in a graft, Br J Ophthalmol 54:361, 1970.

78. Lempert SL et al: A simple technique for removal of recurring granular dystrophy in corneal grafts, Am J Ophthalmol 86:89, 1978.

79. Witschel H and Sundmacher R: Bilateral recurrence of granular dystrophy in the grafts. Graefes Arch Clin Exp Ophthalmol 209:179, 1979.

80. Klintworth GK: Lattice corneal dystrophy: an inherited variety of amyloidosis restricted to the cornea, Am J Pathol 50:371, 1967.

81. Rabb MR, Blodi F, and Boniuk M: Unilateral lattice dystrophy of the cornea, Trans Am Acad Ophthalmol Otolaryngol 78:440, 1974.

82. Reshmi CS and English FP: Unilateral lattice dystrophy of the cornea, Med J Aust 1:966, 1971.

83. Mehta RF: Unilateral lattice dystrophy of the cornea, Br J Ophthalmol 64:53, 1980.

84. Stansbury FC: Lattice type of hereditary corneal degeneration: report of five cases, including one of a child of two years, Arch Ophthalmol 40:189, 1974.

85. Dubord PF and Krachmer JH: Diagnosis of early lattice corneal dystrophy, Arch Ophthalmol 100:788, 1982.

86. Kani A et al: Clinical and histopathological studies of the lattice dystrophy of the cornea, Acta Soc Ophthalmol Jpn 17:357, 1973.

87. Yanoff M et al: Lattice corneal dystrophy: report of an unusual case, Arch Ophthalmol 95:651, 1977.

88. Fogle JA et al: Defective epithelial adhesion in anterior corneal dystrophies, Am J Ophthalmol 79:925, 1975.

89. Zechner EM, Croxatto JO, and Malbran ES: Superficial involvement in lattice corneal dystrophy, Ophthalmolgica 193:193, 1986.

90. François J and Fehér J: Light microscopical and polarization optical study of lattice dystrophy of the cornea, Ophthalmologica 164:1, 1972.

91. Hogan M and Alvarado S: Ultrastructure of lattice dystrophy of the cornea: a case report, Am J Ophthalmol 64:656, 1967.

92. Smith M and Zimmerman L: Amyloid in corneal dystrophies, Arch Ophthalmol 79:407, 1968.

93. Bowen RA et al: Lattice dystrophy of the cornea as a variety of amyloidosis, Am J Ophthalmol 7:822, 1970.

94. McTigue J: The human cornea: a light and electron microscopic study of the normal cornea and its alterations in various dystrophies, Trans Am Acad Ophthalmol Otolaryngol 65:591, 1968.

95. François J, Hanssens M, and Teuchy H: Ultrastructural changes in lattice dystrophy of the cornea, Ophthalmic Res 7:321, 1975.

96. McTigue JW and Fine BS: The stromal lesion in lattice dystrophy of the cornea: a light and electron microscopic study, Invest Ophthalmol 3:355, 1964.

97. McMullan FD et al: Corneal amyloidosis: an immunohistochemical analysis, Invest Ophthalmol Vis Sci 25(suppl):6, 1984.

98. Rodrigues MM et al: Lack of evidence for AA reactivity in amyloid deposits of lattice corneal dystrophy and corneal amyloid degeneration, Invest Ophthalmol Vis Sci 25(suppl):6, 1984.

99. Meretoja J: Familial systemic paramyloidosis with lattice dystrophy of the cornea, progressive cranial neuropathy, skin changes and various internal symptoms: a previously unrecognized heritable syndrome, Ann Clin Res 1:314, 1969.

100. Meretoja J: Comparative histopathological and clinical findings in eyes with lattice corneal dystrophy of two types, Ophthalmologica 165:15, 1972.

101. Meretoja J: Genetic aspects of familial amyloidosis with corneal lattice dystrophy and cranial neuropathy, Clin Genet 4:173, 1973.

102. Purcell JJ et al: Lattice corneal dystrophy associated with familial systemic amyloidosis (Meretoja's syndrome), Ophthalmology 90:1512, 1983.

103. Maury CP et al: Amyloid fibril protein in familial amyloidosis with cranial neuropathy and corneal lattice dystrophy (FAP type IV) is related to transthyretin, Am J Clin Pathol 89:359, 1988.

104. Hida T et al: Clinical features of a newly recognized type of lattice corneal dystrophy, Am J Ophthalmol 104:241, 1987.

105. Hida T et al: Histopathologic and immunochemical features of lattice corneal dystrophy type III, Am J Ophthalmol 104:249, 1987.

106. Mannis MJ et al: Polymorphic amyloid degeneration of the cornea, Arch Ophthalmol 99:1217, 1981.

107. Lorenzetti DWC and Kaufman HE: Macular lattice dystrophies and their recurrences after keratoplasty, Trans Am Acad Ophthalmol Otolaryngol 71:112, 1967.

108. Lanier JD, Fine M, and Togni B: Lattice corneal dystrophy, Arch Ophthalmol 94:921, 1976.

109. Meisler DM and Fine M: Recurrence of the clinical signs of lattice corneal dystrophy (type I) in corneal transplants, Am J Ophthalmol 97:210, 1984.

110. Nakaizumi K: A rare case of corneal dystrophy, Nippon Ganka Gakkai Zasshi 18:949, 1914.

111. Akiya S, Ito I, and Matsui M: Gelatinous drop-like dystrophy of the cornea, Jpn J Clin Ophthalmol 26:815, 1972.

112. Kirk HQ et al: Primary familial amyloidosis of the cornea, Trans Am Acad Ophthalmol Otolaryngol 77:411, 1973.

113. Stock EI and Kielar RA: Primary familial amyloidosis of the cornea, Am J Ophthalmol 82:266, 1976.

114. Nagataki S, Tanishima T, and Sakomoto T: A case of primary gelatinous drop-like corneal dystrophy, Jpn J Ophthalmol 16:107, 1972.

115. Weber FL and Babel J: Gelatinous drop-like dystrophy, Arch Ophthalmol 98:144, 1980.

116. Gartry DS, Falcon MG, and Cox RW: Primary gelatinous drop-like keratopathy, Br J Ophthalmol 73:661, 1989.

117. Ramsey MS and Fine BS: Localized corneal amyloidosis, Am J Ophthalmol 75:560, 1972.

118. Kanai A and Kaufman HE: Electron microscopic studies of primary band-shaped keratopathy and gelatinous drop-like corneal dystrophy in two brothers, Ann Ophthalmol 14:535, 1982.

119. Matsui M, Ito K, and Akiua S: Histochemical and electron microscopic examinations on so-called gelatinous drop-like dystrophy of the cornea, Folia Ophthalmol Jpn 23:466, 1972.

120. Ehlers N and Bramsen T: Central thickness in corneal disorders, Acta Ophthalmol 56:412, 1978.

121. Donnenfeld ED et al: Corneal thinning in macular corneal dystrophy, Am J Ophthalmol 101:112, 1986.

122. Livni N, Abraham FA, and Zauberman H: Groenouw's macular dystrophy: histochemistry and ultrastructure of the cornea, Doc Ophthalmol 37:327, 1974.

123. Snip RC, Kenyon KR, and Green RD: Macular corneal dystrophy: ultrastructural pathology of the corneal endothelium and Descemet's membrane, Invest Ophthalmol 12:88, 1973.

124. Teng CC: Macular dystrophy of the cornea: a histochemical and electron microscopic study, Am J Ophthalmol 62:436, 1966.

125. Morgan G: Macular dystrophy of the cornea, Br J Ophthalmol 50:57, 1966.

126. Klintworth GK and Vogel FS: Macular corneal dystrophy: an inherited acid mucopolysaccharide storage disease of corneal fibroblasts, Am J Pathol 45:565, 1964.

127. François J et al: Ultrastructural findings in macular dystrophy (Groenouw type II), Ophthalmic Res 7:80, 1975.

128. Klintworth GK and Smith CF: Abnormalities of proteoglycans and glycoproteins synthesized by corneal organ cultures derived from patients with macular corneal dystrophy, Lab Invest 48:603, 1983.

129. Hassell JR et al: Macular corneal dystrophy: failure to synthesize a mature keratan sulfate proteoglycan, Proc Natl Acad Sci USA 77:3705, 1980.

130. Hassell JR et al: Defective conversion of a glycoprotein precursor to keratan sulfate proteoglycan in macular corneal dystrophy. In Hawkes S and Wang JL, editors: Extracellular matrix, New York, 1982, Academic Press, Inc.

131. Yang CJ et al: Immunohistochemical evidence of heterogeneity in macular corneal dystrophy, Am J Ophthalmol 106:65, 1988.

132. Edward DP et al: Heterogeneity in macular corneal dystrophy, Arch Ophthalmol 106:1579, 1988.

133. Thonar EJ et al: Absence of normal keratan sulfate in the blood of patients with macular corneal dystrophy, Am J Ophthalmol 102:561, 1986.

134. Sundar-Raj N et al: Macular corneal dystrophy: immu-

nochemical characterization using monoclonal antibodies, Invest Ophthalmol Vis Sci 28:1678, 1987.

135. Robin AL et al: Recurrence of macular corneal dystrophy after lamellar keratoplasty, Am J Ophthalmol 84:457, 1977.

136. Klintworth GK et al: Recurrence of macular corneal dystrophy within grafts, Am J Ophthalmol 95:60, 1983.

137. Streeten BW and Falls HF: Hereditary fleck dystrophy of the cornea, Am J Ophthalmol 51:275, 1961.

138. Collier M: Dystrophie nuageuse centrale et dystrophie ponctiforme prédescemédans une même famille, Bull Soc Ophthalmol Fr 66:575, 1966.

139. Birndoft LA and Ginsberg SP: Hereditary fleck dystrophy associated with decreased corneal sensitivity, Am J Ophthalmol 73:670, 1972.

140. Aracena T: Hereditary fleck dystrophy of the cornea: report of a family, J Pediatr Ophthalmol 12:223, 1975.

141. Patten JT et al: Fleck (Mouchetée) dystrophy of the cornea, Ann Ophthalmol 8:25, 1976.

142. Goldberg MF et al: Variable expression in flecked (speckled) dystrophy of the cornea, Ann Ophthalmol 9:889, 1977.

143. Purcell JJ Jr, Krachmer JH, and Weingeist TA: Fleck corneal dystrophy, Arch Ophthalmol 95:440, 1977.

144. François J and Neetens A: Nouvelle dystrophie hérédo-familiale de parenchyme cornéen (hérédo-dystrophie Mouchetée), Bull Soc Belge Ophthalmol 114:641, 1957.

145. Gillespie F and Covelli B: Fleck (Mouchetée) dystrophy of the cornea: report of a family, South Med J 56:1265, 1963.

146. Stankovic I and Stojanovic D: L'hérédodystrophie Mouchetée du parenchyme cornéen, Ann Oculist (Paris) 197:52, 1964.

147. Nicholson DH, Green WR, and Cross HE: A clinical and histopathological study of François-Neetens speckled corneal dystrophy, Am J Ophthalmol 83:554, 1977.

148. Kiskaddon BM et al: Fleck dystrophy of the cornea: case report, Ann Ophthalmol 12:700, 1980.

149. Van Went JM and Wibaut F: Een zeldzane erfelijke hoornvliesaandoenig, Ned Tijdschr Geenskd 68:2996, 1924.

150. Ehlers N and Matthiessen M: Hereditary crystalline dystrophy of Schnyder, Acta Ophthalmol (Copenh) 51:1, 1967.

151. Luxenburg M: Hereditary crystalline dystrophy of the cornea, Am J Ophthalmol 63:507, 1967.

152. Kaseras A and Price A: Central crystalline corneal dystrophy, Br J Ophthalmol 54:659, 1970.

153. Bron AJ, Williams HP, and Carruthers ME: Hereditary crystalline stromal dystrophy of Schnyder: clinical features of a family with hyperlipoproteinemia, Br J Ophthalmol 56:383, 1972.

154. Grop K: Clinical and histologic findings in crystalline corneal dystrophy, Acta Ophthalmol (Copenh) 51(suppl 120):52, 1973.

155. Delleman JW and Winkelman JE: Degeneratio corneae cristallinea hereditaria: a clinical, genetical, and histological study, Ophthalmologica 155:409, 1968.

156. Lisch W et al: Schnyder's dystrophy: progression and metabolism, Ophthalmic Paediatr Genet 7:45, 1986.

157. Fry WE and Pickett WE: Crystalline dystrophy of the cornea, Trans Am Ophthalmol Soc 48:220, 1950.

158. Weller RO and Rodger FC: Crystalline stromal dystrophy: histochemistry and ultrastructure of the cornea, Br J Ophthalmol 64:46, 1980.

159. Rodrigues MM, et al: Unesterified cholesterol in Schnyder's corneal crystalline dystrophy, Am J Ophthalmol 104:157, 1987.

160. Freddo TF, Polack FM, and Leibowitz HM: Ultrastructural changes in the posterior layers of the cornea in Schnyder's crystalline dystrophy, Cornea 8:170, 1989.

161. Ghosh M and McCulloch C: Crystalline dystrophy of the cornea: a light and electron microscopic study, Can J Ophthalmol 12:321, 1977.

162. Burns RP, Connor W, and Gipson I: Cholesterol turnover in hereditary crystalline corneal dystrophy of Schnyder, Trans Am Ophthalmol Soc 76:184, 1978.

163. Bagolini B and Ioli-Spada G: Bietti's tapetoretinal degeneration with marginal corneal dystrophy, Am J Ophthalmol 65:53, 1968.

164. Harrison RJ, Acheson RR, and Dean-Hart JC: Bietti's tapetoretinal degeneration with marginal corneal dystrophy (crystalline retinopathy): case report, Br J Ophthalmol 71:220, 1987.

165. Wilson DJ et al: Bietti's crystalline dystrophy: a clinicopathologic correlative study, Arch Ophthalmol 107:213, 1989.

166. Strachan IM: Central cloudy corneal dystrophy of François: five cases in the same family, Br J Ophthalmol 53:192, 1969.

167. Bramsen T, Ehlers N, and Baggesen KH: Central cloudy corneal dystrophy of François, Acta Ophthalmol (Copenh) 54:221, 1976.

168. Collier MT: Dystrophie moucheté du parenchyme cornéen avec dystrophie nuageuse centrale, Bull Soc Ophtalmol Fr 64:608, 1964.

169. Collier MT: Elastorrhexie systée et dystrophies cornéennes chez deux soerus, Bull Soc Ophtalmol Fr 65:301, 1965.

170. Pillat A: Zur frage der familiúaren Hornhautentartung: ueber eine einzigartige tiefe scholige und periphere gitterförmige familife Hornhautdystrophie, Klin Monatsbl Augenheilkd 104:571, 1939.

171. Strachan IM: Pre-Descemetic corneal dystrophy, Br J Ophthalmol 52:716, 1968.

172. Thomsitt J and Bron AJ: Polymorphic stromal dystrophy, Br J Ophthalmol 59:125, 1975.

173. Carpel EF, Sigelman RJ, and Doughman DJ: Posterior amorphous corneal dystrophy, Am J Ophthalmol 83:629, 1977.

174. Dunn SP, Krachmer JH, and Ching SS: New findings in posterior amorphous dystrophy, Arch Ophthalmol 102:236, 1984.

175. Collier M: Caracére hérédo-familial de la dystrophie ponctiforme prédescemétique, Bull Soc Ophtalmol Fr 64:731, 1964.

176. Collier M: Dystrophie nuageuse centrale et dystrophie ponctiforme prédescemétique, Bull Soc Ophtalmol Fr 64:1034, 1964.

177. Fernandez-Sasso D, Acosta JEP, and Malbran E: Punctiform and polychromatic pre-Descemet's domi-

nant corneal dystrophy, Br J Ophthalmol 63:336, 1979.

178. Grayson M and Wilbrandt H: Pre-Descemet dystrophy, Am J Ophthalmol 64:276, 1967.

179. Curran RE, Kenyon KR, and Green WR: Pre-Descemet's membrane corneal dystrophy, Am J Ophthalmol 77:711, 1974.

180. Maeder G and Danis P: Surune nouvelle forme de dystrophie cornéene (dystrophia filiformis profunda corneae) associé à un kératocône, Ophthalmologica 114:246, 1947.

181. Franceschetti A and Maeder G: Dystrophie profonde de la cornée dans un cad d'ichtyose congénitale, Bull Mem Soc Fr Ophthalmol 67:146, 1954.

182. Franceschetti A and Schlaeppi V: Dégénérescence en bandelettes et dystrophie prédescemétique de la cornée dans un cas d'ichyhyose congénitale, Dermatologica 115:217, 1957.

183. Sever RJ, Frost P, and Weinstein G: Eye changes in ichthyosis, JAMA 206:2283, 1968.

184. Falls HF and Allen AW: Dominantly inherited keratoconus: report of a family, J Genet Hum 17:317, 1969.

185. Redmond KB: The role of heredity in keratoconus, Trans Ophthalmol Soc NZ 27:52, 1968.

186. Rudemann AD: Clinical course of keratoconus, Trans Am Acad Ophthalmol Otolaryngol 74:384, 1970.

187. Hammerstein W: Zur Genetik des Keratoconus, Graefes Arch Clin Exp Ophthalmol 190:293, 1974.

188. Hallermann W and Wilson EJ: Genetische betrachtugen uber den keratokonus, Klin Monatsbl Augenheilkd 170:906, 1977.

189. Rabinowitz YS et al: Corneal topography in family members of patients with keratoconus using computer-assisted corneal topography analysis, Invest Ophthalmol Vis Sci 30(suppl):188, 1989.

190. Ihalainen A: Clinical and epidemiological features of keratoconus: genetic and external factors in the pathogenesis of the disease, Acta Ophthalmol [Suppl] (Copenh) 178:1, 1986.

191. Rowsey JJ, Reynold AE, and Brown R: Corneal topography, Arch Ophthalmol 99:1093, 1981.

192. Maguire LJ and Bourne WD: Corneal topography of early keratoconus, Am J Ophthalmol 108:107, 1989.

193. Rabinowitz YS and McDonnell PJ: Computer-assisted corneal topography in keratoconus, J Refract Corneal Surg 5:400, 1989.

194. Shapiro MB et al: Anterior clear spaces in keratoconus, Ophthalmology 93:1316, 1986.

195. Zabala M and Archila EA: Corneal sensitivity and topogometry in keratoconus, CLAO J 14:210, 1988.

196. Cullen TF and Butler HG: Mongolism (Down's syndrome) and keratoconus, Br J Ophthalmol 47:321, 1963.

197. Slusher MM, Laibson PR, and Mulberger KD: Acute keratoconus in Down's syndrome, Am J Ophthalmol 63:1137, 1968.

198. Pierse D and Eustace P: Acute keratoconus in mongols, Br J Ophthalmol 55:50, 1971.

199. Walsh SZ: Keratoconus and blindness in 469 institutionalized subjects with Down's syndrome and other causes of mental retardation, J Ment Defic Res 25:243, 1981.

200. Gonzales JJ: Keratoconus consecutive to vernal conjunctivitis, Am J Ophthalmol 3:127, 1920.

201. Copeman PWM: Eczema and keratoconus, Br Med J 2:977, 1965.

202. Tabbara K and Butrus S: Vernal conjunctivitis and keratoconus, Am J Ophthalmol 95:704, 1983.

203. Bereston ES and Baer RL: Keratoconus associated with atopic dermatitis: report of two cases, Arch Dermatol Syphilol 46:358, 1942.

204. Spencer WH and Fisher JJ: The association of keratoconus with atopic dermatitis, Am J Ophthalmol 47:332, 1959.

205. Galin MR and Berger R: Atopy and keratoconus, Am J Ophthalmol 45:904, 1958.

206. Sabiston DW: The association of keratoconus, dermatitis, and asthma, Trans Ophthalmol Soc NZ 18:66, 1966.

207. Gasset AR, Hison WA, and Frias JL: Keratoconus and atopic disease, Ann Ophthalmol 10:991, 1978.

208. Bietti GB and Ferraboschi C: Sur l'association de keratone avec le catarrhe printanier et sur son evidence statistique, Bull Mem Soc Fr Ophtalmol 71:185, 1958.

209. Rahi A et al: Keratoconus and coexisting atopic disease, Br J Ophthalmol 61:761, 1977.

210. Shapiro MB and France T: The ocular features of Down's syndrome, Am J Ophthalmol 99:659, 1985.

211. Beardsley SL and Foulks GN: An association of keratoconus and mitral valve prolapse, Ophthalmology 89:35, 1982.

212. Caffi M: Histopathology of keratoconus, Ann Oftalmol Clin Ocul 92:429, 1966.

213. McPherson SD and Kiffney GT: Some histologic findings in keratoconus, Arch Ophthalmol 79:669, 1968.

214. Pataa C, Joyon L, and Roucher RF: Ultra-structure du keratoconus. Arch Ophthalmol (Paris) 30:403, 1970.

215. Pouliquen Y: Les fibrocytes dans le keratocone. Aspect morphologique et modification de L'espace extracellulaire. Etude en microscopie optique et electronique, Arch Ophtalmol (Paris) 32:571, 1972.

216. Teng CC: Electron microscopic study of the pathology of keratoconus. I, Am J Ophthalmol 55:18, 1963.

217. Gottinger W and Aubock L: Elektronmikroskopische Benfunde bei Keratoconus, Klin Monatsbl Augenheilkd 157:762, 1970.

218. Pouliquen Y et al: Les dépots extracellulaires du stroma corneen dans le keratocone. Etude au microscope electronique, Arch Ophtalmol (Paris) 28:282, 1968.

219. Iwamoto R and DeVoe GA: Electron microscopic study of the Fleischer ring, Arch Ophthalmol 94:1579, 1976.

220. Barraquer-Somers E, Chan CC, and Green WR: Corneal epithelial iron deposition, Ophthalmology 90:729, 1983.

221. Stone DK, Kenyon KR, and Stark WJ: Ultrastructure of keratoconus with healed hydrops, Am J Ophthalmol 82:450, 1976.

222. Waring G, Laibson P, and Rodriques M: Clinical and pathologic alterations of Descemet's membrane with emphasis on endothelial metaplasia, Surv Ophthalmol 18:325, 1974.

223. Pouliquen Y: Keratoconus: Doyne lecture, Eye 1:1, 1987.

224. Newsome DA et al: Detection of specific collagen types in normal and keratoconus corneas, Invest Ophthalmol Vis Sci 20:738, 1981.

225. Nakayasu K et al: Distribution of types I, II, III, IV, and V collagen in normal and keratoconus corneas, Ophthalmic Res 18:1, 1986.

226. Zimmerman DR et al: Comparative studies of collagens in normal and keratoconus corneas, Exp Eye Res 46:431, 1988.

227. Cannon DT and Foster CS: Collagen cross-linking in keratoconus, Invest Ophthalmol Vis Sci 17:63, 1978.

228. Oxlund H and Simonsen AH: Biochemical studies of normal and keratoconus corneas, Acta Ophthalmol (Copenh) 63:666, 1985.

229. Critchfield JW et al: Keratoconus. I. Biochemical studies, Exp Eye Res 46:953, 1988.

230. Yue BY, Sugar J, and Benveniste K: RNA metabolism in cultures of corneal stromal cells from patients with keratoconus, Proc Soc Exp Biol Med 178:126, 1985.

231. Kao WW et al: Increased collagenase and gelatinase activities in keratoconus, Biochem Biophys Res Commun 107:929, 1982.

232. Rehany U, Lehay M, and Shoshan S: Collagenolytic activity in keratoconus, Ann Ophthalmol 14:751, 1982.

233. Robert L et al: Etude morphologique et biochemique du keratocone. II. Etude biochemique, Arch Ophtalmol (Paris) 30:589, 1970.

234. Bleckman G and Kresse H: Studies on the glycosaminoglycan metabolism of cultured fibroblasts from human keratoconus corneas, Exp Eye Res 30:215, 1980.

235. Yue BY et al: Glycoconjugate abnormalities in cultured keratoconus stromal cells, Arch Ophthalmol 106:1709, 1988.

236. Yue BY, Sugar J, and Schrode K: Histochemical studies of keratoconus, Curr Eye Res 7:81, 1988.

237. Meek KM et al: The structure of normal and keratoconus human corneas, Ophthalmic Res 19:6, 1987.

238. Bron AJ: Keratoconus, Cornea 7:163, 1988.

239. Yue BY, Sugar J, and Benveniste K: Heterogenicity in keratoconus: possible biochemical basis, Proc Soc Exp Biol Med 175:336, 1984.

240. Hartstein J: Keratoconus that developed in patients wearing corneal contact lenses, Arch Ophthalmol 80:345, 1968.

241. Hartstein J and Becker B: Research into the pathogenesis of keratoconus. A new syndrome: low ocular rigidity, contact lenses, and keratoconus, Arch Ophthalmol 84:728, 1970.

242. Brady HR: Keratoconus development in a contact lens wearer, Contact Lens Med Bull 5:23, 1972.

243. Steahly LP: Keratoconus following contact lens wear, Ann Ophthalmol 10:1177, 1978.

244. Nauheim JS and Perry AD: A clinicopathologic study of contact lens–related keratoconus, Am J Ophthalmol 100:543, 1985.

245. Gasset AR, Houde WL, and Garcia-Bengochea M: Hard contact lens wear as an environmental risk in keratoconus, Am J Ophthalmol 85:339, 1978.

246. Brightbill FS and Stainer GA: Previous hard contact lens wear in keratoconus, Contact Intraocular Lens Med J 5:43, 1979.

247. Levenson DS: Changes in corneal curvature with long-term PMMA contact lens wear, CLAO J 9:121, 1983.

248. Hartstein J: Corneal warping, Am J Ophthalmol 60:1103, 1965.

249. Levenson DS and Berry CV: Findings on followup of corneal warpage patients, CLAO J 9:126, 1983.

250. Gritz DC and McDonnell PJ: Keratoconus and ocular massage, Am J Ophthalmol 106:757, 1988.

251. Hoefle FB, Kooerman JJ, and Buxton J: The use of contact lenses in patients with keratoconus, Contact Lens Med Bull 5:52, 1972.

252. Kastl PR et al: A 20-year retrospective study of the use of contact lenses in keratoconus, CLAO J 13:102, 1987.

253. Fowler WC, Belin MW, and Chambers WA: Contact lenses in the visual correction of keratoconus, CLAO J 14:203, 1988.

254. Smiddy WE et al: Keratoconus: contact lens or keratoplasty, Ophthalmology 95:487, 1988.

255. Hartstein J: Basics of contact lenses, ed 3, San Francisco, 1979, American Academy of Ophthalmology.

256. Buxton JN, Keates RH, and Hoefle FB: The contact lens correction of keratoconus. In Dabezies OH, editor: Contact lenses: the CLAO guide to basic science and clinical practice, Orlando, Fla, 1984, Grune & Stratton, Inc.

257. Soper JW and Jarrett A: Results of a systematic approach to fitting keratoconus and corneal transplants, Contact Lens J 9:12, 1975.

258. Baldone JA: Piggyback fitting. In Dabezies OH, editor: Contact lenses: the CLAO guide to basic science and clinical practice, Orlando, Fla, 1984, Grune & Stratton, Inc.

259. Kennedy RH, Bourne WM, and Dyer JA: A 48-year clinical and epidemiologic study of keratoconus, Am J Ophthalmol 101:267, 1986.

260. Anseth A: Keratoplasty for keratoconus: a report of 50 operated eyes, Acta Ophthalmol (Copenh) 45:684, 1967.

261. Keates RH and Falkenstein S: Keratoplasty in keratoconus, Am J Ophthalmol 74:442, 1972.

262. Donshik PC et al: Effect of bilateral and unilateral grafts on the incidence of rejections in keratoconus, Am J Ophthalmol 87:823, 1979.

263. Troutman RC and Gaster RN: Surgical advances and results of keratoconus, Am J Ophthalmol 90:131, 1980.

264. Payne JW: Primary penetrating keratoplasty for keratoconus: a long-term follow-up, Cornea 1:21, 1982.

265. Paglen PG et al: The prognosis for keratoplasty in keratoconus, Ophthalmology 89:651, 1982.

266. Matusda M et al: The effect of hard contact lens wear on the keratoconic corneal endothelium after penetrating keratoplasty, Am J Ophthalmol 107:246, 1989.

267. Abelson MB et al: Recurrent keratoconus after keratoplasty, Am J Ophthalmol 90:672, 1980.

268. Nirinkari VS et al: Recurrence of keratoconus in donor cornea 22 years after successful keratoplasty, Br J Ophthalmol 67:32, 1983.

269. Urrets-Zavalia A: Fixed, dilated pupil, iris atrophy, and secondary glaucoma: a distinct clinical entity following penetrating keratoplasty in keratoconus, Am J Ophthalmol 56:257, 1963.

270. Davies PD and Ruben M: The paretic pupil: its incidence and etiology after keratoplasty for keratoconus, Br J Ophthalmol 59:223, 1975.

271. Richard J, Paton D, and Gasset A: A comparison of penetrating keratoplasty and lamellar keratoplasty in the surgical management of keratoconus, Am J Ophthalmol 86:807, 1978.

272. Malbran E and Stefani C: Lamellar keratoplasty in corneal ectasia, Ophthalmologica 164:59, 1972.

273. Wood TO: Lamellar transplants in keratoconus, Am J Ophthalmol 83:543, 1977.

274. Gasset AR: Lamellar keratoplasty in the treatment of keratoconus: conectomy, Ophthalmic Surg 10:26, 1979.

275. Kaufman HE and Werblin TP: Epikeratophakia for the treatment of keratoconus, Am J Ophthalmol 93:342, 1982.

276. McDonald MB et al: Onlay lamellar keratoplasty for the treatment of keratoconus, Br J Ophthalmol 67:615, 1983.

277. McDonald MB et al: Epikeratophakia for keratoconus: the nationwide study, Arch Ophthalmol 104:1294, 1986.

278. Steinert RF and Wagoner MD: Long-term comparison of epikeratoplasty and penetrating keratoplasty for keratoconus, Arch Ophthalmol 106:493, 1988.

279. Frantz JM, McDonald MB, and Kaufman HE: Results of penetrating keratoplasty after epikeratophakia for keratoconus in the nationwide study, Ophthalmology 96:1151, 1989.

280. Aquavella JV: Thermokeratoplasty, Ophthalmic Surg 4:39, 1974.

281. Gasset AR and Kaufman HE: Thermokeratoplasty for keratoconus, Am J Ophthalmol 79:226, 1975.

282. Rowsey JJ and Ross JD: Preliminary report of Los Alamos keratoplasty techniques, Ophthalmology 88:755, 1981.

283. Aquavella JV, Smith RS, and Shaw EL: Alterations in corneal morphology following thermokeratoplasty, Arch Ophthalmol 94:2082, 1976.

284. Fogle JA, Kenyon KR, and Stark WJ: Damage to epithelial basement membrane by thermokeratoplasty, Am J Ophthalmol 83:392, 1977.

285. McClellan KA and Billson FA: Acute hydrops in keratoglobus, Arch Ophthalmol 105:1432, 1987.

286. Stein R, Lazar M, and Adam A: Brittle cornea: a familial trait associated with blue sclera, Am J Ophthalmol 66:67, 1968.

287. Hymas SE, Dar H, and Newman E: Blue sclera keratoglobus, Br J Ophthalmol 53:53, 1969.

288. Gregoratos N, Bartoscocas C, and Papas K: Blue sclera with keratoglobus and brittle cornea, Br J Ophthalmol 55:424, 1971.

289. Biglan AW, Brown SI, and Johnson BL: Keratoglobus and blue sclera, Am J Ophthalmol 83:225, 1977.

290. Jacobs D, Green R, and Maumenee AE: Acquired keratoglobus, Am J Ophthalmol 77:393, 1975.

291. Waardenberg PJ: Does agenesis or dysgenesis neuroepithelialis retinae, whether or not related to keratoglobus, exist? Ophthalmologica 133:454, 1957.

292. Gillespie FD: Congenital amaurosis of Leber, Am J Ophthalmol 61:874, 1966.

293. Cavara V: Keratoglobus and keratoconus: a contribution to nosological interpretation of keratoglobus, Br J Ophthalmol 34:621, 1950.

294. Greenfield G et al: Blue sclera and keratoconus: key features of a distinct heritable disorder of connective tissue, Clin Genet 4:8, 1973.

295. Haney WP and Falls HF: The occurrence of congenital keratoconus posticus circumscriptus (in two siblings presenting a previously unrecognized syndrome), Am J Ophthalmol 52:53, 1961.

296. Karlin DB and Wise GN: Keratoconus posticus, Am J Ophthalmol 52:119, 1961.

297. Schocket GS, Phelps WL, and Pettit TH: Bilateral posterior circumscribed keratoconus, Am J Ophthalmol 57:840, 1964.

298. Lorfel RS and Sugar S: Keratoconus associated with retrolental fibroplasia, Ann Ophthalmol 8:449, 1976.

299. Bermúdez FJ et al: Association of keratoconus and false chordae tendineae in the left ventricle, Am J Ophthalmol 108:93, 1989.

300. Austin MG and Schaefer RF: Marfan syndrome with unusual blood vessel manifestations: primary medionecrosis, dissection of the right innominate, Arch Pathol Lab Med 64:205, 1957.

301. Storch H: Ein fall von arachnodaktylie (dystrophia mesodermalis congenita), typus Marfan, Dermatologica 104:322, 1952.

302. McKusick VA: Heritable disorders of connective tissue, ed 4, St Louis, 1972, The CV Mosby Co.

303. Judisch F, Wariri M, and Krachmer J: Ocular Ehlers-Danlos syndrome with normal lysyl hydroxylase activity, Arch Ophthalmol 94:1489, 1976.

304. Geeraets W: Ocular syndromes, Philadelphia, 1976, Lea & Febiger.

305. Schwartz DE: Noonan's syndrome associated with ocular abnormalities, Am J Ophthalmol 73:995, 1972.

306. Wolter Jr: Bilateral keratoconus in Crouzon's syndrome with unilateral hydrops, Ann Ophthalmol 14:141, 1976.

307. Holtz JS: Congenital ocular anomalies associated with Duane's retraction syndrome, Am J Ophthalmol 77:729, 1974.

308. Blanksma LJ, Donders PC, and van Voorst Vader PC: Xeroderma pigmentosum and keratoconus, Doc Ophthalmol 64:97, 1986.

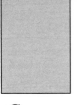

18 DISORDERS OF THE ENDOTHELIUM

ENDOTHELIAL DYSTROPHIES

FUCHS' ENDOTHELIAL DYSTROPHY

Abnormality or loss of endothelial cells occurs with aging and a variety of injuries, such as trauma, inflammation, drugs, and glaucoma. In many cases the manifestations are similar: The earliest sign, corneal guttae, can progress to stromal edema, epithelial edema, and corneal scarring. When these changes are seen in the absence of contributory injury the condition is called Fuchs' dystrophy. Some of these cases may be a result of unrecognized injury; many are related to normal aging or an accelerated aging of the endothelium; and some appear to be true dystrophies, with early onset and hereditary transmission.

Fuchs' dystrophy is a bilateral condition that usually is noted in the elderly and is more common in women.[1] Autosomal dominant transmission has been demonstrated in some cases.[2-6] Some reports have suggested an association between Fuchs' dystrophy and open angle glaucoma,[7] but others have not found this to be the case.[8,9]

Clinical manifestations

Cornea guttata. Vogt used this term, derived from Latin, to describe corneas containing multiple droplike excrescences, or guttae, on the posterior surface. The condition usually is seen in middle-aged or older patients. Corneal guttae have been noted in as many as 70% of patients over 40 years of

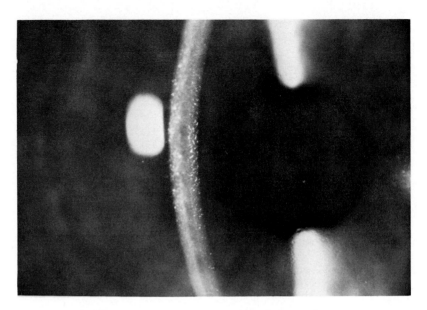

Fig. 18-1. Endothelial guttae seen with slit-lamp microscopy.

age.[10,11] In addition to aging, they can be associated with corneal trauma and inflammation.[12-14] Guttae do not interfere with vision.

Guttae are seen as dewdroplike, wartlike, endothelial excrescences. With direct illumination they appear as refractile circular excavations in the endothelial surface (Figs. 18-1 and 18-2). On specular reflection they are black holes in the endothelial mosaic (Fig. 18-3). They develop first in the central cornea and gradually spread peripherally and become more numerous. Fine pigment deposition is often seen diffusely on the posterior corneal surface. With time Descemet's membrane can develop a beaten-metal appearance.

In some instances the endothelial change is not in guttate form, but rather the endothelium becomes increasingly diffusely relucent, giving the appearance of a grayish membrane.[15,16] In severe inflammation, edema of the endothelial cells can resemble a guttate cornea, but the condition is transient.[17]

Stromal and epithelial edema. If endothelial cell function is sufficiently compromised, stromal edema occurs. Stromal edema is more likely to occur with decreased endothelial cell density, but the density may vary. The number of corneal guttae also does not correlate well; stromal edema can occur in the absence of guttae.[15] With further impairment of endothelial function, epithelial edema develops. Epithelial edema can occur at different stages depending on the intraocular pressure. Elevations of intraocular pressure more readily cause epithelial edema in a cornea with compromised endothelium and stromal edema.

Some reduction of vision occurs with marked stromal edema (approximately > 0.65 mm), but usually it is not until epithelial edema develops that the patient becomes very symptomatic. Epithelial edema causes surface irregularity and haze and recurrent epithelial erosions. At first epithelial edema occurs only in the morning and clears as the day goes on. This is related to the decreased evaporation of fluid from the surface of the eye during sleep as a result of lid closure. Humid weather can similarly affect vision.

When there is early or moderate stromal edema it is difficult to perceive any changes other than a widening of the slit beam. Therefore, pachometry is useful to detect its presence. In more advanced

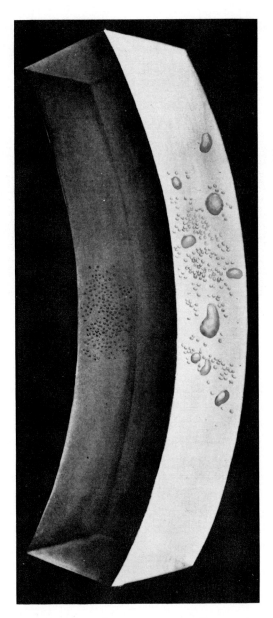

Fig. 18-2. Diagrammatic representation of wartlike excrescences on Descemet's membrane and epithelial bullae seen in advanced Fuchs' dystrophy.

edema, the stroma can become slightly hazy, the posterior corneal surface is pushed posteriorly, and Descemet's membrane can be thrown into folds. The central cornea can become thicker than the peripheral cornea. The posterior stroma and fluid clefts may become increasingly relucent.

Epithelial edema appears first as fine, clear cysts producing nodular elevations of the surface (bedewing). Topical fluorescein can be helpful in demonstrating bedewing, by producing dark gaps in the fluorescein film ("negative" staining). On retroillumination the bedewing appears as a fine patina. Fingerprint-like patterns and other linear opacities may be seen in the deep epithelium, probably caused by shifting of the overlying epithelium. With coalescence of the microcysts, epithelial bullae develop (Fig. 18-2). These markedly reduce vision and can rupture, causing pain and foreign body

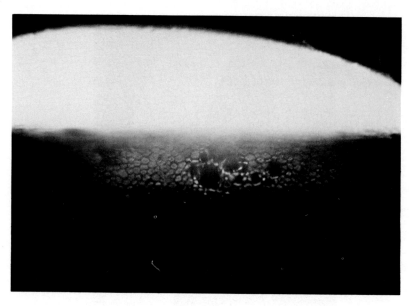

Fig. 18-3. Specular micrograph of endothelium showing guttae (dark holes in endothelial mosaic).

sensation. Subepithelial fibrosis and vascularization can occur in more advanced cases, particularly with recurrent epithelial breakdown (Figs. 18-4 and 18-5).

Histopathology. As noted previously, the main pathologic condition is in the endothelium.[18-20] Guttae are seen as nodular thickenings of Descemet's membrane (Fig. 18-6). They are composed of collagen and most likely are abnormal products of the endothelial cells.[19]

The cell density progressively decreases and cell size increases, with thinning over the Descemet's warts. Some of the endothelial cells take on morphologic features of fibroblasts and produce collagen.[19,20] Other cells show tonofilaments, surface microvilli, and desmosomes, similar to epithelial cells.[21] Descemet's membrane becomes diffusely thickened because of deposition of collagenous basement membranelike material on the posterior surface (see Fig. 1-25).[19,22-24] The anterior banded portion is relatively normal, but the posterior nonbanded layer is thinned or absent and is replaced by a posterior banded layer.[19,23] The thinness of the posterior nonbanded layer suggests that endothelial cell function becomes abnormal at an early age.

Epithelial edema appears first intracellularly in the basal cells (Fig. 18-7). Later, interepithelial and subepithelial pockets of fluid are seen. Bowman's layer usually remains intact. Subepithelial deposition of collagen and basement membranelike material can be noted (Fig. 18-8).

Treatment. Patients with early epithelial edema may benefit from hyperosmotic drops and ointment (Fig. 18-9). Usually 5% NaCl drops are given four to eight times daily and 5% NaCl ointment at bedtime. These may reduce epithelial edema and improve both comfort and vision. A hair dryer, held at arm's length or directed across the face, may help "dry out" the corneal surface, and can be repeated two or three times a day. Lowering of intraocular pressure is useful in some cases. Topical corticosteroids are not beneficial.

A bandage contact lens is beneficial in alleviating discomfort resulting from bullae formation and rupture. It is particularly useful in making life more pleasant for patients for whom corneal transplantation is not desired or recommended. Cautery of Bowman's layer or a conjunctival flap are other alternatives for these patients.

Penetrating keratoplasty is indicated once visual acuity is decreased to the point of impairing nor-

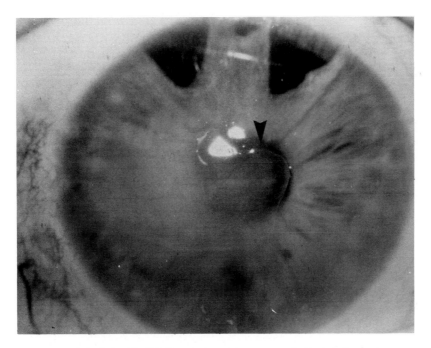

Fig. 18-4. Subepithelial fibrosis *(arrow)* can occur in Fuchs' dystrophy.

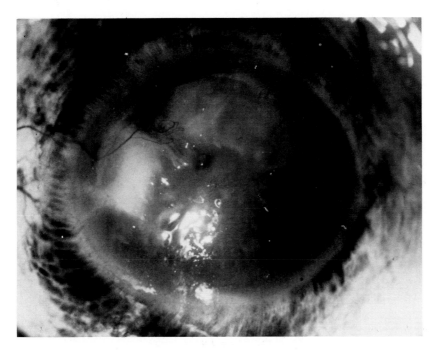

Fig. 18-5. Fuchs' dystrophy with epithelial bullae, scarring, and vascularization.

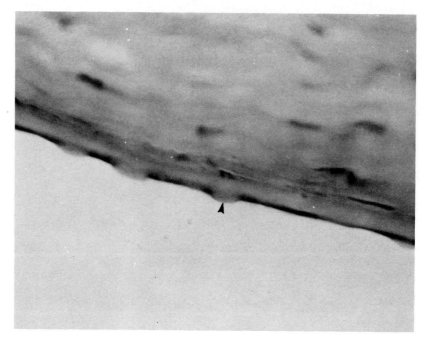

Fig. 18-6. Cornea guttata. Descemet's warts are noted with loss of endothelial cells *(arrow)*.

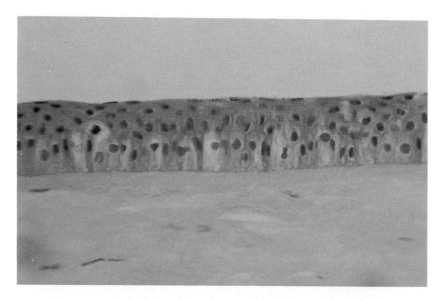

Fig. 18-7. Early epithelial edema in Fuchs' dystrophy, clinically seen as bedewing of epithelium. (From Grayson M and Keates RH: Manual of diseases of the cornea, Boston, 1969, Little, Brown & Co.)

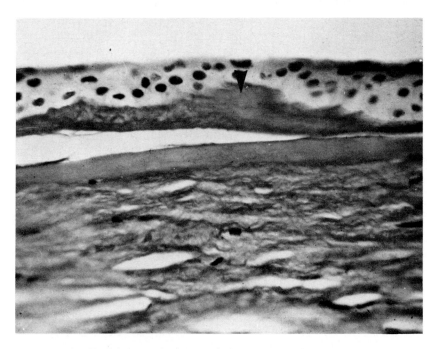

Fig. 18-8. In long-standing Fuchs' dystrophy increase in basement membrane substance *(arrow)* and alterations in Bowman's layer may be seen.

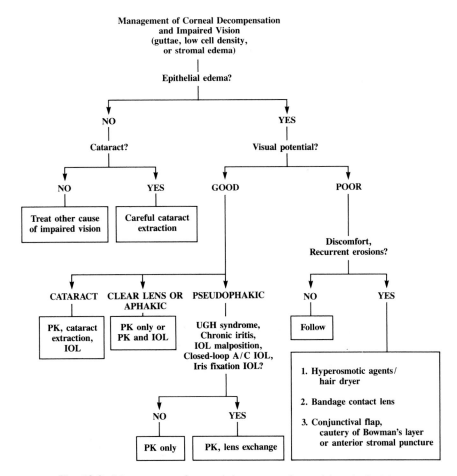

Fig. 18-9. Management of corneal decompensation and impaired vision.

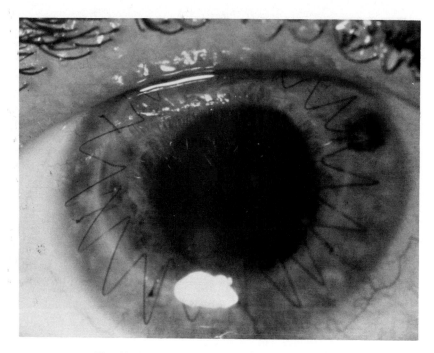

Fig. 18-10. Penetrating graft for Fuchs' dystrophy.

mal activities. The short-term results are quite good (Fig. 18-10),[26] but long-term survival of these grafts is questionable. Some studies have found a relatively high incidence of graft failure.[27,28] Cataracts are often present, and combined keratoplasty and cataract extraction can be performed.[29-32] The relative value of separate vs. combined procedures has not yet been determined, but most surgeons now perform combined procedures.[33] In the presence of a cataract, the indications for keratoplasty are not well defined. Some have recommended keratoplasty whenever the corneal thickness is greater than 0.60 mm,[34] but I proceed with cataract extraction alone unless epithelial edema is present.

CONGENITAL HEREDITARY ENDOTHELIAL DYSTROPHY

Congenital hereditary endothelial dystrophy (CHED) can be inherited in both autosomal dominant or autosomal recessive forms. The recessive form is more common and more severe, whereas the dominant form can be associated with deafness.[35-43] The recessive form is present at birth or develops in the neonatal period and is often associated with nystagmus. Patients with dominantly inherited disease have clear corneas early in life, but within a few years they develop slowly progressive opacification.[41,44-46] They do not develop nystagmus.

The essential feature of CHED is bilateral diffuse corneal edema, unrelated to commonly known etiologic factors, such as congenital glaucoma, intrauterine infections, or mucopolysaccharidosis. The clinical picture can vary from a mild haziness to a moderately severe, diffuse, homogeneous, gray-white, ground-glass appearance of the central cornea that extends to the periphery (Fig. 18-11). The corneal thickness is two to three times greater than normal, but corneal diameter is not enlarged. Macular or dot stromal opacities are sometimes present. Diffuse stromal cloudiness often prevents clinical evaluation of the endothelium and Descemet's membrane, but the latter can sometimes be seen as thickened and gray. Guttae are not present, there is no vascularization, and corneal sensation and intraocular pressure are normal.

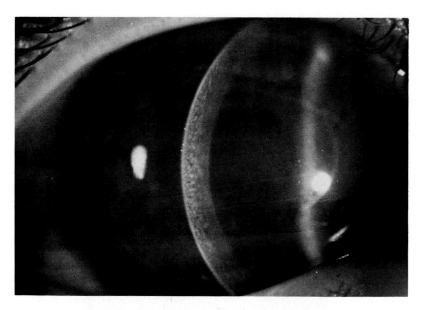

Fig. 18-11. Congenital hereditary endothelial dystrophy.

The corneal opacity may be stationary or show slow progression. Epithelial edema and bedewing can develop, but bullae and discomfort are rarely seen.

This condition appears to result from a degeneration of the endothelium, which may occur in utero or within the first year of life. The anterior banded portion of Descemet's membrane is normal, indicating that the endothelium is functionally normal at least through the fifth month of gestation. However, sometime after the fifth month a defective endothelium secretes abnormal and excessive basement membrane, which accumulates as an aberrant, nonbanded posterior portion of Descemet's membrane.[39,46-51] Endothelial cells are absent or atrophic. In one study the endothelial cells did not grow when placed in culture media.[51] Secondary changes, related to the stromal and epithelial edema, are also noted.

Asymptomatic relatives of patients with CHED can manifest corneal changes resembling those of posterior polymorphous dystrophy.[52] These individuals appear to have a higher risk of producing offspring with CHED.[53]

Treatment. Keratoplasty in such young children is considerably more difficult than in adults, but good results can be obtained in some cases.[54-56]

POSTERIOR POLYMORPHOUS DYSTROPHY

Posterior polymorphous dystrophy (PPD) is usually transmitted as a dominant trait, but recessive patterns of inheritance have been demonstrated in some pedigrees.[57-59] It is most often bilateral, but can be asymmetric and, rarely, unilateral.[60] Some cases are clearly congenital, with cloudy corneas at birth. However, patients with PPD usually demonstrate normal vision and are asymptomatic, so the age of onset can be difficult to determine. Most cases are nonprogressive or very slowly progressive, but in some patients endothelial decompensation can develop, reducing visual acuity.[21]

As indicated by its name, PPD is characterized by deep corneal lesions of various shapes. Nodular, grouped vesicular and blisterlike lesions commonly occur (Figs. 18-12 and 18-13).[61] Gray-white halos often surround the vesicular lesions. Flat gray-white opacities, gray thickenings of Descemet's membrane, sinuous broad bands (Fig. 18-14), or clear bands with white scalloped margins also can

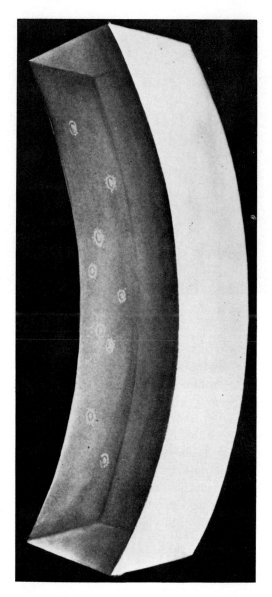

Fig. 18-12. Blisterlike lesions of posterior polymorphous dystrophy.

be present.[21] The latter can be oriented vertically or horizontally and are often confused with Descemet's tears.[62] The lesions stand out on retroillumination. With specular microscopy the lesions are seen to contain abnormal, pleomorphic cells, with indistinct borders and increased reflective highlights.[63,64]

PPD can be associated with anterior segment dysgenesis, with prominent Schwalbe's ring, iridocorneal adhesions, abnormal iris processes, iris atrophy, corectopia, and ectropion uveae (Fig. 18-15).[21] Intraocular pressure elevation occurs in approximately 15% of cases.[21,60,65,66] Band keratopathy,[21] calcium deposition in the deep stroma,[58] and posterior keratoconus[21] also can be seen.

Electron microscopic studies have revealed the main abnormality to be in the endothelial cell.[21,49,60,67-73] Islands of epithelial-like endothelial cells are found, which are larger than normal endothelial cells. They can be multilayered and have extensive microvilli, desmosomal junctions, in-

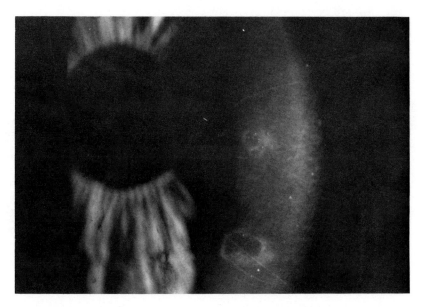

Fig. 18-13. Endothelial lesions in posterior polymorphous dystrophy.

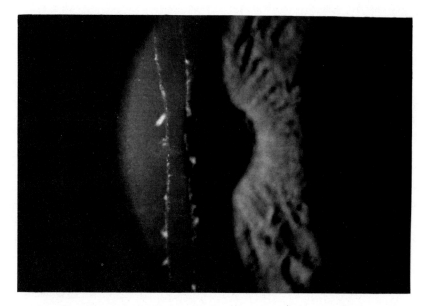

Fig. 18-14. Endothelial bands in posterior polymorphous dystrophy.

tracytoplasmic filaments, and a decreased number of organelles (Figs. 18-16 to 18-19). The abnormal endothelium can extend across the trabecular meshwork and onto the iris.[68,74] The abnormal endothelial cells can be grown in culture and maintain the abnormal characteristics observed in pathologic specimens.[75] The anterior banded layer of Descemet's membrane is normal, but the posterior portion may be thickened by abnormal multilaminate, basement membrane material. Corneal guttae and excavations of Descemet's membrane have been described.

The pathogenesis of PPD is unknown, but it has been suggested that the endothelial cells undergo

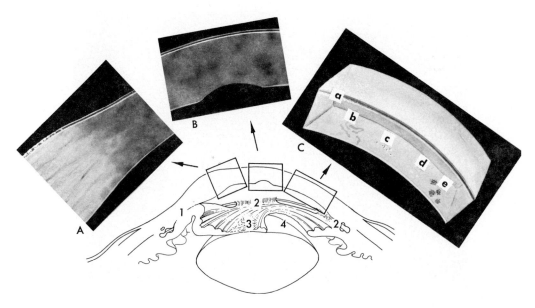

Fig. 18-15. A, Posterior polymorphous dystrophy. Diagrammatic representation of biomicroscopic findings: *(1)* iridocorneal adhesions obliterating trabeculum, *(2)* abnormal iris processes, and *(3)* patchy iris atrophy involving iris stroma. **B,** Area of circumscribed posterior keratoconus. **C,** Section en bloc showing *(a)* calcific deposition in Bowman's membrane, *(b)* "sinuous" opacities, *(c)* vesicular lesions, *(d)* flat, gray-white macular lesions, and *(e)* aggregations of guttae. (From Grayson M: Trans Am Ophthalmol Soc 72:516, 1974.)

transformation into epithelial-like cells, or that their embryonal precursors undergo abnormal differentiation. The angle and iris abnormalities may represent spread of these abnormal cells from the cornea, or they may be a broader reflection of the mesenchymal dysgenesis. Because the anterior banded portion of Descemet's membrane is normal, the abnormality probably develops late in gestation or shortly after birth.

Differential diagnosis. PPD can present as a cloudy cornea at birth and, therefore, must be differentiated from CHED and congenital hereditary stromal dystrophy (CHSD), as well as other etiologies (Table 18-1). Glaucoma, iridocorneal adhesions, and corneal edema can be present in both PPD and Chandler's (iridocorneal endothelial) syndrome. The differentiating features are given in Table 18-2.

Treatment. In most cases no treatment is necessary, but occasionally keratoplasty is required for corneal edema. In two cases histologic changes typical of PPD were observed in failed grafts 7 to 9 years after penetrating keratoplasty was performed for PPD.[76] The authors hypothesized that abnormal cells from the periphery of the host cornea repopulated the posterior graft surface, possibly after destruction of the donor endothelium. In rare instances corneal edema developing in adulthood has improved spontaneously.[57] If extensive angle and iris involvement is present, the resultant glaucoma can be very difficult to manage, and the prognosis for successful keratoplasty is much worse.

IRIDOCORNEAL ENDOTHELIAL SYNDROME

Three different clinical conditions, Chandler's syndrome, essential (or progressive) iris atrophy, and Cogan-Reese iris nevus syndrome, have been grouped together into a single syndrome because the pathologic processes appear to be quite similar.[77] Iridocorneal endothelial (ICE) syndrome is a nonfamilial unilateral disease more common in women and usually diagnosed between 30 and 50 years of age.

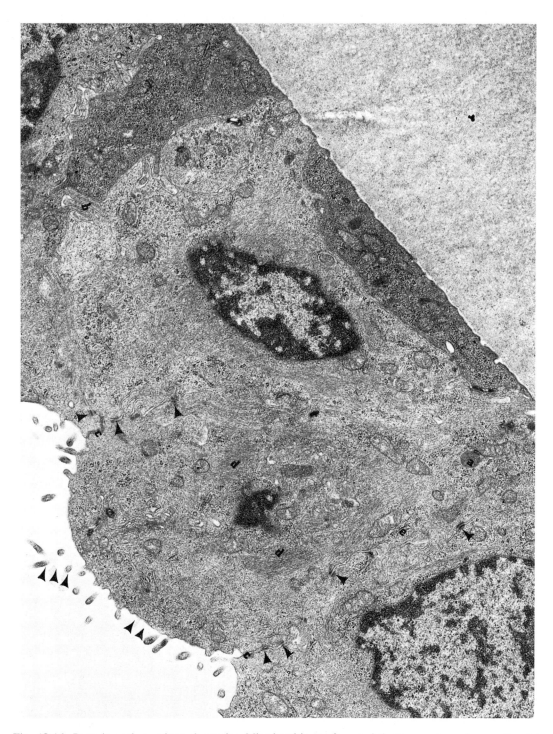

Fig. 18-16. Posterior polymorphous dystrophy. Mitochondria are few, and those present are degenerating *(a)*. Desmosomes *(single arrows)* are abundant, and microvilli are numerous *(triple arrow)*. Extensive interdigitation between cells *(b)* and zonulae occludens are noted *(c)*. Extensive intracytoplasmic filaments *(d);* elongated endoplasmic reticulum *(e)*. Double arrows indicate rounded edge or elevated apices of altered cells. (×8714.5) (From Grayson M: Trans Am Ophthalmol Soc 72:516, 1974.)

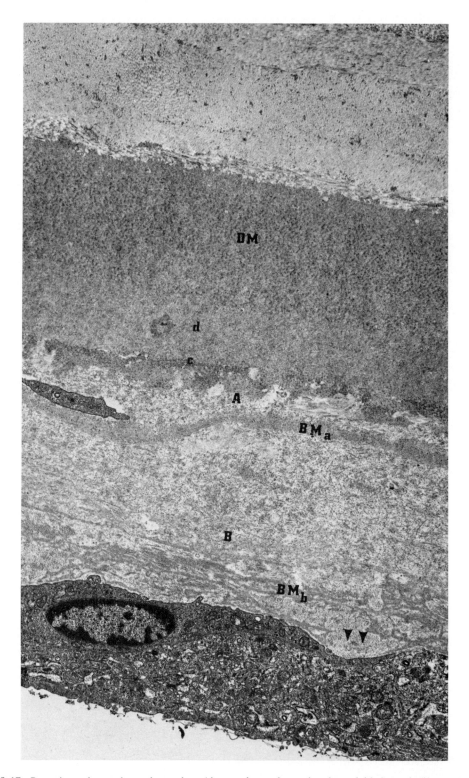

Fig. 18-17. Posterior polymorphous dystrophy. Abnormal membrane has been laid down in layers *A* and *B*. Abnormal membrane consists of collagen fibers and laminated areas of basement membrane *(BMa* and *BMb).* Demarcation line *(c)* is visible. *BMa* separates collagen fiber layers *A* and *B*. Double arrow indicates area in which indentations are made into the posterior cellular layer, possibly representing early guttate lesions. Descemet's membrane *(DM)* shows narrow nonbanded zone *(d)* (×6394.5). (From Grayson M: Trans Am Ophthalmol Soc 72:516, 1974.)

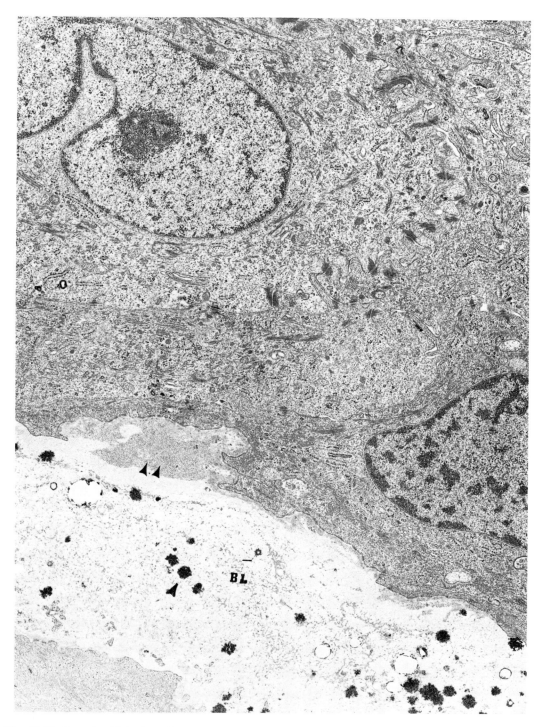

Fig. 18-18. Irregular thickening of basement membrane *(double arrow)* of epithelium is present. Calcium deposits *(single arrow)* are noted in Bowman's layer *(BL)*. Note normal presence of many desmosomes and cytoplasmic filaments in epithelial cells (×8714.5). (From Grayson M: Trans Am Ophthalmol Soc 72:516, 1974.)

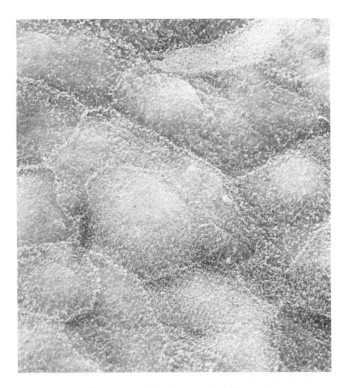

Fig. 18-19. Posterior polymorphous dystrophy. Myriads of microvilli can be seen on scanning electron microscopy.

TABLE 18-1. Comparison of Diffuse Congenital Dystrophies Appearing in the First Year of Life

CHARACTERISTIC	POSTERIOR POLYMORPHOUS DYSTROPHY (CONGENITAL CORNEAL EDEMA)	CONGENITAL HEREDITARY STROMAL DYSTROPHY	CONGENITAL HEREDITARY ENDOTHELIAL DYSTROPHY
Inheritance	Autosomal dominant	Autosomal dominant	Autosomal recessive
Laterality	Bilateral	Bilateral	Bilateral
Time of appearance of opacity	At birth or within first year	At birth	At birth or within first year
Progression	Slowly progressive	None	Minimal
Corneal thickness	Probably normal	Normal	Severely increased
Location of opacity	Diffuse	Central, fades peripherally	Diffuse
Appearance of opacity	Ground glass	Ground glass, flaky, feathery	Ground glass, few white maculae
Histopathology	Abnormal, atrophic endothelium	Abnormal stromal collagen fibrils	Absent or atrophic endothelium

TABLE 18-2. Comparison of Posterior Polymorphous Dystrophy and Chandler's Syndrome

FEATURE	PPD	CHANDLER'S SYNDROME
Laterality	Bilateral	Unilateral
Heredity	Autosomal dominant	None
Sex distribution	Males = females	Females > males
Onset of symptoms	Any age	Second and third decades
Corneal edema	Occasionally	Usually
Endothelium	Ridges, vesicles, plaques	Fine guttaelike changes
Iridocorneal adhesions	25% (usually microscopic)	100%
Iris stromal atrophy	Absent or minimal	Mild-marked (essential iris atrophy)
Ectropion uveae	Infrequent	Frequent
Glaucoma	Infrequent	100%
Progression	May slowly progress	Fairly rapid

Adapted from Rodrigues MM et al: Arch Ophthalmol 98:688, 1980.

CLINICAL MANIFESTATIONS

The chief characteristics of ICE syndrome are corneal endothelial abnormalities, peripheral anterior synechiae, glaucoma, iris atrophy and hole formation, and iris nodules. The relative prominence of these different features varies widely, and is the reason for the original distinction among three different clinical diseases. In essential iris atrophy, the earliest described condition,[78] the iris features predominate, particularly atrophy, hole formation, and corectopia (Figs. 18-20 and 18-21). In Chandler's syndrome iris atrophy and corectopia are mild or absent, and corneal endothelial changes and stromal edema are prominent.[79] In the iris nevus syndrome, nodular, pigmented elevations are present on the surface of the iris (Fig. 18-22).[80] Other corneal and iris abnormalities may or may not be present.

The most common corneal abnormality is a fine hammered-metal appearance of the endothelium.[81] Stromal or epithelial edema commonly develops, with or without an abnormal appearance of the endothelium. Specular examination of the endothelium reveals pleomorphism, polymegathism, and intracellular dark areas.[82-84] Usually the endothelium is diffusely affected, but in some cases focal areas of normal and abnormal cells are seen, and the normal areas disappear with time.[85] The fellow eyes are clinically unaffected, but decreased endothelial cell density and pleomorphism have been noted on specular microscopy.[86]

In some cases there is progressive atrophy of the iris stroma, peripheral anterior synechiae, and stretching of the iris, with corectopia, ectropion uvea, and hole formation (previous called progressive or essential iris atrophy).[81,87] The peripheral anterior synechiae extend to or beyond Schwalbe's line and are usually visible without gonioscopy. The pupil is usually eccentric in the direction of the most prominent synechiae, and the majority of iris holes are found in the opposite side. As many as several hundred fine, yellow to brown pedunculated nodules can be present on the iris surface.[80,88] In some cases these iris nodules are the most prominent feature; in others they develop many years after other iris and corneal changes.[89,90] Elevated intraocular pressure is common and often requires surgical intervention.

HISTOPATHOLOGY

Abnormal endothelial cells are present on the trabecular meshwork, the anterior surface of the iris, and the posterior corneal surface.[77,91-95] The corneal endothelial cells are decreased in number and irregular in shape. They can have epithelial features, including desmosomal junctions, surface microvilli, and increased intracytoplasmic filaments.[92-95] Descemet's membrane can be thickened or

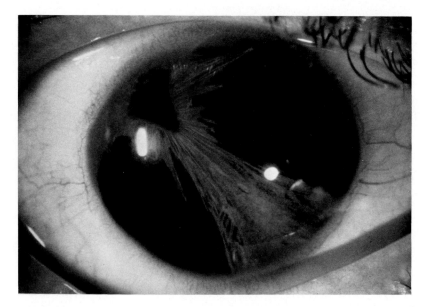

Fig. 18-20. Essential iris atrophy. (Courtesy of Vicente Jocson, Pittsburgh.)

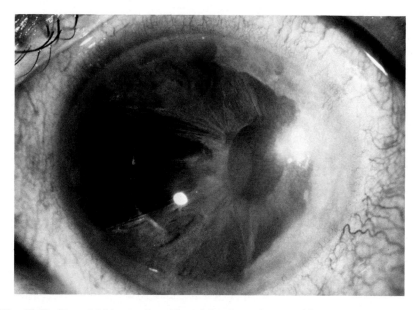

Fig. 18-21. Essential iris atrophy with peripheral anterior synechiae and corneal edema.

normal, but contains an abnormal posterior collagenous layer. The abnormal endothelial cells, together with a basement membrane, extend over the peripheral anterior synechiae and open anterior chamber angle onto the iris surface. Most commonly the membrane covers the iris quadrant toward which the pupil is distorted, and not quadrants containing holes.[77,87] Iris nodules are localized protrusions of normal iris stroma through the cellular sheet, which may later become covered by the sheet.[87,94,96,97]

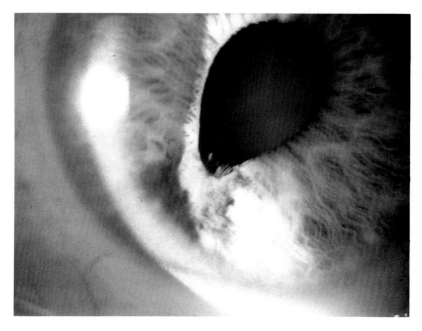

Fig. 18-22. Cogan-Reese iris nevus syndrome. (Courtesy of Massimo Busin, Bonn, Germany.)

PATHOGENESIS

The primary abnormality is most likely a defect in the corneal endothelium.[87] The endothelium may be abnormal congenitally because of an anomalous differentiation of the neural crest mesenchyme, which forms the endothelium.[98] This abnormal endothelium, which cannot maintain normal corneal hydration, grows over the angle and iris surface, forming a membrane that can contract, causing corectopia, ectropion uvea, and stretch holes in the iris. Localized gaps in the membrane create the appearance of iris nevi. Iris ischemia has been noted,[89] but its etiology is unclear.

TREATMENT

Control of intraocular pressure usually can be achieved medically. Drugs that lower aqueous production are more effective. Laser trabeculoplasty usually is not effective.[99] Filtering surgery is reasonably successful,[89] but endothelialization of the bleb can occur.

Lowering intraocular pressure can reduce corneal edema, but penetrating keratoplasty is often required. Two groups have reported good results with keratoplasty,[100,101] but our results at the University of Pittsburgh have been more mixed, with relatively high incidences of graft reaction and rejection.

ENDOTHELIITIS

A linear pattern of endothelial inflammation and destruction can occur in nongrafted corneas. The appearance and the process appear to be similar to those of allogeneic corneal graft rejection. A line of keratic precipitates progresses across the cornea, destroying the endothelium and leaving stromal edema in its wake. Herpes simplex can cause such a picture, unilaterally (see Chapter 12).[102,103] It can also be seen as a recurrent, bilaterally symmetric process in otherwise healthy eyes[104,105] or associated with active pars planitis.[106] The etiology is unknown, but an autoimmune process has been proposed.[104]

Single or multiple inflammatory endothelial plaques are another form of endothelial inflammation seen with herpes simplex.

One pedigree has been described in which there appeared to be a dominantly inherited form of recurrent keratoendotheliitis.[107] Attacks usually began around age 10 and recurred two to three times per year, lasting days to weeks. Corneal edema, guttae, and mild anterior chamber reaction were noted during attacks; and some patients developed stromal opacities after multiple attacks.

REFERENCES

1. Krachmer JH et al: A study of 64 families with corneal endothelial dystrophy, Arch Ophthalmol 96:2036, 1978.
2. Mortelmans L: Forme familiale de la dystrophie cornéene de Fuchs, Ophthalmologica 123:88, 1952.
3. Cross HE, Maumenee AE, and Cantolino SJ: Inheritance of Fuchs' endothelial dystrophy, Arch Ophthalmol 85:268, 1971.
4. Krachmer JH et al: Inheritance of endothelial dystrophy of the cornea, Ophthalmologica 181:301, 1980.
5. Rosenblum P et al: Hereditary Fuchs' dystrophy, Am J Ophthalmol 90:455, 1980.
6. Magovern M et al: Inheritance of Fuchs' combined dystrophy, Ophthalmology 86:1897, 1979.
7. Buxton JN et al: Tonography in cornea guttata: a preliminary study, Arch Ophthalmol 77:602, 1967.
8. Roberts CW et al: Endothelial guttata and facility of aqueous outflow, Cornea 3:5, 1984.
9. Krachmer JH et al: Corneal endothelial dystrophy, Arch Ophthalmol 96:2036, 1978.
10. Goar EL: Dystrophy of the corneal endothelium (cornea guttata), with a report of a histological examination, Am J Ophthalmol 17:215, 1934.
11. Lorenzetti DW et al: Central cornea guttata: incidence in the general population, Am J Ophthalmol 64:1155, 1967.
12. Zeporkes J: Glassy network in the anterior chamber: report of a case, Arch Ophthalmol 10:517, 1933.
13. Wolter JR and Larson BF: Pathology of cornea guttata, Am J Ophthalmol 48:161, 1959.
14. Forgács J: Stries hyalines rétrocornéennes postinflammatories en toiles araignées, Ophthalmologica 145:301, 1963.
15. Abbott RL et al: Specular microscopic and histologic observations in non-guttate corneal endothelial degeneration, Ophthalmology 88:788, 1981.
16. Chi HH, Teng CC, and Katzin HM: Histopathology of primary endothelial-epithelial dystrophy of the cornea, Am J Ophthalmol 45:518, 1958.
17. Krachmer JH, Schnitzer JI, and Fratkin J: Cornea pseudoguttata: a clinical and histopathologic description of endothelial cell edema, Arch Ophthalmol 99:1377, 1981.
18. Irvine AR: The role of the endothelium in bullous keratopathy, Arch Ophthalmol 56:338, 1956.
19. Iwamoto T and DeVoe AG: Electron microscopic studies on Fuchs' combined dystrophy. I. Posterior portion of the cornea, Invest Ophthalmol 10:9, 1971.
20. Hogan MJ, Wood I, and Fine M: Fuchs' endothelial dystrophy of the cornea, Am J Ophthalmol 78:363, 1974.
21. Grayson M: The nature of hereditary deep polymorphous dystrophy of the cornea: its association with iris and anterior chamber dysgenesis, Trans Am Ophthalmol Soc 72:516, 1974.
22. Waring GO: Posterior collagenous layer (PCL) of the cornea, Arch Ophthalmol 100:122, 1982.
23. Bourne WM, Johnson DH, and Campbell RJ: The ultrastructure of Descemet's membrane. III. Fuchs' dystrophy, Arch Ophthalmol 100:1952, 1982.
24. Kenney MC et al: Characterization of the Descemet's membrane isolated from Fuchs' endothelial dystrophy corneas, Exp Eye Res 39:267, 1984.
25. Wilson SE and Bourne WM: Effect of dexamethasone on corneal endothelial function in Fuchs' dystrophy, Invest Ophthalmol Vis Sci 28(suppl):326, 1987.
26. Olson RJ et al: Visual results after penetrating keratoplasty for aphakic bullous keratopathy and Fuchs' dystrophy, Am J Ophthalmol 88:1000, 1979.
27. Stocker FW and Irish A: Fate of successful corneal graft in Fuchs' endothelial dystrophy, Am J Ophthalmol 68:820, 1969.
28. Olson T, Ehlers N, and Favini E: Long-term results of corneal grafting in Fuchs' endothelial dystrophy, Acta Ophthalmol (Copenh) 62:445, 1984.
29. Aquavella JV, Shaw EL, and Rao GN: Intraocular lens implantation combined with penetrating keratoplasty, Ophthalmic Surg 8:113, 1977.
30. Lindstrom RL, Harris WS, and Doughman DJ: Combined penetrating keratoplasty, extracapsular cataract extraction, and posterior chamber intraocular lens implantation, Am Intraocular Implant Soc J 7:130, 1981.
31. Binder PS: Intraocular lens powers used in the triple procedure, Ophthalmology 92:1561, 1985.
32. Busin M et al: Combined penetrating keratoplasty, extracapsular cataract extraction, and posterior chamber intraocular lens implantation, Ophthalmic Surg 18:272, 1987.
33. Arentsen JJ and Laibson PR: Penetrating keratoplasty and cataract extraction: combined vs nonsimultaneous surgery, Arch Ophthalmol 96:75, 1978.
34. Miller CA and Krachmer JH: Endothelial dystrophies. In Kaufman HE et al, editors: The cornea, New York, 1988, Churchill Livingstone.
35. Pietruschka G: Ueber eine Familiäre Endotheldystrophie der Hornhaut (in Kombination met Glaukom, Vitilgo, und Otosklerose), Klin Monatsbl Augenheilkd 136:794, 1960.
36. Maumenee AE: Congenital hereditary corneal dystrophy, Am J Ophthalmol 50:1114, 1960.
37. Pearce WG, Tripathi RC, and Morgan G: Congenital endothelial corneal dystrophy: clinical, pathological and genetic study, Br J Ophthalmol 53:477, 1969.
38. Harboyan G et al: Congenital corneal hereditary dys-

trophy: progressive sensorineural deafness in a family, Arch Ophthalmol 85:27, 1971.

39. Kanai A: Further electron microscopic study of hereditary corneal edema, Invest Ophthalmol 10:545, 1971.

40. Kanai A et al: Electron microscopic study of hereditary corneal edema, Invest Ophthalmol 2:197, 1971.

41. Judisch GF and Maumenee IH: Clinical differentiation of recessive congenital hereditary endothelial dystrophy and dominant hereditary endothelial dystrophy, Am J Ophthalmol 85:606, 1978.

42. Waring GO, Rodrigues MM, and Laibson PR: Corneal dystrophies: II. Endothelial dystrophies, Surv Ophthalmol 23:147, 1978.

43. Kirkness CM et al: Congenital hereditary corneal oedema of Maumenee: its clinical features, management, and pathology, Br J Ophthalmol 71:130, 1987.

44. Antine BE: Congenital corneal dystrophy, Am J Ophthalmol 70:656, 1970.

45. Antine BE: Congenital hereditary corneal dystrophy (CHCD), South Med J 63:946, 1970.

46. Antine, BE: Histology of congenital hereditary corneal dystrophy, Am J Ophthalmol 69:964, 1970.

47. Kenyon KR and Antine B: The pathogenesis of congenital hereditary endothelial dystrophy of the cornea, Am J Ophthalmol 72:787, 1971.

48. Kenyon KR and Maumenee AE: The histological and ultrastructural pathology of congenital hereditary corneal dystrophy: a case report, Invest Ophthalmol 7:475, 1968.

49. Rodrigues MM et al: Endothelial alterations in congenital corneal dystrophy, Am J Ophthalmol 80:678, 1975.

50. Kenyon KR and Maumenee AE: Further studies of congenital hereditary corneal dystrophy of the cornea, Am J Ophthalmol 76:419, 1973.

51. Stainer GA et al: Correlative microscopy and tissue culture of congenital hereditary endothelial dystrophy, Am J Ophthalmol 93:456, 1982.

52. Pearce WG, Tripathi RC, and Morgan G: Congenital endothelial corneal dystrophy: clinical, pathological and genetic study, Br J Ophthalmol 53:477, 1969.

53. Levenson JE, Chandler JW, and Kaufman HE: Affected asymptomatic relatives in congenital hereditary endothelial dystrophy, Am J Ophthalmol 76:976, 1973.

54. Waring GO and Laibson PR: Keratoplasty in infants and children, Trans Am Acad Ophthalmol Otolaryngol 83:283, 1977.

55. Stulting RD et al: Penetrating keratoplasty in children, Ophthalmology 91:1222, 1984.

56. Dreizen NG, Stulting RD, and Cavanagh HD: Penetrating keratoplasty and cataract surgery in children. In Reinecke R, editor: Ophthalmology annual: nineteen eighty-seven, Norwalk, CT, 1987, Appleton-Century Crofts.

57. Cibis GW et al: The clinical spectrum of posterior polymorphous dystrophy, Arch Ophthalmol 95:1529, 1977.

58. Hogan MJ and Bietti G: Hereditary deep dystrophy of the cornea (polymorphous), Am J Ophthalmol 65:777, 1968.

59. Hansen TE: Posterior polymorphous corneal dystrophy, Acta Ophthalmol (Copenh) 61:454, 1983.

60. Boruchoff SA and Kuwabara T: Electron microscopy of posterior polymorphous degeneration, Am J Ophthalmol 72:879, 1971.

61. Snell AC Jr and Irwin ES: Hereditary deep dystrophy of the cornea, Am J Ophthalmol 45:636, 1958.

62. Cibis GW and Tripathi RC: The differential diagnosis of Descemet's tears and posterior polymorphous dystrophy bands, Ophthalmology 89:614, 1982.

63. Hirst LW and Waring GO III: Clinical specular microscopy of posterior polymorphous endothelial dystrophy, Am J Ophthalmol 95:143, 1983.

64. Mashima Y et al: Specular microscopy of posterior polymorphous endothelial dystrophy, Ophthalmic Pediatr Genet 7:101, 1986.

65. Pratt AW, Saheb ME, and Leblanc R: Posterior polymorphous corneal dystrophy in juvenile glaucoma, Can J Ophthalmol 11:180, 1976.

66. Rubenstein RA and Silverman JJ: Hereditary deep dystrophy of the cornea associated with glaucoma and ruptures in Descemet's membrane, Arch Ophthalmol 79:123, 1968.

67. Polack FM et al: Scanning electron microscopy of posterior polymorphous corneal dystrophy, Am J Ophthalmol 89:575, 1980.

68. Rodriques MM et al: Glaucoma due to endothelialization of the anterior chamber angle: a comparison of posterior polymorphous dystrophy of the cornea and Chandler's syndrome, Arch Ophthalmol 98:688, 1980.

69. Rodrigues MM et al: Epithelialization of the corneal endothelium in posterior polymorphous dystrophy, Invest Ophthalmol Vis Sci 19:832, 1980.

70. Tripathi RC, Casey TA, and Wise EG: Hereditary posterior polymorphous dystrophy: an ultrastructural and clinical report, Trans Ophthalmol Soc UK 94:211, 1974.

71. Chan CC et al: Similarities between posterior polymorphous and congenital hereditary endothelial dystrophies: a study of 14 buttons of 11 cases, Cornea 1:155, 1982.

72. Presberg SE et al: Posterior polymorphous corneal dystrophy, Cornea 4:239, 1985.

73. Richardson WP and Hettinger ME: Endothelial and epithelial-like cell formations in a case of posterior polymorphous dystrophy, Arch Ophthalmol 103:1520, 1985.

74. Krachmer JH: Posterior polymorphous corneal dystrophy: a disease characterized by epithelial-like endothelial cells which influence management and prognosis, Trans Am Ophthalmol Soc 83:413, 1985.

75. Rodrigues MM et al: Posterior polymorphous dystrophy of the cornea: cell culture studies, Exp Eye Res 33:535, 1981.

76. Boruchoff SA, Weiner MJ, and Albert DM: Recurrence of posterior polymorphous corneal dystrophy after penetrating keratoplasty, Am J Ophthalmol 109:323, 1990.

77. Eagle RC et al: Proliferative endotheliopathy with iris abnormalities: the iridocorneal endothelial syndrome, Arch Ophthalmol 97:2104, 1979.

78. Harms C: Einseitige spontane Luckenbildung der iris durch atrophie ohne mechanische Zerrung, Klin Monatsbl Augenheilkd 41:522, 1903.

79. Chandler PA: Atrophy of the stroma of the iris: endothelial dystrophy, corneal edema, and glaucoma, Am J Ophthalmol 41:607, 1956.

80. Cogan DG and Reese AB: A syndrome of iris nodules, ectopic Descemet's membrane, and unilateral glaucoma, Arch Ophthalmol 93:963, 1975.

81. Shields MB, Campbell DG, and Simmons RJ: The essential iris atrophies, Am J Ophthalmol 85:749, 1978.

82. Setala K and Vannas A: Corneal endothelial cells in essential iris atrophy: a specular microscopic study, Acta Ophthalmol 57:1020, 1979.

83. Hirst LW et al: Specular microscopy of iridocorneal endothelial syndrome, Am J Ophthalmol 89:1980.

84. Neubauer L, Lund O-E, and Leibowitz HM: Specular microscopic appearance of the corneal endothelium in iridocorneal endothelial syndrome, Arch Ophthalmol 101:916, 1983.

85. Bourne WM: Partial corneal involvement in the iridocorneal endothelial syndrome, Ophthalmology 94:774, 1982.

86. Kupfer C et al: The contralateral eye in the iridocorneal endothelial (ICE) syndrome, Ophthalmology 90:1343, 1983.

87. Campbell DG, Shields MB, and Smith TR: The corneal endothelium and the spectrum of essential iris atrophy, Am J Ophthalmol 86:317, 1978.

88. Scheie HG and Yanoff M: Iris nevus (Cogan-Reese) syndrome: a cause of unilateral glaucoma, Arch Ophthalmol 93:963, 1975.

89. Shields MB et al: Iris nodules in essential iris atrophy, Arch Ophthalmol 94:406, 1976.

90. Daicker B, Sturrock G, and Guggenheim R: Clinicopathological correlation in Cogan-Reese syndrome, Klin Monatsbl Augenheilkd 180:531, 1982.

91. Shields MB et al: Corneal edema in essential iris atrophy, Ophthalmology 86:1533, 1979.

92. Quigley HA and Forster RF: Histopathology of cornea and iris in Chandler's syndrome, Arch Ophthalmol 96:1878, 1978.

93. Richardson RM: Corneal decompensation in Chandler's syndrome: a scanning and transmission electron microscopic study, Arch Ophthalmol 97:2112, 1979.

94. Patel A et al: Clinicopathologic features of Chandler's syndrome, Surv Ophthalmol 27:327, 1983.

95. Hirst LW et al: Epithelial characteristics of the endothelium in Chandler's syndrome, Invest Ophthalmol Vis Sci 24:603, 1983.

96. Eagle RC et al: The iris nevus (Cogan-Reese) syndrome: light and electron microscopic observations, Br J Ophthalmol 64:446, 1980.

97. Radius RL and Herschler J: Histopathology in the iris-nevus (Cogan-Reese) syndrome, Am J Ophthalmol 89:780, 1980.

98. Bahn CF et al: Classification of corneal endothelial disorders based on neural crest origin, Ophthalmology 91:558, 1984.

99. Shields MB: Textbook of glaucoma, ed 2, Baltimore, 1987, Williams & Wilkins.

100. Buxton JN and Lash RS: Results of penetrating keratoplasty in the iridocorneal endothelial syndrome, Am J Ophthalmol 98:297, 1984.

101. Crawford GJ et al: Penetrating keratoplasty in the management of iridocorneal endothelial syndrome, Cornea 8:34, 1989.

102. Vannas A and Ahonen R: Herpetic endothelial keratitis: a case report, Acta Ophthalmol (Copenh) 59:296, 1981.

103. Robin JB, Steigner JB, and Kaufman HE: Progressive herpetic corneal endotheliitis, Am J Ophthalmol 100:336, 1985.

104. Khodadoust AA and Attarzadeh A: Presumed autoimmune corneal endotheliopathy, Am J Ophthalmol 93:718, 1982.

105. Ohashi Y et al: Idiopathic corneal endotheliopathy, Arch Ophthalmol 103:1666, 1985.

106. Khodadoust AA et al: Pars planitis and autoimmune endotheliopathy, Am J Ophthalmol 102:633, 1986.

107. Ruusuvaara P and Setäläka K: Keratoendotheliitis fugax hereditaria: A clinical and specular microscopic study of a family with dominant inflammatory corneal disease, Acta Ophthalmol (Copenh) 65:159, 1987.

IMMUNOLOGIC DISORDERS

IMMUNOLOGIC CHARACTERISTICS OF THE OCULAR SURFACE

The immunology of the eye is influenced by its unique anatomy and physiology. The surface of the eye is protected by several different mechanisms. Nonimmunologic mechanisms include physical protection and removal of foreign material by the lids and the tears, the normal bacterial flora, mucus, tear proteins (for example, lactoferrin and lysozyme), and the barrier function of the epithelium (see Chapter 6). Several current general reviews[1-4] of the immune system provide a review of the basic mechanisms of immunology.

CONJUNCTIVA

The conjunctiva, like other mucosa in the body, is exposed to the external environment and is constantly barraged with foreign antigens. The mucosa are all colonized by commensal organisms, to which they must be relatively unresponsive, while at the same time responding vigorously to pathogenic organisms. They must serve as barriers to the penetration of external antigens and limit the immune response to common environmental antigens.

The mucosa of the gastrointestinal, respiratory, and urogenital tracts are associated with lymphoid tissues, which together are referred to as the *mucosal immune system*. These lymphoid tissues are considered a distinct immunologic entity because they exhibit several unique characteristics that distinguish them from the systemic immune system: They contain some mucosa-specific cell types, such as the mucosal mast cell, and specialized immunoregulatory cells. The lymphocytes of mucosal follicles are a subpopulation that remains largely confined to mucosal tissues; even after release into the circulation they home to mucosal tissues and often specifically to the organ from which they originated. In some cases the epithelium over the lymphoid tissue is composed of specialized cells that transfer antigens to the lymphocytes and can transform into class II MHC antigen-presenting cells.

The mast cells present in mucosa are distinct from mast cells found in other body tissues. They are important in immediate type hypersensitivity reactions; they contain a number of inflammatory mediators, such as histamine, proteases, prostaglandins, and leukotrienes, which are released in response to activation of IgE by an allergen.

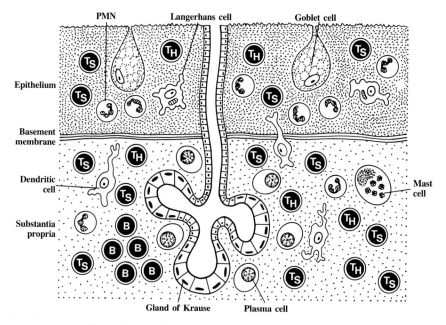

Fig. 19-1. Immunologic cell population of the conjunctiva (see text). *TH,* Helper T lymphocyte; *TS,* suppressor T lymphocyte; *B,* B lymphocyte. (Modified from Sacks EH et al: Ophthalmology 93:1276, 1986.)

The lymphocyte population of the conjunctiva is analogous to the gut-associated lymphoid tissues (GALT) and bronchus-associated lymphoid tissue (BALT), and has been referred to as the conjunctival-associated lymphoid tissue (CALT).[5] Lymphocytes are interspersed in the epithelial layer and form a distinct layer within the substantia propria (Fig. 19-1). Those in the epithelium are mainly cytotoxic-suppressor T cells, and a nearly equal proportion of cytotoxic/suppressor and helper/inducer T cells are found in the substantia propria.[6] A smaller population of B cells is present in the substantia propria, arranged in aggregates, and localized to the fornices. This distribution of T and B cells is similar to that seen in the intestinal mucosa.[7]

Mast cells are also present in the substantia propria, but they are seen in the epithelium only in disease states, such as vernal keratoconjunctivitis and giant papillary conjunctivitis. Small numbers of neutrophils may be present in the epithelium and substantia propria, but eosinophils and basophils are not found in normal conjunctiva. Langerhans cells, which function as antigen-presenting cells, are found in large numbers in the epithelium. They are most plentiful in the bulbar and forniceal conjunctiva. Dendritic antigen-presenting cells are present in the substantia propria.

The lymphoid tissue of the conjunctiva is able to acquire and process antigens. After interaction of the lymphocytes with antigen the activated lymphoblasts are thought to travel to the local lymph nodes, the preauricular and submandibular nodes. From there they are probably released into the blood, and through an unknown mechanism, migrate back to the ocular tissues, and to a lesser extent, to other mucosal tissue.

LACRIMAL TISSUE

The lacrimal gland and accessory lacrimal glands also belong to the mucosal-associated lymphoid tissue system. Their chief contribution appears to be the production of secretory IgA, which is released into the tears. IgA-producing plasma cells are found in the lymphoid aggregates associated with the intralobular ducts, both in the main and accessory lacrimal glands. These cells produce J-linked dimeric IgA, which is taken up by the overlying acinar cells, bound to a secretory component, and released into the gland lumen. Secretory IgA is relatively resistant to proteolysis and is a relatively poor activator of complement (possibly to decrease the inflammatory response and lessen damage to the epithelial surface). IgA appears to be important in protecting against microbial infection by promoting microbial phagocytosis, inhibiting microbial binding to surface epithelium, interfering with bacterial exotoxins, and enhancing antibody-dependent cell-mediated cytotoxicity.

CORNEA

Although the cornea is normally devoid of blood vessels, lymphatics, and inflammatory cells, a number of immunologically active cells and substances are present in the cornea. Immunoglobulins and complement components are present, probably through diffusion from the limbal vessels. C3, C4, and C5 are found throughout the corneal stroma; but the larger C1q molecule is localized to the corneal periphery.[8-10] IgG and IgA are also present throughout the stroma, but at levels much lower than in the serum.[11] The much larger IgM is found only in the peripheral cornea. Langerhans cells, antigen-presenting cells, are found in the corneal epithelium; their density is greatest at the limbus and decreases markedly toward the central cornea.[12]

The cornea enjoys a relative "immune privilege," meaning that foreign antigens, such as a corneal graft, are tolerated much more readily in the cornea than at other sites, partly because of the absence from the cornea of blood vessels and lymphatics, impairing both the afferent and efferent limbs of the immune system. It also may be related to the relative lack of antigen-presenting cells, or the development of anterior chamber–associated immune deviation (ACAID) (see next section).

In pathologic states vascularization of the cornea can occur and is accompanied by the development of lymphoid channels and an increase in the number of Langerhans cells. Their presence diminishes the relative immune privilege of the cornea.

ANTERIOR CHAMBER

The anterior chamber also appears to enjoy a relative immune privilege. When certain foreign antigens are introduced into the anterior chamber a selective suppression of delayed hypersensitivity occurs, which is referred to as anterior chamber–associated immune deviation (ACAID).[13,14] ACAID appears to be an active process, related to secretion of immunosuppressive factors, such as transforming growth factor beta, by cells lining the anterior chamber. Development of ACAID may influence the ability of the immune system to respond to virus or tumor in the anterior chamber or to corneal allografts. Systemic production of antigen-specific antibodies and cytotoxic T cells appears to be normal, and antigen-specific suppressor T cells are also induced. It has been hypothesized that delayed hypersensitivity is selectively suppressed to avoid the amount of innocent bystander tissue destruction that often accompanies it.

DISORDERS OF IMMUNE-MEDIATED INJURY
MECHANISMS OF IMMUNE-MEDIATED INJURY (HYPERSENSITIVITY RESPONSES)

The immune response can cause injury to the host if it is excessive or inappropriate. Such reactions are called hypersensitivity reactions, and four different mechanisms have been described.[15] The types of hypersensitivity reactions believed to be responsible for different ocular disease are listed in Table 19-1.

Type I: anaphylaxis or immediate hypersensitivity. Antigen (allergen) reacts with IgE (and possibly IgG_4) antibody bound to mast cells or circulating basophils. This reaction leads to degranulation of the mast cells or basophils, with the release of inflammatory mediators. The mediators include histamine, serotonin, heparin, eosinophil chemotactic factors of anaphylaxis (ECF-A), slow-reacting substance of anaphylaxis, prostaglandins, and proteases. The levels of intracellular cyclic adenosine monophosphate (cAMP) and cyclic guanine monophosphate (cGMP) influence the release of these mediators from the mast cells and basophils. Elevation of intracellular cAMP inhibits the release of mediators, whereas elevation of cGMP enhances their release.

The diagnosis can be inferred from a history of atopy, development of reactions after contact with an allergen, and itching. Further evidence can be obtained by observation of eosinophils in conjunctival scrapings, reaction to intradermal challenge with the allergen, or detection of specific IgE in serum (radioallergosorbent technique [RAST] or enzyme-linked immunoadsorbent assay [ELISA]).

TABLE 19-1. Types of Hypersensitivity Reactions Associated with Ocular Disease

TYPE I (ANAPHYLACTIC)	TYPE II (CYTOTOXIC)	TYPE III (IMMUNE COMPLEX)	TYPE IV (CELL-MEDIATED)
Allergic conjunctivitis	Cicatricial pemphigoid	Stevens-Johnson syndrome	Contact dermatitis
Vernal keratoconjunctivitis	Bullous pemphigoid	Sjögren's syndrome	Phlyctenulosis
Atopic keratoconjunctivitis	Pemphigus vulgaris	Reiter's syndrome	Allograft reaction
?Giant papillary conjunctivitis	?Mooren's ulcer	Other connective tissue diseases and vasculitis syndromes, including Wegener's granulomatosis, SLE, polyarteritis nodosa	Herpetic disciform keratitis
		?Mooren's ulcer	?Giant papillary conjunctivitis
			?Vernal keratoconjunctivitis
			?Atopic keratoconjunctivitis
			?Stevens-Johnson syndrome

Type II: cytotoxic hypersensitivity. Antibodies are formed and are directed against antigens present on cells. Once bound, the antibodies can activate complement, stimulate mediator release and/or phagocytosis by macrophages and other leukocytes, or activate killer cells (antibody-dependent cell-mediated cytotoxicity [ADCC]). Only complement-fixing antibodies (IgG_1, IgG_3, or IgM) are capable of eliciting these reactions.

To establish the existence of a type II reaction, fixed antitissue antibodies must be present at the disease site and in vitro killer cell activity against the tissue must be demonstrated. Biopsies can be examined for the presence of antibodies and complement.

Type III: immune complex hypersensitivity. Circulating antigen-antibody complexes become deposited in tissues, where they activate complement, cause platelet aggregation, and stimulate mediator release and/or phagocytosis by macrophages and other leukocytes. The antigen can be microbial, environmental, pharmaceutical, or autologous. Development of immune complex disease requires a particular size complex, which is determined by the character of the antigen and the relative amounts of antibody and antigen in circulation; increased vascular permeability; and, probably, decreased clearance of the complexes by phagocytosis.

Circulating immune complexes can be detected in serum, and antigen-antibody-complement complexes can be detected in tissue biopsies.

Type IV: cell-mediated hypersensitivity. Antigen-specific T lymphocytes are stimulated by contact with macrophage-bound antigen. They release mediators and, in some cases, transform into blast cells, which can kill cells bearing the sensitizing antigen. The mediators, called lymphokines, attract and stimulate other mononuclear cells and may play a role in direct cytotoxicity. Type IV reactions are delayed in onset because time is required for synthesis of lymphokines and for their effects to become evident.

Cell-mediated hypersensitivity is most commonly demonstrated by skin testing, either intradermal injection or topical application (patch testing). If the patient is sensitized, a reaction occurs in 24 to 48 hours. In addition, a number of in vitro tests can be performed to demonstrate the presence of specifically sensitized lymphocytes in the serum (for example, antigen stimulation, macrophage migration inhibition, and cell-mediated lympholysis).

APPROACHES TO TREATMENT

Type I. If the offending antigen can be identified, exposure to it can be avoided or reduced. Applying cool compresses and topical vasoconstrictors, such as naphazoline, provides symptomatic relief. Systemic antihistamines are sometimes helpful, particularly in hay fever and dust and grass allergies, but topical antihistamines are rarely beneficial. Topical disodium cromoglycate (Opticrom, Fisons, Bedford, MA) reduces degranulation of mast cells and basophils and is often effective to treat allergic and vernal conjunctivitis. Topical corticosteroids are very effective in decreasing the inflammatory response, but the risks of their chronic use limit their application.

Desensitization immunotherapy is often effective in type I reactions. It involves repeated injections or oral doses of allergen extracts in slowly increasing amounts. Its mechanism of action is uncertain, but it is associated with increased blocking IgG antibody titers, generation of specific suppressor T cells, and nonspecific target cell desensitization.[16]

Types II, III, IV. Although our knowledge of the processes involved in these types of reactions has become much more sophisticated, the means of treatment remain limited to generalized immunosuppression with corticosteroids or other immunosuppressive agents. Cyclosporine is the only exception to this practice because it acts primarily on T cells and T cell–produced mediators, although it appears to have some direct B cell activity.

Corticosteroids. Corticosteroids have both immunosuppressive and antiinflammatory effects. The mechanism of their immunosuppressive action is poorly understood, but they appear to exert direct effects on all inflammatory cells. Corticosteroids decrease the production of inflammatory mediators, including prostaglandins, and interleukin (IL)-1 and IL-2.

Cytotoxic agents. These agents interfere with the synthesis of proteins and nucleic acids, inhibiting cell replication and preferentially killing dividing cells; therefore, they kill B and T cells stimulated to divide. However, this is probably not the only mechanism for their action. Alkylating agents such as cyclophosphamide and chlorambucil alkylate DNA of both resting and dividing cells, resulting in cross linkage of double-stranded DNA, and leading to cell death during mitosis. Purine analogs, such as azathioprine and mercaptopurine inhibit DNA synthesis by interfering with purine metabolism. Folic acid analogs such as methotrexate impair DNA synthesis by inhibiting formation of folic acid, which is important in the synthesis of thymidine. The use of these agents should be undertaken only in conjunction with someone who is familiar with them, such as an oncologist, and with careful monitoring of their systemic effects.

Cyclosporine. Cyclosporine is a relatively new immunosuppressive agent that relatively selectively suppresses T cell function. It appears to act by interfering with the interaction of T cells with antigen-presenting cells.

DISEASES OF IMMEDIATE TYPE HYPERSENSITIVITY

Each of the following diseases appears to be related, at least in part, to a type I hypersensitivity reaction. The term "atopy" is used to describe a number of conditions that tend to occur together in the same family and in the same individual: asthma, allergic rhinitis and conjunctivitis, urticaria, and atopic dermatitis. The tendency to atopy is inherited, probably on a multifactorial basis. Between 10% and 20% of the population are affected by atopy.

Allergic conjunctivitis. This common condition results from a type I reaction to an airborne allergen. The most common allergen is ragweed (hay fever), but a wide variety of antigens can be responsible, including other plant pollens, dust, animal danders, and mold spores. Shortly after exposure, the patient develops itching, burning, and tearing. Rhinitis or sinusitis is commonly present. Many of

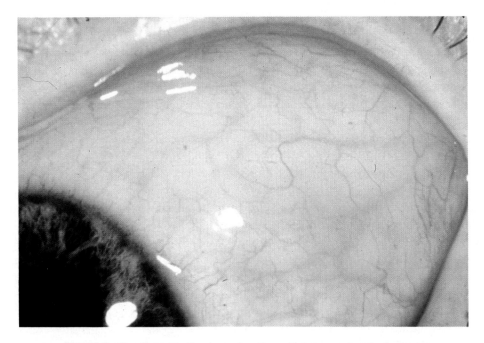

Fig. 19-2. Hay fever reaction in conjunctiva with large conjunctival wheal.

these patients manifest other forms of immediate hypersensitivity, such as asthma, atopic dermatitis, food and drug allergies, and urticaria-angioedema. The symptoms are often seasonal, related to the amount of allergen present in the air.

Signs include conjunctival hyperemia, edema, and chemosis (Fig 19-2), a mild papillary response, lid edema, and mucoid discharge. The diagnosis can usually be made on the basis of history and examination. Conjunctival scrapings often demonstrate eosinophils; however, their absence does not exclude the diagnosis.[17,18] A rapid response to appropriate therapy, such as antihistamines or corticosteroids, is also suggestive. Some special tests are particularly useful for identifying the specific allergen(s): intradermal skin testing and identification of specific serum IgE (RAST, ELISA). A diluted preparation of an allergen can be instilled in the conjunctival sac, and the reaction observed, although this method is seldom practical.

Exposure to the allergen(s) should be reduced as much as possible. Cool compresses and topical vasoconstrictors provide some symptomatic relief. In one study the combination of a vasoconstrictor and a topical antihistamine was superior to either treatment alone.[19] Oral antihistamines are often useful. Topical cromolyn sodium 4% (Opticrom, Fisons, Bedford, MA) can be effective in patients with chronic disease.[20,21] It is given four times daily, and often its effect is not evident until after 2 to 3 weeks of treatment. Topical corticosteroids are very effective in relieving symptoms, but the risks of chronic treatment usually outweigh the benefits. Desensitizing immunotherapy may be a useful approach to patients with severe disease, particularly if it is accompanied by rhinitis or sinusitis. Recently, oral immunotherapy was reported to be effective in alleviating the symptoms of hay fever conjunctivitis.[22]

Vernal keratoconjunctivitis. Vernal keratoconjunctivitis (VKC) is a bilateral, seasonal inflammation caused by allergy and usually seen in young patients.[4,23-25] It occurs most often between the ages of 6 and puberty.[26] Before puberty boys are affected two to three times as often as girls, but the prevalence in girls rises after puberty, so by the age of 20 the sexes are affected almost equally. The disease usually diminishes in severity during the teens and disappears in the early twenties, but it can persist for decades in some individuals.

VKC affects all races and occurs in all parts of the world. The limbal form appears to be more common in blacks and American Indians. The disease is more common in dry, warm climates, such as the Middle East, the Mediterranean basin, and Central America. In more temperate climates, VKC tends to be seasonal, occurring with the onset of spring and decreasing in the fall. During the colder months the symptoms decrease, but the conjunctival changes usually persist with only slight regression. The signs of the limbal form of the disease are more likely to regress, and in mild cases they can resolve completely. In tropical climates the seasonal variation is often less marked.

Clinical manifestations. Itching, the most outstanding symptom, is usually the earliest symptom and may precede all conjunctival signs of disease. Photophobia is also often prominent, and the child responds by continually keeping the face turned toward the ground. Other symptoms include burning, lacrimation, and foreign body sensation. These symptoms are often associated with a thick, sticky, mucoid discharge.

The earliest sign of vernal conjunctivitis may be a simple hyperemia, which is quickly followed by a more marked response characterized by conjunctival thickening or hyperplasia. Hyperplasia can be most prominent either in the superior tarsal conjunctiva (palpebral form) or around the limbus (limbal form). In the palpebral form, the tarsal conjunctiva initially appears dull and pale and may have a milky-blue hue. Later, papillae are the most prominent finding. They can be small and few in number early; but with progression they become larger, more elevated, polygonal, and flat-topped (Fig. 19-3). When they are numerous and tightly packed, the tarsal conjunctiva can have the classic cobblestone appearance. The weight of the papillae can cause a mechanical ptosis. The lower tarsal conjunctiva can also demonstrate papillary hypertrophy, but it is less severely affected, and giant pa-

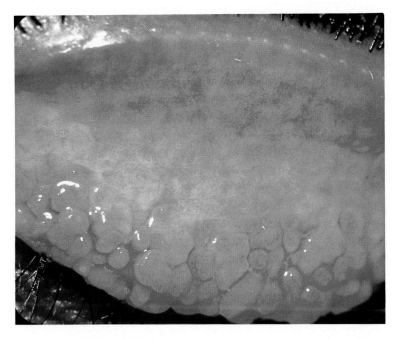

Fig. 19-3. Giant papillary hypertrophy (cobblestone appearance) of upper tarsal conjunctiva.

pillae are rarely seen. (Giant papillae are more often seen in this location in atopic keratoconjunctivitis.)

Limbal involvement appears as semitransparent, smooth, gelatinous elevations (Fig. 19-4), which may be broad and uniform or may form distinct nodules. Their corneal edge is sharp, but they blend gradually into the conjunctiva. They can involve any portion of the limbus or its entire circumference; some authors say that the interpalpebral limbus is most commonly affected, whereas others implicate the superior limbus. The limbal elevations can extend onto the peripheral cornea, often leaving focal areas of opacity and micropannus after their regression (Fig. 19-5). Small epithelial cysts and marginal pits can occur. The pits are translucent, round, nondepressed areas within the opaque limbus and represent localized resolution of limbal infiltration.

Small, flat or mildly elevated, grayish-white to yellow dots, called *Trantas' dots,* can be present on the limbal elevations (Fig. 19-6). These structures are usually seen only at the upper limbus, but they can appear on the bulbar conjunctiva, semilunar folds, and very rarely on the tarsal conjunctiva or cornea. The dots consist of degenerating eosinophils and epithelial cells. They are transient, usually not lasting longer than a week. The dots may be seen in the deep layers of the epithelium; however, they gradually become more superficial and break through to the surface. (Trantas dots also can occur in chronic atopic keratoconjunctivitis and soft contact lens wear.)

Corneal involvement in VKC can take several forms. As mentioned previously, a micropannus can occur. Another form is a farinaceous epitheliopathy (keratitis epithelialis vernalis of Tobgy), which consists of tiny, gray-white, intraepithelial corneal opacities (Fig. 19-7).[27,28] The opacities are most prominent in the superior cornea, with relative sparing of the periphery, and they stain with fluorescein and rose bengal red. A more intense form of farinaceous keratitis can occur, with degeneration and shrinkage of the epithelial cells, producing the appearance of a cobweb or syncytium (Fig. 19-8). This form is more common in patients with palpebral vernal keratitis and tends to be transient, lasting days to weeks.

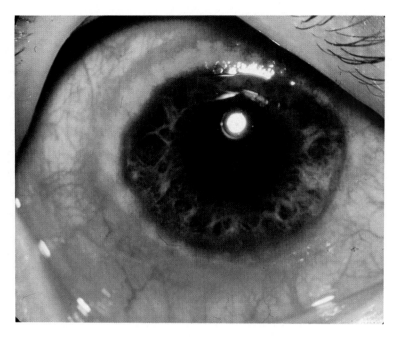

Fig. 19-4. Limbal vernal catarrh exhibiting gelatinous elevations.

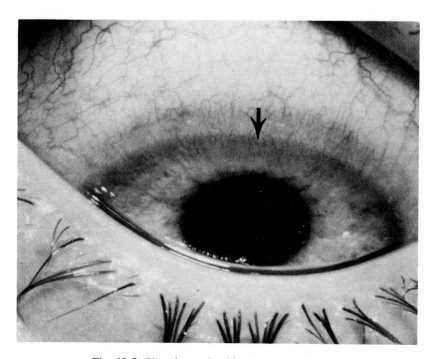

Fig. 19-5. Vernal catarrh with micropannus *(arrow).*

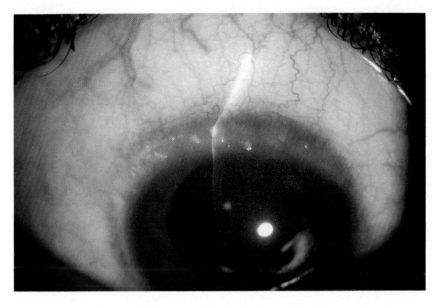

Fig. 19-6. Gelatinous superior limbal elevations, with overlying fine white plaques (Trantas' dots) in limbal vernal.

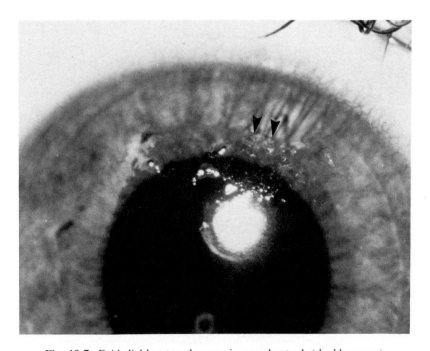

Fig. 19-7. Epithelial keratopathy seen in vernal catarrh *(double arrow)*.

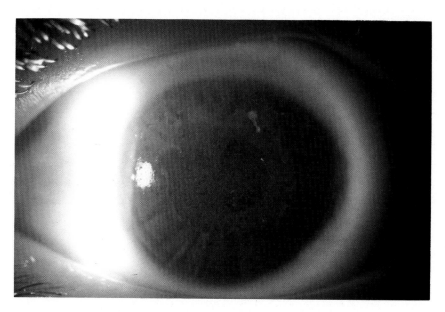

Fig. 19-8. Farinaceous epithelial keratopathy in vernal keratoconjunctivitis.

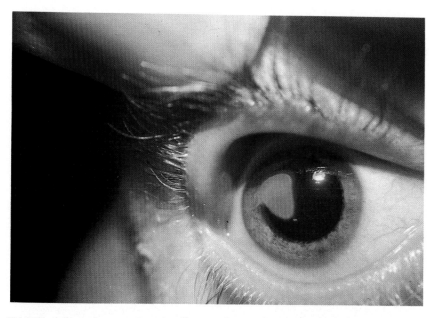

Fig. 19-9. Shieldlike ulcer of cornea occasionally seen in vernal catarrh. (From Grayson M and Keates RH: Manual of diseases of the cornea, Boston, 1969, Little, Brown & Co.)

Characteristic corneal ulcers also can occur (in about 3% to 4% of patients). These are horizontally oval or shield-shaped and are usually located in the superior half of the cornea (Fig. 19-9). (Inferior ulcers were reported in one case.[29]) These ulcers are shallow and have thickened opaque edges and a grayish base, which may be infiltrated. They are usually indolent and do not vascularize. As they heal a gray plaque can form in the bed, which gradually shrinks, leaving an oval or ring opacity in the superficial stroma. Shield ulcers are most common in very young patients, particularly those with large papillae. The ulcers and the other epithelial findings may result from mechanical irritation of the corneal surface by the abnormal palpebral conjunctiva or the toxicity of the inflammatory mediators.

Less often, a deep, fascicular keratitis can be seen. An arclike or annular opacity can be seen in the peripheral stroma, separated by a clear zone from the limbus (vernal pseudogerontoxon). There appears to be a higher incidence of keratoconus in patients with VKC,[30] although the reason for this relationship is not clear. Corneal involvement appears to be less common in patients with purely limbal VKC.[31]

The most characteristic feature of conjunctival scrapings in VKC is the presence of eosinophils and free eosinophilic granules (Fig. 19-10). In addition, fibrin, mucus, epithelial cells, polymorphonuclear leukocytes, and basophils may be present.

VKC generally abates in the teens and disappears in the twenties. Eventually there is complete resolution of all conjunctival signs; there is no residual scarring unless it has been inappropriately treated by radiation or surgery. The corneal involvement usually does not result in changes that reduce vision; however, myopic astigmatism or keratoconus may require optical correction. Excessive steroid treatment can lead to cataract formation or secondary infection.

Histopathology. In early VKC new vessels and cellular infiltration are seen in the conjunctival substantia propria (see Fig. 3-6). Large numbers of eosinophils are accompanied by polymorphonuclear leukocytes, basophils, and mast cells and in later stages by lymphocytes and macrophages.[4,32-34] An increased amount of connective tissue is seen in the substantia propria; it becomes hyalinized and

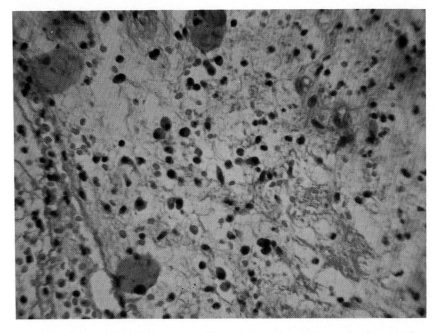

Fig. 19-10. Fragmented and nonfragmented eosinophils seen in conjunctival scraping in case of vernal catarrh.

forms the fibrous core of the papillae. The overlying conjunctival epithelium becomes thickened, increasing from the normal two layers to five to ten layers of irregular, edematous cells. Mast cells, eosinophils, and basophils also are present in the epithelium. In advanced cases the epithelium atrophies to one cell layer and can become keratinized.

Pathogenesis. Strong evidence suggests a role for type I hypersensitivity, but type IV hypersensitivity also may be involved. Evidence for the role of type I hypersensitivity includes a frequent personal or family history of allergies and other forms of atopy; a high concentration of eosinophils in the conjunctiva; a relatively high incidence of systemic eosinophilia[35]; elevated tear IgE and IgG antibodies, including specific antibodies to allergens such as grass and ragweed[25,36-39]; elevated tear histamine[40] and complement[41]; and response to agents that inhibit mast cell degranulation. In patients with specific IgE antibodies against house dust mites, symptoms of VKC correlated well with the quantity of dust mites in their homes.[42]

Several other findings, however, are not explained by this mechanism. Some patients do not have elevated tear IgE[28,31] (although at least some of these patients have elevated IgG_4 antibody, which also may participate in type I reactions). There is proliferation of connective tissue and mixed cellular infiltrate. Occasionally there is no association with other atopic diseases, and high numbers of basophils are present in the conjunctiva. The latter suggests that cutaneous basophil hypersensitivity, a type IV reaction, may play a role.[43,44]

Differential diagnosis. The keratoconjunctivitis associated with atopic dermatitis, atopic keratoconjunctivitis (AKC), can be confused with VKC (Table 19-2). Both occur in atopic individuals, are associated with itching, and may be exacerbated by warm weather. Patients with VKC may have atopic dermatitis, and certainly both VKC and AKC can occur simultaneously. The papillae associated with AKC are usually small and involve the upper tarsal conjunctiva. The discharge is meager and watery, and there are few eosinophils and minimal or no free eosinophilic granules in scrapings. Conjunctival scarring and shrinkage of the inferior fornix are common in AKC, but do not occur in VKC.

Trachoma should also be considered in the differential diagnosis. Trachoma produces round, translucent limbal follicles of uniform size; however, they may be accompanied by true pits (Herbert pits), tarsal follicles, or conjunctival scarring. Conjunctival scrapings in trachoma may contain polymorphonuclear cells, plasma cells, lymphocytes, Leber cells, and epithelial inclusions, but no eosinophils.

Treatment. Fortunately VKC is self-limiting and only rarely causes permanent decrease in vision. Nevertheless, it can be quite disabling. The objective of treatment is to reduce symptoms to permit the child to function as normally as possible, while avoiding iatrogenic complications.

A number of general measures can improve symptoms and may be sufficient in mild cases. Moving to a cooler climate is the most effective form of management, but it clearly is not often practical. Attempts should be made to identify and limit exposure to allergens. Air-conditioning is helpful because it decreases room temperature and filters out airborne allergens. Cool compresses, irrigation with cold saline, and patching provide immediate but transient relief. Desensitization has not proved beneficial.

Topical vasoconstrictors, such as naphazoline, can be applied up to four times daily and are helpful in some cases. A mucolytic agent (for example, acetylcysteine 10% four times daily) is often beneficial when mucous discharge is prominent. Systemic and topical antihistamines are not useful.

If these measures are not sufficient, cromolyn sodium 4% is given four times daily. This treatment is beneficial in most cases, but may require 2 to 3 weeks before the effect is evident.[45-49] Patients with a history of atopic disease have a greater response. Cromolyn sodium must be used continuously, at least during the appropriate seasons; it is not effective when applied only during exacerbations.

TABLE 19-2. Diseases of Immediate-Type Hypersensitivity

	ALLERGIC CONJUNCTIVITIS (HAYFEVER)	VERNAL KERATO-CONJUNCTIVITIS	ATOPIC KERATO-CONJUNCTIVITIS	GIANT PAPILLARY CONJUNCTIVITIS
Hypersensitivity type	I	I, ?IV	I, ?IV	?I, IV
Conjunctiva				
Scarring	−	−	Inferior fornix and papillae	−
Chemosis	+	+	+ (acute)	−
Papillae	Mild diffuse	Medium-giant upper lid	Usually small lower lid	Medium-giant upper lid
Limbus	Normal	Gelatinous elevations Trantas' dots Cysts Marginal pits "Pseudogerontoxon"	Gelatinous elevations Trantas' dots Cysts	CLIK* Superior injection Gelatinous elevations Trantas' dots
Cornea		Micropannus Epitheliopathy "Shield" ulcer	Punctate keratitis Vascularization Opacification Marginal ulceration	Micropannus Superior keratopathy Filaments
Conjunctival scrapings	Eosinophils	Eosinophils Free eosinophilic granules Basophils	Eosinophils Basophils	Eosinophils

*Contact lens–induced keratoconjunctivitis (see Chapter 7).

Topical corticosteroids can provide dramatic relief, but because of the chronic nature of the disease and the risks of prolonged steroid use, steroid treatment is kept to a minimum. In most cases intermittent pulse therapy is sufficient. During severe exacerbations prednisolone acetate 1% or dexamethasone phosphate 0.1% is given every 2 hours during the day, for 4 days, and then rapidly tapered. This regimen may need to be repeated three to four times per year. If necessary, oral steroids can also be given in a 1 to 2 week pulse. In the most persistent cases, daily doses of dilute steroid may be necessary. Topical cyclosporine 2% has been reported to improve signs and symptoms during use, but further evaluation is required.[50] Cryotherapy of the superior tarsal conjunctiva can give short-term relief, possibly by degranulating large numbers of mast cells.[51] Superior tarsal excision and replacement with mucous membrane was helpful in some severe cases, but sometimes large papillae formed at the superior edge of the graft.[52]

Atopic dermatitis with keratoconjunctivitis. Atopic dermatitis is an inflammatory skin disease usually found in patients with other forms of atopy. It appears to have a genetic basis, probably via multifactorial inheritance. Atopic dermatitis also can be seen in some immunodeficiency disorders, for example, Wiskott-Aldrich syndrome and ataxia-telangiectasia.

Clinical manifestations. Atopic dermatitis can begin at any age, but onset during infancy is most common. The duration and severity are quite variable; after infantile onset it can resolve by 2 years of age or persist into adulthood. The skin lesions are dry, erythematous, vesicular, and pruritic. Scratching leads to excoriations, weeping, scaling, and crusting. In infants the forehead, cheeks, and extensor surfaces of the extremities are most involved, and in older patients the antecubital and popliteal areas, neck, wrists, and ankles are more likely to be affected (Fig. 19-11, *A*).

The face and eyelids are often affected in the more severe cases. The lids can become thickened, indurated, and lichenified (Fig. 19-11, *B*). Weeping fissures often occur at the lateral canthi, and punctal eversion or stenosis can occur. Staphylococcal superinfections are common.[53]

Conjunctival involvement occurred in 16% of patients in one series from the Mayo Clinic.[53a] The conjunctival inflammation is accompanied by itching, burning, and mucoid discharge. The conjunctiva often appears hyperemic and chemotic during active disease. In chronic cases the conjunctiva is pale and congested, with a papillary response. Medium or giant papillae can be present, usually inferiorly; the upper tarsal conjunctiva often appears milky, without formation of large papillae. Gelati-

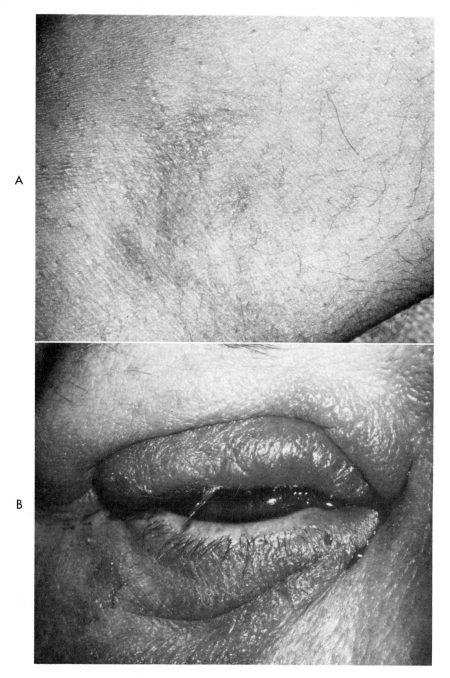

Fig. 19-11. **A,** Antecubital skin lesions in atopic dermatitis. Skin in eczema can be weeping and crusting or dry and lichenified. **B,** Eyelids may be thick and lichenified in atopic dermatitis with keratoconjunctivitis.

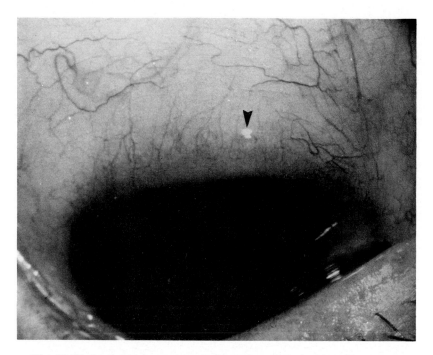

Fig. 19-12. Limbal bleb may be seen in atopic conjunctival keratitis *(arrow)*.

nous elevations, thick broad opacifications (usually superior), epithelial cysts (Fig. 19-12), and Trantas' dots can be seen at the limbus. Scarring can occur and tends to be focal and to develop in the centers of the papillae (Fig. 19-13, *A*) and in the inferior fornix (Fig. 19-13, *B*). It can be severe enough to cause symblepharon, entropion, and trichiasis.

The most common corneal finding is punctate keratitis, which is most prominent inferiorly. Marginal ulceration, vascularization, and stromal opacification can occur (Fig. 19-14). Secondary infection with bacteria or herpes simplex (Fig. 19-15) is common. Keratoconus is also more common in these patients.[54]

Anterior and posterior subcapsular cataracts (Fig. 19-16) occur in approximately 8% of patients.[54,55] The opacities usually begin between 16 and 18 years of age and can progress rapidly.

Pathogenesis. The pathogenesis is unknown, but patients have evidence of both immediate-type hypersensitivity and abnormal cell-mediated immunity. The role of immediate-type hypersensitivity is suggested by a frequent family history of atopy, a high incidence of positive immediate skin test reactions, elevated serum IgE levels in more than 80% of patients, and frequent eosinophilia.[56] However, there is little correlation between allergic disease or serum IgE and clinical findings.

Impaired cell-mediated immunity is suggested by the increased susceptibility of these patients to skin infections by viruses, bacteria, and fungi and decreased delayed-type skin test reactivity.[49,57] The number of circulating T cells, particularly suppressor T cells, is decreased in patients with active disease,[58] and in vitro studies have demonstrated decreased suppression of IgE synthesis by T cells from patients with atopic dermatitis.[59] Therefore, an impairment of suppressor T-cell function may lead to the elevation of IgE production.

Treatment. The treatment of AKC is similar to that of vernal keratoconjunctivitis, but patients with AKC can develop scarring and are more susceptible to superinfection, particularly with herpes simplex, and cataract formation. Symptomatic treatment with cool compresses, topical vasoconstrictors,

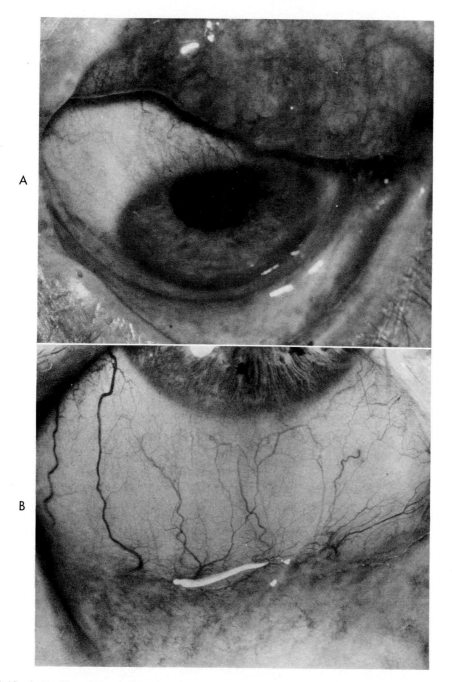

Fig. 19-13. A, Papillary hypertrophy of conjunctiva in case of atopic keratoconjunctivitis. **B,** Atopic keratoconjunctivitis with cicatrization of cul-de-sac.

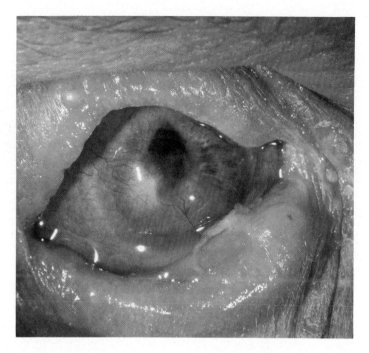

Fig. 19-14. Extensive corneal thinning, scarring, and vascularization in atopic keratoconjunctivitis.

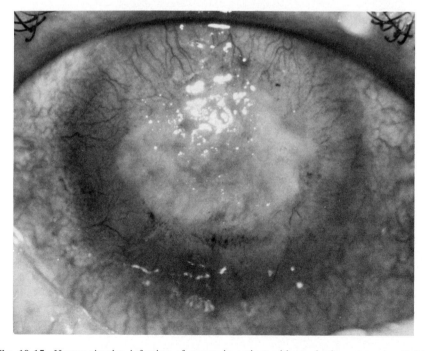

Fig. 19-15. Herpes simplex infection of cornea in patient with atopic dermatoconjunctivitis.

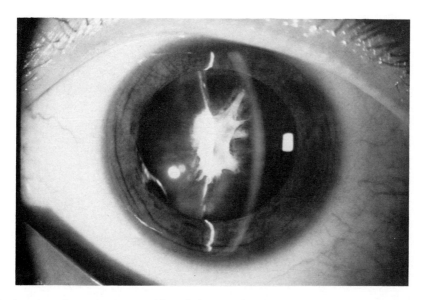

Fig. 19-16. Anterior subcapsular cataract of atopic keratoconjunctivitis. (From Wiley L, Arffa R, and Fireman P: Allergic and immunologic ocular diseases. In Fireman P and Slavin, editors: Atlas of allergic and immunologic diseases, New York, Gower, in press.)

and antihistamines may be helpful. Cromolyn sodium (4% four times daily) is often effective in severe cases.[13,60-62]

Topical corticosteroids are very effective for decreasing inflammation and relieving symptoms, but their use increases the risk of superinfection and cataract. They are certainly indicated when inflammation is producing ectropion, symblepharon, or corneal scarring, but even in these cases the lowest possible dose should be used for the shortest possible time.

Some patients with atopic dermatitis have the hyper-IgE syndrome. This syndrome includes the following features: chronic atopic dermatitis, recurrent pyogenic skin and lung infection, markedly elevated serum IgE, and sometimes defective neutrophil chemotaxis. In some of these patients eye disease was markedly improved by plasmapheresis.[63]

Giant papillary conjunctivitis. Giant papillary conjunctivitis (GPC), a condition initially described in contact lens wearers, is characterized by increased mucus, mild itching, and the development of giant papillae in the upper tarsal conjunctiva.[64,65] A spectrum of clinical findings is associated with this disease; giant papillae are present only in the more advanced cases. Identical findings can be found in association with ocular prostheses,[66,67] corneal shells, exposed nylon sutures,[68,69] cyanoacrylate glue,[70] and extruded scleral buckles.[71]

Clinical manifestations. The earliest symptoms of GPC associated with contact lens wear are itching after removal of the lens and mild mucoid discharge. With progression, itching and then pain occur while the lens is in the eye. Mucous discharge increases, which can coat the lens rapidly after insertion and decrease vision or cause the lids to stick together in the morning. The conjunctival findings often lag behind the symptoms.[72]

Enlarged papillae (>0.3 mm) develop on the upper tarsal surface, and the conjunctiva loses its transparency (Fig. 19-17). In soft contact lens wearers, the papillae tend to affect the middle and superior portions of the tarsus most. They gradually enlarge (to >1 mm) and can become flat-topped and densely packed, creating a cobblestone appearance. In hard contact lens wearers, the papillae

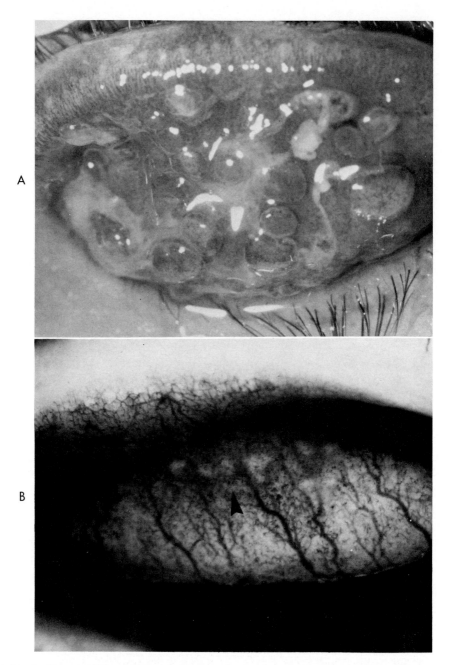

Fig. 19-17. A, Giant papillary reaction of upper tarsal plate in soft contact lens wearer. **B,** Milder reaction in wearer of soft contact lens *(arrow).*

tend to be smaller, more widely separated, and concentrated in the middle or inferior tarsal conjunctiva.

Fluorescein staining of the tops of the papillae can be seen and is a sign of disease activity.[73] Coating of the contact lens surface is often noted and can become quite heavy. Mucous globs or strands may be found on the conjunctival surface or at the canthi. Advanced cases are characterized by gelatinous limbal nodules and Trantas' dots.[74]

Histopathology. Histopathologically, GPC appears similar to vernal conjunctivitis, except that the number of eosinophils and basophils is less in GPC.[65] The papillae represent thickened substantia propria, filled with a normal density of lymphocytes and plasma cells. The overlying epithelium is thickened and irregular. In addition, mast cells are often found in the epithelium, and eosinophils or basophils can be present in the epithelium or the substantia propria.

Pathogenesis. That this condition can result from chronic trauma by prostheses, sutures, or scleral buckles indicates that trauma alone can be sufficient stimulus. However, most contact lens wearers do not develop GPC, suggesting that some additional mechanism is involved. The lens coating appears to play a role: Increased coatings on lenses exacerbate GPC,[72] and when lenses from GPC patients were placed in eyes of monkeys they induced a GPC-like reaction, whereas virgin lenses did not.[75] Many authors have concluded that there is a humeral or cell-mediated allergic reaction to antigens present on the lens, and that trauma may facilitate the exposure of the conjunctival lymphoid system to the antigens. To date, however, specific sensitivity to any of the antigens on these lenses has not been demonstrated.

Treatment. Although cessation of exposure to the foreign body is the most effective treatment, patients are often unwilling to discontinue contact lens wear. In these cases it is frequently possible to continue contact lens wear if certain measures are taken. First, lens wear should be discontinued until the eye is quiet; symptoms such as hyperemia and discharge should resolve, but conjunctival papillae resolve very slowly or not at all. Mild topical steroids can be given to speed this process.

If the patient was wearing a hydrogel lens, switching to a gas-permeable lens often increases lens tolerance. However, continued hydrogel lens wear is sometimes achieved through the following steps:

1. Reduce lens coatings as much as possible through good lens hygiene, regular enzymatic cleaning, and replacement of lenses that do become heavily coated.
2. Avoid the use of sensitizing chemicals (for example, thimerosal).
3. Switch to a smaller diameter, thinner edged lens.
4. Use cromolyn sodium (4% four times daily) regularly to reduce or prevent exacerbation of the disease.[13] (The package insert states that the medication should not be given while the lens is in the eye, but I am not aware of any ill effects from this practice.)

Systemic Lupus Erythematosus

Systemic lupus erythematosus (SLE) is a chronic multisystem disease related to immunologic dysfunction and characterized by the production of autoantibodies. It is seen more frequently in women, with the peak age of onset in the twenties to thirties.

Pathogenesis. SLE appears to result from a dysfunction in immunoregulation: Impaired suppressor T-cell function allows for production of autoantibodies, such as antinuclear antibodies, anticell membrane antibodies, and antithyroid antibodies. Immune complexes are formed, which become deposited in many tissues, causing local inflammation and damage (a type III hypersensitivity reaction). A similar condition can develop in patients on certain drugs, such as hydralazine, procainamide, isoniazid, methyldopa, and hydantoins, through production of autoantibodies.

Clinical manifestations. The most common cutaneous feature of SLE is an erythematous rash, which can appear on the nose and cheeks in a "butterfly" distribution, and on the neck and extremities, especially the tips and dorsa of the fingers, palms, and areas of skin above the elbows. Discoid rashes, alopecia, and mucosal ulcers also can be seen. Other findings include arthritis, polyarthralgia, pleuritis, pericarditis, myocarditis, lymphadenopathy, splenomegaly, nephritis, and hematologic and neurologic disease.

The most common findings in the eye involve the retina: cotton-wool spots, retinal hemorrhages, and edema of the retina and disc, all probably related to a retinal vasculitis. The lids may exhibit

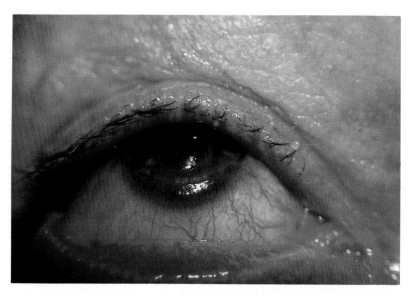

Fig. 19-18. Noninfiltrative marginal melt of cornea seen in case of lupus erythematosus. The eye is also dry, with lusterless appearance.

telangiectasia just above the lid margins. Episcleritis or scleritis can occur and can be the presenting sign of the disease.[76,77] Anterior uveitis can also be seen, usually in association with scleritis.

Keratoconjunctivitis sicca is common in SLE.[78,79] Patients also exhibit punctate keratitis unrelated to dryness.[80-82] Interstitial keratitis[83,84] and quiet, relatively noninfiltrated marginal melts (Fig. 19-18) can be seen. Infiltrative lesions also occur and respond to topical steroid therapy (Fig. 19-19).

Discoid Lupus Erythematosus

Discoid lupus erythematosus (DLE) refers to the presence of characteristic skin lesions that may be seen in isolation or in association with SLE. The lesions are sharply demarcated, raised, erythematous, and scaly and may exhibit telangiectasia and follicular plugging. Central scarring produces depigmentation and permanent loss of appendages. The lesions can affect any part of the body but are most common in light-exposed areas, especially the face and scalp. Approximately 5% of patients with DLE progress to SLE; however, 20% of patients with SLE have DLE lesions. Immunoglobulin, complement, and a mononuclear infiltrate are present at the dermal-epidermal junction in involved areas.

DLE skin lesions may affect the eyelid skin (Fig. 19-20).[85] The lesions can extend over the lid margins and into the conjunctival sac. Conjunctival scarring and lid margin distortion can result.[77]

Superficial punctate keratitis, recurrent epithelial erosions, neovascularization, and marginal corneal infiltrates occasionally occur[86-88] (Fig. 19-21). The inferior, light-exposed portion of the cornea is more affected. In one patient the ocular lesions responded to systemic treatment with quinacrine hydrochloride.[87] Two other patients responded to topical corticosteroid therapy.[88]

Rheumatoid Arthritis

Rheumatoid arthritis is a multisystem, inflammatory autoimmune disorder that primarily affects the joints. It is found more frequently in women, with an average age of onset of 30 to 40 years. The onset of the arthritis is usually gradual, but acute, fulminant cases occur. The small joints of the hands and feet are most commonly involved, followed by the wrists, elbows, ankles, knees, and hips.

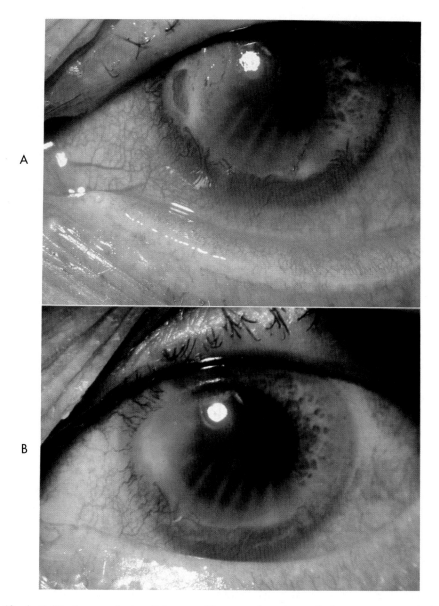

Fig. 19-19. A, Infiltrative marginal melt in case of lupus erythematosus. **B,** Its response to topical steroid medication.

The appearance of the hands is characteristic (Fig. 19-22). Many extraarticular manifestations can be seen, and their presence correlates with the chronicity and severity of the articular disease.[89] Affected tissues include the skin, lungs, heart, lymphatic system, peripheral nervous system, and eye. A generalized vasculitis can occur, manifested by peripheral neuropathy, cutaneous lesions, and gastrointestinal ulcers.

Rheumatoid arthritis appears to be caused by a chronic T-lymphocyte and macrophage-dependent response to foreign or autoantigens present in synovial tissue.[90] Immune complexes are often found in serum, joints, and other tissues, and although they can contribute to the disease, they are probably not the primary cause. IgG and IgM antiimmunoglobulin antibodies are formed (rheumatoid factors), which react with immunoglobulins and fix complement.

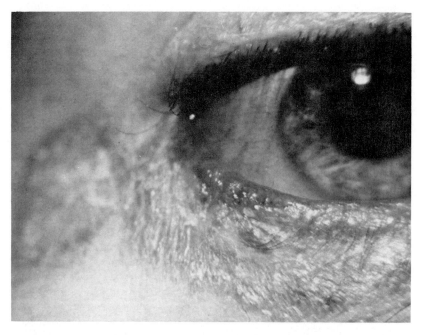

Fig. 19-20. Discoid lupus. (From Grayson M and Keates RH: Manual of diseases of the cornea, Boston, 1969, Little, Brown & Co.)

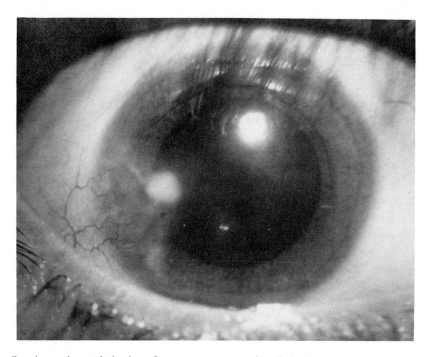

Fig. 19-21. Scarring and vascularization of cornea occurs occasionally in discoid lupus. (From Grayson M and Keates RH: Manual of diseases of the cornea, Boston, 1969, Little, Brown & Co.)

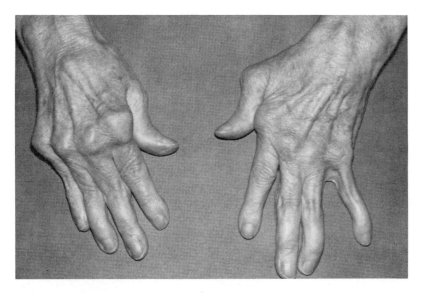

Fig. 19-22. Characteristic appearance of hands in rheumatoid arthritis.

The ocular complications usually occur in patients with severe disease, especially those who have other extraarticular complications.[91] The most common ophthalmic finding is keratoconjunctivitis sicca, which occurs in approximately 15% to 25% of patients.[92,93] Xerophthalmia is also present in some cases (see Sjögren's syndrome, Chapter 14).

Episcleritis and scleritis, which are due to an immune complex vasculitis of the conjunctival or scleral vessels,[99] are also commonly seen.[94-98] The scleritis can take any of the typical forms: diffuse anterior, nodular anterior, necrotizing with inflammation, posterior scleritis, or scleromalacia perforans. Rheumatoid arthritis, the most common disease associated with scleritis, is present in nearly all cases of scleromalacia perforans.[100] The presence of necrotizing scleritis in a patient with rheumatoid arthritis indicates systemic disease activity and a poor overall prognosis; without aggressive treatment a majority of the patients die within 5 years.[101,102]

The most common corneal manifestations of rheumatoid arthritis are those due to keratitis sicca (see Chapter 14). The cornea is also affected in approximately 50% to 70% of patients with scleritis.[89,90,103] Corneal involvement usually occurs as a direct extension of perilimbal scleritis onto the peripheral cornea (sclerokeratitis). Watson has divided the corneal changes in scleritis into four types: sclerosing keratitis, acute stromal keratitis, marginal furrowing, and keratolysis; each can occur in rheumatoid arthritis.[90,92] (These types are described in the section on scleritis.) Episcleritis can also be associated with peripheral corneal lesions, most commonly peripheral stromal infiltration and edema.[90,104]

Peripheral corneal melting also can occur in the absence of scleritis.[82,105] The cornea may show a noninfiltrative, slowly melting lesion either at the limbus or 1 to 2 mm inside the limbus (Fig. 19-23). Infiltrative peripheral cornea lesions also occur (Fig. 19-24). Occasionally the furrows or melting areas perforate (Figs. 19-25 and 19-26).

Some of the drugs used in treating rheumatoid arthritis, such as systemic corticosteroids, gold salts, and antimalarials, can produce ocular complications (see Chapter 27). Antimalarial agents, such as hydroxychloroquine sulfate (Plaquenil), can cause a whorllike pattern of intraepithelial deposits, resembling the keratopathy of Fabry's disease (verticillate or vortex dystrophy). Lens pigmentation and peripheral corneal infiltration (Fig. 19-27) and ulceration can result from gold therapy.

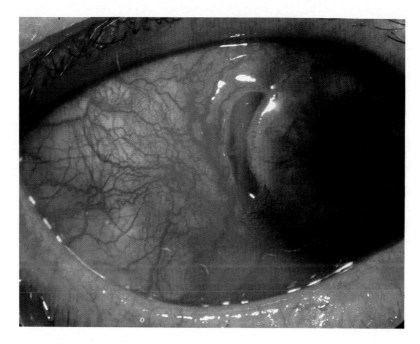

Fig. 19-23. Marginal noninfiltrative melting of limbal tissues in rheumatoid arthritis.

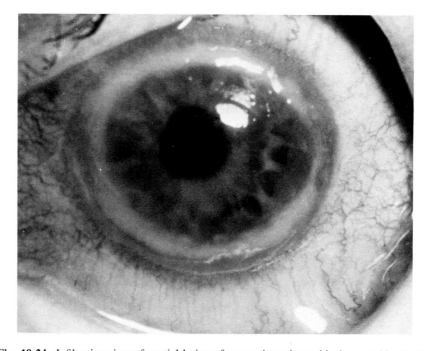

Fig. 19-24. Infiltrative circumferential lesion of cornea in patient with rheumatoid arthritis.

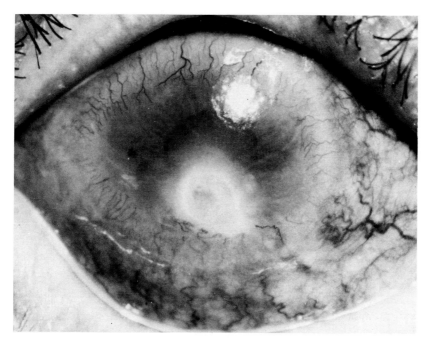

Fig. 19-25. Central corneal perforation in rheumatoid arthritis.

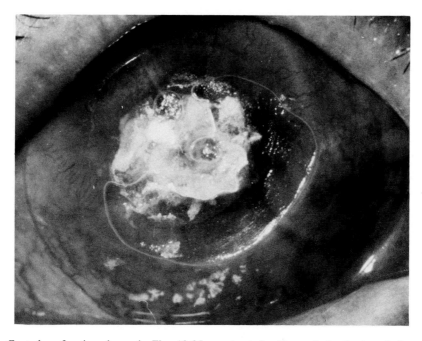

Fig. 19-26. Central perforation shown in Fig. 19-25 was treated with surgical adhesive. Soft contact lens is applied over adhesive.

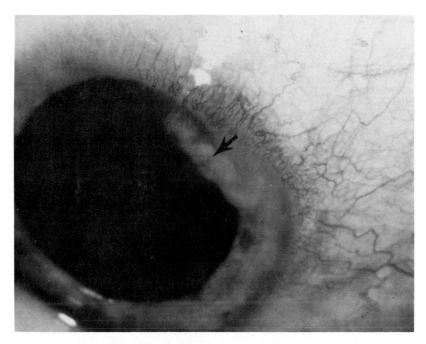

Fig. 19-27. Marginal infiltration noted in patient treated with gold for rheumatoid arthritis *(arrow).*

Juvenile rheumatoid arthritis can be associated with chronic iritis, and band keratopathy is a relatively common complication.[106] Keratoconjunctivitis sicca also has been reported.[107]

PROGRESSIVE SYSTEMIC SCLEROSIS (SCLERODERMA)

Progressive systemic sclerosis (PSS) is a multisystem disorder characterized by inflammatory, fibrotic, degenerative, and vascular changes in the skin and in some internal organs, particularly the gastrointestinal tract, lungs, heart, and kidney. Women are more often affected than men, with an onset typically in the third or fourth decade. The hallmark of PSS is induration of the skin (scleroderma), most commonly over the digits, resulting from collagen deposition in the dermis (Fig. 19-28). Raynaud's phenomenon (present in 90% of cases), arthritis, pulmonary fibrosis, impaired gastrointestinal motility (particularly esophageal), calcinosis, renal failure, and telangiectasia are other manifestations.

The pathogenesis is unknown. There appears to be early vascular endothelial injury; some have suggested that this is the primary event.[108] Much indirect evidence supports a role for the immune system, including the presence of perivascular cellular infiltrates in patients with active disease, the high incidence of antinuclear and other autoantibodies in the serum, and the occurrence of scleroderma-like changes in graft-versus-host disease, a condition known to be related to cell-mediated immunity.[99,109]

Both keratoconjunctivitis sicca[110,111] and conjunctival fornix foreshortening[112,113] occur in the majority of patients. One may find lid distortions from involvement of the skin of the lid and lid telangiectasias. Corneal involvement is rare, but one may find infiltration and vascularization (Fig. 19-29).[114]

RELAPSING POLYCHONDRITIS

This disease, characterized by recurrent inflammation of cartilaginous tissues, occurs equally in men and women, with onset usually between 40 and 60 years of age. The pathogenesis is unknown,

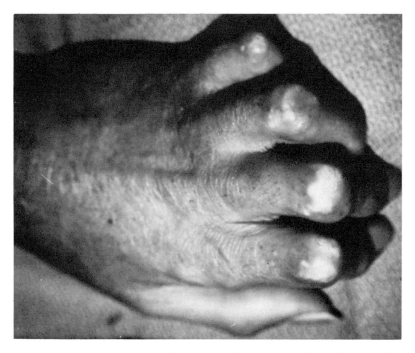

Fig. 19-28. Progressive systemic sclerosis. Tightening of skin and contraction of fingers with Raynaud's phenomenon is seen. (From Grayson M: The cornea in systemic disease. In Duane TD, editor: Clinical ophthalmology, vol 4, Hagerstown, MD, 1976, Harper & Row.)

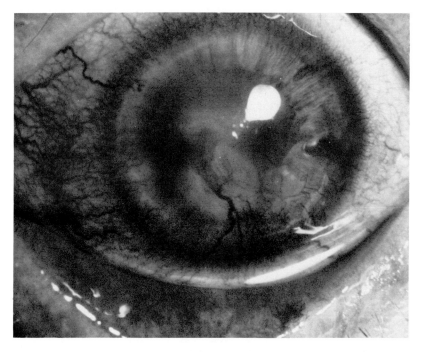

Fig. 19-29. Marked injection, vascularization, and infiltration of cornea in progressive systemic sclerosis. (From Grayson M: The cornea in systemic disease. In Duane TD, editor: Clinical ophthalmology, vol 4, Hagerstown, MD, 1976, Harper & Row.)

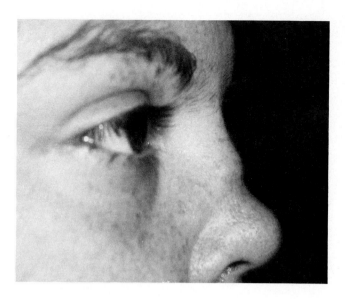

Fig. 19-30. Collapse of nose in relapsing polychondritis.

but both humeral and cell-mediated immunities are thought to bring about tissue damage. Also, anti-cartilage antibodies have been found in patients with relapsing polychondritis,[115] and polychondritis can occur in patients with connective tissue disorders (for example, Wegener's granulomatosis, rheumatoid arthritis, and systemic lupus erythematosus).

Inflammation in the cartilage of the pinnae of the ears, nose (Fig. 19-30), larynx, trachea, and joints occurs, as well as heart valve disease, vasculitis, and glomerulonephritis.[116]

Eye involvement occurs in approximately 60% of patients and includes episcleritis (40% of patients), conjunctivitis (25% of patients), scleritis, keratitis, and iritis.[117-121] Episcleritis or conjunctivitis may be the presenting sign of the disease. Corneal involvement usually occurs as a result of adjacent scleritis, but isolated marginal keratitis also can occur.[108,122,123] Peripheral corneal infiltration and noninfiltrated marginal melts can be seen. The latter can extend circumferentially to encircle the cornea and can lead to perforation.

INFLAMMATORY BOWEL DISEASE

Inflammatory bowel diseases (IBD) are idiopathic disorders in which there is chronic gastrointestinal inflammation. The two forms of IBD are ulcerative colitis and Crohn's disease. Ulcerative colitis affects only the large bowel and is characterized by ulceration and relatively superficial inflammation. Crohn's disease can affect any portion of the gastrointestinal tract, but typically involves the terminal ileum and ascending colon. The inflammation involves the entire intestinal wall and contains granulomas.

Crohn's disease may be associated with retinal edema, neuroretinitis, periorbital edema, and recurrent iridocyclitis. Episcleritis, scleritis, sclerokeratitis, and scleromalacia[124] have been reported.[125,126] Infiltrative marginal ulcerations of the cornea occur. In addition, small white nonfluorescein-staining opacities can be seen in the midperipheral superficial stroma.[126,127]

Episcleritis and scleritis also can occur in ulcerative colitis. Necrotizing infiltrative marginal corneal melting and marginal infiltrates may be present.[128,129]

BEHÇET'S SYNDROME

Behçet's syndrome is a rare, idiopathic, multisystem inflammatory disease associated with prominent mucocutaneous and ocular findings. The underlying pathologic condition appears to be an in-

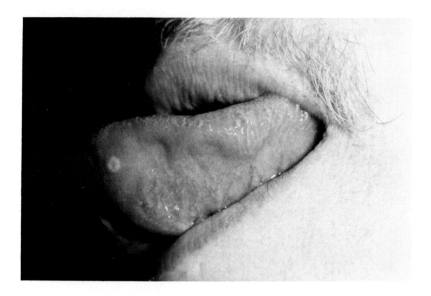

Fig. 19-31. Aphthous ulcer of tongue in Behçet's disease.

flammatory obliterative vasculitis, particularly involving the venous system. The presence of vasculitis and abnormal humoral and cell-mediated immunities in patients with this syndrome suggests an immune pathogenesis. Circulating antibodies to human oral mucous membrane and immune complexes in involved tissues are found in approximately 50% of patients.[130] Destruction of mucous membranes by the patient's lymphocytes has been demonstrated in vivo.[131] The incidence of histocompatibility antigen HLA-B5 is greater than expected in these patients.[132]

The hallmarks of Behçet's syndrome are recurrent aphthous (Fig. 19-31) and genital ulceration and uveitis. One can also find pustular skin lesions, polyarthritis, thrombophlebitis, involvement of the central nervous system, and gastrointestinal disturbances. The conjunctiva may exhibit inflammation, ulcerations (Fig. 19-32), edema, and hemorrhages. These lesions may be recurrent. Corneal opacification, vascularization, ulceration, and punctate keratopathy can occur. Cyclosporine appears to be the most effective treatment.[133]

VASCULITIS SYNDROMES

Vasculitis syndromes are a heterogeneous group of disorders characterized by inflammation of blood vessels. They are generally believed to be caused by a type III hypersensitivity reaction due to the deposition of immune complexes in the vessel walls. The nature of the antigen is not known, but in some cases it appears to be microbial. Cell-mediated immune mechanisms may also be involved, particularly in those diseases where granuloma formation is observed (for example, Wegener's granulomatosis).[134]

Cranial arteritis. Cranial arteritis, also referred to as giant cell arteritis or temporal arteritis, is an inflammatory disorder of large- and medium-sized arteries, occurring mostly in the elderly. Multiple arteries can be affected, but it characteristically affects branches of the carotid artery, particularly the temporal artery. Ocular findings include ischemic optic neuropathy, central retinal artery occlusion, cranial nerve palsies, uveitis, and scleritis.[135] Although rare, marginal corneal ulceration has been reported in this condition. In addition, both corneal and conjunctival ulceration was seen in one patient.[136]

Polyarteritis nodosa. Polyarteritis nodosa is a systemic necrotizing vasculitis of small- and medium-sized muscular arteries, particularly the renal and visceral arteries. Men are affected more than twice

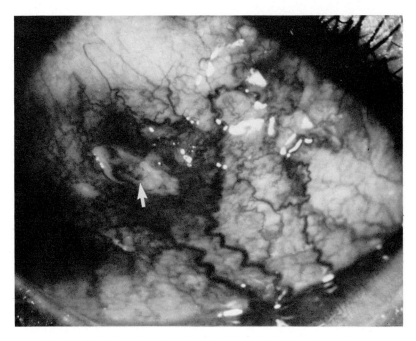

Fig. 19-32. Ulceration of conjunctiva *(arrow)* in Behçet's syndrome.

as often as women, and the average age at onset is 45 years. Because the blood vessels of any organ system of the body can be involved, the systemic manifestations are quite variable. Patients often present with nonspecific signs and symptoms, such as fever, weight loss, weakness, abdominal pain, and myalgia, alone or in addition to complaints related to dysfunction of a specific organ.

Ophthalmic involvement occurs in approximately 20% of patients, most commonly as choroidal vasculitis.[137] Other findings include choroiditis, retinal vasculitis, optic atrophy, papilledema, exudative retinal detachment, central retinal artery occlusion, iritis, and cranial nerve palsies.[126]

The conjunctiva can be hyperemic and may contain subconjunctival hemorrhages. Pale yellow, waxy, raised, and very friable conjunctival lesions can occur,[138] which are associated with edema and necrosis and a surrounding inflammatory reaction. Nodular episcleritis and nodular, diffuse or necrotizing scleritis can be seen (Fig. 19-33).

Melting of the margins of the cornea, with or without infiltration, can be seen. It can appear similar to a Mooren's ulcer, and can be the presenting sign of the disease.[139-143] However, unlike Mooren's ulcer, in most cases it is associated with an adjacent scleritis. The ulcers can spread circumferentially or centrally and can form a ring ulcer.[131] The keratitis is associated with marked injection of the eye and severe pain. The final result may be scarring, vascularization, or perforation of the globe.

Polyarteritis nodosa is present in approximately 25% of patients with Cogan's syndrome. In this condition one sees an interstitial keratitis characterized by deep yellowish stromal infiltration and vascularization (see Chapter 11). Vestibuloauditory disease, such as tinnitus, vertigo, and deafness, are often present.

Allergic angiitis and granulomatosis (Churg-Strauss syndrome). Allergic angiitis and granulomatosis is a form of necrotizing systemic vasculitis, which is similar to polyarteritis nodosa. However, unlike polyarteritis nodosa, pulmonary involvement is the dominant manifestation; the vasculitis affects veins and capillaries, as well as arteries. Granulomas and eosinophils are found in affected tissues, and there is a strong association with severe asthma and peripheral eosinophilia.

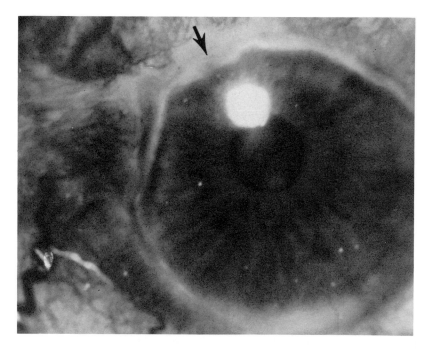

Fig. 19-33. Marginal melt in periarteritis *(arrow).*

Ocular complications include conjunctival granulomas,[144,145] episcleritis,[146] and marginal corneal ulceration.[147,148]

Systemic corticosteroid treatment is used in most cases. In fulminant or resistant cases a combined regimen of cyclophosphamide and alternate-day prednisone may be necessary.[149]

Wegener's granulomatosis. This disease is a distinct form of vasculitis that mostly affects the upper and lower respiratory tracts and the renal glomeruli. It can be seen at any age, but has a peak incidence in the third and fourth decades. Patients typically present with upper respiratory tract findings, such as recurrent epistaxis, chronic rhinorrhea, sinus pain and drainage, or chronic otitis media. Pulmonary involvement may be manifested on chest x-ray as chronic cough, hemoptysis, dyspnea, or asymptomatic infiltrates. Many other tissues can be involved, particularly the kidneys, skin, peripheral and central nervous system, and heart. The main pathologic features are a necrotizing vasculitis of small arteries and veins with granuloma formation and focal and segmental glomerulonephritis. The pathogenesis of Wegener's granulomatosis is unknown, but it is reasonable to suspect that it occurs as an aberrant immunologic reaction to an antigen that enters through or resides in the upper airway.

Ocular involvement occurs in approximately 60% of patients and is the presenting sign in 16%.[150-153] Orbital inflammation, which often occurs as a result of extension from adjacent sinus disease, commonly causes proptosis and can be severe enough to cause corneal exposure, restricted motility, and papilledema.[154] Retinal vasculitis, uveitis, optic neuropathy, episcleritis, scleritis, and conjunctivitis also can occur.

The cornea in patients with Wegener's granulomatosis may exhibit a necrotizing infiltrative marginal ulcer (Fig. 19-34),[155-158] which is usually associated with adjacent nodular or necrotizing scleritis. Localized conjunctivitis or episcleritis is often the initial sign, followed by development of scleritis and adjacent keratitis.[128] Peripheral intrastromal infiltrates form, and, with progression, the overlying epithelium breaks down, leading to formation of a crescentic ulcer. This ulcer extends both

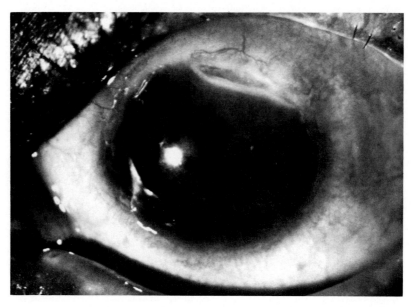

Fig. 19-34. Infiltrative peripheral corneal lesion in Wegener's granulomatosis. (Courtesy of Bartly J. Mondino, Los Angeles.)

centrally and circumferentially and can have an overhanging edge, making the corneal appearance indistinguishable from that of Mooren's ulcer, although, the sclera is usually not involved in Mooren's ulcer. Perforation of these ulcers can occur.[146,159]

Systemic immunosuppression is indicated for treatment of both the ocular and the systemic disease. Combined therapy with corticosteroids and cyclophosphamide has lengthened the survival from an average of 5 months to more than 4 years.[141]

TREATMENT

Many of the diseases just described have similar external ocular manifestations: episcleritis, scleritis, and marginal corneal infiltration and ulceration (Table 19-3). The approach to treatment differs, depending on whether the patient has an identified immunologic disease. If a patient with no previous history of immunologic disease presents with scleritis, marginal corneal ulceration or infiltration, or severe or recurrent episcleritis, a systemic evaluation should be performed, including a thorough history and examination by an internist or rheumatologist, an erythrocyte sedimentation rate, antinuclear antibody titer, rheumatoid factor assay, complete blood count, blood urea nitrogen, creatinine, chest x-ray, and possibly serum complement levels and biopsy of skin lesions.

If the patient is known to have an immunologic disease, such as rheumatoid arthritis, the physician managing the systemic disease should be notified of the ocular involvement and informed that it is a sign of activity of the systemic disease, requiring systemic treatment. Usually treatment entails initiation or enhancement of immunosuppression. Management of episcleritis and marginal corneal ulceration and infiltration is discussed in the next two sections. Scleritis is discussed in a later section.
Episcleritis. In most cases episcleritis can be managed either with observation or with topical corticosteroids. Oral, nonsteroidal, antiinflammatory agents (NSAIA) can be used in recalcitrant cases.
Marginal corneal infiltration or ulceration. Local ocular therapy is usually insufficient for marginal corneal infiltration and ulceration. However, some measures can help to limit corneal damage while waiting for systemic immunosuppression to take effect. Use of topical corticosteroids can

TABLE 19-3. Anterior Segment Involvement in Immune-Mediated Diseases

	LID DISEASE	K SICCA	CONJUNCTIVITIS	CONJUNCTIVAL SCARRING	EPISCLERITIS	SCLERITIS	MARGINAL INFILTRATES	ULCERATIVE KERATITIS
Systemic lupus erythematosus	+	++			+	+	+	+
Discoid lupus erythematosus		(?)+		+		+		
Rheumatoid arthritis		++			+	+	+	+
Progressive systemic sclerosis	+	+++		+++			+	
Relapsing polychondritis			++		++	+	+	+
Crohn's disease					++	++	++	++
Ulcerative colitis					++	++	++	++
Behçet's syndrome					++	++		
Polyarteritis nodosa			+		++	++	?+	++
Wegener's granulomatosis					+	++	+	+

lessen corneal infiltration, but in general, they should be applied only when the epithelium is intact. Topical lubrication and bandage contact lenses can help promote epithelial healing, particularly when keratoconjunctivitis sicca is present. Topical cyclosporine 2% has been reported to be effective in a few cases,[160-163] but this drug is not commercially available and experience has been quite limited.

If there is no history of systemic disease and no contraindication to systemic corticosteroids, I treat initially with prednisone (1 mg/kg/day). If the patient has been diagnosed with a systemic inflammatory disease, such as rheumatoid arthritis, the managing physician is contacted and an immediate increase in immunosuppression arranged. In general this regimen allows healing of the ulceration within 1 week. First the perilimbal injection and edema is reduced, and ulceration is slowed or halted; then the epithelium gradually closes over the ulcer bed.

Sometimes this treatment is not sufficient or rapid enough and progressive ulceration occurs. In these cases, or where systemic immunosuppression is not possible, resection of adjacent conjunctiva is often helpful.[164-166] The conjunctiva may be a source of inflammatory cells and destructive enzymes, such as collagenase. Limbal conjunctivectomy is a simple procedure that can be performed in the office with the use of topical anesthetic drops and a subconjunctival injection of 1% lidocaine in the area of the limbal melt. The conjunctiva is excised for 3 to 4 mm from the limbus, extending circumferentially past the margins of the ulceration. The conjunctiva is not sutured.

Application of cyanoacrylate tissue adhesive can also retard ulceration and seal perforations. I use it if the ulceration is approaching Descemet's membrane or progressing rapidly. Lamellar or penetrating keratoplasty may be necessary to restore integrity to the globe or to clear the visual axis. Scleral reinforcement may be necessary for advanced thinning. Pretibial periosteum is probably the optimum tissue; eye bank sclera can provide temporary support, but it is more likely to melt away in the same manner as the patient's own sclera.

If both prednisone and local therapy are insufficient, immunosuppression with cyclophosphamide or cyclosporine can be used. It can take 2 to 3 weeks before the effect of these medications is evident, so the disease must be controlled by other means until that time.

DISORDERS OF THE IMMUNE SYSTEM
WISKOTT-ALDRICH SYNDROME

The classic findings in Wiskott-Aldrich syndrome, an X-linked recessive immune disease, are eczema, thrombocytopenia, and susceptibility to bacterial, viral, fungal, and protozoal infections. Defects in both the cellular and humoral immune systems are present. Most patients die from bleeding or infection. Autoimmune disorders also are common, and more than 20% of patients develop malignancy, most often lymphoma or leukemia.

Although the numbers of lymphocytes are normal, patients cannot mount delayed hypersensitivity responses. Serum IgM is reduced, IgA and IgE are elevated, and catabolism of all immunoglobulins is increased. Antibody production to microbial antigens is reduced, particularly to polysaccharide antigens, such as those present in the capsules of pneumococci.[167] These findings may be related to a deficiency of a cell-membrane glycoprotein normally present on T lymphocytes and platelets.[168]

Conjunctivitis, conjunctival bleeding, necrotizing lid ulcers (Fig. 19-35), blepharitis, and episcleritis can occur. In addition, ulcerative keratitis and chronic or recurrent viral infection can be seen.

ACQUIRED IMMUNE DEFICIENCY SYNDROME

Acquired immune deficiency syndrome is an immunodeficiency disease due to infection with a T-cell lymphotrophic virus (HIV). The major clinical manifestations are related to deficiencies of cell-mediated immunity and include a variety of opportunistic infections and malignancies. The most frequent ocular manifestations are related to chorioretinal infection, especially with cytomegalovirus and *Candida* and *Toxoplasma* species. The cornea and conjunctiva can be affected by herpes zoster or

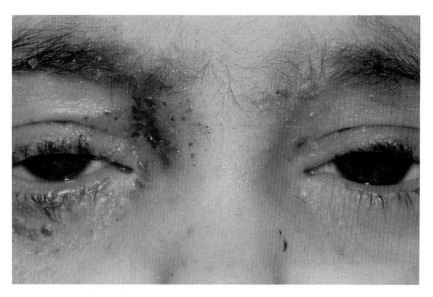

Fig. 19-35. Wiskott-Aldrich syndrome with ulcerative lid lesions.

herpes simplex infection, and Kaposi's sarcoma can occur in the lids and conjunctiva (see Chapter 30).

MULTIPLE MYELOMA AND DYSPROTEINEMIAS

Multiple myeloma is a malignant proliferation of plasma cells. It results in bone pain, anemia, bleeding, susceptibility to infection, hypercalcemia, renal failure, neurologic symptoms, amyloidosis, and serum hyperviscosity. Age of onset is usually between 50 and 70 years of age.

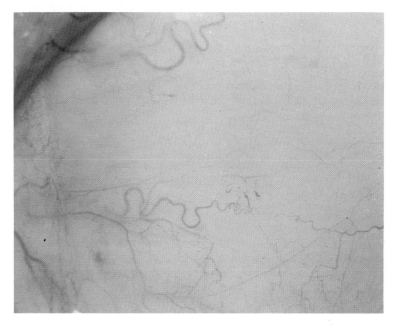

Fig. 19-36. Conjunctival vessel tortuosity in multiple myeloma.

Ocular manifestations. Lytic lesions of the orbital bones, nerve palsies, papilledema, and visual field defects occur in multiple myeloma.[169] In addition, one may find infiltration of adnexal tissue by myeloma cells, proteinaceous cysts of the nonpigmented ciliary epithelium, and hyperviscosity retinopathy.

Marked tortuosity of the conjunctival vessels, with sludging of the circulation, can result from increased blood viscosity (Fig. 19-36). Crystals can be seen in the conjunctiva, cornea (Fig. 19-37, *A*), and retina (Fig. 19-37, *B*).[170] Fine, punctate or needlelike, multicolored crystals occur in the corneal epithelium or anterior stroma.[160,171] A diffuse stromal haze may be noted (Fig. 19-37, *A*). In some cases amorphous gray-white epithelial and subepithelial deposits are seen in the corneal periphery[172-174] that can extend like fingers from the superior cornea. In most cases vision is only mildly reduced.

Histologically, corneal crystals have been found in keratocytes and epithelium.[175,176] They are

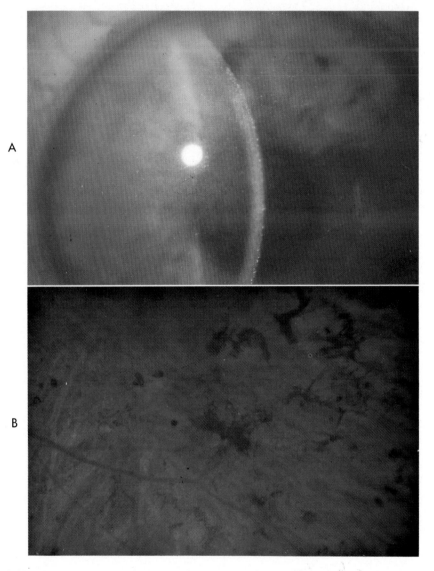

Fig. 19-37. Multiple myeloma. **A,** Crystals in corneal epithelium and stromal haze. **B,** Retinal crystals.

composed of immunoglobulin-related proteins; immunoperoxidase staining has been most strongly positive for IgG and IgA kappa and lambda light chains.[177]

A polychromatic, dustlike deposition of copper can occur in central Descemet's membrane, with sparing of the peripheral cornea. This deposition also is seen in the anterior lens capsule. Both appear to be related to the ability of some myeloma proteins to bind copper.[178]

Similar changes can be seen in patients with other forms of dysproteinemia, such as benign monoclonal gammopathy[175,176] (Figs. 19-38 and 19-39) and essential cryoglobulinemia.[173] In addition, patches of myeloma cells can be deposited on the corneal endothelium, and calcific band keratopathy can result from the hypercalcemia often present in multiple myeloma. Dystrophic corneal changes

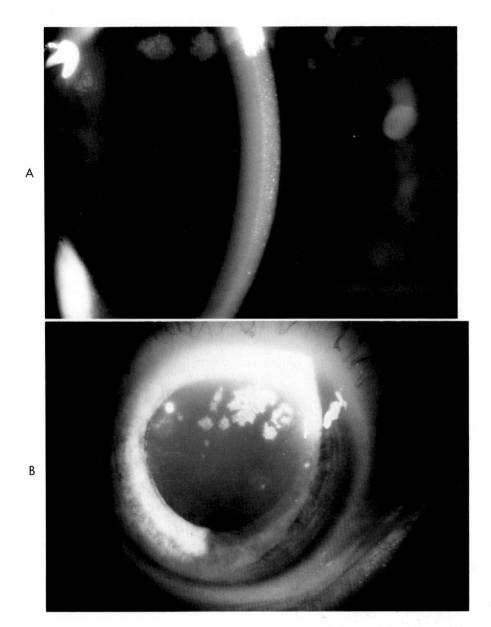

Fig. 19-38. Benign monoclonal gammopathy. **A,** Subepithelial glistening deposits. **B,** Large geographic crystalline patches involving full thickness of cornea. (From Miller KH et al: Ophthalmology 87:944, 1980.)

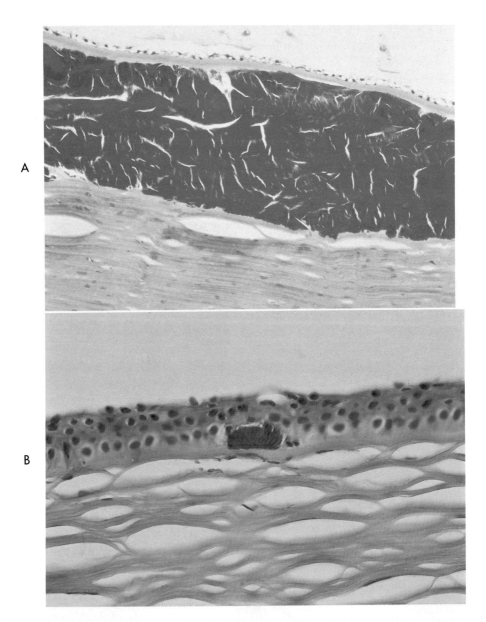

Fig. 19-39. Benign monoclonal gammopathy. **A,** Large deposits in posterior corneal stroma. Descemet's membrane and endothelium are normal (Masson's trichrome, original magnification ×400). **B,** Subepithelial corneal deposit and surrounding normal epithelium, Bowman's membrane, and stroma (Van der Grift, original magnification ×100). (From Miller KH et al: Ophthalmology 87:944, 1980.)

have been reported in multiple myeloma, Waldenström's macroglobulinemia, and cryoglobulinemia.[179,180] These dystrophic changes appear as reticulated and undulating patterns of opacification in the posterior stroma.[180]

LANGERHANS CELL GRANULOMATOSIS (EOSINOPHILIC GRANULOMA, HAND-SCHÜLLER-CHRISTIAN SYNDROME)

This group of diseases involve proliferation of Langerhans cells. Hand-Schüller-Christian syndrome includes exophthalmos, diabetes insipidus, and destructive bone lesions and is seen in 25% of

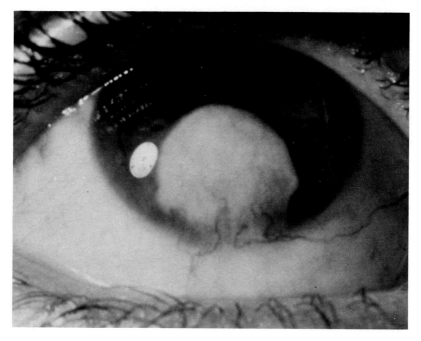

Fig. 19-40. Yellow infiltrate involving all layers of the cornea in Hand-Schüller-Christian disease. (Courtesy L. Calkins, Kansas City, MO.)

cases of multifocal eosinophilic granuloma. Large xanthelasmas of the lids can be seen. Yellow-white infiltration of the corneal limbus and peripheral stroma can occur (Fig. 19-40), possibly representing a nodular xanthoma.

GRAFT-VERSUS-HOST DISEASE

Graft-versus-host disease is the major complication of bone marrow transplantation. T lymphocytes in the transplanted marrow recognize antigens of the host as foreign, become sensitized, and attack the host tissue. The major targets are the skin, gastrointestinal tract, and liver.[181]

The most frequent ocular manifestations are keratoconjunctivitis sicca, cicatricial lagophthalmos, and sterile conjunctivitis and uveitis.[182,183] Persistent epithelial defects and stromal ulceration, both sterile and infectious, can result from the dry eye and lagophthalmos. The amount of conjunctival inflammation appears to be a good indicator of the severity of the graft-versus-host reaction and the prognosis for survival.[184]

SCLERITIS

The eye can be likened to a ball-and-socket joint, and many of the conditions that affect the joints can also affect the sclera.[100] Scleritis occurs most often in women during the fourth to sixth decades of life. The most common systemic disease associated with scleritis is rheumatoid arthritis, but a wide variety of inflammatory diseases also can be seen[96,97,104] (see box on p. 480).

Histologically, scleritis is seen as a granulomatous reaction (Fig. 19-41). The sclera is infiltrated with plasma cells, lymphocytes, and mast cells. In areas of necrosis there is perivascular cuffing with lymphocytes and medial necrosis, leading to vascular thrombosis, occlusion, or aneurysm formation.[185-188] Recently, vasculitis was demonstrated immunopathologically in biopsies from patients with scleritis.[99] Clinically, scleritis is accompanied by pain, lacrimation, and photophobia. There is dilation of the deep episcleral vessels, giving the eye a bluish-red hue, which is best appreciated in

DISEASES ASSOCIATED WITH SCLERITIS AND EPISCLERITIS

EPISCLERITIS	SCLERITIS
SYSTEMIC INFLAMMATORY DISEASES	
Rheumatoid arthritis	Rheumatoid arthritis
Relapsing polychondritis	Ankylosing spondylitis
Rheumatic heart disease	Psoriatic arthritis
Inflammatory bowel disease	Systemic lupus erythematosus
	Polyarteritis nodosa
	Wegener's granulomatosis
	Relapsing polychondritis
	Rheumatic heart disease
	Inflammatory bowel disease
	Behçet's syndrome
	Cranial arteritis
	Cogan's intersitial keratitis
INFECTIOUS DISEASES	
Tuberculosis	Tuberculosis
Syphilis	Syphilis
Herpes simplex	Herpes simplex
Herpes zoster	Herpes zoster
METABOLIC DISORDERS	
Gout	Gout
	Thyrotoxicosis
SKIN DISEASES	
Erythema nodosum	Erythema nodosum
Erythema multiforme	Acne rosacea
Acne rosacea	

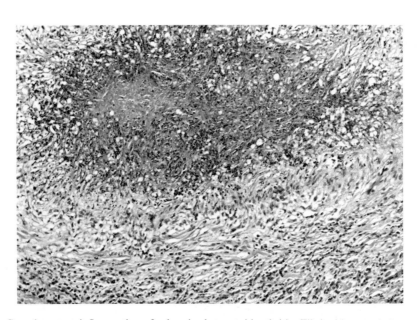

Fig. 19-41. Granulomatous inflammation of sclera in rheumatoid arthritis. Fibrinoid necrosis is surrounded by a zone of palisading epithelioid cells and lymphocytes (hematoxylin-eosin stain, ×200). (Courtesy of Bruce L. Johnson, Pittsburgh.)

TABLE 19-4. Features of Episcleritis and Scleritis

	CONJUNCTIVITIS	EPISCLERITIS	SCLERITIS
Symptoms	Discharge, gritty sensation, itching	Usually none, may have mild discomfort, pricking	Deep, boring pain; may have tearing, photophobia
Injection			
Location	Diffuse, forniceal	Usually sectoral but can be diffuse, nodular	Diffuse or nodular
Hue	Red	Red	Purplish
Tenderness	No	Mild or none	Usually
Blanching with phenylephrine 10%	Yes	Moderate	No
Other findings	Follicles, chemosis, SPK, focal keratitis	Rarely corneal scarring	Scleral edema, scleral thinning (darkening), iritis, keratitis, serous elevation of choroid
Associated disease	Pharyngitis, fever, allergies, urethritis	<30% Herpes zoster, gout, vasculitis	50% Systemic vasculitis, e.g., rheumatoid arthritis, herpes zoster, gout, many others

daylight (Table 19-4). The sclera can be edematous, or necrotic and devoid of overlying vessels. Anterior scleritis can be divided into the following four types[100]:

1. *Diffuse*—Broad area(s) of scleral inflammation, with minimal or diffuse scleral edema, and no necrosis
2. *Nodular*—One or more localized areas of scleral inflammation, with nodular scleral edema and no necrosis (Fig. 19-42)

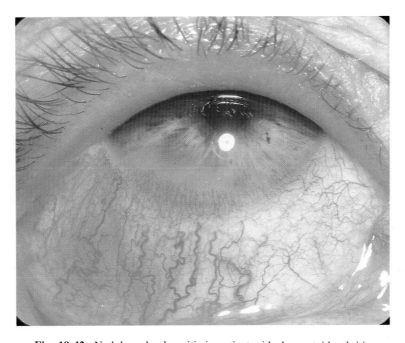

Fig. 19-42. Nodular sclerokeratitis in patient with rheumatoid arthritis.

3. *Necrotizing with inflammation*—One or more avascular patches of necrotic sclera, associated with scleral inflammation and pain (Fig. 19-43)

4. *Necrotizing without inflammation*—Scleral necrosis without surrounding inflammtion or pain; long-standing rheumatoid arthritis (Fig. 19-44)

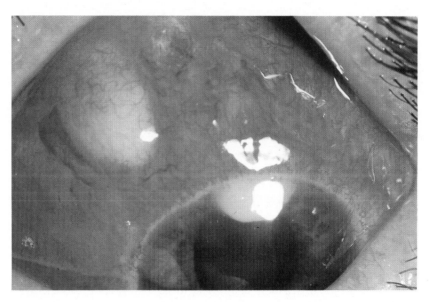

Fig. 19-43. Severe sclerouveitis with large necrotizing granulomas. One lesion extends into anterior chamber.

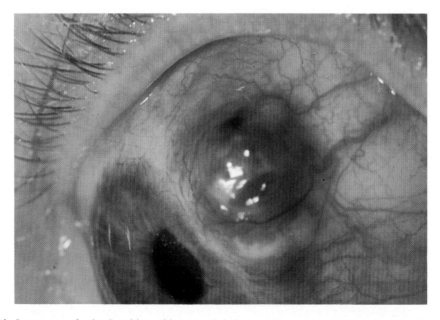

Fig. 19-44. Large area of scleral melting without much inflammatory reaction (scleromalacia perforans) in case of rheumatoid arthritis.

CORNEAL CHANGES IN SCLERITIS

Watson reports that corneal involvement occurs in 37% of patients with scleritis.[100] He has divided corneal involvement into four types: acute stromal keratitis, sclerosing keratitis, limbal guttering, and keratolysis.

Acute stromal keratitis. This can accompany diffuse or nodular nonnecrotizing scleritis. Superficial and midstromal opacities are seen both centrally and near the limbus adjacent to areas of scleral inflammation (Figs. 19-45 and 19-46). The peripheral and central corneal stroma can become diffusely edematous and cloudy. Vascularization and permanent scarring can develop with time.

Sclerosing keratitis. Sclerosing keratitis is the most common form of corneal involvement and can occur in any form of scleritis. The perilimbal corneal becomes thickened and gray; with time the opacification advances toward the central cornea. Crystalline opacities can be seen behind the leading edge. Nodular corneal opacities, ring infiltrates, vascularization, and lipid deposition can develop (Fig. 19-47).

Limbal guttering. Peripheral corneal thinning, similar to that occurring without adjacent scleritis, can occasionally be seen. Healing is accompanied by vascularization, lipid deposition, and, in some cases ectasia, resulting in an appearance similar to that of Terrien's degeneration. Rarely, perforation can occur.

Keratolysis. Keratolysis occurs in severe cases of necrotizing scleritis, with or without inflammation. The previously clear peripheral cornea appears to melt away, leading to a descemetocele or rupture.

EVALUATION

All patients with scleritis should undergo a thorough history and physical examination, preferably by a rheumatologist. If the results of the examination are not suggestive of a systemic inflammatory disease, further evaluation is generally not informative; however, the following tests are suggested: complete blood count with differential, erythrocyte sedimentation rate, serum uric acid, serologic test for syphilis, chest x-ray, and x-ray of sacroiliac joints.

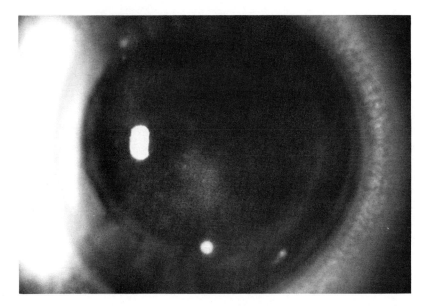

Fig. 19-45. Acute stromal keratitis in scleritis, with central and peripheral stromal infiltration.

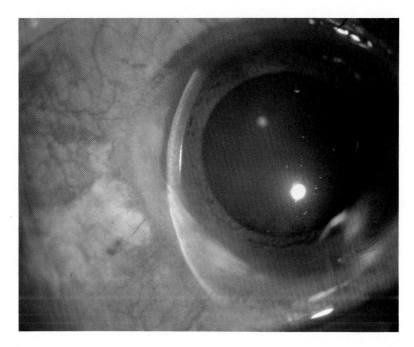

Fig. 19-46. Midstromal peripheral corneal infiltration adjacent to area of scleritis. (Courtesy of Bartly J. Mondino, Los Angeles.)

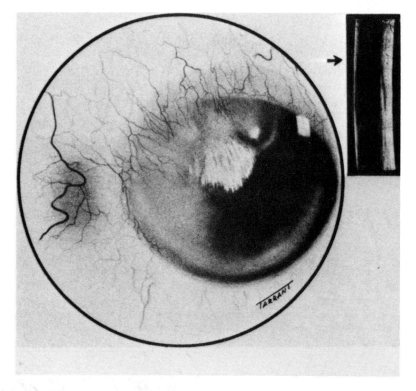

Fig. 19-47. Sclerokeratitis. A diffuse peripheral change affects the whole corneal stroma at the site of the scleritis. Behind the advancing edge the corneal lamellae take on a crystalline appearance like floss candy. A "precipitin ring" has formed around one opacity. (From Watson PG: Diseases of the sclera and episclera. In Duane TD and Jaeger EA, editors: Clinical ophthalmology, vol 4, Philadelphia, 1988, Harper & Row.)

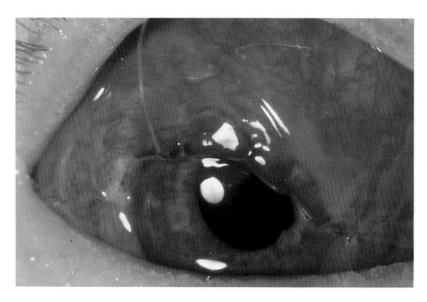

Fig. 19-48. Autogenous tibial periosteum used to reinforce sclera in case seen in Fig. 19-44.

TREATMENT

If a systemic inflammatory disease is present, it should be treated primarily, in conjunction with an internist or rheumatologist. Immunosuppressive therapy is more often indicated for these patients.

Scleritis almost never responds to topical treatment alone; systemic treatment with a NSAIA, corticosteroid, or other immunosuppressive agents is required. In patients with nonsevere, nonnecrotizing scleritis and no evidence of systemic disease, a nonsteroidal antiinflammatory agent (indomethacin 25 mg three times daily, or ibuprofen 400 mg four times daily) is usually tried first. Generally the first response to therapy is relief from pain. Some reduction in injection, tenderness, or corneal disease should be seen within 2 weeks. Once the eye is quiet the dose can be gradually tapered.

If the scleritis is severe or necrotizing or unresponsive to nonsteroidal agents, systemic corticosteroids are indicated. The initial dose of prednisone is approximately 1 mg/kg. Once the inflammation is controlled the dose can be reduced relatively quickly (over about 2 weeks) to 20 to 40 mg/day; thereafter the dose is slowly tapered. If this regimen is not effective, high-dose intravenous pulse therapy can be considered (1 g methylprednisolone intravenously three times during the first 7 days, followed by 1 g weekly, with gradual tapering).[189]

Immunosuppressive therapy is primarily used in patients with a known systemic inflammatory disease, such as Wegener's granulomatosis. However, they also can be used in addition to or instead of corticosteroids in patients who require a high maintenance dose of corticosteroids or who do not respond to corticosteroids. Cyclophosphamide appears to be the most effective agent. Topical or systemic cyclosporine have been used successfully in a few patients.[190]

It is sometimes necessary to surgically reinforce areas of thinning or perforation. The disease process should be controlled, or the patch will melt quickly. Cornea, sclera, or periosteum can be used, depending on the size and location of the defect (Fig. 19-48).

MISCELLANEOUS IMMUNOLOGIC DISEASES OF THE CORNEA

PHLYCTENULOSIS

Phlyctenulosis is an inflammatory disorder involving the cornea or conjunctiva that appears to be caused by cell-mediated hypersensitivity (type IV).[191-194] A phlycten, derived from the Greek word, *phlyctaena,* which means blister, is a small vesicle, blister, or pustule. In the past sensitivity to tuberculoprotein was the most common cause of phlyctenulosis, and it was associated with poor hygiene and poor nutrition. Now phlyctenulosis is most commonly associated with staphylococcal infection. It is most often seen in the first two decades of life.

Clinical manifestations. Phlyctenulosis usually occurs in self-limited attacks, although some cases can persist for many weeks. In purely conjunctival cases the symptoms are mild, but severe photophobia is characteristic when the cornea is involved.

The first attack usually occurs at the limbus; later attacks can occur in the cornea, or on the bulbar (Fig. 19-49) or tarsal conjunctiva. The lesion can be pinpoint in size to several millimeters; in general, the older the child the larger the phlyctenule. In addition, phlyctenules tend to be large and succulent if active tuberculosis is present. Each lesion follows a course of elevation, infiltration, ulceration, and resolution over a total period of 6 to 12 days. The phlyctenule begins as a small round or oval, hard, red, elevated lesion. Within 2 to 3 days a yellowish-white center develops and then ulcerates. When it occurs at the limbus, approximately two thirds of the phlyctenule lies on the conjunctival side and one third on the cornea. The phlyctenule usually leaves a scar only on the corneal side (Fig. 19-50). The scar is typically triangular, with its base at the limbus and its apex toward the central cornea. Although it is usually superficial, deep stromal scarring can also occur.

Later attacks also tend to occur at the limbus; they develop adjacent to the limbus or at the central edge of pannus from previous attacks. In this manner the phlyctenulosis can become confluent at the limbus or march across the cornea ("wandering" phlyctenule). More than one phlyctenule can occur at the same time. Corneal phlyctenules are seen as an amorphous infiltrate (Fig. 19-51), which ulcerates and usually becomes vascularized. A fascicle of vessels can extend to the infiltrate (Fig. 19-52), resembling the ulcer of herpes simplex.

Corneal perforations occur more commonly in tubercular phlyctenulosis, particularly in blacks and Eskimos, but staphylococcal disease also can lead to perforation, usually after many attacks, and with topical steroid use. Old phlyctenular disease is a cause of Salzmann's nodular corneal degeneration.

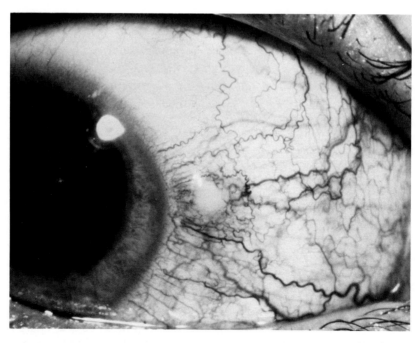

Fig. 19-49. Conjunctival phlyctenule.

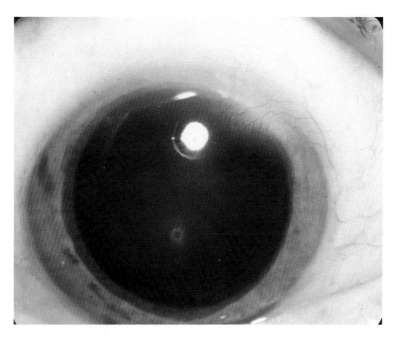

Fig. 19-50. Scarring of cornea with superficial vascularization resulting from limbal phlyctenular disease. (Courtesy F. Wilson II, Indianapolis.)

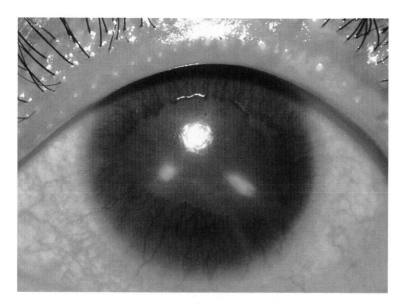

Fig. 19-51. Corneal infiltrate resulting from tuberculous phlyctenular disease.

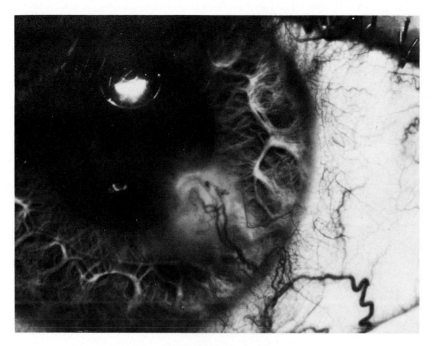

Fig. 19-52. Fascicular type of phlyctenular corneal disease.

Etiology. Phlyctenulosis appears to be a cell-mediated (type IV) hypersensitivity response to a topical foreign antigen. In addition to tuberculosis, phlyctenular disease is associated with staphylococci, *Coccidioides immitis, Candida albicans* (Fig. 19-53), lymphogranuloma venereum, parasites, adenoviruses, and herpes simplex.[193,195] The greatest number of cases today are associated with staphylococcal blepharitis. Phlyctenulosis is also seen occasionally during convalescence from coccidioidomycosis. In coccidioidomycosis there are no corneal stromal phlyctenules; the phlyctenules are confined to the limbal area. Therefore the visual disability that often occurs in tuberculous phlyctenulosis is not seen. The phlyctenulosis of cutaneous candidiasis is recurrent but usually not visually damaging.

Mondino et al.[196-198] were able to create both marginal infiltrates and phlyctenule-like lesions in rabbits, by immunization with *Staphylococcus aureus* followed by topical application of live staphylococci or staphylococcal cell wall antigen (ribitol teichoic acid). The phlyctenules contain plasma cells, lymphocytes, and macrophages, and polymorphonuclear leukocytes invade when necrosis occurs.[4] Helper T cells outnumber suppressor T cells, and mature B cells are also present.[199]

Treatment. The primary treatment is removal of the inciting infection. The lid margins should be cultured and skin testing for tuberculosis performed. Staphylococcal blepharitis should be treated by lid hygiene and topical antibiotics. Tuberculous phlyctenulosis responds extremely well to topical corticosteroids. Staphylococcal phlyctenulosis does not respond as well; often the disease recurs despite apparent elimination of the organism from the lid margin. However, low-dose topical corticosteroid and cycloplegia usually greatly increase comfort and lessen corneal scarring. Keratoplasty may be necessary for treating perforation or central corneal scarring. Penetrating keratoplasty for visual rehabilitation has a favorable prognosis.[200]

Marginal (Catarrhal) Infiltrates and Ulcers

Catarrhal ulcers and infiltrates of the cornea are usually associated with chronic staphylococcal blepharoconjunctivitis. The experimental work in rabbits[196-198] has suggested that it is caused by an

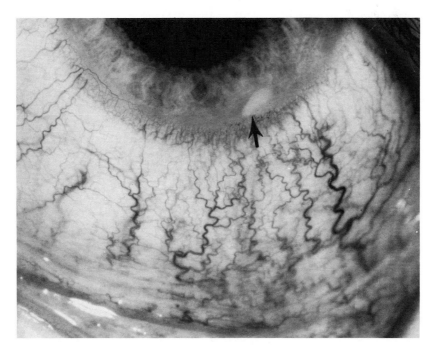

Fig. 19-53. *Candida albicans* phlyctenulosis *(arrow).*

antibody response to *S. aureus* cell wall antigen, with immune complex formation in the peripheral corneal stroma. However, many of these patients have only non-aureus staphylococci on their lids.[201]

The catarrhal infiltrate or ulcer is a gray-white, painful lesion that is circumferential with the limbus. A lucid corneal interval usually is seen between the lesion and the limbus (Fig. 19-54) or the central edge of corneal vessels. It has been hypothesized that the position of the infiltrate is related to the deposition of the immune complexes formed between the corneal staphylococcal antigen and the antibodies entering from the limbal vessels.[194]

The lesions can be single or multiple, narrow or broad; they are most often located in an area where the lid margin crosses the limbus. Without treatment they usually clear within 2 to 3 weeks. Catarrhal infiltrates can also be caused by the following: (1) *Haemophilus aegyptius,* (2) *Moraxella lacunata,* (3) beta-hemolytic streptococci, (4) bacillary dysentery, (5) food or drug allergy, (6) lymphogranuloma, (7) *Neisseria gonorrhoeae,* (8) *Escherichia coli,* and (9) actinomyces.[202-204]

Treatment. Clinically, these lesions cannot be definitely distinguished from peripheral corneal infection, infiltrates, and ulcers associated with rheumatoid arthritis and other collagen vascular diseases and peripheral herpes simplex infection. Therefore it is important to consider these possibilities, particularly when taking a history; to obtain a bacterial and, in some cases, a viral culture; and to look for scleritis.

In most cases lid scrubs and antibiotic ointment (bacitracin, erythromycin, or gentamicin) are initiated and a bacterial culture is performed. If the culture is negative after 48 hours, topical corticosteroid (for example, prednisolone acetate two to four times daily) is begun. Oral tetracycline is sometimes necessary for control of meibomitis.

STERILE CORNEAL INFILTRATES ASSOCIATED WITH CONTACT LENSES

Conjunctival hyperemia and anterior stromal infiltrates can develop in contact lens wearers, especially those wearing hydrophilic contact lenses. The cause of these infiltrates is unclear. Delayed hy-

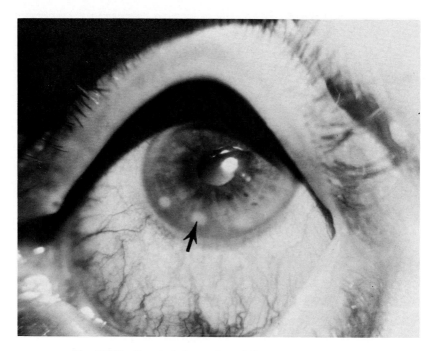

Fig. 19-54. Catarrhal ulcers of staphylococcal origin *(arrow)*.

persensitivity to thimerosal may be responsible in some cases (see Fig. 9-5).[205] Most infiltrates now are unrelated to thimerosal and may be caused by a reaction to other chemicals absorbed by the lens, to microbes or their products in the lenses, to protein deposits on the lenses, or to foreign material trapped under the lens.

Differentiating these infiltrates from infectious infiltrates can be difficult. Sterile infiltrates tend to be smaller (< 1 mm), multiple or arcuate in shape, and not associated with significant pain, discharge, epithelial defect, or anterior chamber reaction.[206] However, it is not possible to clinically differentiate sterile and infectious ulcers with certainty. Therefore it is best to discontinue lens wear, culture the infiltrate, not patch the eye, and follow the patient closely. Depending on the degree of suspicion of infection and the severity of the infiltrate, regular strength or fortified antibiotics should be administered.

MOOREN'S ULCER

Mooren's ulcer is a localized disease of the cornea characterized by chronic ulceration. It can develop at any age but is rare in individuals younger than 20 years of age. It is bilateral in 25% to 50% of cases. Mooren's ulcer tends to occur in two clinical types (Table 19-5).[207] A relatively benign, unilateral form usually occurs in older people (past the fourth decade) and is more responsive to therapy. The more severe, atypical, bilateral form is found in younger patients (third decade), and is much more difficult to treat. The latter form appears to be more common in African men.[208,209] Physical or chemical trauma may antedate the development of Mooren's ulcers.

Clinical findings. Patients usually complain of severe pain, redness, and light sensitivity. The first sign is an infiltrate in the peripheral anterior stroma, most often located in the interpalpebral space. Within a few weeks, the overlying epithelium is lost and stromal thinning begins (Fig. 19-55), which slowly deepens and spreads centrally and circumferentially (Fig. 19-56). The central margin often has an overhanging edge; the peripheral edge extends to the limbus and occasionally onto the sclera.

TABLE **19-5.** Clinical Features of Two Types of Mooren's Ulcer

FEATURE	TYPE I	TYPE II
Prevalence	Common form	Atypical form; common in Africa
Pathogenic factors	Trauma	Trauma, (?)helminthiasis
Age	Usually >40	Usually 20-30
Sex	M > F	M > F
Laterality	25% bilateral	75% bilateral
Pain	Moderate to severe	Variable
Course	Slowly progressive	May be rapid
Response to treatment	Moderate	Poor
Perforation	Uncommon	One third

Modified from Schanzlin D: Mooren's ulceration. In Smolin G and Thoft RA, editors: The cornea: scientific foundations and clinical practice, Boston, 1986, Little, Brown & Co.

Some portions of the ulcer can be quiescent, while others are active; the epithelium is absent over areas of activity. In the wake of the ulceration, the stroma is thinned by one half to three quarters and is covered by superficial vascularization.

The ulceration normally runs a course of 3 to 12 months[4]; periods of total remission are not uncommon. In severe cases the entire cornea can be involved and perforation can occur.

Histopathology. Histopathologic examination of the conjunctiva adjacent to Mooren's ulcers shows heavy infiltration with plasma cells and lymphocytes.[164,210,211] The corneal stroma shows active inflammation, particularly in the area of the overhanging edge.[210,212,213] The principal cells are neutrophils, but plasma cells, eosinophils, and lymphocytes are also present.

Etiology. Some have hypothesized that corneal injury, by surgery, infection, or trauma, alters corneal antigens and elicits an autoimmune response.[4] In many cases such an injury can be identified. In

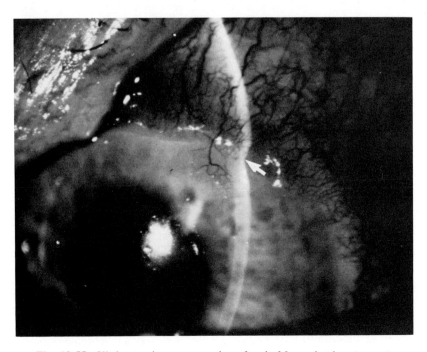

Fig. **19-55.** Slit-lamp microscope section of early Mooren's ulcer *(arrow)*.

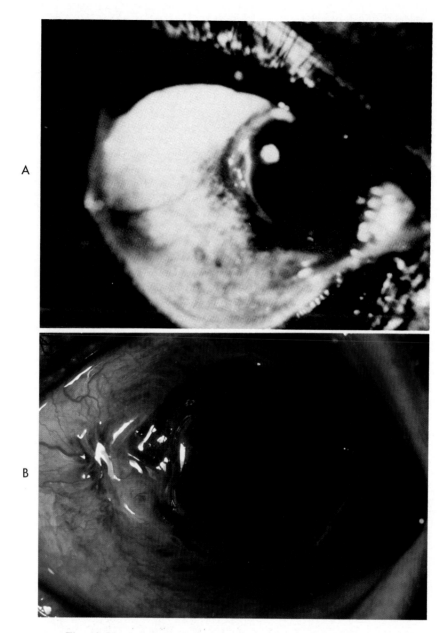

Fig. 19-56. A, Mooren's ulcer. **B,** Progression of ulceration seen in **A.**

Nigeria, Mooren's ulcer is frequently associated with systemic helminth infections[209]; in these cases an immunologic reaction to helminth-related antigens in the cornea or to corneal antigens altered by the infection may be responsible.[214]

Several findings suggest the role of autoimmunity: the high concentration of plasma cells in the adjacent conjunctiva, circulating autoantibodies against corneal and conjunctival tissue,[210,211,215-217] tissue-fixed antibodies and complement in the conjunctiva,[210] elevated circulating immune complex and IgA levels,[216] and reduced suppressor T-cell levels.[211] Cell-mediated immunity against corneal tissue has also been demonstrated in some patients.[212,218] However, these findings can be secondary to the destructive corneal inflammation.

The corneal changes in Mooren's ulcer are very similar to those seen in systemic diseases with vasculitis, such as Wegener's granulomatosis and polyarteritis nodosa. Therefore a perilimbal vasculitis may be able to produce the same manifestations.

The tissue destruction appears to be at least partially mediated by collagenase and other degradative enzymes. Metabolic products from tissue culture of the conjunctiva are able to degrade collagen and corneal proteoglycan.[210]

Diagnosis. The diagnosis of Mooren's ulcer can only be made once these collagen vascular diseases and other causes of vasculitis are excluded. A thorough history, medical examination, chest x-ray, erythrocyte sedimentation rate, complete blood count, rheumatoid factor, antinuclear antibody titer, Venereal Disease Research Laboratory (VDRL), fluorescent-treponemal antibody absorption test (FTA-ABS), blood urea nitrogen level, and creatinine level should be obtained.

In most cases, Mooren's ulcer can be distinguished clinically from other causes of peripheral corneal ulceration. Terrien's marginal degeneration is noninflammatory and nonpainful, and the epithelium is intact (see Table 16-3). Bacterial corneal ulcers usually have more yellowish infiltrate, purulent discharge, and greater anterior chamber, conjunctival, and scleral reaction. Peripheral herpetic ulceration does not exhibit an overhanging central edge and may be associated with decreased corneal sensation. However, bacterial and viral cultures should be performed. Catarrhal ulcers can be distinguished by the presence of blepharitis, the lucid interval between the ulcer and the limbus, the lack of an overhanging central edge, and the lack of severe pain.

Treatment. There is no well-established and generally successful treatment for Mooren's ulcer. Whether the ulceration can be arrested depends largely on the aggressiveness of the disease. In general, unilateral ulcers in elderly individuals tend to respond more than bilateral ulcers in young individuals.[207]

I treat initially with topical and (if possible) systemic corticosteroids: prednisolone acetate 1% (four to eight times a day) and oral prednisone (1 mg/kg/day). Cycloplegics, and sometimes a bandage contact lens, are also given to help relieve discomfort. If progression occurs despite 4 to 5 days

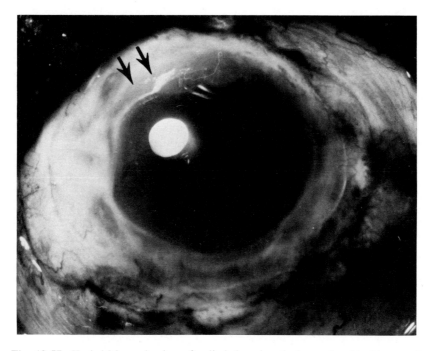

Fig. 19-57. Healed Mooren's ulcer after limbal conjunctival resection *(double arrow)*.

of treatment, or if perforation is threatened, limbal conjunctival excision is performed (Fig. 19-57).[219] The effect of the excision appears to be temporary and can be repeated several times. Cryotherapy of the perilimbal conjunctiva may have a similar effect.[220]

If progression occurs despite these measures and perforation or extensive destruction of the eye is threatened, stronger immunosuppressive agents should be considered. Cyclophosphamide and methotrexate both have been successful in many cases.[221,222] These agents should be administered only after discussing the risks and benefits with the patient and coordinating the therapy with a hematologist or rheumatologist who monitor their systemic effects. Cyclosporin A has recently been reported to be effective in several cases, even when cytotoxic agents were not, and may have a lower risk of systemic complications.[160,161] Very high doses of corticosteroids (1 g methylprednisolone intravenously three times during the first 7 days, followed by 1 g weekly, with gradual tapering) are another option.[189] Cyanoacrylate adhesive can be helpful in sealing small perforations or retarding progression of deep ulceration. Lamellar keratectomy of the central island of remaining stroma can quiet the process and retain some useful vision.[223,224] However, perforation may still occur.

REFERENCES

1. Stites DP, Stobo JD, and Wells JV, editors: Basic and clinical immunology, ed 6, Norwalk, CT, 1987, Appleton & Lange.
2. Roitt I, Brostoff J, and Male D, editors: Immunology, ed 2, New York, 1989, Mosby/Gower.
3. Barrett JT: Textbook of clinical immunology, ed 5, St Louis, 1988, Mosby–Year Book, Inc.
4. Smolin G and O'Connor GR: Ocular immunology, Philadelphia, 1981, Lea & Febiger.
5. Franklin RM and Remus LE: Conjunctival-associated lymphoid tissue: evidence for a role in the secretory immune system, Invest Ophthalmol Vis Sci 25:181, 1983.
6. Sacks EH et al: Lymphocytic subpopulations in the normal human conjunctiva: a monoclonal antibody study, Ophthalmology 93:1276, 1986.
7. Strober W and Brown WR: The mucosal immune system. In Samter M, editor: Immunological diseases, ed 4, Boston, 1988, Little, Brown & Co.
8. Mondino BJ et al: Alternate and classical pathway components of complement in the normal cornea, Arch Ophthalmol 98:346, 1980.
9. Mondino BJ and Hoffman DB: Hemolytic complement activity in normal human donor corneas, Arch Ophthalmol 98:2041, 1980.
10. Mondino BJ and Brady KJ: Distribution of hemolytic complement in the normal cornea, Arch Ophthalmol 99:1430, 1981.
11. Allansmith MR and McClennan B: Immunoglobulins in the human cornea, Am J Ophthalmol 80:125, 1975.
12. Gillete TE, Chandler JW, and Greiner JV: Langerhans cells of the ocular surface, Ophthalmology 89:700, 1982.
13. Streilein JW, Neiderkorn JY, and Shadduck JA: Systemic immune unresponsiveness induced in adult mice by anterior chamber presentation of minor histocompatibility antigens, J Exp Med 152:1121, 1980.
14. Streilein JW: Immune regulation and the eye: a dangerous compromise, FASEB J 1:199, 1987.
15. Gell PGH, Coombs RA, and Lackmann P, editors: Clinical aspects of immunology, ed 3, Oxford, 1974, Blackwell Scientific Publications.
16. Norman PS and Lichtenstein LM: Allergic rhinitis. In Samter M, editor: Immunological diseases, ed 4, Boston, 1988, Little, Brown & Co.
17. Abelson MB, Madiwale N, and Weston JF: Conjunctival eosinophils in allergic ocular disease, Arch Ophthalmol 101:631, 1983.
18. Theodore FH: The significance of conjunctival eosinophilia in the diagnosis of allergic conjunctivitis, Ear Nose Throat J 30:653, 1951.
19. Abelson MB et al: Effects of Vasocon-A in the allergen challenge model of acute allergic conjunctivitis, Arch Ophthalmol 108:520, 1990.
20. Kray KT et al: Cromolyn sodium in seasonal allergic conjunctivitis, J Allergy Clin Immunol 76:623, 1986.
21. Allansmith MR and Ross RN: Ocular allergy and mast cell stabilizers, Surv Ophthalmol 30:229, 1986.
22. Taudorf E et al: Oral immunotherapy in birch pollen hayfever, J Allergy Clin Immunol 80:153, 1987.
23. Neumann E et al: A review of 400 cases of vernal conjunctivitis, Am J Ophthalmol 74:166, 1959.
24. Allansmith MR: Vernal conjunctivitis. In Duane TD, editor: Clinical ophthalmology, vol 5, Philadelphia, 1988, Harper & Row.
25. Buckley RJ: Vernal keratoconjunctivitis, Int Ophthalmol Clin 28:303, 1988.
26. Rice NSC and Jones BR: Vernal keratoconjunctivitis: an allergic disease of the eyes of children, Clin Allergy 3:629, 1973.
27. Togby AF: Keratitis epithelial vernalis, Bull Ophthalmol Soc Egypt 28:104, 1935.
28. Jones BR: Vernal keratitis, Trans Ophthalmol Soc UK 81:215, 1961.
29. Shuler JD, Levenson J, and Mondino BJ: Inferior corneal ulcers associated with palpebral vernal conjunctivitis, Am J Ophthalmol 106:106, 1988.
30. Khan MD et al: Incidence of keratoconus in spring catarrh, Br J Ophthalmol 72:41, 1988.
31. Tuft SJ, Dart JKG, and Kemeny M: Limbal vernal keratoconjunctivitis: clinical characteristics and immunoglobulin E expression compared with palpebral vernal, Eye 3:420, 1989.
32. Collin HB and Allansmith MR: Basophils in vernal

conjunctivitis in humans: an electron microscopic study, Invest Ophthalmol Vis Sci 16:858, 1977.

33. Easty DL et al: Immunological investigations in vernal eye disease, Trans Ophthalmol Soc UK 100:98, 1980.

34. Morgan G: The pathology of vernal conjunctivitis, Trans Ophthalmol Soc UK 91:467, 1971.

35. Alimuddin M: Vernal conjunctivitis, Br J Ophthalmol 39:160, 1955.

36. Samra Z et al: Vernal keratoconjunctivitis: the significance of immunoglobulin E levels in tears and serum, Int Arch Allergy Appl Immunol 74:158, 1984.

37. Ballow M and Mendelson L: Specific immunoglobulin E antibodies in tear secretions of patients with vernal conjunctivitis, J Allergy Clin Immunol 66:112, 1980.

38. Allansmith MR, Hahn GS, and Simon MA: Tissue, tear and serum IgE concentrations in vernal conjunctivitis, Am J Ophthalmol 81:506, 1976.

39. Ballow M et al: IgG specific antibodies to rye grass and ragweed pollen antigens in the tear secretions of patients with vernal conjunctivitis, Am J Ophthalmol 95:161, 1983.

40. Abelson MB, Baird RS, and Allansmith MR: Tear histamine levels in vernal conjunctivitis and other ocular inflammations, Ophthalmology 87:812, 1980.

41. Ballow M, Donshik PC, and Mendelson L: Complement proteins and C3 anaphylatoxin in tears of patients with conjunctivitis, J Allergy Clin Immunol 76:473, 1985.

42. Mumcuoglu YK et al: House dust mites and vernal keratoconjunctivitis, Ophthalmologica 196:175, 1988.

43. Allansmith MR et al: Conjunctival basophil hypersensitivity in the guinea pig, J Allergy Clin Immunol 78:919, 1986.

44. Friedlander MG and Cyr R: Ocular findings in systemic cutaneous basophil hypersensitivity, Invest Ophthalmol Vis Sci 18:964, 1979.

45. Easty DL, Rice NSC, and Jones BR: Disodium cromoglycate (Intal) in the treatment of keratoconjunctivitis, Trans Ophthalmol Soc UK 91:491, 1971.

46. Easty DL, Rice NSC, and Jones BR: Clinical trial of topical disodium cromoglycate in vernal keratoconjunctivitis, Clin Allergy 2:99, 1972.

47. Kazdan JJ et al: Sodium cromoglycate (Intal) in the treatment of vernal keratoconjunctivitis and allergic conjunctivitis, Can J Ophthalmol 11:300, 1976.

48. Foster CS: The cromolyn sodium collaborative study group: evaluation of topical cromolyn sodium in the treatment of vernal keratoconjunctivitis, Ophthalmology 95:194, 1988.

49. Baryishak YR et al: Vernal keratoconjunctivitis in an Israeli group of patients and its treatment with sodium cromoglycate, Br J Ophthalmol 66:118, 1982.

50. Ben Ezra D et al: Cyclosporine eyedrops for the treatment of severe vernal keratoconjunctivitis, Am J Ophthalmol 101:278, 1986.

51. Singh G: Cryosurgery in palpebral vernal catarrh, Ann Ophthalmol 14:252, 1982.

52. Tse DT et al: Mucous membrane grafting for severe palpebral vernal conjunctivitis, Arch Ophthalmol 101:1879, 1983.

53. Rich LF and Hanifin JM: Ocular complications of atopic dermatitis and other eczemas, Int Ophthalmol Clin 25:61, 1985.

53a. Garrity JA and Liesegang TJ: Ocular complications of atopic dermatitis, Can J Ophthalmol 19:21, 1984.

54. Brunsting LA, Reed WB, and Bair HL: Occurrence of cataracts and keratoconus with atopic dermatitis, Arch Dermatol 72:237, 1955.

55. Cowan A, Klauder JV: Frequency of occurrence of cataracts in atopic dermatitis, Arch Ophthalmol 43:759, 1950.

56. Rocklin RE and Pincus S: Atopic dermatitis. In Samter M, editor: Immunological diseases, ed 4, Boston, 1988, Little, Brown & Co.

57. Palacios J, Fuller EW, and Blaylock WK: Immunological capabilities of patients with atopic dermatitis, J Invest Dermatol 47:484, 1966.

58. Leung DYM, Rhodes AR, and Geha RS: Enumeration of T cell subsets in atopic dermatitis using monoclonal antibodies, J Allergy Clin Immunol 67:450, 1981.

59. Hemady Z et al: Abnormal regulation of in vitro IgE synthesis by T cells obtained from patients with atopic dermatitis, Clin Immunol Immunopathol 35:156, 1985.

60. Ostler HB: Acute chemotic reaction to cromolyn, Arch Ophthalmol 100:412, 1982.

61. Jay JL: Clinical features and diagnosis of adult atopic keratoconjunctivitis and the effect of treatment with sodium cromoglycate, Br J Ophthalmol 65:335, 1981.

62. Ariyanayagam M et al: Topical sodium cromoglycate in the management of atopic eczema, Br J Dermatol 112:343, 1985.

63. Aswad MI, Tauber J, and Baum J: Plasmapheresis treatment in patients with severe atopic keratoconjunctivitis, Ophthalmology 95:444, 1988.

64. Spring TF: Reaction to hydrophilic lenses, Med J Aust 1:499, 1974.

65. Allansmith MR, Korb DR, and Greiner JV: Giant papillary conjunctivitis induced by hard or soft contact lens wear: quantitative histology, Ophthalmology 85:766, 1978.

66. Srinivasan DB et al: Giant papillary conjunctivitis with ocular prosthesis, Arch Ophthalmol 97:892, 1979.

67. Meisler DM, Krachmer JH, and Goeken JA: An immunopathologic study of giant papillary conjunctivitis associated with an ocular prosthesis, Am J Ophthalmol 92:368, 1981.

68. Jolson AS and Jolson SC: Suture barb giant papillary conjunctivitis, Ophthalmic Surg 15:139, 1984.

69. Sugar A and Meyer RF: Giant papillary conjunctivitis after keratoplasty, Am J Ophthalmol 91:239, 1981.

70. Carlson AN and Wilhelmus KR: Giant papillary conjunctivitis associated with cyanoacrylate glue, Am J Ophthalmol 104:437, 1987.

71. Robin JB et al: Giant papillary conjunctivitis associated with an extruded scleral buckle, Arch Ophthalmol 105:619, 1987.

72. Allansmith MR and Ross RN: Giant papillary conjunctivitis, Int Ophthalmol Clin 28:309, 1988.

73. Abelson MB and Allansmith MR: Ocular allergies. In Smolin G and Thoft RA, editors: The cornea: scientific foundations and clinical practice, Boston, 1983, Little, Brown & Co.

74. Meisler DM, Zaret CR, and Stock EL: Trantas' dots and limbal inflammation associated with soft contact lens wear, Am J Ophthalmol 89:66, 1980.

75. Ballow M et al: An animal model for contact lens-induced giant papillary conjunctivitis, Invest Ophthalmol Vis Sci 28:39, 1987.

76. Foster CS: Immunosuppressive therapy in external ocular inflammatory disease, Ophthalmology 87:140, 1980.

77. Frith P et al: External ocular findings in lupus erythematosus: a clinical and immunopathological study, Br J Ophthalmol 74:163, 1990.

78. Ramos-Niembro F and Alarcon-Segovia D: Development of sicca symptoms in SLE patients with existing subclinical abnormalities, Arthritis Rheum 22:935, 1979.

79. Dubois EI and Tuffanelli DL: Clinical manifestations of SLE: analysis of 520 cases, JAMA 190:104, 1964.

80. Gold DH, Morris DA, and Henkind P: Ocular findings in SLE, Br J Ophthalmol 56:800, 1972.

81. Pillat A: Uber das vorkommen von choroiditis bei lupus erythematodes, Graefes Arch Clin Exp Ophthalmol 133:566, 1934.

82. Spaeth GL: Corneal staining in systemic lupus erythematosus, N Engl J Med 276:1168, 1967.

83. Halmay O and Ludwig K: Bilateral band-shaped deep keratitis and iridocyclitis in systemic lupus erythematosus, Br J Ophthalmol 48:558, 1964.

84. Reeves JA: Keratopathy associated with systemic lupus erythematosus, Arch Ophthalmol 74:159, 1965.

85. Huey C et al: Discoid lupus erythematosus of the eyelids, Ophthalmology 90:1389, 1983.

86. Doesschat JT: Corneal complications in lupus erythematosus discoidus, Ophthalmologica 132:153, 1956.

87. Foster CS: Ocular surface manifestations of neurological and systemic diseases, Int Ophthalmol Clin 19:207, 1979.

88. Raizman MB and Baum J: Discoid lupus keratitis, Arch Ophthalmol 107:545, 1989.

89. Gordon DA, Stein JL, and Border I: The extra-articular features of rheumatoid arthritis: a systemic analysis of 127 cases, Am J Med 54:445, 1973.

90. Decker JL et al: Rheumatoid arthritis: evolving concepts of pathogenesis and treatment, Ann Intern Med 101:810, 1984.

91. Jayson MIV and Easty DL: Ulceration of the cornea in rheumatoid arthritis, Ann Rheum Dis 36:428, 1977.

92. Ericson S and Syndmark E: Studies on the sicca syndrome in patients with rheumatoid arthritis, Acta Rheum Scand 16:60, 1970.

93. Talal N: Sjögren's syndrome. In Samter M, editor: Immunological diseases, ed 4, Boston, 1988, Little, Brown & Co.

94. Jayson MI and Jones DEP: Scleritis and rheumatoid arthritis, Ann Rheum Dis 30:343, 1971.

95. Gardner KM, Rajacich GM, and Mondino BJ: Ophthalmological manifestations of adult rheumatoid arthritis and cicatricial pemphigoid, Int Ophthalmol Clin 25:1, 1985.

96. Lyne AJ and Pitkeathley DA: Episcleritis and scleritis: association with connective tissue diseas   Arch Ophthalmol 80:171, 1968.

97. McGavin DDM et al: Episcleritis and scleritis: a study of their clinical manifestations and associations with rheumatoid arthritis, Br J Ophthalmol 60:192, 1976.

98. Watson PG and Hazelman BL: The sclera and systemic disorders, London, 1976, WB Saunders.

99. Fong LP, Foster CS, and Sainz de la Maza M: Vascular immunopathology in scleritis, Ophthalmology 95(suppl):160, 1988.

100. Watson PG: Diseases of the sclera and episclera. In Duane TD and Jaeger EA, editors: Clinical ophthalmology, vol 4, Philadelphia, 1988, Harper & Row.

101. Foster CS, Forstot SL, and Wilson LA: Mortality rate in rheumatoid arthritis patients developing necrotizing scleritis or peripheral ulcerative keratitis. Effects of systemic immunosuppression, Ophthalmology 90:175, 1980.

102. Erhardt CC et al: Factors predicting a poor life prognosis in rheumatoid arthritis: an eight year prospective study. Ann Rheum Dis 48:7, 1989.

103. Sevel B: Rheumatoid nodule of the sclera, Trans Ophthalmol Soc UK 85:357, 1965.

104. Watson PG and Hayreh SS: Scleritis and episcleritis, Br J Ophthalmol 60:163, 1976.

105. Brown SI and Grayson M: Marginal furrows: a characteristic corneal lesion of rheumatoid arthritis, Arch Ophthalmol 79:563, 1968.

106. Chylack LT Jr et al: Ocular manifestations of juvenile rheumatoid arthritis, Am J Ophthalmol 79:1026, 1975.

107. Jackson J et al: Sjögren's syndrome in juvenile rheumatoid arthritis (JRA) (abstract), Arthritis Rheum 16:122, 1973.

108. Gilliland BC: Progressive systemic sclerosis (diffuse scleroderma). In E Braunwald, et al, editors: Harrison's principles of internal medicine, ed 11, New York, 1987, McGraw-Hill.

109. Silver RM and Leroy EC: Systemic sclerosis (scleroderma). In Samter M, editor: Immunological diseases, ed 4, Boston, 1988, Little, Brown & Co.

110. Alarcón-Segovia D et al: Sjögren's syndrome and progressive systemic sclerosis (scleroderma), Am J Med 57:78, 1974.

111. Kirkham TH: Scleroderma and Sjögren's syndrome, Br J Ophthalmol 53:131, 1969.

112. Horan EC: Ophthalmic manifestations of progressive systemic sclerosis, Br J Ophthalmol 53:388, 1969.

113. Stucci CA and Geiser JD: Manifestations oculares de la sclérodermie generalisée (points communs avec le syndrome de Sjögren), Doc Ophthalmol 22:72, 1967.

114. Manschot S: Über die pathologie und pathogenese von sclerodermia universalis, Mitt Med Fakult Kaiserl Univ Tokyo 31:55, 1924.

115. Meyer O et al: Relapsing polychondritis: pathogenic role of anti-native collagen type II antibodies, J Rheumatol 8:820, 1981.

116. Herman JH: Polychondritis. In WN Kelly et al, editors: Textbook of rheumatology, Philadelphia, 1985, WB Saunders.

117. Barth WF and Berson EF: Relapsing polychondritis, rheumatoid arthritis and blindness, Am J Ophthalmol 66:890, 1968.

118. McKay DAR, Watson PG, and Lyne AJ: Relapsing polychondritis and eye disease, Br J Ophthalmol 58:600, 1974.

119. Dolan DL, Lemmon GB, and Teitelbaum FR: Relapsing polychondritis: analytical literature review and studies on pathogenesis, Am J Med 41:285, 1966.

120. Anderson B: Ocular lesions in relapsing polychondritis and other rheumatoid syndromes, Trans Am Acad Ophthalmol Otolaryngol 71:227, 1967.

121. Rucker CW and Ferguson RH: Ocular manifestations of relapsing polychondritis, Trans Am Ophthalmol Soc 62:167, 1979.

122. Matoba A et al: Keratitis in relapsing polychondritis, Ann Ophthalmol 16:367, 1984.

123. Zion VM, Brackup AH, and Weingeist S: Relapsing polychondritis, erythema nodosum, and sclerouveitis: a case report with anterior segment angiography, Surv Ophthalmol 19:107, 1974.

124. Evans JP and Eustace P: Scleromalacia perforans associated with Crohn's disease treated with sodium versenate (EDTA), Br J Ophthalmol 57:330, 1973.

125. Hopkins DJ et al: Ocular disorders in a series of 332 patients with Crohn's disease, Br J Ophthalmol 58:732, 1974.

126. Macoul KL: Ocular changes in granulomatous ileocolitis, Arch Ophthalmol 84:95, 1970.

127. Schulman MF and Sugar A: Peripheral corneal infiltrates in inflammatory bowel disease, Ann Ophthalmol 13:109, 1981.

128. Ellis PP and Gentry JH: Ocular complications of ulcerative colitis, Am J Ophthalmol 58:779, 1964.

129. Billson FA et al: Ocular complications of ulcerative colitis, Gut 8:102, 1967.

130. Gamble CN et al: The immune complex pathogenesis of glomerulonephritis and pulmonary vasculitis in Behçet's disease, Am J Med 66:1031, 1979.

131. Rogers RS, Sams WM, and Shorter RG: Lymphocytotoxicity for oral epithelial cells in recurrent aphthous stomatitis and Behçet syndrome, Arch Dermatol 109:361, 1974.

132. Lehner T et al: An immunogenetic basis for the tissue involvement in Behçet's syndrome, Immunology 37:895, 1979.

133. Nussenblatt RB and Palestine AG: Uveitis: fundamentals and clinical practice, Chicago, 1989, Mosby–Year Book, Inc.

134. Katz P and Fauci AS: Systemic vasculitis. In Samter M, editor: Immunological diseases, 4th ed, Boston, 1988, Little, Brown & Co.

135. Gold DH: Ocular manifestations of connective tissue (collagen) diseases. In Duane T, editor: Clinical ophthalmology, vol 5, Philadelphia, 1988, Harper & Row.

136. Gerstle CS and Friedman AH: Marginal corneal ulceration (limbal guttering) as a presenting sign of temporal arteritis, Ophthalmology 87:1173, 1980.

137. Foster CS: Ocular manifestations of the nonrheumatic acquired collagen vascular diseases. In Smolin G and Thoft RA, editors: The cornea: scientific foundations and clinical practice, Boston, 1983, Little, Brown & Co.

138. Purcell JJ, Birkenkamp R, and Tsai CC: Conjunctival lesions in periarteritis nodosa, Arch Ophthalmol 102:736, 1984.

139. Cogan DG: Corneoscleral lesions in periarteritis and Wegener's granulomatosis, Trans Am Ophthalmol Soc 53:321, 1955.

140. Moore JG and Sevel D: Corneoscleral ulceration in periarteritis nodosa, Br J Ophthalmol 50:651, 1966.

141. Foster CS: Systemic immunosuppressive therapy for progressive bilateral Mooren's ulcer, Ophthalmology 92:1436, 1985.

142. Harbart F and McPherson SD: Scleral necrosis in periarteritis nodosa, Am J Ophthalmol 30:727, 1947.

143. Wise GN: Ocular periarteritis nodosa, Arch Ophthalmol 48:1, 1952.

144. Meisler DM et al: Conjunctival inflammation and amyloidosis in allergic granulomatosis and angiitis (Churg-Strauss syndrome), Am J Ophthalmol 91:216, 1981.

145. Shields CL, Shields JA, and Rozanski TI: Conjunctival involvement in Churg-Strauss syndrome, Am J Ophthalmol 102:601, 1986.

146. Cury D, Breakey AS, and Payne BF: Allergic granulomatous angiitis associated with uveoscleritis and papilledema, Arch Ophthalmol 55:261, 1966.

147. Chumbley LC, Harrison EG, and DeRemee RA: Allergic granulomatosis and angiitis (Churg-Strauss syndrome): report and analysis of 30 cases, Mayo Clin Proc 52:477, 1977.

148. Robin JB et al: Ocular involvement in the respiratory vasculitides, Surv Ophthalmol 30:127, 1985.

149. Fauci AS: The vasculitis syndromes. In Braunwald E et al, editors: Harrison's principles of internal medicine, ed 11, New York, 1987, McGraw-Hill.

150. Fauci AS et al: Wegener's granulomatosis: prospective clinical and therapeutic experience with 85 patients for 21 years, Ann Intern Med 98:76, 1983.

151. Bullen CL et al: Ocular complications of Wegener's granulomatosis, Ophthalmology 90:270, 1983.

152. Haynes BF et al: The ocular manifestations of Wegener's granulomatosis: fifteen years experience and review of the literature, Am J Med 63:131, 1977.

153. Straatsma BR: Ocular manifestations of Wegener's granulomatosis, Am J Ophthalmol 44:789, 1957.

154. Weith J and Farkos TG: Pseudotumor of the orbit as a presenting sign in Wegener's granulomatosis, Surv Ophthalmol 17:106, 1970.

155. Austin P et al: Peripheral corneal degeneration and occlusive vasculitis in Wegener's granulomatosis, Am J Ophthalmol 85:311, 1978.

156. Brady HR, Israel MR, and Lewin WH: Wegener's granulomatosis and corneoscleral ulcer, JAMA 193:148, 1965.

157. Ferry AP and Leopold IH: Marginal (ring) corneal ulcer as a presenting manifestation of Wegener's granuloma: a clinicopathologic study, Trans Am Acad Ophthalmol Otolaryngol 74:1276, 1970.

158. Sevel D: Necrogranulomatous keratitis associated with Wegener's granulomatosis and rheumatoid arthritis, Am J Ophthalmol 63:250, 1967.

159. Biglan AW et al: Corneal perforation in Wegener's granulomatosis treated with corneal transplantation, Ann Ophthalmol 9:799, 1979.

160. Hill JC and Potter P: Treatment of Mooren's ulcer with cyclosporin A: report of three cases, Br J Ophthalmol 71:11, 1987.

161. Wakefield D and Robinson LP: Cyclosporin therapy in Mooren's ulcer, Br J Ophthalmol 71:415, 1987.

162. Zierhut M et al: Topical treatment of severe corneal ulcers with cyclosporin A, Graefes Arch Clin Exp Ophthalmol 227:30, 1989.

163. Kruit PJ, van Balen AT, and Stilma JS: Cyclosporin A treatment in two cases of corneal peripheral melting syndrome, Doc Ophthalmol 59:33, 1985.

164. Wilson FM, Grayson M, and Ellis FD: Treatment of peripheral corneal ulcers by limbal conjunctivectomy, Br J Ophthalmol 60:713, 1976.

165. Feder RS and Krachmer JH: Conjunctival resection for the treatment of the rheumatoid corneal ulceration, Ophthalmology 91:111, 1984.

166. Eiferman RA, Carother DJ, and Yankeelov JA: Peripheral rheumatoid ulceration and evidence for conjunctival collagenase production, Am J Ophthalmol 87:703, 1979.

167. Waldmann TA: Immunodeficiency diseases: primary and acquired. In Samter M, editor: Immunological diseases, ed 4, Boston, 1988, Little, Brown & Co.

168. Remold-O'Donnell E et al: Characterization of a human lymphocyte surface sialoglycoprotein that is defective in Wiskott-Aldrich syndrome, J Exp Med 159:1705, 1984.

169. Orellana J and Friedman AH: Ocular manifestations of multiple myeloma, Waldenström's macroglobulinemia and benign monoclonal gammopathy, Surv Ophthalmol 26:3, 1981.

170. Pinkerton RMH and Robertson DM: Corneal and conjunctival changes in dysproteinemia, Invest Ophthalmol 8:357, 1969.

171. Aronson SB and Shaw R: Corneal crystals in multiple myeloma, Arch Ophthalmol 61:541, 1959.

172. Beebe WE, Webster RG, and Spencer WB: Atypical corneal manifestations of multiple myeloma: a clinical histopathologic, and immunohistochemical report, Cornea 8:274, 1989.

173. Kremer I et al: Corneal subepithelial monoclonal kappa IgG deposits in essential cryoglobulinaemia, Br J Ophthalmol 73:669, 1989.

174. Hill JC and Mulligan GP: Subepithelial corneal deposits in IgG lambda myeloma, Br J Ophthalmol 73:552, 1989.

175. Rodrigues MM et al: Posterior corneal crystalline deposits in benign monoclonal gammopathy: a clinico-pathologic case report, Arch Ophthalmol 97:124, 1979.

176. Barr CC, Gelender H, and Font R: Corneal crystalline deposits associated with dysproteinemia: report of two cases and review of literature, Arch Ophthalmol 98:884, 1980.

177. Miller KH et al: Immunoprotein deposition in the cornea, Ophthalmology 87:944, 1980.

178. Lewis RA, Falls HF, and Troyer DO: Ocular manifestations of hypercupremia associated with multiple myeloma, Arch Ophthalmol 93:1050, 1975.

179. Gloor B: Diffuse corneal degeneration in a case of Waldenström's macroglobulinemia, Ophthalmologica 155:449, 1968.

180. Oglesby RB: Corneal opacities in a patient with cryoblobulinemia and reticulohistiocytosis, Arch Ophthalmol 65:63, 1961.

181. Thomas ED et al: Bone-marrow transplantation, N Engl J Med 292:832, 1975.

182. Jack M et al: Ocular manifestations of graft-vs-host disease, Arch Ophthalmol 101:1080, 1983.

183. Franklin R et al: Ocular manifestations of graft-vs-host disease, Ophthalmology 90:4, 1983.

184. Jabs DA et al: The eye in bone marrow transplantation. III. Conjunctival graft vs host disease, Arch Ophthalmol 107:1343, 1989.

185. Ferry AP: Histopathology of rheumatoid episcleral nodues: an extra-articular manifestation of rheumatoid arthritis, Arch Ophthalmol 82:77, 1969.

186. Watson PG: The nature and treatment of scleral inflammation (Doyne Memorial Lecture), Trans Ophthalmol Soc UK 102:257, 1982.

187. Fraunfelder FT and Watson PG: Evaluation of eyes enucleated for scleritis, Br J Ophthalmol 60:227, 1976.

188. Rao NA, Marak GE, and Hidayat AA: Necrotizing scleritis: a clinico-pathologic study of 41 cases, Ophthalmology 92:1542, 1985.

189. Wakefield D, McCluskey P, and Penny R: Intravenous pulse methylprednisolone therapy in severe inflammatory eye disease, Arch Ophthalmol 104:847, 1986.

190. Hoffman F and Wiederholt M: Local treatment of necrotizing scleritis with cyclosporin A, Cornea 4:3, 1985.

191. Sorsby A: The aetiology of phlyctenular ophthalmia, Br J Ophthalmol 26:189, 1942.

192. Thygeson P: The etiology and treatment of phylctenular keratoconjunctivitis, Am J Ophthalmol 34:1217, 1951.

193. Thygeson P: Observations on nontuberculous phlyctenular keratoconjunctivitis, Trans Am Acad Ophthalmol Otolaryngol 58:128, 1954.

194. Smolin G and Okumoto M: Staphylococcal blepharitis, Arch Ophthalmol 95:812, 1977.

195. Jeffrey MP: Ocular diseases caused by nematodes, Am J Ophthalmol 40:41, 1953.

196. Mondino BJ and Dethlefs B: Occurrence of phlyctenules after immunization with ribitol teichoic acid of *Staphylococcus aureus,* Arch Ophthalmol 102:461, 1984.

197. Mondino BJ and Kowalski R: Phlyctenulae and catarrhal infiltrates, Arch Ophthalmol 100:1968, 1982.

198. Mondino BJ, Laheji AK, and Adamu SA: Ocular immunity to *Staphylococcus aureus,* Invest Ophthalmol Vis Sci 28:560, 1987.

199. Abu el Asrar AM et al: Immunocytological study of phlyctenular eye disease, Int Ophthalmol 10:33, 1987.

200. Smith RE, Dippe DW, and Miller SD: Phlyctenular keratoconjunctivitis: results of penetrating keratoplasty in Alaskan natives, Ophthalmic Surg 6:62, 1975.

201. Bowers R et al: Non-aureus staphylococcus in corneal disease, Invest Ophthalmol Vis Sci 30(suppl):380, 1989.

202. Thygeson P: Marginal corneal infiltrates and ulcers, Trans Am Acad Ophthalmol Otolaryngol 51:198, 1946.

203. Duke-Elder S, Leigh AG: System of ophthalmology, vol VIII: Diseases of the outer eye, St Louis, 1965, Mosby–Year Book, Inc.

204. Cohn H et al: Marginal corneal ulcers with acute beta streptococcal conjunctivitis and chronic dacryocystitis, Am J Ophthalmol 87:541, 1979.

205. Mondino BJ and Groden LR: Conjunctival hyperemia

and corneal infiltrates with chemically disinfected soft contact lenses, Arch Ophthalmol 98:1767, 1980.

206. Stein RM et al: Infected vs sterile corneal infiltrates in contact lens wearers, Am J Ophthalmol 105:632, 1988.

207. Wood TO and Kaufman HE: Mooren's ulcer, Am J Ophthalmol 71:417, 1971.

208. Kietzman B: Mooren's ulcer in Nigeria, Am J Ophthalmol 65:679, 1968.

209. Majekodunmi AA: Ecology of Mooren's ulcer in Nigeria, Doc Ophthalmol 49:211, 1980.

210. Brown SI: Mooren's ulcer: histopathology and proteolytic enzymes of adjacent conjunctiva, Br J Ophthalmol 59:670, 1975.

211. Murray PE and Rahi AHS: Pathogenesis of Mooren's ulcer: some new concepts, Br J Ophthalmol 68:182, 1984.

212. Foster CS et al: The immunopathology of Mooren's ulcer, Am J Ophthalmol 88:149, 1979.

213. Young RG and Watson PG: Light and electron microscopy of corneal melting syndrome (Mooren's ulcer), Br J Ophthalmol 66:341, 1982.

214. Ban der Gaag R, et al: Circulating antibodies against corneal epithelium and hookworm in patients with Mooren's ulcer from Sierra Leone, Br J Ophthalmol 67:623, 1983.

215. Brown SI, Mondino BJ, and Rabin BS: Autoimmune phenomenon in Mooren's ulcer, Am J Ophthalmol 82:835, 1976.

216. Berkowitz PT et al: Presence of circulatory immune complexes in patients with peripheral corneal diseases, Arch Ophthalmol 101:242, 1983.

217. Schaap OL, Feltkamp TEW, and Breenbart AC: Circulating antibodies to corneal tissue in a patient suffering from Mooren's ulcer (ulcus rodens corneae), Clin Exp Immunol 5:365, 1969.

218. Mondino BJ, Brown SI, and Rabin BS: Cellular immunity in Mooren's ulcer, Am J Ophthalmol 85:788, 1978.

219. Brown SI: Mooren's ulcer: treatment by conjunctival excision, Br J Ophthalmol 59:675, 1975.

220. Aviel E: Combined cryoapplications and peritomy in Mooren's ulcer, Br J Ophthalmol 56:48, 1972.

221. Foster CS: Systemic immunosuppressive therapy for progressive bilateral Mooren's ulcer, Ophthalmology 92:1436, 1985.

222. Brown SI and Mondino BJ: Therapy of Mooren's ulcer, Am J Ophthalmol 98:1, 1984.

223. Brown SI and Mondino BJ: Penetrating keratoplasty in Mooren's ulcer, Am J Ophthalmol 89:255, 1980.

224. Martin NF, Stark WJ, and Maumenee AE: Treatment of Mooren's-like ulcer by lamellar keratectomy: report of six eyes and literature review, Ophthalmic Surg 18:564, 1987.

ENDOCRINE DISORDERS

HYPERTHYROIDISM (GRAVES' DISEASE)

Hyperthyroidism most commonly occurs as part of a syndrome that may include goiter, exophthalmos, and pretibial myxedema. The eye changes seem to be independent of thyroid activity; they can be seen in the hyperthyroid state, or they may appear after a euthyroid or hypothyroid state has been reached. In some patients typical eye changes are present but no clinical history of thyroid dysfunction can be elicited. Graves' disease appears to be an autoimmune condition,[1,2] but the mechanism of the ocular changes is unclear.

Ophthalmic involvement occurs in approximately 50% of patients. Patients may complain of a sandy feeling in the eyes, lacrimation, photophobia, decreased vision, or double vision. The most common signs are lid retraction, lid lag, conjunctival injection and chemosis, and proptosis. There is often a fullness and edema of the lids (Fig. 20-1). The conjunctival vessels are most dilated over the muscle insertions, and marked hyperemia and chemosis can occur (Fig. 20-2). The lids occasionally show increased pigmentation (Fig. 20-3).

Corneal involvement is related to exposure from proptosis and lid retraction. The earliest change is punctate staining of the cornea and conjunctiva in the interpalpebral zone. With more severe drying, chemosis, epithelial defects, ulceration, and even perforation can result. Hyperthyroidism may also be associated with superior limbic keratoconjunctivitis (see Chapter 7).

Mild exposure can be treated with lubricants and nocturnal taping of the lids or moisture barriers.

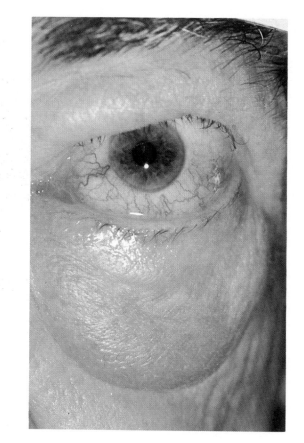

Fig. 20-1. Edema of lids, proptosis, conjunctival injection, and exposure keratitis of lower one fourth of cornea in thyroid orbitopathy.

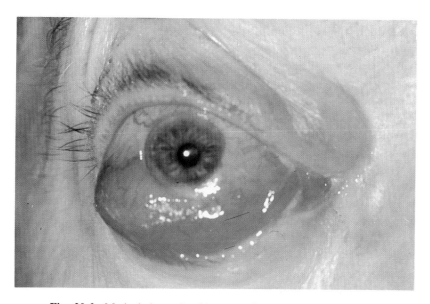

Fig. 20-2. Marked chemosis of lower conjunctiva in Graves' disease.

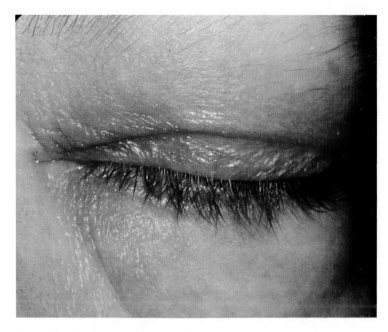

Fig. 20-3. Pigmentation of lids (Jellinek's sign) in case of hyperthyroidism.

In more advanced cases, lid surgery, such as lateral tarsorrhaphy or lid relaxation procedures, may be helpful. Exophthalmos can be reduced with oral corticosteroids, radiation, or surgical decompression.

HYPOTHYROIDISM

Superficial punctate keratopathy can occasionally be seen in hypothyroidism. Some have also suggested that hypothyroidism can cause an increase in tear production.

MULTIPLE ENDOCRINE NEOPLASIA

Multiple endocrine neoplasia is a rare hereditary condition in which neoplasias arise in multiple endocrine glands. Multiple endocrine neoplasia (MEN) type I[3,4] includes the following:
1. Autosomal dominant inheritance
2. Parathyroid adenoma or hyperplasia
3. Pancreatic adenomas
4. Thyroid adenomas
5. Adrenocortical adenomas
6. Subcutaneous lipomas

MEN type IIa (Sipple's syndrome)[5-9] includes the following:
1. Autosomal dominant inheritance
2. Medullary carcinoma of the thyroid
3. Pheochromocytomas
4. Parathyroid adenoma or hyperplasia
5. Multiple mucosal neuromas
6. Marfanoid habitus

MEN type IIb (Froboese's syndrome)[10] includes the following:
1. Sporadic or autosomal dominant inheritance
2. Medullary carcinoma of the thyroid

3. Pheochromocytomas
4. Parathyroid adenomas
5. Skeletal anomalies
6. Abnormal facies: thick lips, soft tissue prognathism (Fig. 20-4)
7. Multiple mucosal neuromas
8. Thickened peripheral nerves

The only ocular involvement in type I is visual field defects caused by pituitary adenomas. Prominent corneal nerves are rarely present in type IIa. Ophthalmic signs are relatively common in MEN type IIb (Table 20-1).[11,12] Thickened nerves are seen in the cornea (Fig. 20-5), iris, and conjunctiva. The nerve fibers form an irregular lattice pattern across the entire cornea. They are seen as large white trunks entering the stroma, with smaller branches into the anterior and posterior stroma. Enlarged nerves can also be seen in the bulbar or tarsal conjunctiva. The nerves frequently appear as flat, poorly circumscribed bundles. They also can be smooth, yellow, and elevated and can resemble pingueculae. Multiple white cords may be seen radiating from the cornea. Paralimbal nerve bundles may be associated with dilated conjunctival vessels.

Less commonly, thickening of the lids or irregular prominences along the free margins are seen (Fig. 20-6), which also are caused by abnormal nerves. Nasal displacement of the puncta, everted eyelids, decreased tear formation, and poor pupillary dilation can also be seen.

The nerves in the cornea do not appear to be myelinated; they contain numerous closely packed axons and Schwann cells. The latter have abundant basal lamina material but do not ensheathe the axons with myelin. The nodules of the conjunctiva and lid are composed of coiled myelinated nerves, with thickened perineurium and sometimes ganglion cells.

The ophthalmologist may have the opportunity to make the diagnosis of MEN by recognizing the prominent corneal nerves and other ocular findings. The differential diagnosis of increased visibility of the corneal nerves is discussed in Chapter 3. Investigation for MEN and medullary carcinoma of the thyroid is very important. Serum concentration of calcitonin is elevated in medullary carcinoma of the thyroid and is a useful diagnostic test.

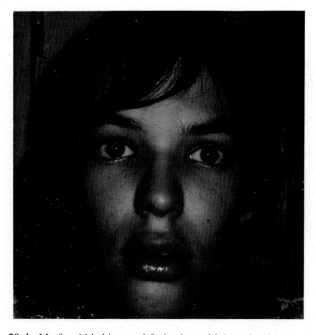

Fig. 20-4. Marfanoid habitus and facies in multiple endocrine neoplasia.

TABLE 20-1. Comparison of MEN Type IIb and Neurofibromatosis

	MEN TYPE IIB	VON RECKLINGHAUSEN'S NEUROFIBROMATOSIS
Basic defect	Disorder of neural crest derivatives	Disorder of neural crest derivatives
Mode of inheritance	Sporadic or autosomal dominant	Autosomal dominant
General appearance	Marfanoid habitus; characteristic facies	Hemihypertrophy of face or extremity (occasional)
		Lip hypertrophy (occasional)
Skeleton	Various anomalies	Various anomalies
Mucocutaneous	Multiple mucosal neuromas	Multiple neurofibromas
	Cafe-au-lait spots	Cafe-au-lait spots
		Molluscum fibrosum
		Freckling, especially in armpits
		General hyperpigmentation
Alimentary tract	Ganglioneuromatosis (diffuse hyperplasia of nerves	Neurofibromas (specific localized tumors)
Neural	Thickened peripheral nerves	Increased incidence of tumors of the central and peripheral nervous systems (neurofibromas, gliomas, meningiomas, ependymomas)
Other tumors	Increased incidence of pheochromocytomas (56%)	Increased incidence of pheochromocytomas (1% to 5%)
	Medullary carcinoma of the thyroid	
Ocular signs	Prominent corneal nerves	Prominent corneal nerves (questionable)
	Ocular neuromas	Ocular neurofibromas
	Thickened eyelids	Thickened eyelids
	Increased intraocular pressure (rare)	Congenital glaucoma
	Impaired pupillary dilation	Melanocytosis of choroid
	Linear thickening of limbal conjunctiva	Retinal detachment (secondary to choroidal neurofibromatosis)
	Decreased tear formation	Optic nerve gliomas and meningiomas
	Nasal displacement of lacrimal puncta	Ectopic neurons in optic nerve
	Prominent orbital ridges	Orbital bone defects
	Heavy eyebrows	Nonexpansile pulsating exophthalmos
		Myelinated retinal nerve fibers

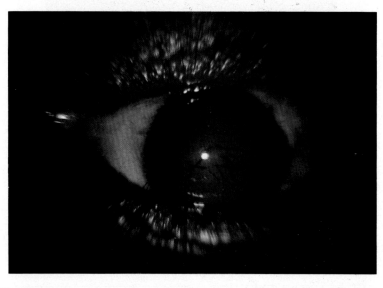

Fig. 20-5. Increased visibility of corneal nerves in multiple endocrine neoplasia.

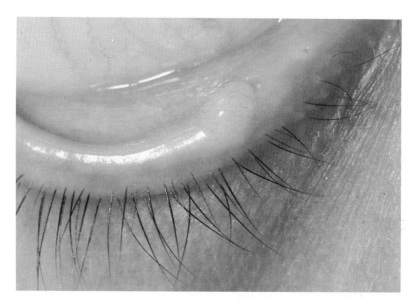

Fig. 20-6. Neuromas of conjunctival lid margin in multiple endocrine neoplasia. (From Grayson M: The cornea in systemic disease. In Duane TD, editor: Clinical ophthalmology, vol 4, Hagerstown, MD, 1976, Harper & Row.)

MEN type IIb and neurofibromatosis have many similarities in their clinical picture, and most likely they have been confused in the past (Table 20-1). It is questionable whether neurofibromatosis is associated with prominent corneal nerves; such cases may have been unrecognized MEN type IIb.

DISORDERS OF CALCIUM METABOLISM

HYPERPARATHYROIDISM

In hyperparathyroidism calcium can be deposited as hydroxyapatite crystals in the corneal (Fig. 20-7) and conjunctival epithelium, corneal endothelium, and anterior sclera.[13,14] The calcium is seen intracellularly in the nucleus and cytoplasm, in contrast to the extracellular deposition seen from most other causes.

CHRONIC KIDNEY FAILURE

Patients with renal failure often develop hypercalcemia or hyperphosphatemia, and calcium phosphate can be deposited in the cornea and conjunctiva.[15-18] The corneal deposits are seen as band keratopathy or a more diffuse limbal opacification (Fig. 20-8). The limbal deposits can resemble Vogt's girdle, but they are chalky white, larger, and coarser, and there is no clear zone at the limbus.[19] Conjunctival calcium deposition gives the limbal deposits a granular appearance. Mild calcification is very common and is usually asymptomatic, but it can be associated with redness and irritation.[15,20] The calcium is deposited extracellularly.[15] Interestingly a kidney transplant will result in resolution of conjunctival and corneal calcification, but hemodialysis does not.[17]

IDIOPATHIC HYPERCALCEMIA OF INFANCY

Idiopathic hypercalcemia of infancy is a rare cause of hypercalcemia that begins between 3 and 9 months of age.[21] The manifestations may include failure to thrive, apathy, polyuria, muscular weakness, hypertension, mental retardation, osteosclerosis, aortic stenosis, dwarfed habitus, and peculiar "elfin" facies (Fig. 20-9). There appears to be abnormal sensitivity to vitamin D and increased cal-

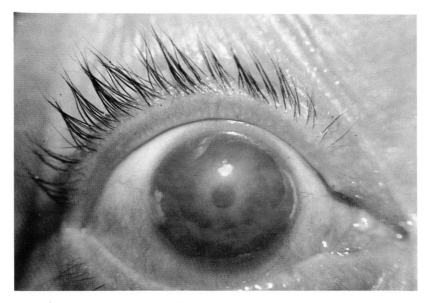

Fig. 20-7. Hyperparathyroidism with calcium deposition in anterior cornea.

cium absorption form the intestines.[22] In addition to corneal calcium deposition, papilledema, strabismus, nystagmus, pupillary changes, and lenticular opacities have been described. Ultrastructurally, the corneal calcium deposition is seen to be intracellular, often confined to the nucleus. Extracellular deposits have also been seen.[23]

HYPOPHOSPHATASIA

Hypophosphatasia is a rare familial disease characterized by multiple skeletal abnormalities and malformations, increased intracranial pressure, failure to thrive, and often early death from nephro-

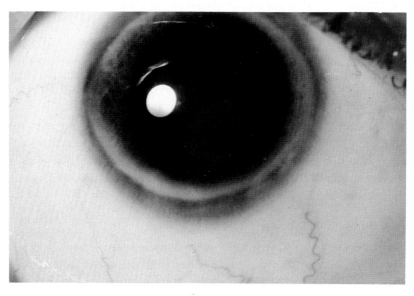

Fig. 20-8. Calcific deposits of calcium in cornea in renal failure.

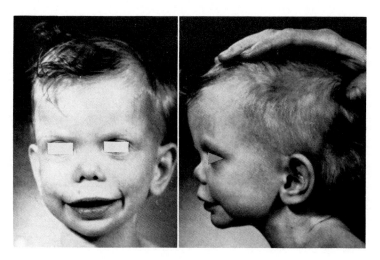

Fig. 20-9. Elfin facies in idiopathic hypercalcemia of infancy. (From Harley RD, DiGeorge AM, and Mabry CC, Apt LL: Trans Am Acad Ophthalmol Otolaryngol 69:997, 1965.)

calcinosis.[24,25] It appears to result from an autosomally inherited deficiency of the tissue nonspecific alkaline phosphatase isoenzyme. Serum calcium is normal or slightly elevated, serum phosphorus is normal, and alkaline phosphatase is low. Urine calcium is high, and all patients excrete excessive amounts of phosphoryl ethanolamine in the urine. The bone disorder is a form of rickets, with severe osteomalacia.

Band keratopathy and conjunctival calcification have been noted, and may be accompanied by blue sclera, a malformation of the orbits (harlequin orbits), cataracts, optic atrophy, and pathologic lid retraction.[24,25]

HYPOPARATHYROIDISM

Acquired hypoparathyroidism is usually related to mechanical injury to or surgical removal of the parathyroid glands. The clinical manifestations are the result of hypocalcemia and include tetany, seizures, mental abnormalities, intestinal upset, and ectodermal abnormalities. A variety of ocular problems can occur, including lenticular abnormalities, blepharospasm, strabismus, nystagmus, papilledema, ptosis, and photophobia. Not as common are corneal vascularization and keratopathy.

Hypoparathyroidism also occurs idiopathically, possibly on a hereditary basis, and can be associated with deficiencies of other organs, such as the adrenals, ovaries, and thymus. In the candidiasis-endocrinopathy syndrome, hypoparathyroidism, Addison's disease, pernicious anemia, ovarian failure, and mucocutaneous candidiasis appear in childhood.[26,27] An autoimmune pathogenesis has been suggested, but the evidence is minimal. Ulcerating vascularization and opacification of the cornea can occur, possibly as a phlyctenular response to candidiasis.

REFERENCES

1. Jacobson DH and Gorman CA: Endocrine ophthalmopathy: current ideas concerning etiology, pathogenesis and treatment, Endocr Rev 5:200, 1984.
2. Burman JD and Baker JR Jr: Immune mechanisms in Graves' disease, Endocr Rev 6:183, 1985.
3. Steiner AL, Goodman AD, and Powers SR: Study of a kindred with pheochromocytoma, medullary thyroid carcinoma, hyperparathyroidism, and Cushing disease: multiple endocrine neoplasia, type 2, Medicine 47:371, 1968.
4. Craven DE, Goodman D, and Carter JH: Familial multiple endocrine adenomatosis: multiple endocrine neoplasia, type I, Arch Intern Med 129:567, 1972.
5. Sipple JH: The association of pheochromocytoma with carcinoma of the thyroid gland, Am J Med 31:163, 1961.
6. Gorlin RJ et al: Multiple mucosal neuromas, pheochromocytoma and medullary carcinoma of thyroid-a syndrome, Cancer 22:293, 1968.
7. Baum JL and Adler ME: Pheochromocytomas, medul-

lary thyroid carcinoma, and multiple mucosal neuroma: a variant of the syndrome, Arch Ophthalmol 87:574, 1972.

8. Gorlin RJ and Menkin BL: Multiple neuromas, pheochromocytoma, medullary carcinoma of the thyroid and marfanoid body build with muscle wasting, Z Kinderheilkd 113:313, 1972.

9. Keiser HR et al: Sipple's syndrome: medullary thyroid carcinoma, pheochromocytoma, and parathyroid disease: studies in a large family, Ann Intern Med 78:561, 1973.

10. Norton JA, Froome LC, Farrell RE, and Wells SA: Multiple endocrine neoplasia type IIb: the most aggressive form of medullary thyroid carcinoma, Surg Clin North Am 59:109, 1979.

11. Robertson DM, Sizemore GW, and Gordon H: Thickened corneal nerves as a manifestation of multiple endocrine neoplasia, Trans Am Acad Ophthalmol Otolaryngol 79:772, 1975.

12. Spector B, Klintworth GK, and Wells SA: Histologic study of the ocular lesions in multiple endocrine neoplasia syndrome type IIb, Am J Ophthalmol 91:204, 1981.

13. Berkow JW, Fine SB, and Zimmerman LE: Unusual ocular calcification in hyperparathyroidism, Am J Ophthalmol 66:812, 1968.

14. Jensen OA: Ocular calcification in primary hyperparathyroidism, Acta Ophthalmol 53:173, 1971.

15. Berlyne GM: Microcrystalline conjunctival calcification in renal failure, Lancet 2:366, 1968.

16. Calderia JAF, Sabbaga E, and Ianhez LE: Conjunctival and corneal changes in renal failure, Br J Ophthalmol 54:399, 1970.

17. Harris LS et al: Conjunctival and corneal calcific deposits in uremic patients, Am J Ophthalmol 72:130, 1971.

18. Porte R and Crombie AL: Corneal and conjunctival calcification in chronic renal failure, Br J Ophthalmol 57:339, 1973.

19. Demco TA, McCormick AQ, and Richards JSF: Conjunctival and corneal changes in chronic renal failure, Can J Ophthalmol 9:208, 1974.

20. Berlyne GM and Shaw AB: Red eyes in renal failure, Lancet 1:4 1967.

21. Fraser D et al: A new look at infantile hypercalcemia, Pediatr Clin North Am 13:503, 1966.

22. Garabédian M et al: Elevated plasma $1,25\text{-}(OH)_2D$ concentrations in infants with hypercalcemia and elfin facies, N Engl J Med 312:948, 1985.

23. Harley RD et al: Idiopathic hypercalcemia of infancy: optic atrophy and other ocular changes, Trans Am Acad Ophthalmol Otolaryngol 69:977 1965.

24. Brenner RL et al: Eye signs of hypophosphatasia, Arch Ophthalmol 81:614, 1969.

25. Fraser D: Hypophosphatasia, Am J Ophthalmol 22:730, 1957.

26. Richman RA et al: Candidiasis and multiple endocrinopathy, Arch Dermatol 111:625, 1975.

27. Whitaker J et al: The syndrome of juvenile hypoadrenocorticism, hypoparathyroidism and superficial moniliasis, J Clin Endocrinol Metab 16:1374, 1956.

DISORDERS OF LIPID METABOLISM

Sphingolipidoses
- Fabry's disease
- Gaucher's disease
- Metachromatic leukodystrophy
- GM$_1$ gangliosidosis I
- Other diseases
Hyperlipoproteinemias
- Type I
- Type IIa
- Type IIb
- Type III

- Type IV
- Type V
Apoprotein A-1 deficiency
Lecithin-cholesterol acyltransferase deficiency
Tangier disease
Fish-eye disease
Refsum's disease
Cerebrotendinous xanthomatosis
Phytosterolemia
Farber's disease

SPHINGOLIPIDOSES

Sphingolipids are lipids that contain a long chain base, such as ceramides, cerebrosides, glanglio-sides, and sphingomyelins. The sphingolipidoses are disorders of sphingolipid catabolism; enzymatic defects result in intracellular accumulation of the lipid enzyme substrates. Depending on the specific enzymatic defect, nervous tissue, reticuloendothelial cells, viscera, or vascular tissue can be affected.

FABRY'S DISEASE

Fabry's disease, also known as angiokeratoma corporis diffusum, results from deficiency of ceramide trihexosidase (an alpha-galactosidase).[1,2] It is transmitted as an X-linked recessive trait. Trihexosylceramide accumulates in vascular endothelium and smooth muscle cells, heart muscle, renal glomeruli, sweat glands, central nervous system, spleen, liver, lymph nodes, and bone marrow. It is characterized clinically by telangiectatic skin lesions, hypohidrosis, febrile episodes, peripheral neuropathy, renal failure, cardiovascular disease, gastrointestinal symptoms, and central nervous system disturbances. The skin eruptions appear in childhood or around puberty and consist of small (pinpoint to several millimeters), round, red to blue-black spots (Fig. 21-1), some of which become hyperkeratotic (Fig. 21-2). They are noted particularly on the breast, glutea, hips, thighs, and upper extremities.

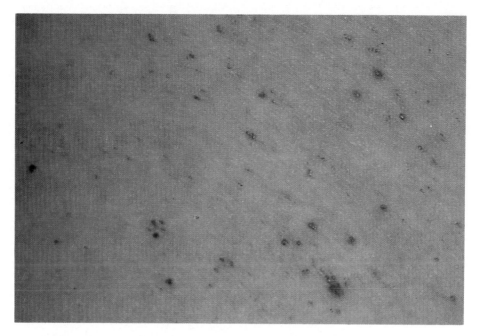

Fig. 21-1. Skin lesions in Fabry's disease.

Fig. 21-2. Skin lesions in Fabry's disease may become hyperkeratotic.

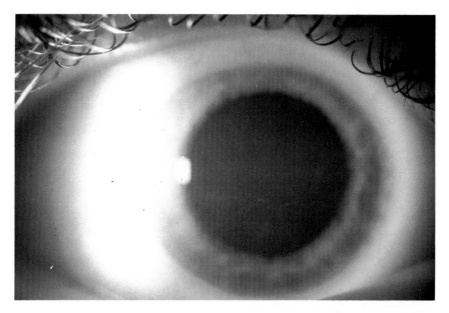

Fig. 21-3. Whorl-like opacification of epithelium in Fabry's disease.

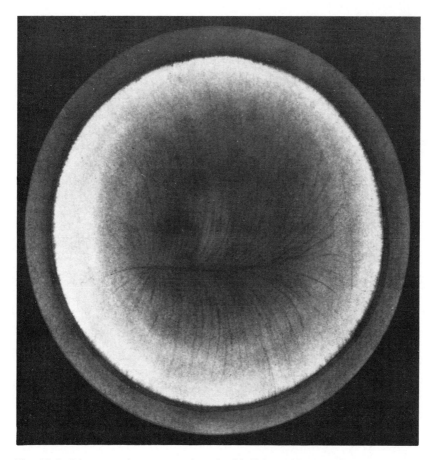

Fig. 21-4. Diagrammatic representation of epithelial opacification in Fabry's disease.

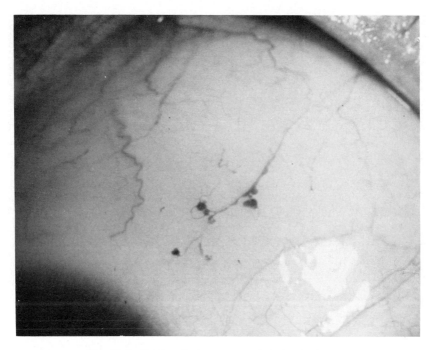

Fig. 21-5. Conjunctival aneurysms in Fabry's disease.

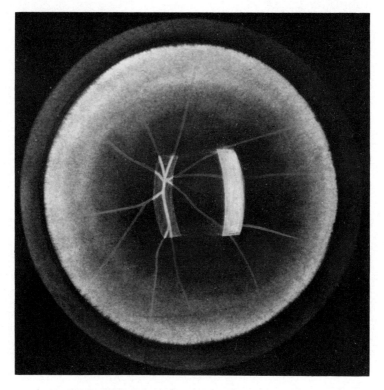

Fig. 21-6. Spokelike cataract in Fabry's disease.

Ocular findings occur in the majority of patients.[3-6] The most common finding is corneal opacification, which is present in nearly all affected males, as well as in 90% of female carriers.[7] They consist of fine, superficial, white, yellow, or brown dots, distributed in a vortex pattern (Figs. 21-3 and 21-4). The opacities can be seen only with the aid of a slit-lamp microscope and do not affect vision. They appear to result from accumulation of sphingolipid in the epithelium. Histologically, intracytoplasmic lamellar inclusions are noted, especially in the basal epithelial cells.[8,9] Similar inclusions can also be present in stromal keratocytes, Bowman's layer, endothelium, and conjunctival epithelium.[10-12]

Other causes of opacities in a vortex distribution (cornea verticillata) are deposition of chloroquine, amiodarone and other drugs, Tangier disease, striate melanokeratosis, and Melkersson-Rosenthal syndrome (see Chapter 3).

Dilation and tortuosity of the conjunctival vessels, sometimes with aneurysm formation, occurs in approximately 60% of patients (Fig. 21-5). Posterior spokelike sutural cataracts, consisting of 9 to 12 spokes (Fig. 21-6) occur in about 50% of patients. Sphingolipid is probably deposited in the lens suture line. Cream-colored anterior capsular deposits, sometimes in a propellar-like pattern, also may be noted. Vision is not affected. Other ocular manifestations include periorbital edema (25% of cases), papilledema, retinal edema, optic atrophy, and dilation and tortuosity of the retinal vessels.

GAUCHER'S DISEASE

Gaucher's disease is an inherited deficiency of beta-glucosidase, the glucocerebroside-cleaving enzyme, resulting in accumulation of glucocerebrosides in reticuloendothelial cells throughout the body, particularly the liver and spleen. Three different forms are recognized: (1) an adult form with liver and spleen enlargement, bone lesions, and skin pigmentation; (2) an infantile form, with severe neurologic abnormalities, and usually death by 3 years of age; and (3) a juvenile form, combining the features of the adult form with milder, slowly progressive neurologic impairment. All are inherited as an autosomal recessive trait.

The adult form of the disease may exhibit prominent, dark yellow pingueculae,[13] which are noted nasally and occur in approximately 25% of cases. Histologically they contain foamy epithelioid cells (Gaucher cells) instead of the elastosis seen in the usual pingueculum. White deposits were observed in the peripheral corneal endothelium, chamber angle, and pupillary margin in one patient.[14] Occasionally, a cherry-red spot can be seen in the macula. Perimacular degeneration and ring granular opacities around the fovea occasionally occur. Retinal hemorrhages, edema, and nystagmus are seen in juveniles.

METACHROMATIC LEUKODYSTROPHY

Metachromatic leukodystrophy is a disorder of myelin metabolism with progressive neurologic deterioration, affecting both the central and peripheral nervous systems.[15] It occurs in several forms, including congenital, late infantile, juvenile, and adult, and all appear to be related to abnormalities of arylsulfatase A (cerebroside sulfatase). In the congenital and infantile forms, corneal clouding can occur,[16,17] as well as optic atrophy, abnormal extraocular movements, pupillary abnormalities, and graying of the macula.[15,18]

GM₁ GANGLIOSIDOSIS

This rare autosomal recessive disease occurs in congenital, juvenile, and adult forms, all caused by a deficiency of beta-galactosidase.[19] The infantile form is characterized by coarse facies, hepatosplenomegaly, a macular cherry-red spot (50% of cases), developmental delay, and skeletal changes resembling those of the mucopolysaccharidoses. The infant is affected at birth or shortly thereafter and survives only 1 to 2 years. Mild diffuse corneal clouding and conjunctival microvascular abnor-

TABLE 21-1. Sphingolipidoses with Anterior Segment Findings*

	FABRY'S DISEASE	GAUCHER'S DISEASE	METACHROMATIC LEUKODYSTROPHY†	GM_1 GANGLIOSIDOSIS	NIEMANN-PICK DISEASE
Heredity	Sex-linked recessive	Autosomal recessive	Autosomal recessive	Autosomal recessive	Autosomal recessive
Enzyme defect	Ceramide trihexosidase; (alpha-galactosidase)	Beta-glucocerebrosidase	Arylsulfatase A	Beta-galactosidase	Sphingomyelinase
Tissue storage	Trihexosylceramide	Glucosylceramide	Cerebroside sulfate	G_{M1} ganglioside Glycoproteins Keratan sulfate	Sphingomyelin and cholesterol
Corneal clouding	+	−	+	±	+ (rare)
Macular grayness or cherry-red spots	−	±	+	+	+ (neuropathic forms)
Optic atrophy	−	−	+	−	−
Conjunctiva	Vascular dilation and tortuosity	Dark yellow pingueculae (25%)	−	−	−

*Corneal clouding has also been reported in one case of Sandhoff's disease (G_{M1} gangliosidosis II).
†Congenital and infantile forms.

malities are present in some patients.[20-22] In the adult form, corneal clouding can occur, as well as spondyloepiphyseal dysplasia, similar to that seen in mucopolysaccharidosis IV, spasticity and ataxia, but intelligence is normal.[23] No ocular abnormalities have been reported in patients with the juvenile form.

OTHER DISEASES

Niemann-Pick disease may rarely be associated with clouding of the corneas.[24] In the Niemann-Pick group of diseases (sphingomyelin-cholesterol lipidoses), lamellar and membranous cytoplasmic inclusions are found in epithelium, keratocytes, and endothelium.[24-27] In one case of Sandhoff's disease (GM_2 gangliosidosis) corneal clouding was present.[28] In others the corneas are clear, but on pathologic examination single membrane-bound vacuoles are seen in keratocytes.[29] Table 21-1 summarizes the enzymatic defects and ocular signs in the sphingolipidoses that affect the anterior segment.

HYPERLIPOPROTEINEMIAS

Hyperlipoproteinemia is commonly associated with earlier onset of corneal arcus, xanthelasma (Fig. 21-7), and occasionally with xanthomas and other external ocular disease. Lipoproteins are divided into pre-beta-, or very low–density lipoproteins (VLDL), beta- or low density–lipoproteins (LDL), alpha- or high-density lipoproteins (HDL), and chylomicrons. Six patterns of serum lipoprotein elevation were distinguished by Freidrickson in 1967 (Table 21-2).[30]

More recently it has become apparent that most of the lipoprotein patterns are not specific to a single disease, but can be caused by several different genetic diseases, as well as by other metabolic diseases. In addition, some specific genetic diseases can produce more than one lipoprotein type. However, past descriptions of ocular complications have referred only to Freidrickson types and have not distinguished between the different causes, so the ophthalmic findings are discussed here in terms

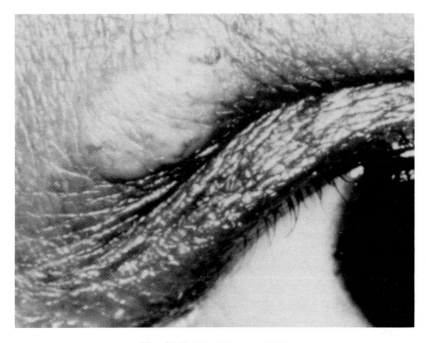

Fig. 21-7. Xanthelasma of lid.

TABLE 21-2. Major Hyperlipoproteinemias

TYPE	PRIMARY DISORDERS	MAJOR ELEVATION IN PLASMA		PREMATURE CORNEAL ARCUS	LID/CONJUNCTIVA	LIPEMIA RETINALIS
		LIPOPROTEIN	LIPID			
I	Familial lipoprotein lipase deficiency Familial apoprotein CII deficiency	Chylomicrons	Triglycerides	−	Eruptive xanthomata in lids	+
IIa	Familial hypercholesterolemia Multiple lipoprotein-type hyperlipidemia Polygenic/exogenous hypercholesterolemia	LDL	Cholesterol	+	Xanthelasma Lid and conjunctival xanthomata	−
IIb	Multiple lipoprotein-type hyperlipidemia Familial hypercholesterolemia	LDL and VLDL	Cholesterol and triglycerides	+	− (Xanthomata)	−
III	Familial dysbetalipoproteinemia	VLDL remnants	Triglycerides and cholesterol	+	Xanthelasma (lid xanthomata)	+
IV	Familial hypertriglyceridemia (mild form) Multiple lipoprotein-type hyperlipidemia Sporadic hypertriglyceridemia Tangier disease	VLDL	Triglycerides	−	(Lid xanthomata)	+
V	Familial hypertriglyceridemia (severe form) Familial apoprotein CII deficiency Multiple lipoprotein-type hyperlipidemia	VLDL and chylomicrons	Triglycerides and cholesterol	−	Eruptive xanthomata (rare)	+

of Freidrickson types. In general premature arcus and xanthelasma occur in types with hypercholesterolemia, and eruptive xanthomas occur in types with hypertriglyceridemia (Table 21-2).

TYPE I (HYPERCHYLOMICRONEMIA, OR BUERGER-GRUTZ DISEASE)

Hyperlipoproteinemia type I is rare and can be caused by either of two autosomal recessive disorders: familial lipoprotein lipase deficiency and familial apoprotein CII deficiency. The serum is creamy white because of an accumulation of chylomicrons, containing mainly triglyceride; this can be seen as lipemia retinalis when plasma levels exceed 2000 mg/ml. In familial lipoprotein lipase deficiency, eruptive xanthomata, which are small, yellow-orange papules surrounded by an erythematous halo, can develop when the lipemia is severe. They are most commonly seen on the face, buttocks, and limbs and can involve the lids. Hepatomegaly, splenomegaly, and foam cell infiltration of the bone marrow also develop. In familial apoprotein CII deficiency, VLDL is also elevated, and a type V lipoprotein pattern can be present. Eruptive xanthomata are rare. Rarely lipid keratopathy occurs in type I lipoproteinemia, but premature corneal arcus usually does not.[31]

TYPE IIA (HYPERBETALIPOPROTEINEMIA, HYPERCHOLESTEROLEMIA)

Most individuals with this lipid profile have polygenic hypercholesterolemia as a result of an interaction between multiple genetic factors and environmental factors, such as diet and obesity. Type IIa can be related to single gene mutations, as in familial hypercholesterolemia and multiple lipoprotein-type hyperlipidemia, common autosomal dominant disorders, or secondary to a variety of systemic conditions, including Cushing's syndrome, hypothyroidism, Werner's syndrome, acute intermittent porphyria, and nephrotic syndrome. It is characterized by increased LDL of normal composition. In familial hypercholesterolemia heterozygous individuals have a higher than normal incidence of premature coronary disease and peripheral atherosclerotic occlusive disease. Xanthomatous lesions develop in the tendons, particularly the Achilles, plantar, patellar, and digital extensors of the hands. In individuals homozygous for familial hypercholesterolemia, the disease is much more severe, and death from myocardial infarction usually occurs before age 20.[32,33] Patients with multiple lipoprotein-type hyperlipidemia tend to have mild and variable elevations of plasma lipids. Premature atherosclerosis and coronary artery disease are more common than normal, but xanthomata do not occur. In familial cases corneal arcus develops at an earlier age: It is present in 50% of heterozygotes over the age of 30, and in 75% over age 40;[34] in homozygotes it usually appears in the first decade. In familial hypercholesterolemia xanthelasmas, raised yellow plaques near the inner canthus of the eyelids (Fig. 21-7), occur frequently, and conjunctival xanthomata and lipid keratopathy can also occur.

TYPE IIB

Type IIb is characterized by elevated VLDL and LDL. Both total serum cholesterol and serum triglyceride are elevated. It may be hereditary, most commonly caused by multiple lipoprotein-type hyperlipidemia, and rarely by familial hypercholesterolemia. This pattern also can be seen in Cushing's syndrome and the nephrotic syndrome. Corneal arcus is more common, and xanthomata can be seen in familial hypercholesterolemia cases.

TYPE III (DYSBETALIPOPROTEINEMIA)

Type III is rare and is usually inherited as an autosomal recessive trait. Serum triglyceride and cholesterol levels are elevated as a result of accumulation of abnormal beta-lipoproteins derived from partial catabolism of VLDL (VLDL remnants or intermediary density lipoprotein). Two types of xanthomata are seen: xanthoma striata palmaris, orange or yellow discolorations of the palmar and digital creases; and tuberous xanthomata, nodular elevations most often seen on the elbows and knees. Premature coronary vascular disease and peripheral vascular disease are common. Obesity, diabetes mellitus, and hypothyroidism are often present. Premature corneal arcus, xanthelasma, and lipemia retinalis can be seen.

TYPE IV (HYPERPREBETALIPOPROTEINEMIA)

Type IV can be inherited, due to familial hypertriglyceridemia, a common autosomal dominant disorder; idiopathic; or related to any of multiple systemic conditions, including diabetes mellitus, oral contraceptives, alcoholism, uremia, emotional stress, acromegaly, and von Gierke's disease. Typically, patients with familial and sporadic hypertriglyceridemia exhibit obesity, hyperglycemia, and hyperinsulinemia. Serum VLDL and triglyceride are usually mildly to moderately elevated; but severe exacerbations occur with excessive alcohol consumption, use of oral contraceptives, hypothyroidism, poorly controlled diabetes, or other precipitating factors. During such exacerbations chylomicrons are also elevated (type V pattern), and eruptive xanthomata and pancreatitis can occur. Lipemia retinalis can be seen.

TYPE V (HYPERPREBETALIPOPROTEINEMIA AND HYPERCHYLOMICRONEMIA)

Type V is a rare type in which VLDL and chylomicrons accumulate in the blood on a normal diet. The serum is creamy, and the triglyceride level is high. It typically results from familial apoprotein CII deficiency and rarely occurs in familial hypertriglyceridemia (as described previously) or multiple lipoprotein-type hyperlipidemia. Homozygous individuals with familial apoprotein CII deficiency present in adolescence or early adult life with recurrent attacks of pancreatitis. Eruptive xanthomata rarely occur. Heterozygotes do not develop pancreatitis. Patients with familial hypertriglyceridemia who develop a type V pattern can develop pancreatitis and eruptive xanthomata. Lipemia retinalis is common, but corneal arcus is not.

A number of other, relatively rare disorders of lipid metabolism can affect the cornea, and are discussed in the rest of this chapter and summarized in Table 21-3.

APOPROTEIN A-1 DEFICIENCY

Only four patients with apoprotein A-1 deficiency have been described; they are divided into three types.[35] Diffuse corneal clouding was present in all four cases. HDL was very low, and early coronary artery disease occurred in all cases. Planar xanthomata and hepatosplenomegaly were also present in some cases.

LECITHIN-CHOLESTEROL ACYLTRANSFERASE DEFICIENCY

Lecithin-cholesterol acyltransferase deficiency is a rare autosomally inherited deficiency of plasma lecithin-cholesterol acyltransferase (LCAT), an enzyme that normally esterifies cholesterol. Serum-unesterified cholesterol and VLDL are increased, and esterified cholesterol and lysolethicin are reduced. The structures of all lipoproteins are abnormal.

Corneal opacities consisting of many small gray dots can be seen throughout the stroma, beginning in early childhood. The opacities can become dense in the periphery resembling a corneal arcus.[36-41] There is a lucid interval at the limbus, but occasionally crystals, presumably cholesterol, are seen near Descemet's membrane. Visual acuity is not affected. Vacuoles containing membranous deposits are present in keratocytes.

TANGIER DISEASE (FAMILIAL HIGH-DENSITY LIPOPROTEIN DEFICIENCY)

Tangier disease is transmitted as an autosomal recessive trait.[42] In homozygotes a complete absence of plasma high-density alpha-lipoprotein (HDL) is noted; in its place an abnormal high-density lipoprotein is found. There may be an abnormally low level of LDL, cholesterol, and phospholipids and elevated levels of VLDL and triglycerides in the plasma. Cholesterol esters are diffusely depos-

TABLE **21-3.** Other Disorders of Lipid Metabolism

DISEASE	INHERITANCE	SERUM	CORNEA	LID/CONJUNCTIVA
Apoprotein A-1 deficiency	Unknown	Low HDL	Diffuse clouding	
LCAT deficiency	AR*	High VLDL, unesterified cholesterol	Diffuse dotlike opacities, arcus-like	
Tangier disease	AR	Absent HDL	Stromal clouding, vision normal	Yellowish orange conjunctival tinge
Fish-eye disease	Unknown	Increased LDL, triglyceride, VLDL, low HDL	White-yellow dotlike opacities; increased thickness	
Refsum's disease	AR	Increased phytanic acid	Thickened epithelium, pannus; increased visibility of nerves; guttae, edema	
Cerebrotendinous xanthomatosis	AR	Increased cholestanol		Xanthelasma
Phytosterolemia	AR	Increased phytosterols	Premature arcus	Xanthelasma
Farber's disease	AR	Increased tissue ceramide	Clouding	Conjunctival granulomas (type I)

*AR, autosomal recessive.

ited in reticuloendothelial cells. One sees a yellowish orange tinge of the tonsils, tonsil beds, rectal mucosa, and conjunctiva. There is enlargement of the liver, spleen, and lymph nodes and peripheral neuropathy and coronary artery disease.

The cornea shows stromal clouding caused by the deposition of cholesterol esters.[43] Many small dots are seen throughout the stroma, sometimes in a whorl-like fashion, densest posteriorly and in the horizontal meridian. A lipid arcus is not present, and vision is not affected.

FISH-EYE DISEASE

Fish-eye disease is a rare inherited disorder in which marked corneal clouding is the most prominent finding. The eyes are said to resemble those of boiled fish. LDL, triglyceride, and VLDL levels are elevated, and HDL is reduced.[38,44] Corneal clouding begins late in the second decade and can become sufficiently dense as to require keratoplasty. Gray-white-yellow dots are seen throughout the stroma and are densest in the periphery. Corneal thickness is increased. On histopathologic examination, numerous extracellular vacuoles made of a cholesterol-containing lipid are seen throughout the stroma.[44]

REFSUM'S DISEASE

Refsum's disease is an autosomal recessive disease of lipid metabolism that results in accumulation of phytanic acid, a C_{20} branched-chain fatty acid. The enzymatic defect is in the alpha-oxidation of beta-methylated fatty acids. It is an important disease to recognize because dietary restriction of phytols and plasmapheresis therapy can significantly improve the outcome.

The major manifestations are neurologic (caused by demyelination) and retinal. Common findings include peripheral neuropathy, cerebellar ataxia, nerve deafness, anosmia, pupillary abnormalities, retinal pigmentary degeneration, ichthyosis, and skeletal abnormalities. Irregular, thick, hazy corneal epithelium; fibrovascular pannus; and increased visibility of the corneal nerves can be present.[45] Corneal guttae, stromal edema, and cataracts can also occur.

CEREBROTENDINOUS XANTHOMATOSIS

Cerebrotendinous xanthomatosis is a rare autosomal recessive disorder of sterol metabolism caused by a deficiency of hepatic mitochondrial 26-hydroxylase, which is involved in the synthesis of bile acids. Cholesterol and cholestanol are stored in most tissues, and particularly in xanthomata, bile, and brain.[46] The manifestations include dementia, cerebellar ataxia, tuberous and tendon xanthomata, spinal cord paresis, and early atherosclerosis. Patients have a high incidence of xanthelasmas and cataracts and should be treated with chenodeoxycholic acid.

PHYTOSTEROLEMIA

Phytosterolemia is another rare, inherited sterol storage disease. It is inherited as an autosomal recessive trait and is characterized by tendon and tuberous xanthomata and premature coronary artery disease.[46] Increased amounts of phytosterols (plant sterols) are found in serum, erythrocytes, and in some tissues. Premature corneal arcus and xanthelasmas are seen. Patients are treated with diets low in plant and shellfish sterols, and cholestyramine.

FARBER'S DISEASE

Farber's disease is a genetic disorder of lipid metabolism, associated with deficiency of lysosomal acid ceramidase and tissue accumulation of ceramide. The manifestations include painful and progressively deformed joints, subcutaneous nodules, hoarseness, nervous system dysfunction, lung, heart, and lymph node involvement, and usually death within a few years. Corneal opacities have been noted in these patients[47]; granulomatous, xanthoma-like conjunctival lesions occur in type I.[48]

Macular cherry-red spots also are found in some patients. Histologically, granulomas and accumulation of lipid-laden macrophages are noted in affected tissues. Round inclusions, surrounded by a bilaminar membrane, are seen in conjunctival and corneal epithelium and in keratocytes.[49]

REFERENCES

1. Hashimoto K, Lieberman P, and Lamkin N: Angiokeratoma corporis diffusum (Fabry disease), Arch Dermatol 112:1416, 1976.
2. Karr WJ Jr: Fabry's disease (angiokeratoma corporis diffusum universale), Am J Med 7:829, 1959.
3. Grace EV: Diffuse angiokeratosis (Fabry's disease), Am J Ophthalmol 62:139, 1966.
4. Sher NA, Letson RD, and Desnick RJ: The ocular manifestations in Fabry's disease, Arch Ophthalmol 97:671, 1979.
5. Spaeth GL and Frost P: Fabry's disease: its ocular manifestations, Arch Ophthalmol 74:760, 1965.
6. Franceschetti AT: Fabry's disease: ocular manifestations, Birth Defects 12:195, 1976.
7. Weingeist TA and Blodi FC: Fabry's disease: ocular findings in a female carrier, Arch Ophthalmol 85:169, 1971.
8. Font RL and Fine BS: Ocular pathology in Fabry's disease, Am J Ophthalmol 73:419, 1973.
9. Francois J, Hanssens M, and Teuchy H: Corneal ultrastructural changes in Fabry's disease, Ophthalmologica 176:313, 1978.
10. Frost P, Tamala Y, and Spaeth GL: Fabry's disease-glycolipid lipidosis: histochemical and electronmicroscopic studies of two cases, Am J Med 40:618, 1966.
11. Weingeist TA and Blodi FC: Fabry's disease. Ocular findings in a female carrier: a light and electron microscopic study, Arch Ophthalmol 85:169, 1971.
12. Riegel EM et al: Ocular pathology of Fabry's disease in a hemizygous male following renal transplantation, Surv Ophthalmol 26:247, 1982.
13. Petrohelos M et al: Ocular manifestations of Gaucher's disease, Am J Ophthalmol 80:1006, 1975.
14. Sasaki T and Tsukahara S: New ocular findings in Gaucher's disease: a report of two brothers, Ophthalmologica 191:206, 1985.
15. Kolodny EH: Metachromatic leukodystrophy and multiple sulfatase deficiency: sulfatide lipidosis. In Scriver CR et al, (editors): The metabolic basis of inherited disease, ed 6, New York, 1989, McGraw-Hill.
16. Quigley HA and Green RW: Clinical and ultrastructural ocular histopathologic studies of adult onset metachromatic leukodystrophy, Am J Ophthalmol 82:471, 1976.
17. Francois J: Metabolic disorders and corneal changes, Dev Ophthalmol 4:1, 1981.
18. Libert J et al: Ocular findings in metachromatic leukodystrophy, Arch Ophthalmol 97:1495, 1979.
19. O'Brien J: Generalized gangliosidosis: J Pediatr 75:167, 1969.
20. Emery JM et al: GM1 gangliosidosis: ocular and pathological manifestations, Arch Ophthalmol 85:177, 1971.
21. Weiss MJ et al: GM1 gangliosidosis type I, Am J Ophthalmol 76:999, 1973.
22. Sorcinelli R, Sitzia A, and Loi M: Cherry-red spot, optic atrophy and corneal cloudings in a patient suffering from GM1 gangliosidosis type I, Metab Pediatr Syst Ophthalmol 10:62, 1987.
23. Beaudet AL: Lysosomal storage diseases. In Braunwald E, et al, editors: Harrison's principles of internal medicine, ed 11, New York, 1987, McGraw-Hill.
24. Robb RM and Kuwabara T: The ocular pathology of type A Niemann-Pick disease: a light and electron microscopic study, Invest Ophthalmol 12:366, 1973.
25. Howes EL et al: Ocular pathology of infantile Niemann-Pick disease: study of fetus of 23 weeks' gestation, Arch Ophthalmol 93:494, 1975.
26. Libert J, Toussaint D, and Guiselings R: Ocular findings in Niemann-Pick Disease, Am J Ophthalmol 80:991, 1975.
27. Walton DS, Robb RM, and Crocker AC: Ocular manifestations of group A Niemann-Pick disease, Am J Ophthalmol 84:174, 1978.
28. Tremblay M and Szots F: GM$_2$ Type 2-gangliosidosis (Sandhoff's disease)—ocular and pathological manifestations, Can J Ophthalmol 9:338, 1974.
29. Brownstein S et al: Sandhoff's disease (G$_{M2}$ gangliosidosis type 2): histopathology and ultrastructure of the eye, Arch Ophthalmol 98:1089, 1980.
30. Freidrickson DS, Levy RI, and Lees RS: Fat transport in lipoproteins: an integrated approach to mechanisms and disorders, N Engl J Med 276:34, 1967.
31. Vinger PF and Sacks BA: Ocular manifestations of hyperlipoproteinemia, Am J Ophthalmol 70:563, 1970.
32. Brown MS and Goldstein JL: The hyperlipoproteinemias and other disorders of lipid metabolism. In Braunwald, et al, editors: Harrison's principles of internal medicine, ed 11, New York, 1987, McGraw-Hill.
33. Spaeth GL: Ocular manifestations of lipoprotein disease, JCE Ophthalmol 41:11, 1979.
34. Jaeger W and Eisenhauer GG: Der diagnostische wert des arcus cornae als hinsweis auf lipoidstoff-wechselstorungen, Klin Monatsbl Augenheilkd 171:321, 1977.
35. Breslow JL: Familial disorders of high density lipoprotein metabolism. In Scriver CR et al, editors: The metabolic basis of inherited disease, ed 6, New York, 1989, McGraw-Hill.
36. Gjone E and Bergaust B: Corneal opacity in familial plasma cholesterol ester deficiency, Acta Ophthalmol (Copenh) 47:222, 1969.
37. Horven I, Effe K, and Gjone E: Corneal and fundus changes in familial LCAT deficiency, Acta Ophthalmol (Copenh) 52:201, 1974.
38. Bron AJ: Corneal changes in the dyslipoproteinemias, Cornea 8:135, 1989.
39. Bron AJ et al: Primary LCAT deficiency disease, Lancet 1:929, 1975.
40. Bethell W, McCullocoh C, and Ghosh M: Lethicin cholesterol acyltransferase deficiency: light and electron microscopic finding from 2 corneas, Can J Ophthalmol 10:494, 1975.

41. Vrabec MP et al: Ophthalmic observations in lecithin cholesterol acyltransferase deficiency, Arch Ophthalmol 106:225, 1988.

42. Hoffman H II, and Freidrickson DS: Tangier disease (familial high density lipoprotein deficiency): clinical and genetic features in two adults, Am J Med 39:582, 1965.

43. Chu FC et al: Ocular manifestations of familial high-density lipoprotein deficiency (Tangier disease), Arch Ophthalmol 97:1926, 1979.

44. Philipson BT: Fish eye disease, Birth Defects 18:441, 1982.

45. Baum JL, Tannenbaum M, and Kolodny EH: Refsum's syndrome with corneal involvement, Am J Ophthalmol 60:699, 1965.

46. Björkhem I and Skrede S: Familial diseases with storage of sterols other than cholesterol: cerebrotendinous xanthomatosis and phytosterolemia. In Scriver CR et al, editors: The metabolic basis of inherited disease, ed 6, New York, 1989, McGraw-Hill.

47. Ozaki H et al: Farber's disease (disseminated lipogranulomatosis): the first case reported in Japan, Acta Med Okayama 32:69, 1978.

48. Zetterstrom R: Disseminated lipogranulomatosis (Farber's disease), Acta Paediatr 47:501, 1958.

49. Zarbin MA et al: Farber's disease. Light and electron microscopic study of the eye, Arch Ophthalmol 103:73, 1985.

DISORDERS OF
CARBOHYDRATE METABOLISM

SYSTEMIC MUCOPOLYSACCHARIDOSES

The extracellular matrix plays a vital role in the maintenance and regulation of cellular function, as well as in intercellular support. It is composed primarily of macromolecules of carbohydrate and protein. Mucopolysaccharides, also called glycosaminoglycans (GAGs), are components of the extracellular matrix in many tissues, including the cornea. They are complexes of carbohydrate and protein in which the polysaccharide component is more prominent than the protein. (The terms "mucoprotein" or "glycoprotein" are used when the protein component predominates.)

The major acid mucopolysaccharides found in the corneal stroma are keratan sulfate 1, chondroitin, and chondroitin sulfate and dermatan sulfate. Keratan sulfate 1 is found exclusively in the cornea. Heparan sulfate, another major mucopolysaccharide, is not present in the cornea, but is found in the retina, the central nervous system, and the aorta.

The mucopolysaccharidoses are recessively inherited deficiencies of enzymes that degrade mucopolysaccharides.[1-5] Degradation of the polysaccharide chain is catalyzed by glycosidases, hydrolytic enzymes present in lysosomes.[6] The absence or abnormal structure of a lysosomal hydrolase leads to accumulation of its substrates intracellularly. The specific enzyme defect determines which mucopolysaccharides accumulate and which tissues are affected. Deficiencies in enzymes that normally degrade dermatan sulfate or keratan sulfate lead to accumulation of these substances in the cornea, resulting in corneal clouding. Accumulation of heparan sulfate can cause retinopathy and optic atrophy.

TABLE 22-1. Ocular and Systemic Features of Mucopolysaccharidoses

DISEASE	CORNEA OPACIFICATION	RETINAL PIGMENTARY DEGENERATION	OPTIC ATROPHY	MENTAL RETARDATION	CARDIOVASCULAR	SKELETAL DYSPLASIA
MPS IH Hurler's syndrome	+	+	+	+	+	+
MPS IS Scheie's syndrome	+	+	+	−	+	+
MPS IH/S Hurler-Scheie compound	+	+	+	±	+	+
MPS IIA Hunter's syndrome, severe	−*	+	+	+	+	+
MPS IIB Hunter's syndrome, mild†	+	+	+	±	+	+
MPS III Sanfilippo's syndrome A-D	−	+	+	+	−	+
MPS IV Morquio's syndrome	+‡	−	+	−	+	+
MPS VI Maroteaux-Lamy syndrome, severe§	+	−	+	−	+	+
MPS VI Maroteaux-Lamy syndrome, mild	+	−	−	−	−	−
MPS VII Sly's syndrome	+§	?	?	+	?	+

*Ciliary body involved. Subclinical corneal clouding is demonstrable histochemically.
†Sclera involved.
‡Corneal clouding may not be grossly evident until after age 10, extent variable.
§Corneal clouding present in infantile type and in some cases of adult form.

TABLE 22-2. Heredity and Enzymatic Defects in Systemic Mucopolysaccharidoses

	SYNDROME	ENZYMATIC DEFECT	EXCESSIVE URINARY MPS	INHERITANCE
MPS IH	Hurler	Alpha-L-Iduronidase	Dermatan sulfate* Heparan sulfate	Recessive
MPS IS	Scheie	Alpha-L-Iduronidase	Dermatan sulfate Heparan sulfate	Recessive
MPS II	Hunter A-B	Sulfoiduronate sulfatase	Dermatan sulfate Heparan sulfate	X-linked recessive
MPS IIIA	Sanfilippo A	Heparan sulfate sulfatase	Heparan sulfate	Recessive
MPS IIIB	Sanfilippo B	N-Acetyl-alpha-D-glucosaminidase	Heparan sulfate	Recessive
MPS IIIC	Sanfilippo C	Acetyl-CoA: glucosaminide N-acetyltransferase	Heparan sulfate	Recessive
MPS IIID	Sanfilippo D	N-acetylglucosamine 6-sulfate sulfatase	Heparan sulfate	Recessive
MPS IV	Morquio	N-acetylgalactosamine 6-sulfate sulfatase	Keratan sulfate	Recessive
MPS VI	Maroteaux-Lamy	Arylsulfatase B	Dermatan sulfate	Recessive
MPS VII	Sly	Beta-Glucuronidase	Dermatan sulfate (?)Heparan sulfate	Recessive

*Dermatan sulfate was previously called chondroitin sulfate B.

In both cases the stored mucopolysaccharides apparently also spill out of the cells into the blood, from which they can be deposited in reticuloendothelial cells, blood vessels, and heart valves, or excreted in the urine.

The clinical characteristics of the mucopolysaccharidoses are summarized in Table 22-1 and the heredity and enzymatic defects in Table 22-2.

HURLER'S SYNDROME

Hurler's syndrome (MPS IH) is characterized by gargoylelike facies, marked skeletal abnormalities (dysostosis multiplex), and progressive mental retardation. Skeletal abnormalities include dorsal and lumbar kyphosis with gibbus, short stature (Fig. 22-1), flaring of the lower ribs, and broad hands with stubby fingers (Fig. 22-2). Hepatosplenomegaly and cardiac problems are common. Those affected can appear normal at birth, but the disease becomes evident during the first 1 to 2 years of life. Death usually occurs during the teenage years as a result of cardiorespiratory complications. There is a deficiency of alpha-L-iduronidase, resulting in accumulation of heparan sulfate and dermatan sulfate.

The cornea can be clear at birth, but soon after becomes characterized by an avascular noninflammatory clouding (Fig. 22-3). Fine, gray, punctate opacities are first seen in the anterior stroma, then in the posterior stroma and endothelium, resulting in a diffuse, ground-glass haze. Corneal thickness may be increased. Pigmentary retinopathy and optic atrophy also commonly occur.[7] Glaucoma due to trabecular involvement has been reported.[8] Short-term success of corneal transplantation in Hurler's syndrome also has been reported.[9]

SCHEIE'S SYNDROME

Scheie's syndrome (MPS IS) is caused by a different defect in the same enzyme affected in Hurler's syndrome, alpha-L-iduronidase. Hurler's and Scheie's syndromes are caused by allelic mutations of the same gene; the disease is demonstrated when patients are homozygous for the abnormal allele. Systemically, Scheie's syndrome is less severe; growth and intelligence are usually near normal.

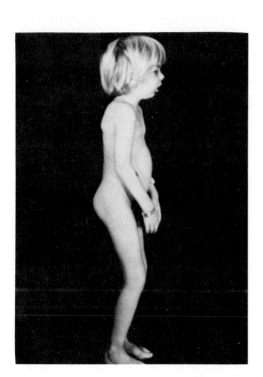

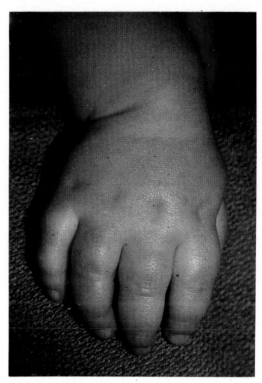

Fig. 22-1   **Fig. 22-2**

Fig. 22-1. Physical stature in Hurler's disease. (From Grayson M and Keates RH: Manual of diseases of the cornea, Boston, 1969, Little, Brown & Co.)

Fig. 22-2. Deformity of hands in Hurler's disease. (From Grayson M and Keates RH: Manual of diseases of the cornea, Boston, 1969, Little, Brown & Co.)

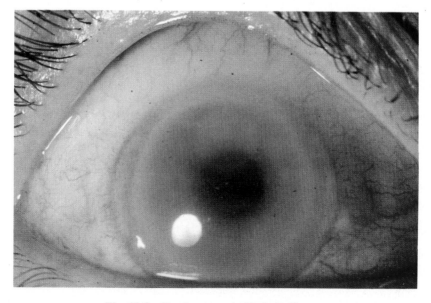

Fig. 22-3. Cloudy cornea in Hurler's disease.

Claw hand, coarse facial features, joint stiffness, hepatomegaly, and aortic regurgitation can be present.

Severe progressive corneal clouding occurs, which is more marked in the periphery.[10] It may be present at birth or develop early in life. Pigmentary retinopathy, optic atrophy, and glaucoma also occur. Acute narrow-angle glaucoma has been seen as a result of limbal corneal thickening from mucopolysaccharide deposition.[11]

Penetrating keratoplasty can remove the corneal opacity, but vision may be limited by retinal or optic nerve disease.[10,12-14]

HURLER-SCHEIE COMPOUND

Rarely, a patient has one Hurler allele and one Scheie allele. This Hurler-Scheie compound (MPS IH/S) results in a phenotype halfway between the two diseases. Corneal clouding, abnormal facies, skeletal deformities, moderate mental retardation, and aortic valve disease occur.[15,16]

HUNTER'S SYNDROME

Hunter's syndrome (MPS II) is the only one of the mucopolysaccharidoses transmitted as an X-linked recessive trait. It is caused by a deficiency of iduronate sulfate sulfatase, resulting in accumulation of heparan sulfate and dermatan sulfate.[17] Severe and mild forms occur, and both are similar to Hurler's syndrome, with skeletal dysplasia (dysostosis multiplex), mental retardation, deafness, and cardiovascular changes. The severe form is still milder than Hurler's syndrome, but death usually occurs before age 15. Patients with the mild form have fair intelligence and live 30 to 50 years. Gross corneal clouding is not seen; however, in patients with the mild form, a corneal opacity can occur later in life. Retinal pigmentary changes and optic atrophy occur, and involvement of the sclera and cilia may be present.[18,19]

It has been stated that the lack of early corneal clouding can be used to discriminate clinically between Hunter's and Hurler's syndromes,[20] but this may not always be true; cases of Hurler's syndrome with clear corneas up to 14 years of age have been reported.[21]

SANFILIPPO'S SYNDROME

Sanfilippo's syndrome (MPS III) can be caused by any of four different enzymatic defects, with the same phenotype (but not all involving the same gene).[5] All of the enzymes are involved in the degradation of heparan sulfate (Table 22-2). These patients have progressive severe mental retardation, but less severe hepatosplenomegaly and skeletal and facial abnormalities (Fig. 22-4). They usually live only into the teens. The corneas are grossly clear, but some opacity may be evident on slit-lamp microscope examination.[22,23] Pigmentary retinal degeneration and optic atrophy occur.

MORQUIO'S SYNDROME

Morquio's syndrome (MPS IV) occurs in severe and mild types (types A and B, respectively), with different enzymatic defects (Table 22-2). Both defects result in accumulation of keratan sulfate. Characteristic facies, marked dwarfism, and skeletal dysplasia occur, but not mental retardation. Spinal cord or medullary compression can develop from vertebral dysplasia, as well as deafness, hepatosplenomegaly, and cardiac disease. Corneal clouding commonly develops, but is variable. It may not be grossly evident until after 10 years of age; it can exhibit only a mild diffuse stomal haze; or it can be severe at any age.[24] Optic atrophy is common, but not retinopathy.

MAROTEAUX-LAMY SYNDROME

Maroteaux-Lamy syndrome (MPS VI) exhibits many of the skeletal anomalies seen in Hurler's syndrome, but intelligence is normal and aortic disease is absent. Arylsulfatase B deficiency leads to

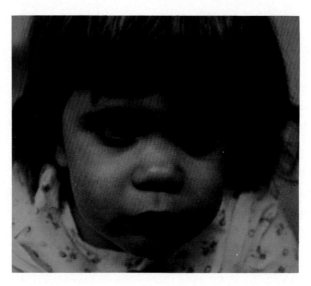

Fig. 22-4. Characteristic facial appearance in case of Sanfilippo's syndrome. (From Grayson M and Keates RH: Manual of diseases of the cornea, Boston, 1969, Little, Brown & Co.)

accumulation of dermatan sulfate. Corneal opacities are present in all cases, although a slit-lamp microscope is sometimes needed to see them.[25] Optic atrophy and hydrocephalus may be seen, but there is no retinal degeneration. Successful corneal transplantation has been reported in one case,[26] but in another case recurrence of deposition clouded the graft in less than 1 year.[27]

SLY'S SYNDROME

Individuals with Sly's syndrome, also known as beta-glucuronidase deficiency and MPS VII, exhibit mental retardation, skeletal dysplasia, and hepatosplenomegaly. Corneal clouding is present in the infantile type, which appears between 7 months and 8 years of age.[28-30] Corneal clouding also can be present in the milder adult form.

HISTOPATHOLOGY

The corneal findings in all of the mucopolysaccharidoses are similar.[31-34] Vacuolization of the cytoplasm affects conjunctival and corneal epithelium, endothelium, and keratocytes (Fig. 22-5). Ultrastructurally the vacuoles are either single membrane-bound structures containing fibrillogranular material or membranous lamellar inclusions (Fig. 22-6). Extracellular mucopolysaccharide deposition also can be found in the stroma or subepithelially.[18] The changes are noted in all cases with clinically cloudy corneas. Less marked changes are also found in patients with MPS II and MPS III and clear corneas.[35,36]

TREATMENT

As mentioned earlier, corneal transplantation has resulted in at least short-term clear corneas, but vision still may be limited by optic nerve or retinal disease. Bone marrow transplantation can correct the enzymatic deficiency by providing cells with normal enzyme activity.[37] Early results suggest that corneal clouding and retinal function can stabilize or even improve[38]; however, there is no improvement in central nervous system function.

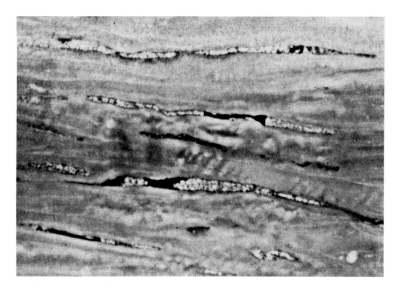

Fig. 22-5. Vacuolization of keratocyte cytoplasm in case of Maroteaux-Lamy syndrome. (From Kenyon KR et al: Am J Ophthalmol 73:718, 1972.)

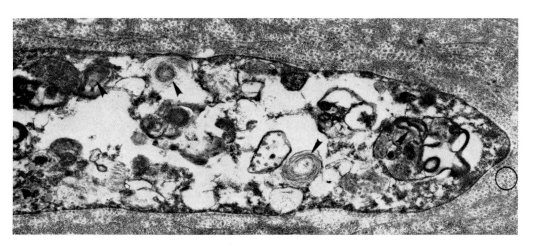

Fig. 22-6. Higher magnification of keratocyte, showing membranous lamellar inclusions and fibrillogranular material. (From Kenyon KR et al: Am J Ophthalmol 73:718, 1972.)

LOCAL CORNEAL MUCOPOLYSACCHARIDOSES
MACULAR CORNEAL DYSTROPHY

Macular dystrophy is a hereditary disorder of keratan sulfate synthesis (see Chapter 17). Mucopolysaccharide accumulates in stromal keratocytes and endothelial cells and is deposited between the stromal lamellae, resulting in corneal clouding. The accumulated mucopolysaccharide appears to be related to keratan sulfate, and in some patients keratan sulfate is absent from the serum and cartilage; however, no systemic manifestations have been observed.

MUCOPOLYSACCHARIDOSES OF BOWMAN'S LAYER

Several cases of isolated conjunctival and corneal clouding caused by acid mucopolysaccharide deposition have been described in infants and in a 20-year-old patient.[39] The corneal deposits were limited to Bowman's layer. Systemic mucopolysaccharidosis was not evident, but in one case cardiovascular anomalies and telangiectasias involving multiple organ systems were present. In addition, peripheral edema, cyanosis, and inguinal hernia have been seen.

DIABETES MELLITUS

Patients with diabetes mellitus can have decreased corneal sensation and decreased epithelial adhesion. The sensation is usually only mildly reduced,[40-42] but neurotrophic ulcers have been reported.[43,44] Decreased adhesion of the corneal epithelium and delayed epithelial wound healing are often noted in diabetics.[45,46] Thickening of the epithelial basement membrane and reduced penetration of anchoring fibrils into Bowman's layer may be responsible.[47] More rapid epithelial clouding during intraocular surgery, decreased epithelial barrier function,[48] decreased tear production,[41] and intraepithelial fructose and sorbitol (normally not present)[49] have been noted in diabetic patients. Endothelial abnormalities, such as a decreased percentage of hexagonal endothelial cells and a higher coefficient of variation of cell size, have also been reported.[50,51]

GLYCOGEN STORAGE DISEASE
TYPE 1A (VON GIERKE'S DISEASE)

Von Gierke's disease, also known as glucose-6-phosphatase deficiency, is an autosomal recessive disorder marked by hypoglycemia, hepatomegaly, bleeding diathesis, hyperlipidemia, and short stature. A faint brown peripheral corneal clouding may be noted. Lipemia retinalis and eruptive xanthomas can occur with hyperlipidemia, and multiple yellowish, discrete paramacular lesions can be seen.

TYPE II (POMPE'S DISEASE)

Pompe's disease is relatively common, has no ocular manifestations, but distinctive pathologic findings were present in a conjunctival specimen.[52] Glycogen-engorged fibroblasts were seen in the substantia propria. In addition, membrane-bound inclusions containing glycogen particles were found in the corneal epithelium and endothelium.

REFERENCES

1. Neufeld EF and Muenzer J: The mucopolysaccharidoses. In Scriver CR et al, editors: The Metabolic basis of inherited disease, ed 6, New York, 1989, McGraw-Hill.
2. Brown SI and Kuwabara T: Peripheral corneal opacification and skeletal deformities: a newly recognized acid mucopolysaccharidosis simulating rheumatoid arthritis, Arch Ophthalmol 83:667, 1970.
3. Jeanloz RW: The nomenclature of acid mucopolysaccharides, Arthritis Rheum 3:233, 1960.
4. Kenyon KR: Ocular manifestations and pathology of systemic mucopolysaccharidoses, Birth Defects 12:133, 1976.
5. Spranger J: The mucopolysaccharidoses. In Emery AEH and Rimoin DL, editors: Principles and practice of medical genetics, New York, 1983, Churchill Livingstone,
6. Van Hoof F and Hers HG: The abnormalities of lysosomal enzymes in mucopolysaccharidoses, Eur J Biochem 7:34, 1968.
7. Gills PF, Hobson R, Hanley B, and McKusick V: Electroretinography and fundus oculi findings in Hurler's disease and allied mucopolysaccharidoses, Arch Ophthalmol 74:596, 1965.
8. Spellacy E et al: Glaucoma in a case of Hurler disease, Br J Ophthalmol 64:773, 1980.
9. Rosen DA et al: Keratoplasty and electron microscopy of the cornea in systemic mucopolysaccharidosis (Hurler's disease), Can J Ophthalmol 3:218, 1968.
10. Scheie HG, Hambrick GW, and Barnes LA: A newly recognized form of Hurler's disease (gargoylism), Am J Ophthalmol 53:753, 1962.
11. Quigley HA, Maumenee AE, and Stark WJ: Systemic mucopolysaccharidosis, Am J Ophthalmol 80:1, 1975.
12. Canstantopoulas B, Dekaban AS, and Scheie HG: Heterogeneity of disorders in patients with corneal clouding, normal intellect, and mucopolysaccharidosis, Am J Ophthalmol 72:1106, 1971.
13. Quigley HA and Goldberg MF: Scheie syndrome and macular corneal dystrophy: an ultrastructural comparison of conjunctiva and skin, Arch Ophthalmol 85:553, 1971.
14. Sugar J: Corneal manifestations of the systemic mucopolysaccharidoses, Ann Ophthalmol 11:531, 1979.

15. Chijiiwa T et al: Ocular manifestations of Hurler/Scheie phenotype in two sibs, Jpn J Ophthalmol 27:54, 1983.

16. Kajii T et al: Hurler/Scheie genetic compounds (mucopolysaccharidosis IH/IS) in Japanese brothers, Clin Genet 6:394, 1974.

17. Bach G et al: The defect in Hunter syndrome: deficiency of sulfoiduronate sulfatase, Proc Natl Acad Sci USA 70:2134, 1973.

18. Goldberg MF and Duke JR: Ocular histopathology in Hunter's syndrome: systemic mucopolysaccharidosis, type II, Arch Ophthalmol 77:503, 1967.

19. Winchester P et al: A new acid mucopolysaccharidosis with skeletal deformities simulating rheumatoid arthritis, Am J Roentgenol Radium Ther Nucl Med 106:121, 1961.

20. DiFerrante H et al: Mucopolysaccharide storage diseases: corrective activity of normal human serum and lymphocyte extracts, Birth Defects 9:31, 1973.

21. Gardner RJM and Hay JR: Hurler's syndrome with clear corneas, Lancet 2:845, 1974.

22. Sanfilippo SJ et al: Mental retardation associated with acid mucopolysacchariduria (heparitin sulfate type), J Pediatr 63:837, 1963.

23. Bartsocas C et al: San Filippo type C disease: clinical findings in four patients with a new variant of mucopolysaccharidosis III, Eur J Pediatr 130:251, 1979.

24. Van Noorden GK, Zellweger H, and Ponseti I: Ocular findings in Morquio-Ullrich's disease, Arch Ophthalmol 64:585, 1960.

25. Goldberg MF, Scott CI, and McKusick VA: Hydrocephalus and papilledema in Maroteaux-Lamy syndrome (mucopolysaccharidosis type VI), Am J Ophthalmol 69:969, 1970.

26. Suveges I: Histological and ultrastructural studies of the cornea in Maroteaux-Lamy syndrome, Graefes Arch Clin Exp Ophthalmol 212:29, 1979.

27. Schwartz MF, Werblin TP, and Green WR: Occurrence of mucopolysaccharide in corneal grafts in the Maroteaux-Lamy syndrome, Cornea 4:58, 1985.

28. Hoyme HE et al: Presentation of mucopolysaccharidosis VII (β-glucuronidase deficiency) in infancy, J Med Genet 18:237, 1981.

29. Beaudet AL et al: Variation in the phenotypic expression of beta glucuronidase deficiency, J Pediatr 86:388, 1975.

30. Sly WS: The mucopolysaccharidoses. In Bondy PK and Rosenberg LE, editors: Metabolic control and disease, ed 8, Philadelphia, 1980, WB Saunders.

31. Kenyon KR et al: The systemic mucopolysaccharidoses: ultrastructural and histological studies of conjunctiva and skin, Am J Ophthalmol 73:811, 1972.

32. Francois J: Metabolic disorders and corneal changes, Dev Ophthalmol 4:1, 1981.

33. Kenyon KR et al: Ocular pathology of the Maroteaux-Lamy syndrome (systemic mucopolysaccharidosis type VI): histologic and ultrastructural report of two cases, Am J Ophthalmol 73:718-741, 1972.

34. McDonnell JM, Green WR, and Maumenee IH: Ocular histopathology of systemic mucopolysaccharidosis, type II-A (Hunter syndrome, severe), Ophthalmology 92:1772, 1985.

35. DelMonte MA et al: Histopathology of Sanfilippo's syndrome, Arch Ophthalmol 101:1255, 1983.

36. Lavery MA et al: Ocular histopathology and ultrastructure of Sanfilippo's syndrome, type III-B, Arch Ophthalmol 101:1263, 1983.

37. Krivit W et al: Bone-marrow transplantation in the Maroteaux-Lamy syndrome (mucopolysaccharidosis type VI), N Engl J Med 311:1606, 1984.

38. Summers CG et al: Ocular changes in the mucopolysaccharidoses after bone marrow transplantation: a preliminary report, Ophthalmology 96:977, 1989.

39. Rodrigues MM, Calhoun J, and Harley RD: Corneal clouding with increased acid mucopolysaccharide accumulation in Bowman's membrane, Am J Ophthalmol 79:916, 1975.

40. Schwartz DE: Corneal sensitivity in diabetics, Arch Ophthalmol 91:174, 1974.

41. Schultz RO et al: Diabetic keratopathy, Trans Am Ophthalmol Soc 79:180, 1981.

42. Schultz RO et al: Diabetic keratopathy as a manifestation of peripheral neuropathy, Am J Ophthalmol 96:368, 1983.

43. Hyndiuk R et al: Neurotrophic corneal ulcers in diabetes mellitus, Arch Ophthalmol 95:2193, 1977.

44. Olsen T, Busted N, and Schmitz O: Corneal thickness in diabetes mellitus, Lancet 1:883, 1980.

45. Perry HD et al: Corneal complications after closed vitrectomy through the pars plana, Arch Ophthalmol 96:401, 1978.

46. Foulks GN et al: Factors related to corneal epithelial complications after closed vitrectomy in diabetics, Arch Ophthalmol 97:1076, 1979.

47. Kenyon KR: Recurrent corneal erosion: pathogenesis and therapy, Int Ophthalmol Clin 19:169, 1979.

48. Göbbels M, Spitznas M, and Oldendoerp J: Impairment of corneal epithelial barrier function in diabetics, Graefe's Arch Clin Exp Ophthalmol 227:142, 1989.

49. Schultz RO et al: Diabetic keratopathy, Trans Am Ophthalmol Soc 79:180, 1981.

50. Schultz RO et al: Corneal endothelial changes in type I and type II diabetes mellitus, Am J Ophthalmol 98:401, 1984.

51. Itoi M et al: Specular microscopic studies of the corneal endothelium of Japanese diabetics, Cornea 8:2, 1989.

52. Libert J et al: Ocular ultrastructural study in a fetus with type II glycogenosis, Br J Ophthalmol 61:476, 1977.

DISORDERS OF COMBINED CARBOHYDRATE AND LIPID METABOLISM

Mucolipidoses
- Mucolipidosis I
- Mucolipidosis II (I-cell disease)
- Mucolipidosis III (pseudo-Hurler polydystrophy)
- Mucolipidosis IV (Berman syndrome)

Glycoprotein storage disorders
- Sialidosis
- Mannosidosis
- Fucosidosis

MUCOLIPIDOSES

Mucolipidoses are lysosomal storage diseases involving some combination of mucopolysaccharide, glycoprotein, glycolipid, and oligosaccharide metabolism (Table 23-1). Some forms exhibit features of both mucopolysaccharidoses (MPS) and sphingolipidoses. Corneal clouding is seen in several of the disorders.

MUCOLIPIDOSIS I

Most of the patients previously categorized as having mucolipidosis I actually have a specific glycogen storage disease, so it has been recommended that this term be abandoned.[1] Some of these patients have sialidosis or mannosidosis.

MUCOLIPIDOSIS II (I-CELL DISEASE)

Mucolipidosis II is characterized by gargoylelike facies, severe growth and psychomotor retardation, thickened skin, and MPS-like skeletal dysplasia (dysostosis multiplex).[2,3] Mild hepatomegaly, progressive corneal clouding, glaucoma, and megalocornea can occur as well. Cherry-red spots are not seen.[4,5]

Striking granular inclusions are seen in fibroblasts and keratocytes (I-cells), and this can be dem-

TABLE 23-1. Disorders of Combined Carbohydrate and Lipid Metabolism

	ENZYME DEFECT	STORED	HEREDITY	CORNEAL CLOUDING	RETINOPATHY	RETARDATION	SKELETAL DYSPLASIA
MUCOLIPIDOSES							
MLS II (I cell disease)	UDP-N-acetylglucosamine (GlcNAc1): glycoprotein GlcNAc 1-phototransferase	Mucopolysaccharides, lipids	AR*	Common	+†	+	+
MLS III (pseudoHurler polydystrophy)	UDP-N-acetylglucosamine (GlcNAcl): glycoprotein GlcNAc 1-phototransferase	Mucopolysaccharides, lipids	AR	+ (mild)	+	+ (mild)	+
MLS IV (Berman's syndrome)	Unknown	Gangliosides phospholipids, acid MPS	AR	+	-	+	-
GLYCOPROTEIN STORAGE DISORDERS							
Goldberg-Cotlier syndrome (sialidosis)	Glycoprotein neuraminidase ± beta-galactosidase	Sialoglycopeptides +/or N-glycosidically linked oligosaccharides	AR	+	Cherry-red spot	-	±
Mannosidosis	Alpha-D-mannosidase	N-glycosidically linked oligosaccharides	AR	+ Superficial	-	+	+
Fucosidosis	Alpha-L-fucosidase	Oligosaccharides and glycoasparagines	AR	+ Superficial	+	+	+

*Autosomal recessive.
†One case described.

onstrated in conjunctival biopsy specimens.[5,6] The disease is caused by a defect in the posttranslational processing of lysosomal enzymes. Both types II and III are deficiencies of the same enzyme, UDP-N-acetylglucosamine (GLcNAc):glycoprotein GLcNAc 1-phosphotransferase, which is involved in posttranslational synthesis of the oligosaccharide portion of many lysosomal enzymes. This enzyme synthesizes a recognition marker, which normally binds to a receptor in the lysosome. In the absence of this marker the lysosomal enzymes are not bound by the lysosomes, resulting in their secretion into the extracellular space.[7]

MUCOLIPIDOSIS III (PSEUDOHURLER POLYDYSTROPHY)

Mucolipidosis III is a milder disorder than type II, but patients also exhibit many of the manifestations of the mucopolysaccharidoses, particularly dysostosis multiplex. During the first decade, restricted joint mobility, small stature, claw hand deformity, hip dysplasia, and scoliosis develop. Mild mental retardation and cardiac valve disease are also present. Corneal clouding is consistently present by age 10.[8,9] Fine, discrete opacities are seen initially in the anterior or posterior stroma and progress to involve the entire stroma. The inclusions in fibroblasts, including conjunctival fibroblasts, are similar to those in mucolipidosis type II, but less marked.[10]

MUCOLIPIDOSIS IV (BERMAN'S SYNDROME)

Berman's syndrome is manifested by mental retardation, retinal degeneration, and corneal clouding without other somatic features.[11] It has been reported mainly in Ashkenazi Jews. The exact enzyme deficiency is not known. Bilateral diffuse corneal haze is usually evident at birth or by 6 weeks of age.[12-14] Multiple dotlike opacities are present in all layers of the stroma, homogeneously from the center to the periphery. On histologic examination characteristic inclusions are found in the epithe-

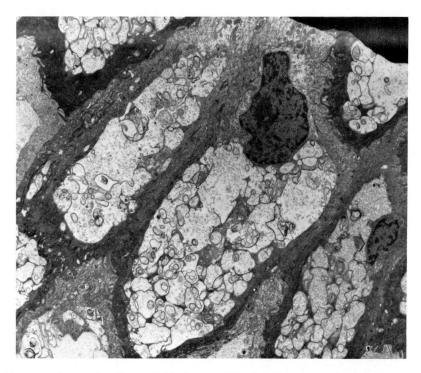

Fig. 23-1. Electron micrograph of mucolipidosis type IV, showing membrane-bound vesicles containing whorled membranous inclusions and granular material. (Courtesy Bruce L. Johnson, Pittsburgh.)

lium of the cornea and conjunctiva and, to a much lesser extent, in keratocytes and conjunctival substantia propria.[15-17] Two types of single membrane-bound vesicles are seen: Some contain whorled membranous inclusions, thought to represent phospholipids, and others contain granular material, consistent with mucopolysaccharides (Fig. 23-1).

Because the corneal clouding is largely caused by epithelial disease, conjunctival transplantation (with donor conjunctiva from an unaffected sibling) was performed in one patient.[18] The central cornea remained clear at 1 year, but extensive peripheral vascularization occurred.

GLYCOPROTEIN STORAGE DISORDERS

These are rare autosomal recessive disorders involving enzymes that hydrolyze polysaccharide linkages. All are characterized by mental retardation, coarse facies, and skeletal dysplasia.

SIALIDOSIS

Sialidosis is caused by deficiency of glycoprotein neuraminidase, sometimes in association with beta-galactosidase deficiency. Patients have a cherry-red spot in the macula, spokelike lens opacities, mental retardation, myoclonus, hepatosplenomegaly, and MPS-like skeletal dysplasia. Progressive stromal and epithelial corneal clouding occurs in some patients.[19] On histopathologic examination single membrane-bound inclusions are found in corneal epithelial cells and keratocytes, as in the mucopolysaccharidoses, and rare lamellar bodies, as seen in the sphingolipidoses, are also present.

Goldberg-Cotlier syndrome is a sialidosis with combined deficiency of neuraminidase and beta-galactosidase. The characteristics are the same as in neuraminidase deficiency alone, and corneal clouding is present.[20,21]

MANNOSIDOSIS

Individuals with mannosidosis demonstrate coarse facies, cardiac dysfunction, hepatosplenomegaly, gingival hyperplasia, and skeletal dysplasia. It is most often lethal in childhood. Due to a deficiency of alpha-mannosidase, glycoprotein-derived, mannose-containing oligosaccharides accumulate in tissues and are excreted in the urine. Spokelike posterior cortical cataracts are commonly seen.[22] They consist of numerous punctate vacuoles arranged in a cartwheel-like or spokelike configuration. Superficial corneal opacities have been reported in a few cases.

FUCOSIDOSIS

Patients with fucosidosis differ from those with mannosidosis by the presence of abnormal sweat electrolytes and cutaneous angiokeratomas. Deficiency of alpha-fucosidase leads to tissue accumulation of oligosaccharides, glycolipids, and glycopeptides. Dilated, tortuous conjunctival vessels and central anterior corneal opacification have been reported.[23,24] Cytoplasmic, membrane-bound inclusions, containing fibrillogranular and multilaminated material, are found in corneal, conjunctival, and vascular endothelium.[25,26]

REFERENCES

1. Beaudet AL: Lysosomal storage diseases. In Braunwald E et al, editors: Harrison's principles of internal medicine, ed 11, New York, 1987, McGraw-Hill.
2. Luchsinger U et al: I-cell disease, N Engl J Med 282:1374, 1970.
3. Lightbody J et al: I-cell disease: multiple lysosomal-enzyme defect, Lancet 1:451, 1971.
4. Borit A, Sugarman GI, and Spencer WH: Ocular involvement in I-cell disease (mucolipidosis II) light and electron-microscopic findings, Graefes Arch Clin Ophthalmol 198:25, 1976.
5. Libert J et al: Ocular findings in I-cell disease (mucolipidosis type II), Am J Ophthalmol 83:617, 1977.
6. Kenyon KR and Sensenbrenner JA: Mucolipidosis II (I-cell disease): Ultrastructural observations of conjunctiva and sclera, Invest Ophthalmol 10:555-567, 1971.
7. Nolan CM and Sly CS: I-cell disease and pseudo-Hurler polydystrophy: disorders of lysosomal enzyme phosphorylation and localization. In Scriver CR et al, editors: The metabolic basis of inherited disease, ed 6, New York, 1989, McGraw-Hill.
8. Kelly TE et al: Mucolipidosis III(pseudo-Hurler poly-

dystrophy): clinical and laboratory studies in a series of 12 patients, Johns Hopkins Med J 137:156, 1975.

9. Traboulsi EI and Maumenee IH: Ophthalmic findings in mucolipidosis III (pseudo-Hurler polydystrophy), Am J Ophthalmol 102:592, 1986.

10. Quigley HA and Goldberg MF: Conjunctival ultrastructure in mucolipidosis 3 (pseudo Hurler polydystrophy), Invest Ophthalmol 10:568, 1971.

11. Newell FW, Matalon R, and Meyer S: A new mucolipidosis with psychomotor retardation, corneal clouding and retinal degeneration, Am J Ophthalmol 80:440, 1975.

12. Berman ER et al: Congenital corneal clouding with abnormal systemic storage bodies: a new variant of mucolipidosis, J Pediatr 84:519, 1974.

13. Merin S et al: Mucolipidosis IV: ocular systemic and ultrastructural findings, Invest Ophthalmol Vis Sci 14:437, 1975.

14. Amir N, Zlotogora J, and Bach G: Mucolipidosis type IV: clinical spectrum and natural history, Pediatrics 79:953, 1987.

15. Kenyon KR et al: Mucolipidosis IV: histopathology of conjunctiva, cornea and skin, Arch Ophthalmol 97:1106, 1979.

16. Zwann J and Kenyon KR: Two brothers with presumed mucolipidosis IV, Birth Defects 18:381, 1982.

17. Riedel KG et al: Ocular abnormalities in mucolipidosis IV, Am J Ophthalmol 99:125, 1985.

18. Dangel ME, Bremer DL, and Rogers GL: Treatment of corneal opacification in mucolipidosis IV with conjunctival transplantation, Am J Ophthalmol 99:137, 1985.

19. Cibis GW et al: Mucolipidosis I, Arch Ophthalmol 101:933, 1983.

20. Emery JM et al: Gm$_1$-gangliosidosis: ocular and pathological manifestations, Arch Ophthalmol 85:177, 1971.

21. Goldberg MF et al: Macular cherry-red spot, corneal clouding, and beta-galactosidase deficiency: clinical, biochemical, and electron microscopic study of a new autosomal recessive storage disease, Arch Intern Med 128:387, 1971.

22. Arbisser AI et al: Ocular findings in mannosidosis, Am J Ophthalmol 82:465, 1976.

23. Borrone C et al: Fucosidosis: clinical, biochemical, immunologic, and genetic studies in two new cases, J Pediatr 84:727, 1974.

24. Snyder RO et al: Ocular findings in fucosidosis, Birth Defects 12:241, 1976.

25. Libert J, Van Hoof F, and Tonduer M: Fucosidosis: ultrastructural study of conjunctiva and skin and enzyme analysis of tears, Invest Ophthalmol 15:626, 1976.

26. Hoshino M et al: Fucosidosis: ultrastructural study of the eye in an adult, Graefes Arch Clin Exp Ophthalmol 227:162, 1989.

DISORDERS OF AMINO ACID METABOLISM

Anterior segment involvement in disorders of amino acid metabolism is summarized in Table 24-1.

ALKAPTONURIA

One of the prominent clinical features of this autosomal recessive metabolic disorder is a characteristic bluish gray or black pigmentation of connective tissue, known as *ochronosis*.[1] It is caused by a deficiency of homogentisic acid oxidase, an enzyme normally present in the liver and kidneys. Homogentisic acid is an intermediate in the metabolism of tyrosine and phenylalanine, and homogentisic acid oxidase normally converts it to maleylacetoacetic acid. The enzyme deficiency leads to excessive amounts of homogentisic acid, most of which is excreted in the urine; however, the acid and its oxidized, pigmented, polymers (alkapton) also can bind collagen, leading to their accumulation in connective tissue. In addition, for unknown reasons, degenerative changes occur, particularly in cartilage and intervertebral discs.

TABLE 24-1. Disorders of Amino Acid Metabolism with Corneal Findings

DISORDER	ENZYME DEFICIENCY	ACCUMULATED MATERIAL	HEREDITY	CORNEAL FINDINGS	OTHER OCULAR FINDINGS
Alkaptonuria	Homogentisic acid oxidase	Homogentisic acid	AR*	Ochre-colored deposits in limbal area	Interpalpebral pigmentation of conjunctiva, episclera, sclera, and rectus tendons
Cystinosis	Impaired transport of cystine across lysosomal membranes	Cystine	AR	Diffuse stromal crystals; recurrent erosions (late)	Peripheral retinopathy; crystals in conjunctiva sclera and uvea
Tyrosinemia II (Richner-Hanhart syndrome)	Hepatic tyrosine aminotransferase	Tyrosine	AR	Epithelial deposits, dendritic or sunburst pattern; vascularization	Conjunctival plaques

*Autosomal recessive.

The earliest signs are usually pigmentation of the sclerae and ears (Fig. 24-1), which become manifest between 20 and 40 years of age. One also can see pigmentation of the nose and internal cartilage and ligaments. Degenerative arthropathy, involving mainly the large joints and the spine, develops in the majority of patients. The urine darkens on standing as a result of the oxidation of homogentisic acid; however, in the presence of reducing agents or if the urine has an acid pH, darkening does not occur.

Ocular manifestations. Ocular pigmentation occurs in the interpalpebral fissure. The conjunctiva, episclera, sclera, and the tendons of the horizontal recti can become pigmented with this material[2-6] (Fig. 24-2). In addition, the cornea immediately inside the limbus may exhibit areas of pigmentation. The pigment is usually brownish black, appears like "oil droplets," and is located in the area of Bowman's layer and deep epithelium. Their appearance is similar to the droplets of spheroidal degeneration. Pigmentation of the tarsal plates and lids also can be seen.

Histopathology. The pigment is seen with light microscopy as amber- (ochre) colored globules or fiberlike structures in the peripheral cornea, conjunctiva, and sclera. Ultrastructurally, the pigment is extracellular, attached to collagen fibers and fibrocytes.[7]

Cystinosis

Cystinosis is an autosomal recessive disorder characterized by intralysosomal accumulation of free cystine in body tissues, particularly in the reticuloendothelial cells of the bone marrow, liver, spleen, and lymphatic system. Deposition also can occur in the kidneys, leading to generalized proximal tubular dysfunction (Fanconi syndrome), and in ocular tissues, including the cornea, conjunctiva, and retina. The defect appears to involve impaired efflux of cystine from lysosomes, rather than a defect in catabolism. Cystine and cysteine levels in plasma and urine are not elevated, but increased concentrations can be detected in leukocytes or cultured fibroblasts or in biopsies of rectal mucosa.[8]

Clinical manifestations. Cystinosis occurs in three forms: infantile, adolescent, and adult. The infantile form usually becomes apparent by 4 to 6 months of age. Growth retardation, vitamin D–resistant rickets, hypopigmentation of the skin and hair, and progressive renal failure occur, with death occurring usually before age 10. The adolescent form exhibits less severe renal impairment, which usually becomes apparent in the second decade.[9,10] In the adult form the patients are in good health;

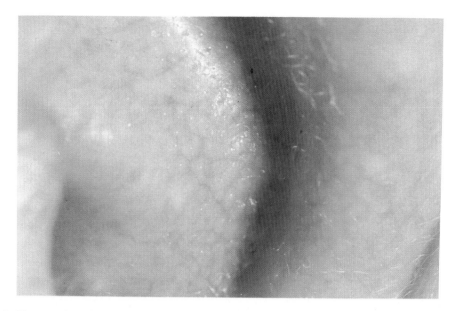

Fig. 24-1. Pigmentation of ear cartilage in alkaptonuria. (From Grayson M: The cornea in systemic disease. In Duane TD, editor: Clinical ophthalmology, vol 4, Hagerstown, MD, 1976, Harper & Row.)

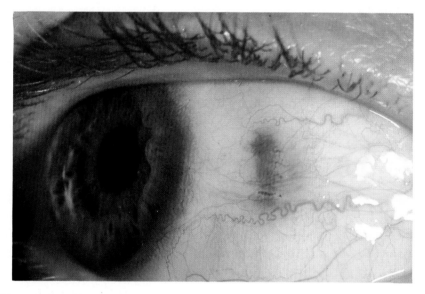

Fig. 24-2. Pigmentation of lateral rectus tendon in alkaptonuria. (From Grayson M: The cornea in systemic disease. In Duane TD, editor: Clinical ophthalmology, vol 4, Hagerstown, MD, 1976, Harper & Row.)

they are usually free of symptoms, except perhaps for photophobia. The only manifestations are corneal; renal function is normal and retinopathy is absent.

Corneal and conjunctival involvement occurs in all three forms of cystinosis, and the appearance is similar. In the cornea, glistening, polychromatic, needlelike to rectangular crystals are seen (Fig. 24-3). They first appear anteriorly and gradually spread posteriorly, always more peripherally than centrally.[11] In the infantile form they first appear from 6 to 15 months of age and involve the entire

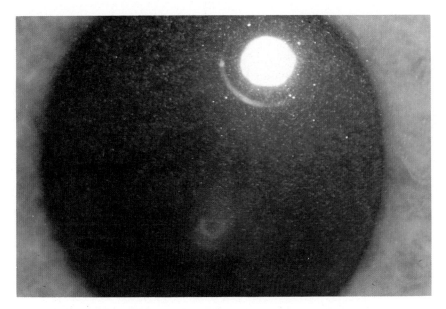

Fig. 24-3. Corneal crystals in cystinosis.

stroma by age 7. In the adult form they may become evident in the teen years or as late as 50 years of age.

The crystals continue to become denser with age.[12,13] They may cause a rather intense photophobia but do not decrease acuity. In advanced cases corneal erosions can occur as often as several times each month, and the cornea can become thickened.[14] Crystal deposition also can be seen on the anterior lens surface and can thicken the iris stroma.[13]

Crystal deposits are also evident in the conjunctiva, particularly in the bulbar and forniceal areas, where they create a ground-glass appearance.[15] Peripheral retinopathy is consistently present only in the infantile form. There is extensive depigmentation in the periphery, with irregular clumps of pigment (Fig. 24-4). The retinal pigmentary changes may precede the corneal and conjunctival changes by many months and rarely may be seen as early as the fifth week of life.[16]

Histopathology. With electron microscopy the corneal crystals are seen to be intracellular, within epithelium and keratocytes, and membrane bound.[8,16-18] Crystal deposition results in thinning and focal breaks in Bowman's membrane, which may be related to the photophobia.[18] Crystals also are present in subepithelial conjunctiva, sclera, iris, ciliary body, choroid, extraocular muscles, and retinal pigment epithelium.[8,16-22] The crystals in the conjunctiva and uvea have been identified as L-cystine by x-ray diffraction.[23]

A conjunctival biopsy specimen can confirm the diagnosis and may be taken fairly easily. It should be fixed in absolute ethanol and examined with polarized light for detection of typical crystals (Fig. 24-5). However, the diagnosis also can be made by leukocyte cystine assay, which is less invasive.

Differential diagnosis. A number of other conditions are associated with crystals in the cornea (see Chapter 3). In most cases corneal appearance, patient age, and systemic findings can differentiate the disorders. However, multiple myeloma and other dysproteinemias can be difficult to distinguish from adult cystinosis. The corneal changes are very similar, and systemic manifestations are often absent. Examination of a conjunctival biopsy specimen or leukocyte cystine assay can indicate the proper diagnosis.

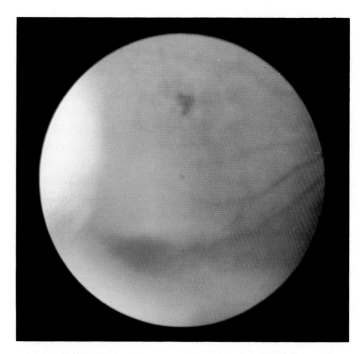

Fig. 24-4. Peripheral retinal depigmentation with irregular clumps of pigment in cystinosis. (From Grayson M: The cornea in systemic disease. In Duane TD, editor: Clinical ophthalmology, vol 4, Hagerstown, MD, 1976, Harper & Row.)

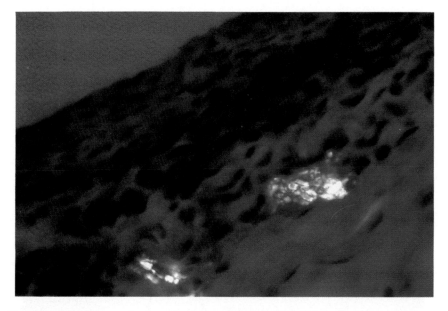

Fig. 24-5. Typical crystals of cystinosis seen with polarized light in biopsy of conjunctiva.

Treatment. Cysteamine (beta-mercaptoethylamine) can be used to reduce corneal crystal content. The cysteamine reacts with intracellular cystine, forming a cysteine-cysteamine disulfide, which resembles lysine and is transported out of the lysosome by the normal lysine transport system. The cysteamine is given as a 10 mM drop, each hour during the day.[24] A corneal transplant was clear after 2 years in one case,[25] but in another crystal deposition recurred in less than 6 weeks.[26]

TYROSINEMIA II (RICHNER-HANHART SYNDROME)

Two major disorders are associated with hypertyrosinemia, tyrosinemia types I and II. Tyrosinemia type I (also known as hereditary tyrosinemia) is a rare autosomal recessive disease characterized by cirrhosis of the liver and renal tubular dysfunction, but there are no ocular manifestations. Patients with tyrosinemia type II (also known as hypertyrosinemia, Richner-Hanhart syndrome) exhibit skin lesions, corneal opacities, and occasionally mental retardation.[27] Autosomal recessively transmitted, it appears to be caused by a deficiency of tyrosine aminotransferase, resulting in high levels of tyrosine in the blood and urine.[28] In most cells, the excess tyrosine is removed by mitochondrial aspartate transaminase (converting it to pHPPA), but this enzyme is not present in cells of ectodermal origin. The palms and soles are affected by hyperhidrosis, blisters, and painful erosions that become crusted and hyperkeratotic (Fig. 24-6).[29] Hyperkeratotic plaques also can be found on the knees and elbows (Fig. 24-7).

Ocular manifestations. Corneal involvement occurs in most cases and usually precedes the skin lesions. In one case, however, ocular involvement developed 17 years after the skin lesions.[30] The patient can develop photophobia, tearing, redness, and pain anywhere from 2 weeks to 8 years of age. Intraepithelial and subepithelial opacification occurs, sometimes with erosions or ulcerations.[28,31-33]

Grayson[34] described a case in which the corneal lesions consisted of dustlike opacities randomly distributed in the lower aspect of the cornea. The lesions did not stain with fluorescein; there was neither vascularization nor decreased sensation. The only complaint was that of photophobia. Similar findings were observed in a premature infant with temporary hypertyrosinemia. Multiple subepithelial

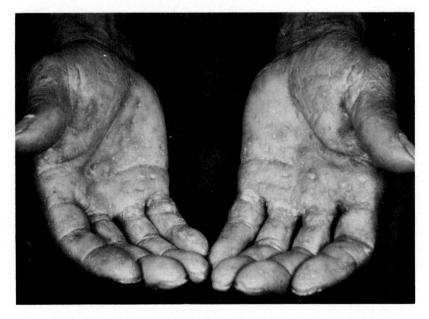

Fig. 24-6. Painful hyperkeratotic lesions on hands in tyrosinemia.

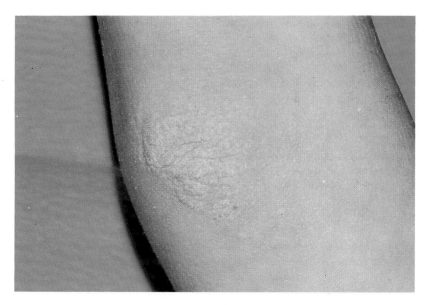

Fig. 24-7. Hyperkeratotic skin lesion in tyrosinemia.

The corneal lesions may have a dendritic or sunburst configuration (Fig. 24-8), with surrounding ground-glass haze.[36] The dendritic lesions often have been confused with herpetic dendrites, but there are distinguishing features: The lesions in tyrosinemia type II are thick and plaquelike; they do not exhibit the fine, delicate club-shaped edges of herpes simplex dendrites; they are bilateral, which is rare in herpes simplex; they do not stain with fluorescein; they are usually not associated with vascularization; and the sensation is intact. Subcapsular lens opacities, conjunctival thickening, and an extensive papillary hypertrophy of the tarsal conjunctiva also have been observed.

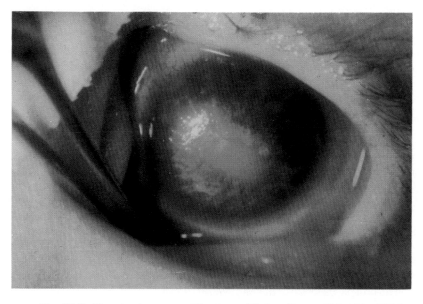

Fig. 24-8. Tyrosine in cornea. (Courtesy of Robert Burns, Columbia, MO.)

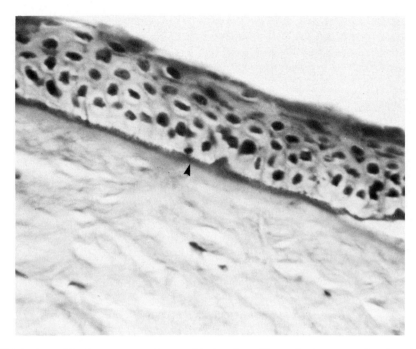

Fig. 24-9. Thickening of the basement membrane with tiny fingerlike projections extending into the basal layer of the epithelium.

Histopathology. In one case the cornea was examined with light microscopy and demonstrated hyperplastic stratified epithelium with intracellular edema.[37] In Grayson's case histologic examination revealed thickening of the basement membrane with tiny fingerlike projections extending into the basal layer of the epithelium[34] (Fig. 24-9). Examination of a conjunctival plaque revealed membrane-bound inclusions in superficial epithelial cells and blood vessel endothelium.[28]

Rats fed a diet high in tyrosine develop snowflakelike corneal opacities and paw erythema.[38] Intracytoplasmic crystals are found in the corneal epithelium.[39]

Treatment. Institution of a diet low in tyrosine and phenylalanine can lead to resolution of the eye and skin lesions. In two cases the cornea lesion recurred after a penetrating graft.[40,41] In one of these cases the recurrence appeared to be related to systemic corticosteroid treatment.[41]

PHENYLKETONURIA

Phenylketonuria (PKU) is a group of disorders characterized by reduced activity of phenylalanine hydroxylase. The most common is classic phenylketonuria, which is inherited as an autosomal recessive trait and results in mental retardation, seizures, hypopigmentation, and eczema. In most cases PKU is diagnosed shortly after birth because of routine testing, and early institution of dietary therapy can prevent complications.

Cataracts, partial albinism, and photophobia can be seen.[42,43] Small corneal opacities were reported in one patient, but the etiology was unclear.[44]

AMYLOIDOSIS

Amyloidosis is a disorder of protein metabolism in which there is tissue deposition of a characteristic extracellular protein material. Amyloid deposits can be localized (for example, corneal amyloid degeneration and lattice dystrophy) or systemic and primary or secondary, and vary accordingly.

Amyloidosis has been classified in many ways, but the following appears to be clinically most useful: (1) association with immunocyte dyscrasia, with or without frank malignancy, such as multiple myeloma, in which the amyloid fibrils are derived from immunoglobulin light chains (AL type); (2) association with chronic inflammatory or infectious disease (AA type); (3) heredofamilial amyloidosis, the type associated with familial Mediterranean fever (AA type) and a variety of neuropathic, nephropathic, cardiomyopathic, and other forms, in which the amyloid fibrils are most commonly derived from serum prealbumin (AF prealbumin type); (4) a common nonhereditary pathologic finding in elderly individuals (AS type); and (5) localized amyloidosis, without evidence of systemic disease. The eye can be affected by primary and secondary localized amyloidosis and in AL and familial types of systemic amyloidosis.

Primary localized amyloidosis. Primary localized amyloidosis can affect the bulbar or palpebral conjunctiva, Tenon's capsule, tarsus, limbus, lacrimal gland, or orbit.[45-48] In the lid and conjunctiva the amyloid appears as a soft, yellow nodule. The conjunctival deposit is usually subepithelial. Lattice corneal dystrophy, types I and III, and gelatinous droplike dystrophy also can be classified as types of primary localized amyloidosis of the cornea.[49]

Secondary localized amyloidosis. Secondary localized amyloidosis of the cornea can occur after trauma or can be associated with a chronic ocular inflammatory disorder (see Amyloid Degeneration, Chapter 16). The amyloid may appear as a small, salmon pink to yellow-white, fleshy, waxy, sometimes nodular mass or masses on the cornea or conjunctiva; as grayish perivascular deposits; as lamellar deposits; or as a subepithelial pannus. Such amyloid deposits are nearly always clinically insignificant and are most often found only on histologic examination.

Primary systemic amyloidosis. Nonfamilial primary systemic amyloidosis is almost always related to an immunocyte disorder, even if one is not clinically apparent.[50] Purpuric and papillary lesions of the eyelids and conjunctiva can be seen (Fig. 24-10). Neurologic involvement can lead to ptosis, ophthalmoplegia, neuroparalytic keratitis, and pupillary abnormalities. In familial forms the findings are similar, but veil-like vitreous opacities, retinal periphlebitis, and glaucoma can occur.[51-53] Scalloped pupils can occur and appear to be diagnostic.[54]

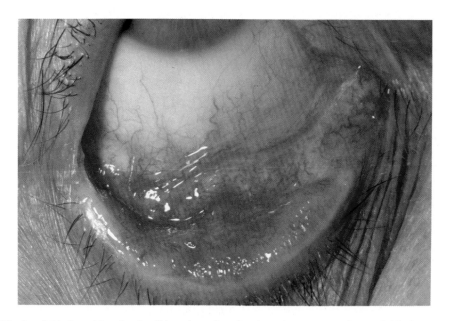

Fig. 24-10. Amyloid deposition in the lid and conjunctiva in primary systemic amyloidosis. (Courtesy of George F. Buerger, Jr, Pittsburgh.)

A rare form of dominantly inherited primary systemic amyloidosis, familial amyloid polyneuropathy type IV, or Meretoja's syndrome, is associated with lattice dystrophy of the cornea.[55-58] The latticelike corneal changes usually become manifest between 20 and 35 years of age; in later decades one sees involvement of the skin, peripheral nerves, and cranial nerves (see Chapter 17). The exact nature of the amyloid protein has not been determined, but it is related to transthyretin, a component of plasma prealbumin.[59]

WILSON'S DISEASE

Wilson's disease is characterized by progressive neurologic impairment and liver dysfunction. Copper is deposited in almost all body tissues, especially in the liver, brain, kidneys, and cornea. The exact metabolic defect has not been identified, but the rate of copper excretion into bile is reduced, with accumulation of copper in the liver, which eventually spills over into the blood, leading to extrahepatic deposition. It is transmitted as an autosomal recessive trait.

Approximately one half of patients present with hepatic involvement: acute hepatitis, cirrhosis, or asymptomatic hepatosplenomegaly. Neurologic or psychiatric disturbances, such as tremors, spasticity, chorea, rigidity and psychoses, are the first clinical signs in most other patients. Occasionally amenorrhea or spontaneous abortions can be the only manifestations.

OCULAR MANIFESTATIONS

In Wilson's disease copper deposition can be seen in the cornea, as the Kayser-Fleischer ring, and in the lens, as "sunflower cataracts"[60] (Table 24-2). The Kayser-Fleischer copper ring is a peripheral band, 1 to 3 mm wide, at the level of Descemet's membrane and extending to the limbus without a lucid interval (Fig. 24-11). It is usually yellow-brown but may appear gold, red, blue, green, or any mixture of these colors.[61-64] The color can change depending on the angle of illumination. On occasion, one can see a double ring, with an outer ruby red ring and a green inner ring.[61] The deposition is first noted as a thin crescent superiorly, then inferiorly, and eventually circumferentially. If posterior embryotoxon is present, a clear space separates the ring from the limbus, since Descemet's membrane ends anteriorly. Gonioscopic examination is sometimes required to detect an early Kayser-Fleischer ring because deposition occurs most peripherally first, and the ring may be obscured by an arcus or wide limbus.

A Kayser-Fleischer ring is seen in approximately 95% of patients with Wilson's disease.[65-67] It is present in all cases with neurologic involvement, and 70% to 90% of hepatic cases; however, it is absent in over 30% of children presenting with acute liver disease and may be absent in those without neurologic or hepatic symptoms.

TABLE 24-2. Other Metabolic Disorders with Anterior Segment Findings

DISORDER	CORNEAL FINDINGS	OTHER OCULAR FINDINGS
Wilson's disease	Kayser-Fleischer ring	Sunflower cataract
Hyperuricemia (gout)	Urate crystal deposition	Conjunctivitis, episcleritis, scleritis
Porphyria cutanea tarda	Blistering and scarring, crystals*[60]	Cicatricial ectropion, punctal stenosis, conjunctival vesicles and scarring, scleral thinning
Congenital erythropoietic porphyria	Scarring	Cicatricial ectropion, keratoconjunctivitis, scleral thinning, optic atrophy, retinal hemorrhages
Hemochromatosis	—	Rusty brown pigmentation of perilimbal conjunctiva
Zellweger's syndrome	Clouding	Cataracts, glaucoma, retinal pigmentary abnormalities, optic disc pallor
Biotinidase deficiency	—	Conjunctivitis

*One case.

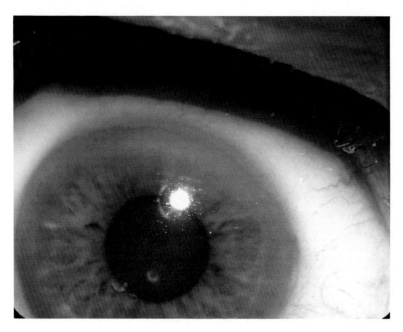

Fig. 24-11. Kayser-Fleischer ring.

A characteristic "sunflower" cataract is also present in 15% to 20% of patients. It is seen as a green or brown pigmentation of the central anterior and posterior lens capsule, in a central and petaloid distribution.[64,68]

The corneal pigmentation is caused by granular copper deposition in peripheral Descemet's membrane.[64,69-72] Using more sensitive means of detection, copper deposition also has been demonstrated centrally, and it appears to be bound to sulfur.[73]

DIFFERENTIAL DIAGNOSIS

The diagnosis of Wilson's disease can be made by demonstration of a serum ceruloplasmin less than 20 mg/dl and either Kayser-Fleischer rings or increased concentration of copper in a liver biopsy. However, approximately 5% of patients with the disease have higher ceruloplasmin levels, and some patients with other liver diseases have both elevated liver copper and pigmented corneal rings. These rings are clinically identical to Kayser-Fleischer rings and have been reported in primary biliary cirrhosis, progressive intrahepatic cholestasis of childhood, chronic active hepatitis with cirrhosis, other cholestatic syndromes, and exogenous chalcosis.[74-76] Patients with Wilson's disease can be differentiated from those with these disorders by their inability to incorporate radioactive copper into ceruloplasmin.[77]

Other conditions that cause pigmentation of the posterior corneal surface and can be mistaken for Wilson's disease are multiple myeloma, extensive copper treatment for trachoma (corneal and lenticular changes), copper intraocular foreign bodies, and carotenemia. In multiple myeloma, copper is deposited centrally in Descemet's membrane, Bowman's layer, and the anterior and posterior lens capsules. In carotenemia golden yellow rings are present at the site of a corneal arcus; in addition, night blindness can be present.

TREATMENT

The most effective treatment of Wilson's disease is removal of deposits with D-penicillamine, which prevents as well as reverses the clinical manifestations. The Kayser-Fleischer rings regress with penicillamine treatment and are a good indicator of the effectiveness of therapy. The most dramatic response is in the neurologic symptoms, but some patients show improvement in their liver disease. The most symptomatic patients may show the most remarkable improvement.[78,79] Lifetime therapy is required. Regression of Kayser-Fleischer rings has also been observed after liver transplantation.[80]

HYPERURICEMIA

Elevation of serum uric acid occurs in a wide variety of disorders. *Gout* is the combination of hyperuricemia with any of the following: characteristic arthritis, urate deposition in joints (tophi), interstitial renal disease, or uric acid nephrolithiasis. It primarily occurs in men, with a peak incidence in the fifth decade. It represent a heterogeneous group of disorders, often caused by a combination of genetic and environmental influences.

OCULAR MANIFESTATIONS

Monosodium urate can be deposited in the cornea, conjunctiva, and sclera. An acute conjunctival inflammation can occur, with marked hyperemia and a scanty foamy discharge (Fig. 24-12). The patient complains of photophobia, burning, and pain.[81-83] Conjunctival tophi also can occur.[81]

Fine, punctate or needlelike, refractile crystals can appear in the anterior corneal stroma and epithelium and are most dense in the palpebral fissure.[84] This deposition can occur in cases of hyperuricemia with or without gouty symptoms. The corneal appearance can be similar to band keratopathy, but is brownish rather than the whitish gray seen with calcium deposition (Fig. 24-13). Urate crystals can be demonstrated in the nuclei of the epithelial cells and in the superficial stroma.[84] Scleritis, episcleritis, and iritis can also be seen.[82]

Identical uric acid crystal deposition also can occur without hyperuricemia or gout, in which case it is called *urate keratopathy*. Urate keratopathy appears to be caused by local disturbance of uric acid metabolism.

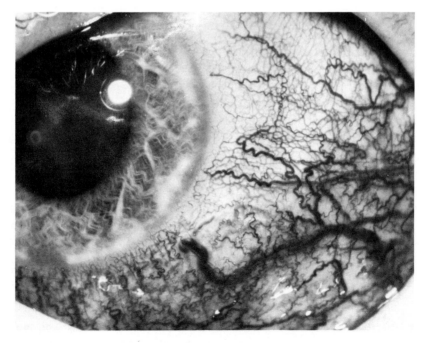

Fig. 24-12. Severe hyperemia of conjunctiva and episclera seen in gout.

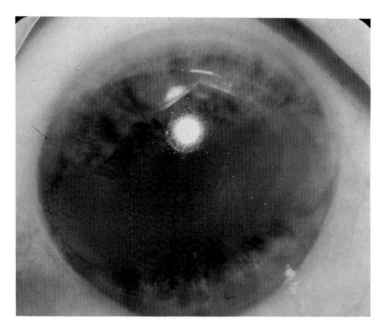

Fig. 24-13. Urate band keratopathy.

TREATMENT

Acute gouty arthritis is treated with antiinflammatory agents, typically colchicine or indomethacin and occasionally corticosteroids. Presumably, acute conjunctivitis, episcleritis, and scleritis could be treated similarly. Antihyperuricemic agents (for example, allopurinol, probenecid, or sulfinpyrazone) are given to prevent further complications. Corneal epithelial deposits can be removed by scraping or superficial keratectomy.[85]

PORPHYRIA

The porphyrias are a group of disorders of heme biosynthesis. Heme functions as a prosthetic, oxygen-carrying group for many proteins in the body, including hemoglobin, cytochromes, and catalase. It is essential for life and is present in all aerobic cells. The two major sites of heme synthesis are the liver and red blood cells, and depending on the specific form of porphyria, the erythropoietic or hepatic site can be predominantly affected, or both can be equally affected. The main clinical symptoms are intermittent attacks of nervous system dysfunction, sensitivity of the skin to light, or both.

PORPHYRIA CUTANEA TARDA

Porphyria cutanea tarda (PCT), also known as symptomatic porphyria, is the most common form of porphyria. It can be inherited or sporadic and is commonly associated with alcoholism and iron overload (hepatic siderosis). PCT is characterized by photosensitive cutaneous lesions, liver disease, and urinary excretion of porphyrins; neurologic symptoms do not occur. It usually becomes manifest between 40 and 60 years of age. Skin abnormalities include increased facial pigmentation, increased fragility to trauma, erythema, scleroderma-like changes, and vesicular and ulcerative lesions.

Recurrent vesication of the lid skin can lead to scarring, with cicatricial ectropion and punctal stenosis.[86-88] The conjunctiva can be hyperemic and chemotic and vesicles can form, leading to necrosis, scarring, and symblepharon formation.[86,87,89,90] The interpalpebral conjunctiva is most affected. Scarring of the cornea can result from blistering or as a complication of cicatricial ectropion. In one case white-tan nonrefractile crystals were present in the peripheral anterior stroma.[60] Scleritis, chiefly interpalpebral scleromalacia has been described, but histologic examination of one such case indicated scleral dehydration and elastotic degeneration, not inflammation or thinning.[87] In one report the scleral lesions showed pink fluorescence with ultraviolet light.[60]

CONGENITAL ERYTHROPOIETIC PORPHYRIA

This rare, recessively inherited form of porphyria affects only erythropoiesis. The exact enzymatic defect is not known. It becomes manifest at or shortly after birth and is recognized by the excretion of pink or red urine. Later, affected individuals develop hemolytic anemia, splenomegaly, and cutaneous photosensitivity, causing bullous eruptions of the skin. Neurologic dysfunction does not occur.

Optic nerve atrophy and retinal hemorrhages may be found on fundus examination. Scarring and depigmentation of the eyelids, ectropion, keratoconjunctivitis, conjunctival necrosis, scleromalacia, and corneal melting and scarring can occur.[86,91]

OTHER FORMS OF PORPHYRIA

Photosensitivity also is a feature of variegate porphyria and erythrohepatic porphyria, and it is likely that similar ocular lesions can occur in these patients. The most extensive report of ocular involvement in the porphyrias was published in 1952,[86] and our understanding and classification of porphyrias was limited at that time. However, conjunctival blistering and scarring was noted in many of their patients with skin involvement.

HEMOCHROMATOSIS

Hemochromatosis is an iron storage disorder in which increased absorption of iron from the intestine results in tissue deposition. It can occur on a genetic basis, with autosomal recessive inheritance, or secondary to other disease, particularly chronic disorders of erythropoiesis such as thalassemia or sideroblastic anemia. The liver, pancreas, and heart are most affected. A rusty brown pigmentation of the perilimbal bulbar conjunctiva, greater inferiorly than superiorly, has been described.[92,93]

ZELLWEGER'S SYNDROME

Zellweger's syndrome is a rare hereditary deficiency of peroxisomes in the liver and kidney, sometimes associated with a mitochondrial defect. It is characterized by severe hypotonia, high forehead, large anterior fontanelle, midface hypoplasia, and hepatomegaly. Affected infants usually die within a few months of birth. Cloudy corneas and cataracts are present in the majority of cases, and glaucoma, Brushfield spots, persistent pupillary membrane, epicanthus, rapidly progressive retinal dystrophy, and optic disc pallor also can be present.[94]

BIOTINIDASE DEFICIENCY

Biotin is a B vitamin that serves as a prosthetic group in carboxylase enzymes involved in gluconeogenesis, fatty acid synthesis, and amino acid catabolism. Biotinidase deficiency is a rare disorder of the recycling of endogenous biotin. It occurs in two forms, neonatal and juvenile. The neonatal form presents in the first few days of life with lactic acidosis, organic acidemia, and hyperammonemia. Children with the juvenile form have seizures, hypotonia, ataxia, breathing problems, developmental delay, skin rash, alopecia, hearing loss, and optic atrophy. Affected individuals present 3 weeks to several years of age, usually with metabolic ketolactic acidosis. Conjunctivitis, which is present in one half of patients, is one of the initial findings in about 10% of patients.[95,96] Corneal ulcers occur rarely.

REFERENCES

1. La Du BN: Alcaptonuria. In Scriver CR et al, editors: The metabolic basis of inherited disease, ed 6, New York, 1989, McGraw-Hill.
2. Smith JW: Ochronosis of the sclera and cornea complicating alkaptonuria: review of the literature and report of four cases, JAMA 120:1282, 1942.
3. Hatch JL: Hereditary alkaptonuria with ochronosis, Arch Ophthalmol 62:575, 1959.
4. Garrett EE: Ocular ochronosis with alkaptonuria, Am J Ophthalmol 55:617, 1963.
5. Rones B: Ochronosis oculi in alkaptonuria, Am J Ophthalmol 49:440, 1960.
6. Wirtschafter JD: The eye in alkaptonuria, Birth Defects 12:279, 1976.
7. Kampik A, Sani JN, and Green WR: Ocular ochronosis: clinicopathological, histochemical and ultrastructural studies, Arch Ophthalmol 98:1441, 1980.
8. Kenyon KR and Sensenbrenner JA: Electron microscopy of cornea and conjunctiva in childhood cystinosis, Am J Ophthalmol 78:68, 1974.
9. Goldman H et al: Adolescent cystinosis: comparison with infantile and adult forms, Pediatrics 47:979, 1971.
10. Zimmerman TJ, Hood CI, and Gasset AR: "Adolescent" cystinosis: a case presentation and review of the recent literature, Arch Ophthalmol 92:265, 1974.
11. Melles RB et al: Spatial and temporal sequence of corneal crystal deposition in nephropathic cystinosis, Am J Ophthalmol 104:598, 1987.
12. Yamamoto GK et al: Long-term ocular changes in cystinosis: observation in renal transplant recipients, J Pediatr Ophthalmol Strabismus 16:21, 1979.
13. Kaiser-Kupfer MI et al: Long-term ocular manifestations in nephropathic cystinosis, Arch Ophthalmol 104:706, 1986.
14. Katz B et al: Corneal thickness in nephropathic cystinosis, Br J Ophthalmol 73:665, 1989.
15. Wong VG: Ocular manifestations in cystinosis, Birth Defects 12:181, 1976.
16. Schneider JA, Wong VG, and Seegmiller JE: The early diagnosis of cystinosis, J Pediatr 74:114, 1969.
17. Sanderson PO, et al: Cystinosis: a clinical, histopathologic, and ultrastructural study, Arch Ophthalmol 91:270, 1974.
18. Kaiser-Kupfer MI et al: Nephropathic cystinosis: immunohistochemical and histopathologic studies of cornea, conjunctiva and iris, Curr Eye Res 6:617, 1987.
19. Wong VG, Lietman PS, and Seegmiller JE: Alterations of pigment epithelium in cystinosis, Arch Ophthalmol 77:361, 1967.
20. Cogan DG and Kuwabara T: Ocular pathology of cystinosis, Arch Ophthalmol 63:51, 1960.
21. Wong VG, Schulman JD, and Seegmiller JE: Conjunctival biopsy for the biochemical diagnosis of cystinosis, Am J Ophthalmol 70:278, 1970.
22. Francois J et al: Cystinosis: a clinical and histopathologic study, Am J Ophthalmol 73:643, 1972.

23. Frazier PD and Wong VG: Cystinosis: histologic and cyrstallographic examination of crystals in eye tissue, Arch Ophthalmol 80:87, 1968.
24. Kaiser-Kupfer MI et al: Removal of corneal crystals by topical cysteamine in nephropathic cystinosis, N Engl J Med 316:775, 1987.
25. Kaiser-Kupfer MI, Datiles MB, and Gahl WA: Clear graft two years after keratoplasty in nephropathic cystinosis, Am J Ophthalmol 105:318, 1988.
26. Katz B, Melles RB, and Schneider JA: Recurrent crystal deposition after keratoplasty in nephropathic cystinosis, Am J Ophthalmol 104:190. 1987.
27. Goldsmith LA and Laberge C: Tyrosinemia and related disorders. In Scriver CR et al, editors: The metabolic basis of inherited disease, ed 6, New York, 1989, McGraw-Hill.
28. Bienfang DC, Kuwabara T, and Pueschel SM: The Richner-Hanhart syndrome: report of a case with associated tyrosinemia, Arch Ophthalmol 94:1133, 1976.
29. Goldsmith LA and Reed J: Tyrosine-induced eye and skin lesions: a treatable genetic disease, JAMA 236:382, 1976.
30. Colditz PB et al: Tyrosinaemia II, Med J Aust 141:244, 1984.
31. Burns RP: Soluble tyrosine aminotransferase deficiency: an unusual cause of corneal ulcers, Am J Ophthalmol 73:400, 1972.
32. Sandberg HO: Bilateral keratopathy in tyrosinosis, Acta Ophthalmol 53:760, 1975.
33. Jaeger W et al: Herpetiform bilateral epithelial corneal dystrophy caused by tyrosinemia (Richner-Hanhart syndrome), Klin Monatsbl Augenheilkd 173:506, 1978.
34. Grayson M: Corneal manifestations of keratosis plantaris and palmaris, Am J Ophthalmol 59:483, 1965.
35. Driscoll DJ et al: Corneal tyrosine crystals in transient neonatal tyrosinemia, J Pediatr 113:91, 1988.
36. Charlton KH et al: Pseudodendritic keratitis and systemic tyrosinemia, Ophthalmology 88:355, 1981.
37. Zaleski WA, Hill A, and Murray RG: Corneal erosions in tyrosinosis, Can J Ophthalmol 8:556, 1973.
38. Rich LF, Beard ME, and Burns RP: Excess dietary tyrosine and corneal lesions, Exp Eye Res 17:87, 1973.
39. Gipson IK, Burns RP, and Wolfe-Lande JD: Crystals in corneal epithelial lesions of tyrosine-fed rats, Invest Ophthalmol 14:937, 1975.
40. Larregue M et al: Syndrome du Richner-Hanhart ou tyrosinose oculo-cutanee, Ann Dermatol Venereol 106:53, 1979.
41. Sayar RB et al: Clinical picture and problems of keratoplasty in Richner-Hanhart syndrome, Ophthalmologica 197:1, 1988.
42. Zwaan J: Eye findings in patients with phenylketonuria, Arch Ophthalmol 101:1236, 1983.
43. Cottilicelli L et al: Ophthalmological findings of phenylketonuria: a survey of 14 cases, J Pediatr Ophthalmol Strabismus 22:78, 1985.

44. Penrose LS: Two cases of phenylpyruvic amentia, Lancet 1:23, 1935.

45. Brownstein MH, Elliott R, and Helwig EB: Ophthalmologic aspects of amyloidosis, Am J Ophthalmol 69:423, 1970.

46. Knowles DM II et al: Amyloidosis of the orbit and adnexae, Surv Ophthalmol 19:367, 1975.

47. Smith ME and Zimmerman LE: Amyloidosis of the eyelid and conjunctiva, Arch Ophthalmol 75:42, 1966.

48. Blodi FC and Apple DJ: Localized conjunctival amyloidosis, Am J Ophthalmol 88:346, 1979.

49. Ramsey MS and Fine BS: Localized corneal amyloidosis: case report with electromicroscopic findings, Am J Ophthalmol 75:560, 1972.

50. Pepys MB: Amyloidosis. In Samter M, editor: Immunological diseases, ed 4, Boston, 1988, Little, Brown & Co.

51. Ferry AP and Lieberman TW: Bilateral amyloidosis of the vitreous body: report of a case without systemic or familial involvement, Arch Ophthalmol 94:982, 1976.

52. Kaufman HE and Thomas IB: Vitreous opacities diagnostic of familial primary amyloidosis, N Engl J Med 261:1267, 1959.

53. Kaufman HE: Primary familial amyloidosis, Arch Ophthalmol 60:1036, 1958.

54. Lessell S et al: Scalloped pupils in familial amyloidosis, N Engl J Med 293:914, 1975.

55. Meretoja J: Familial systemic paramyloidosis with lattice dystrophy of the cornea, progressive cranial neuropathy, skin changes and various internal symptoms: a previously unrecognized heritable syndrome, Ann Clin Res 1:314, 1969.

56. Meretoja J: Comparative histopathological and clinical findings in eyes with lattice corneal dystrophy of two types, Ophthalmologica 165:115, 1972.

57. Meretoja J: Genetic aspects of familial amyloidosis with corneal lattice dystrophy and cranial neuropathy, Clin Genet 4:173, 1973.

58. Purcell JJ et al: Lattice corneal dystrophy associated with familial systemic amyloidosis (Meretoja's syndrome), Ophthalmology 90:1512, 1983.

59. Maury CP et al: Amyloid fibril protein in familial amyloidosis with cranial neuropathy and corneal lattice dystrophy (FAP type IV) is related to transthyretin, Am J Clin Pathol 89:359, 1988.

60. Chumbley LC: Scleral involvement in symptomatic porphyria, Am J Ophthalmol 84:729, 1977.

61. Froment J, Bonnet P, and Paufique L: Anneau pigmenté de Kayser-Fleischer dans la pseudosclérose, Bull Soc Ophtalmol Fr 2:713, 1937.

62. Manschot WA: Ring of Kayser and Fleischer, Ophthalmologica 132:164, 1956.

63. Slovis TL et al: The varied manifestations of Wilson's disease, J Pediatr 78:578, 1971.

64. Tso MOM, Fine BS, and Thorpe HE: Kayser-Fleischer ring and associated cataract in Wilson's disease, Am J Ophthalmol 79:479, 1975.

65. Scheinberg IH: Wilson's disease. In Braunwald E et al, editors: Harrison's principles of internal medicine, ed 11, New York, 1987, McGraw-Hill.

66. Wiebers DO, Hollenhorst RW, and Goldstein NP: The ophthalmological manifestations of Wilson's disease, Mayo Clin Proc 52:409, 1977.

67. Dobyns WB, Goldstein NP, and Gordon H: Clinical spectrum of Wilson's disease (hepatolenticular degeneration), Mayo Clin Proc 54:35, 1979.

68. Cairns JE, Williams HP, and Walshe JM: Sunflower cataract in Wilson's disease, Br Med J 3:95, 1969.

69. Uzman LL and Jakus MA: The Kayser-Fleischer ring: a histochemical and electron microscope study, Neurology 7:341, 1957.

70. Ellis PP: Ocular deposition of copper in hypercupremia, Am J Ophthalmol 68:423, 1969.

71. Harry J and Tripathi R: Kayser-Fleischer ring: a pathological study, Br J Ophthalmol 54:794, 1970.

72. Johnson BL: Ultrastructure of the Kaiser-Fleischer ring, Am J Ophthalmol 76:455, 1973.

73. Johnson RE and Campbell RJ: Wilson's disease: electron microscopic, x-ray energy spectroscopic, and atomic absorption spectroscopic studies of cornea copper deposition and distribution, Lab Invest 46:564, 1982.

74. Fleming CR et al: Pigmented rings in non-Wilsonian liver disease, Ann Intern Med 86:285, 1977.

75. Frommer D et al: Kayser-Fleischer-like rings in patients without Wilson's disease, Gastroenterology 72:1331, 1977.

76. Kaplinsky C et al: Familial cholestatic cirrhosis associated with Kayser-Fleischer rings, Pediatrics 65:782, 1980.

77. Scheinberg IH: Wilson's disease. In Braunwald E et al, editors: Harrison's principles of internal medicine, ed 11, New York, 1987, McGraw-Hill.

78. Mitchell AM and Heller GL: Changes in Kayser-Fleischer ring during treatment of hepatolenticular degeneration, Arch Ophthalmol 80:622, 1968.

79. Sussman W and Scheinberg IH: Disappearance of Kaiser-Fleischer rings: effects of penicillamine, Arch Ophthalmol 82:738, 1969.

80. Schoenberger M and Ellis PP: Disappearance of Kayser-Fleischer rings after liver transplantation, Arch Ophthalmol 97:1914, 1979.

81. Hutchinson J: The relation of certain diseases of the eye to gout, Br Med J 2:995, 1884.

82. McWilliams JR: Ocular findings in gout, Am J Ophthalmol 35:1778, 1952.

83. Ferry AP, Safir A, and Melikan HE: Ocular abnormalities in patients with gout, Ann Ophthalmol 17:632, 1985.

84. Slansky HH and Kuwabara T: Intranuclear urate crystals in corneal epithelium, Arch Ophthalmol 80:338, 168.

85. Fishman RS and Sunderman FW: Band keratopathy in gout, Arch Ophthalmol 75:367, 1967.

86. Barnes HD and Boshoff PH: Ocular lesions in patients with porphyria, Arch Ophthalmol 48:567, 1952.

87. Sevel D and Burger D: Ocular involvement in cutaneous porphyria. A clinical and histological report, Arch Ophthalmol 85:580, 1970.

88. Sober AJ, Grove AS Jr, and Muhlbauer JE: Cicatricial ectropion and lacrimal obstruction associated with sclerodermoid variant of porphyria cutanea tarda, Am J Ophthalmol 91:400, 1981.

89. Duke-Elder S and Leigh AG: System of Ophthalmology, vol VIII: Diseases of the outer eye, St Louis, 1965, Mosby–Year Book, Inc.

90. Stokes WH: Ocular manifestations in hydroa vacciniforme, Arch Ophthalmol 23:1131, 1940.

91. Mohan M et al: Corneoscleral ulceration in congenital erythropoietic porphyria (a case report), Jpn J Ophthalmol 32:21, 1988.

92. Cibis PA, Brown EB, and Hong WM: Ocular aspects of systemic siderosis, Am J Ophthalmol 44:158, 1957.

93. Davies G et al: Deposition of melanin and iron in ocular structures in haemochromatosis, Br J Ophthalmol 56:338, 1972.

94. Cohen SMZ et al: Ocular histopathologic and biochemical studies of the cerebrohepatorenal syndrome (Zellweger's syndrome) and its relationship to neonatal adrenoleukodystrophy, Am J Ophthalmol 96:488, 1984.

95. Campana G et al: Ocular aspects in biotinidase deficiency: clinical and genetic original studies, Ophthalmic Paediatr Genet 8:125, 1987.

96. Wolf B and Heard GS: Disorders of biotin metabolism. In Scriver CR et al, editors: The metabolic basis of inherited disease, ed 6, New York, 1989, McGraw-Hill.

DISEASES OF THE SKIN

BULLOUS OCULOCUTANEOUS DISEASES

The conjunctiva or cornea can be involved in a wide variety of blistering skin diseases (Table 25-1). Most of these cause conjunctival inflammation, and secondary conjuctival and corneal scarring is the main complication.

CICATRICIAL PEMPHIGOID

Pemphigoid diseases of the skin are a group of disorders characterized by subepidermal bulla formation and deposition of immunoglobulins within the lamina lucida of the epithelial basement membrane in skin and mucous membrane. This group includes cicatricial pemphigoid, bullous pemphigoid, herpes gestationis, and localized scarring pemphigoid. Only cicatricial pemphigoid and bullous pemphigoid affect the eye.

Cicatricial pemphigoid (CP) is a cicatricial disease of the conjunctiva and, to a lesser extent, other mucous membranes and skin, presumed to be of autoimmune origin. It also has been called benign mucous membrane pemphigoid, ocular pemphigoid, and essential shrinkage of the conjunctiva. It is generally believed to result from a type II hypersensitivity reaction.

Clinical manifestations. CP is a disease of older people; it seldom develops before age 50, and it is more common in women. Oral mucosal lesions (Fig. 25-1) occur in approximately 90% of patients, and lesions of the nose, larynx, anus, esophagus, and vagina also can be seen.[1,2] Skin lesions (Fig. 25-2) occur in approximately 25% of patients.[3] Ocular involvement occurs in the majority of cases and can be the only manifestation of the disease. The most serious complications of CP result from the ocular involvement, except for rare cases of death due to esophageal strictures.

The onset is usually insidious with recurrent attacks of mild and clinically nonspecific conjunctival inflammation. On occasion, mucopurulent discharge occurs, and erroneous diagnoses of bacterial conjunctivitis are not uncommon. During these early episodes conjunctival hyperemia, edema, ulceration, and vesicles can be present. In the absence of coexisting vesiculobullous inflammation of the skin or other mucosa, usually the first clinical clue to the true nature of the problem is slight fore-

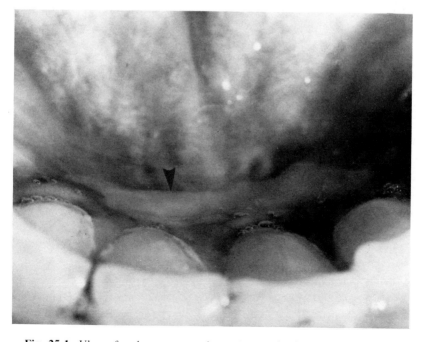

Fig. 25-1. Ulcer of oral mucous membrane *(arrow)* in cicatricial pemphigoid.

TABLE 25-1. Bullous Skin Diseases

	AGE (MOST COMMON)	SKIN LESIONS	COURSE	SITE OF BLISTER FORMATION
Cicatricial pemphigoid	> 60 yrs; F > M	Vesiculobullous 25%-50%	Chronic	SE*
Stevens-Johnson syndrome	10-30 yrs	Multiforme: target lesions, macules, papules, bullae	4-6 wks (rarely recurrent)	SE
Toxic epidermal necrolysis				
Staphylococcal	<10 yrs	Flaccid, necrotic sheets	4-6 wks (rarely recurrent)	IE†
DTEN	10-30 yrs	Flaccid, necrotic sheets	4-6 wks (rarely recurrent)	IE (basal)
Bullous pemphigoid	40-60 yrs	Large, tense bullae	Usually self-limited	SE
Pemphigus vulgaris	30-50 yrs	Bullae, Nikolsky sign	Chronic	IE
Dermatitis herpetiformis	20-40 yrs	Pruritic, vesicles, papules, bullae	Chronic	SE
Linear IgA disease	30-50 yrs	Tense bullae	?Usually self-limited	SE
Epidermolysis bullosa‡	Varies with type	Blisters after trauma	Chronic	IE or SE
Chronic bullous disease of childhood	<5 yrs	Large tense bullae	<10 yrs	SE

*SE, Subepidermal.
†IE, Intraepidermal.
‡See Table 25-2.

shortening of the inferior conjunctival fornices (Fig. 25-3). Gossamer subepithelial scarring of the conjunctiva also may be found. These subtle conjunctival signs should be sought in any older patient with chronic or recurrent red eyes of unknown origin.

CP occasionally presents with severe acute inflammation. The patient suddenly develops lid swelling, intense conjunctival hyperemia and edema, and infiltration with rapid scarring to the subepithelial conjunctiva. Bullae are encountered only rarely.

The disease is nearly always bilateral, although it may be very asymmetric, and activity may be present in only one eye. CP is a chronic disease, with exacerbations and remissions. Progressive conjunctival scarring occurs and can lead to symblepharon (Fig. 25-4), misdirected lashes (Fig. 25-5), entropion, and keratoconjunctivitis sicca. Tear deficiency occurs as a result of closure of the tear ductules, and loss of goblet cells leads to mucus deficiency. The lids can become fixed to the globe, with constant exposure of the cornea and conjunctiva (Fig. 25-6). The cornea is remarkably spared except in the late stages, when it may be seriously compromised by the secondary effects of cicatrization, drying, and trichiasis. The compromised cornea is then subject to superficial scarring and vascularization, persistent epithelial defects, sterile ulceration, and bacterial infection (Fig. 25-7).

Foster et al.[4] have divided CP into four stages:

Stage 1—Conjunctival inflammation, mucoid discharge, rose bengal staining of the conjunctiva, and subtle subepithelial fibrosis (fine striae)

IMMUNOPATHOLOGY		CONJUNCTIVAL INVOLVEMENT		
IG DEPOSITION	**LOCALIZATION**	**FREQUENCY**	**SCARRING**	**OTHER**
Linear IgG	Lamina lucida	70%-90%	+	
C3 protein ±IgM	Superficial microvessels; ± dermoepidermal junction	Frequent	+	Entropion, trichiasis, dry eye, secondary corneal disease
		Common	+	
		Common	+	Sjögren's syndrome
Linear IgG	Lamina lucida	Infrequent	−	
Linear IgG	Intercellular spaces	16%	−	Palpebral conjunctiva
Granular IgA	Tips of dermal papillae	Rare	+	Jejunal disease
Linear IgA	Basal lamina, lamina lucida		+	
Varies	Varies	Frequent	+	Blepharitis corneal erosion, vesicles, ulcers
Linear IgA	Lamina lucida	?Common	+	

Stage 2—Conjunctival shrinkage, with foreshortening of the inferior fornix

Stage 3—More advanced shrinkage, with symblepharon formation; keratopathy, corneal pannus, trichiasis, and dry eye

Stage 4—End-stage disease, with severe dry eyes, ankyloblepharon, and ocular surface keratinization

One series found a relatively high incidence of glaucoma in CP patients.[5] Most of these patients had a long history of glaucoma before CP was diagnosed, and it is possible that the glaucoma medication played a role in the development of the disease. Those CP patients with a history of glaucoma were more likely to have persistent inflammation despite treatment.

Histopathology. During active disease subepithelial bullae may be seen. There is an inflammation in the epithelium and substantia propria of the conjunctiva, with lymphocytes, plasma cells, polymorphonuclear leukocytes (PMNs) and eosinophils.[6,7] Later subepithelial fibrosis, loss of goblet cells,[8,9] and keratinization of the epithelium occur.[7,10] Increased numbers of desmosomes and tonofilaments have been observed in the conjunctival epithelium[11] and have reverted to normal with immunosuppression.[12]

Pathogenesis. The formation of the bullae appears to be caused by an autoimmune response against components of the basement membrane. During active disease immunoglobulins (IgG and sometimes IgA and IgM) and complement components can often be found along the epithelial basement mem-

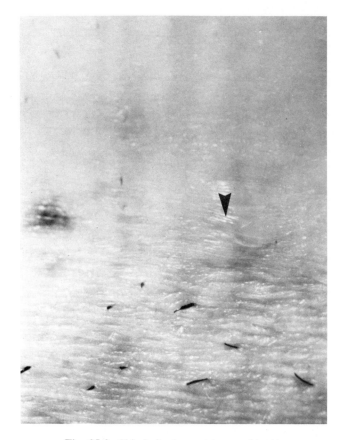

Fig. 25-2. Skin bulla *(arrow)* in pemphigoid.

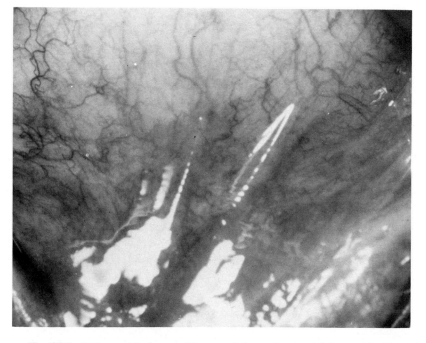

Fig. 25-3. Early symblepharon of lower cul-de-sac in cicatricial pemphigoid.

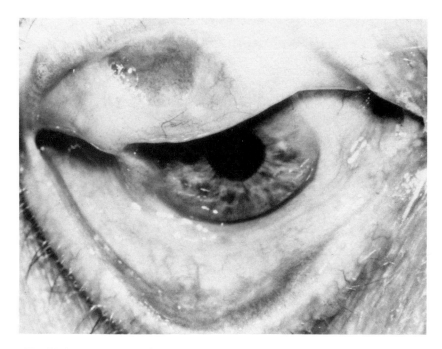

Fig. 25-4. Extensive scarring of upper tarsal conjunctiva in cicatricial pemphigoid.

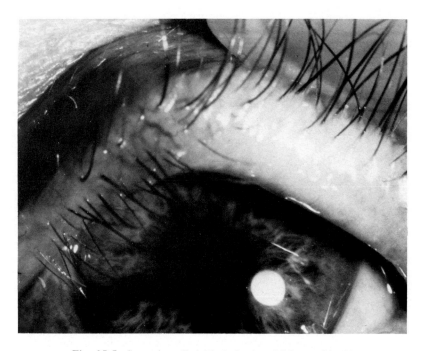

Fig. 25-5. Secondary distichiasis in cicatricial pemphigoid.

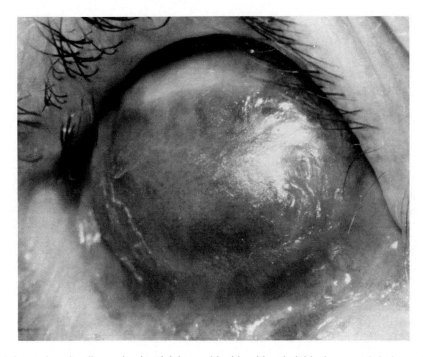

Fig. 25-6. Advanced ocular disease in cicatricial pemphigoid, with ankyloblepharon and drying and keratinization of corneal and conjunctival epithelium.

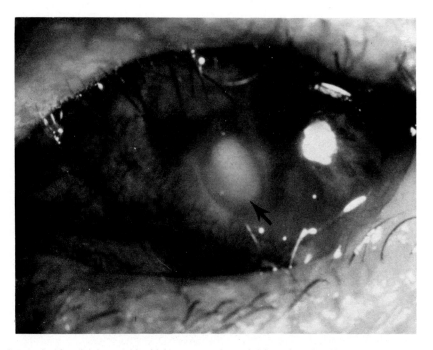

Fig. 25-7. Cornea in cicatricial pemphigoid is prone to bacterial invasion. In this case *Staphylococcus aureus* infection is present *(arrow)*.

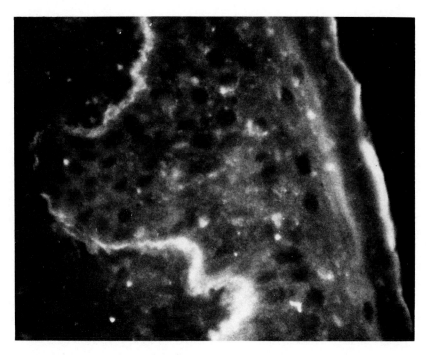

Fig. 25-8. Deposition of immunoglobulin in epithelial basement membrane in case of cicatricial pemphigoid. (Courtesy of S.F. Bean, Houston.)

brane of the conjunctiva[13-16] (Fig. 25-8). However, the presence of circulating antibasement membrane antibodies is uncommon[14,17-19] (in contrast to bullous pemphigoid, in which circulating antibasement membrane antibodies are present in most cases). The exact antigen against which these antibodies are directed has not been identified, but the bulla forms in the lamina lucida.[20]

The mitotic rate of the conjunctival epithelium is higher than normal, suggesting a hyperproliferative state,[21] which may contribute to the disease or occur in response to increased epithelial cell loss. HLA-B12 has been found more frequently in these patients, in 45% compared with 20% of controls.[22] Also, approximately half of patients with CP have elevated serum levels of IgA,[23] and antinuclear antibodies are often present.[24]

Diagnosis. The diagnosis of CP is usually clinical, based on progressive bilateral conjunctival scarring. Further support for the diagnosis often can be obtained by finding a few eosinophils in a conjunctival scraping. The eosinophils are seldom numerous, but the presence of even a single eosinophil in the absence of conjunctival bleeding is significant. Eosinophils are more likely to be found during acute inflammatory exacerbations of the disease.

Immunopathologic examination of a conjunctival biopsy may demonstrate antibodies at the level of the basement membrane. However, biopsy must be obtained from an area of active disease, and the absence of antibodies does not rule out the diagnosis. The biopsy also can exacerbate the disease; scarring is probably less if the biopsy is taken from the bulbar conjunctiva, away from the fornix.

Chronic cicatrization of the conjunctiva also can occur from other causes, and one should particularly think of these in any patient with unilateral disease. Prolonged topical administration of echothiophate iodide, pilocarpine, epinephrine, or idoxuridine (IDU) can cause conjunctival scarring.[25-28] Drug-induced pemphigoid is clinically identical to cicatricial pemphigoid, except that it is often unilateral, and there are no systemic signs. Cicatrization can cease when medication is stopped, or continue to progress. Systemic administration of practolol and D-penicillamine can lead to conjunctival scarring. Other causes include chemical burns, radiation, Stevens-Johnson syndrome, sarcoidosis,[29] infectious conjunctivitis, masquerade syndrome (Fig. 25-9), and trauma.

The other bullous skin diseases, discussed later, should also be considered in the differential diagnosis. The conjunctiva is infrequently involved in bullous pemphigoid. Conjunctival lesions occur in the majority of patients with pemphigus vulgaris, but they produce transient symptoms and rarely cause permanent scarring. Conjunctival involvement can also occur in dermatitis herpetiformis and epidermolysis bullosa.

Treatment. The treatment of CP is disappointing. At this time the most effective means of inhibiting the progression of the disease is immunosuppressive therapy. A combination of prednisone and cyclophosphamide has been demonstrated to quiet ocular inflammation and prevent further scarring in most cases.[4,30] The initial doses are cyclophosphamide 100 to 150 mg/day and prednisone 80 to 120 mg/day. The dose is gradually tapered, as indicated by the patient's clinical response and the occurrence of side effects. As with any immunosuppressive therapy, the patient also should be followed for adverse effects by someone familiar with the use of these agents. Immunosuppression is indicated only for patients with active inflammation and progressive scarring (stages 2 and 3).

Systemic corticosteroid alone can quiet inflammation but is less effective in preventing cicatrization.[31] Dapsone, which interferes with the function of PMNs and inhibits release of lysosomal enzymes, also may be effective.[32] It can be used in conjunction with prednisone and has a lower risk of complications than do cytotoxic agents. Cyclosporine has been used in a few cases with variable results.[33]

Complications of conjunctival scarring must also be addressed. Topical artificial tear solutions are used to alleviate drying and exposure. Electrolysis, cryotherapy, and occasionally lid surgery may be necessary to treat trichiasis. Bandage contact lenses can be used to manage drying, trichiasis, and epithelial defects, but they increase the risk of infection. Prompt diagnosis and treatment of infections are essential.

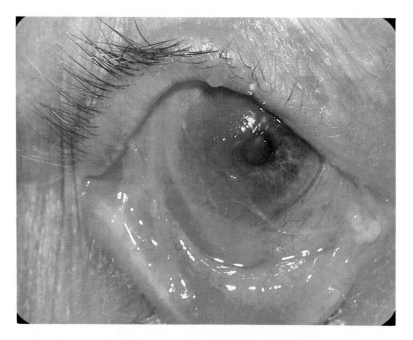

Fig. 25-9. Conjunctival pathologic condition resembling cicatricial pemphigoid. In this case, however, conjunctival carcinoma is present.

Intraocular procedures should be undertaken only when absolutely necessary; many eyes progress to atrophy bulbi after otherwise uncomplicated cataract extraction. If surgery is performed, the patient should be immunosuppressed and quiescent before surgery and probably for at least 2 months after surgery.[34] Penetrating keratoplasty is nearly always unsuccessful.

BULLOUS PEMPHIGOID

Bullous pemphigoid (BP) is another member of the pemphigoid group of diseases. It is characterized by the presence of large, tense, nongrouped blisters occurring mainly on the sides of the neck and axillary and inguinal regions, which resolve without scarring. BP most commonly arises in the fifth and sixth decades of life, although it can occur at any age. It is generally a benign, self-limited disease. The oral mucosa is involved in approximately one third of patients, and the eye is affected only rarely.[35]

Bullous pemphigoid appears to be an autoimmune disease, with autoantibodies directed against an antigen (bullous pemphigoid antigen) in the lamina lucida of basement membranes. Linear deposition of IgG, and occasionally IgA, IgM, or IgE, is seen along the epithelial basement membrane.[36] Circulating antibodies directed against this same antigen are found in the majority of patients.[36,37]

ERYTHEMA MULTIFORME MAJOR (STEVENS-JOHNSON SYNDROME)

Erythema multiforme is an episodic, self-limited, mucocutaneous inflammatory disorder. Clinically, the disease manifests as a spectrum from mild to severe; the severe form is called erythema multiforme major, or Stevens-Johnson syndrome. It is most commonly precipitated by herpes simplex

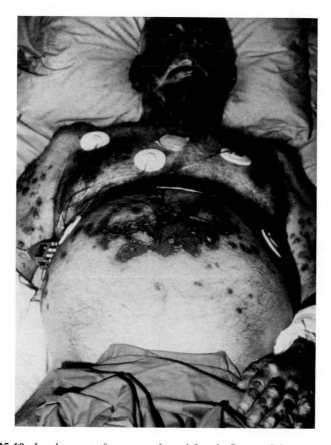

Fig. 25-10. Involvement of arms, trunk, and face in Stevens-Johnson syndrome.

infection or drugs, but it can be associated with other infectious agents or carcinoma, and often no precipitating factor can be identified. The pathogenesis of the mucocutaneous lesions is thought to be related to immune complexes, cell-mediated immunity, or both.[38]

Erythema multiforme major most often affects children and young adults and is seldom encountered in the elderly. A prodrome of fever, malaise, sore throat, and arthralgia may precede the skin eruptions by a few days. The skin lesions can take many forms but are predominantly either "bull's eye" or bullous. The dorsal hands and feet and extensor surfaces of the forearms and legs are most frequently involved, often with a strikingly symmetric distribution (Figs. 25-10 and 25-11). The mucous membranes, especially of the eyes and mouth, are frequently affected by bullous and erosive lesions. Individual skin lesions tend to have life cycles of about 2 weeks. Recurrent cycles of lesions can occur, with most appearing by 6 weeks after onset. Recurrences develop in approximately one third of patients.

Ocular manifestations. Conjunctival inflammation occurs in a large proportion of cases and correlates with systemic severity. The conjunctivitis is diffuse and bilateral (Fig. 25-12) and can be catarrhal, mucopurulent, hemorrhagic, or membranous and ultimately cicatrizing.[39] Conjunctival bullae and ulcerative lesions also can occur. There is a tendency for relative sparing of the cornea until the late complications of conjunctival scarring ensue. However, one can see corneal ulceration, drying, and peripheral vascularization during the acute phase of the disease. Unlike cicatricial pemphigoid, the corneal and conjunctival inflammation does not progress indefinitely. Once the systemic disease has resolved, the ocular inflammation quiets. Rarely, however, recurrent inflammation is observed for many years after the initial episode.[40]

The final result can vary from no visible sequelae to severe scarring, keratoconjunctivitis sicca, corneal vascularization (Fig. 25-13), keratinization of the lid margins (Fig. 25-14), symblepharon (Fig. 25-15), and lid distortions with trichiasis and entropion.[41,42] Iridocyclitis and even panophthalmitis can occur. The subsequent effects of these complications can be disabling and can lead to blindness.

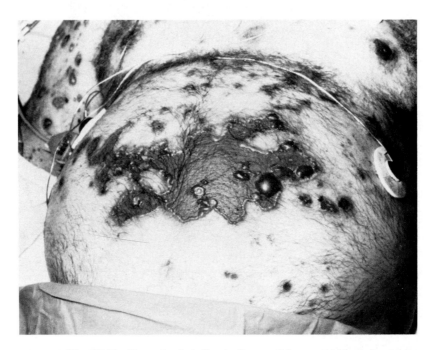

Fig. 25-11. Hemorrhagic bullae in Stevens-Johnson syndrome.

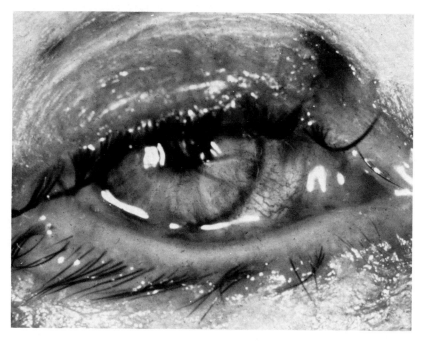

Fig. 25-12. Diffuse mucopurulent and membranous conjunctivitis in Stevens-Johnson syndrome.

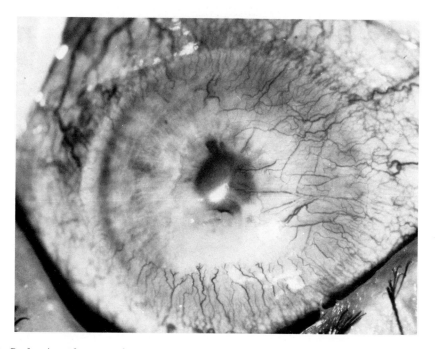

Fig. 25-13. Perforation of cornea after treatment of vascularized and dry cornea of Stevens-Johnson syndrome with frequent topical steroids.

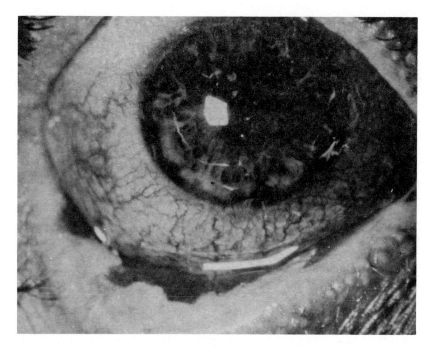

Fig. 25-14. Keratinization of lid margin after Stevens-Johnson syndrome.

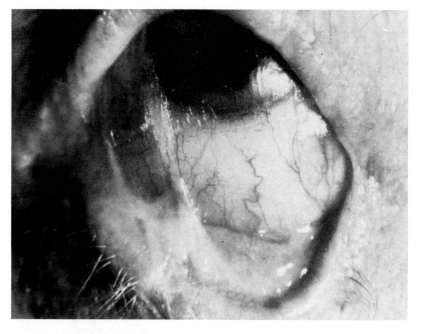

Fig. 25-15. Corneal keratinization, symblepharon formation, dry eye, and corneal vascularization resulting from Stevens-Johnson syndrome.

Treatment. Treatment of the systemic disease is primarily supportive. Suspected etiologic factors are eliminated, fluid balance is maintained, and antipruritics and analgesics are administered. Systemic corticosteroids are generally given, but their efficacy for the systemic disease is unclear, and they appear to have no effect on the ocular disease.

In the presence of conjunctivitis, topical steroids and antibiotic ointment are given, but their effect is questionable. If there is evidence of conjunctival ulceration or synechiae, I take measures to decrease symblepharon formation, although the benefits of this procedure are questionable. Daily lysis of synechiae can be performed, but preventing contact between the bulbar and palpebral conjunctiva appears to be more effective. This can be accomplished with a symblepharon ring, or a plastic wrap can be sutured around the lid; both usually require use of a bandage lens.

The plastic wrap is performed as follows: a piece of plastic wrap is cut to the width of the palpebral fissure. Three 5-0 nylon mattress sutures are placed near the end of the wrap and are passed from the fornix out through the skin. The wrap is then folded over the skin surface, and the sutures are passed through the wrap and tied. The wrap is then trimmed to length.

Management of the complications of Stevens-Johnson syndrome is similar to that described for cicatricial pemphigoid. If lid function and tear production are not very impaired, surgical measures can be successful. Lamellar dissection or keratoepithelioplasty can be performed to remove superficial corneal scarring and improve vision.

TOXIC EPIDERMAL NECROLYSIS (LYELL'S DISEASE, SCALDED SKIN SYNDROME)

Toxic epidermal necrolysis (TEN) may represent a variant of erythema multiforme. It is characterized by broad areas of skin necrosis and sloughing, resembling a thermal burn. Severe cases of erythema multiforme can evolve into a clinical appearance similar to TEN.[43] There are two distinct groups of patients: In children the eruption is most commonly related to staphylococcal infection, usually *Staphylococcus aureus* phage group 2,[44,45] whereas in adults it is usually related to drugs or is idiopathic.[46,47]

TEN begins with a prodrome like that of erythema multiforme. A few days later erythema and bullae of the skin and mucous membranes appear.[48] The bullae become flaccid, and large areas of epidermis fall away, leaving an appearance of scalded skin (Fig. 25-16). Remaining areas of skin are often wrinkled and can be made to slide away like a "slipped rug" when pressure is applied. Mucous membranes of the mouth, genitalia, and rectum are frequently affected. Necrolysis can be generalized within 24 hours, but usually spreads gradually from a Stevens-Johnson syndromelike initial appearance.[49] The mortality is about 20%.[46]

Intraepithelial cleavage accounts for the skin sloughing. The cleavage occurs superficially in the granular layer of the skin in the staphylococcal-related disease, whereas in the drug-induced form cleavage occurs at the basal layer of the epidermis. TEN associated with staphylococcal infection appears to be related to a toxin produced by the bacteria, which alters the intercellular substance between epidermal cells. This toxin can produce an identical syndrome in mice.[50,51] The drug-related and idiopathic forms are probably severe types of erythema multiforme and also are immunologically mediated.[38,52,53]

Ocular manifestations. The ocular findings are the same as those of erythema multiforme, except that they tend to be milder in TEN. Conjunctival involvement is common; mucopurulent conjunctivitis is most frequent, but membranous conjunctivitis with subsequent scarring also can occur. The conjunctival scarring can lead to the same complications as were described for erythema multiforme, including trichiasis, lid distortion, dry eye, and corneal vascularization and opacification.[54] Sjögren's syndrome, with xerostomia and lymphocytic infiltration of the salivary glands, also can occur after TEN.[53]

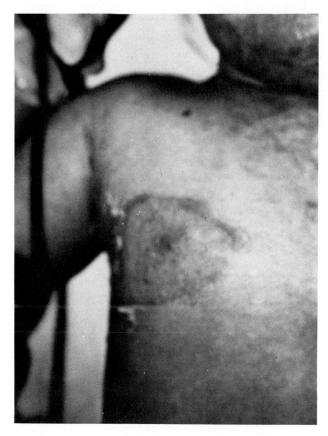

Fig. 25-16. Toxic epidermal necrolysis. Skin bullae become flaccid, and large areas of epidermis fall away, leaving "scalded skin."

Treatment. The treatment is no different from that described for erythema multiforme, except that intensive and immediate antibiotic therapy should be instituted in the staphylococcal form of the disease. Because of the extensive epidermal necrosis, these patients may require the specialized care of a burn unit for control of infection and fluid balance.

Epidermolysis Bullosa

Epidermolysis bullosa (EB) is a group of rare diseases characterized by the formation of bullous lesions after minor mechanical trauma (Figs. 25-17 to 25-19). Dystrophic nail problems also occur. Most of these diseases are hereditary. The pathogenesis is not well understood, but they appear to be disorders of the epithelial cell attachment complex—hemidesmosomes, basement membrane, or anchoring fibrils. The exact layer of separation between the epidermis and dermis differs in the various forms of the disease, probably related to different defects in the components of the epithelial attachment complex (Table 25-2).[55] Autoimmunity against basement membrane components appears to be responsible for epidermolysis bullosa acquisita.[56-58]

Ocular manifestations. Ocular involvement has been reported in most types of EB, including EB simplex-Koebner, EB atrophicans gravis and inversa, recessive dermolytic EB (Hallopeau-Siemens syndrome), and dominant dermolytic EB (Cockayne-Touraine and Pasini albo-papuloid types).[59,60] Blepharitis, bullous lesions of the lids, conjunctival vesicles, and corneal erosions can occur.[2,61-66] Corneal erosions appear to be the most common ocular complication, and their frequency is propor-

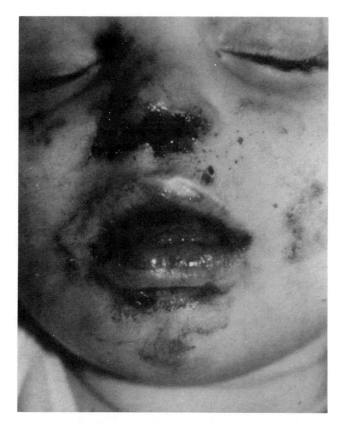

Fig. 25-17. Epidermolysis bullosa with hemorrhagic lesions of mucous membranes.

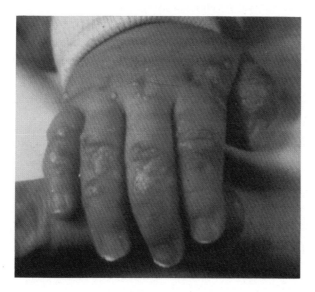

Fig. 25-18. Typical bullous lesions of hand in epidermolysis bullosa.

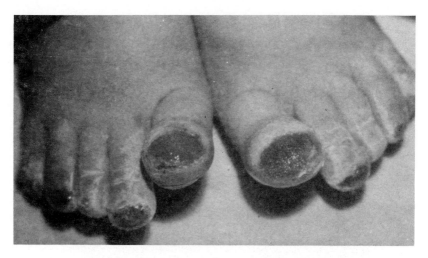

Fig. 25-19. Dystrophic nails in epidermolysis bullosa.

tional to the frequency of blistering of the skin.[60] Conjunctival involvement can lead to ulceration, pseudomembrane formation, and symblepharon. These changes appear to be localized and slowly progressive.[64] Corneal ulceration and scarring can result from the conjunctival changes or from erosions (Fig. 25-20); even perforation can occur. Eyelid scarring develops after blistering in the dermolytic types and can lead to ectropion.

Treatment. Blepharitis is treated with lid hygiene. Antibiotic ointment can be given for corneal erosions, but patching should be avoided because the skin frequently blisters beneath the tape. Bandage contact lenses can be used to decrease recurrences. Lubricants, moisture chambers, or skin grafts may be necessary for treatment of cicatricial ectropion.

DERMATITIS HERPETIFORMIS

Dermatitis herpetiformis is a chronic inflammatory dermatosis with erythematous, papillary vesicular or pustular lesions occurring in groups with a symmetric distribution and accompanied by intense itching. The skin lesions usually heal without scarring. Dermatitis herpetiformis commonly begins in

TABLE 25-2. Epidermolysis Bullosa

TYPE	INHERITANCE	SITE OF BLISTER FORMATION
Epidermolytic epidermolysis bullosa (simplex)	AD*	Within basal epithelial cells
Junctional epidermolysis bullosa (letalis)	AR†	Superficial lamina lucida of basement membrane
Dermolytic epidermolysis bullosa (dystrophic)		
Dominant (hyperplastic, others)	AD	Lamina densa of basement membrane and anchoring fibrils
Recessive (polydysplastic, others)	AR	Lamina densa of basement membrane and anchoring fibrils
Epidermolysis bullosa acquisita	− (Autoimmune)	Linear IgG and C3 along basement membrane

*Autosomal dominant.
†Autosomal recessive.

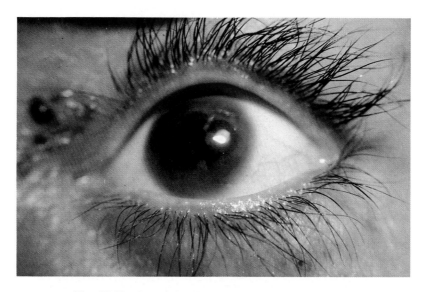

Fig. 25-20. Corneal involvement in epidermolysis bullosa.

the third or fourth decades and undergoes a course of exacerbations and remissions, generally lasting decades. The majority of patients also have jejunal atrophy, which can produce an enteropathy indistinguishable from adult celiac disease. Deposits of immunoglobulin, predominantly IgA, have been observed along the dermal-epidermal junction at the tips of the dermal papillae.[67] A reaction to wheat antigens may play a role in both the bowel and skin disease.

Eye involvement is not very common and usually occurs in severe cases. Shrinkage of the conjunctiva and conjunctival eosinophilia can occur.[68]

LINEAR IgA DISEASE (LINEAR IgA BULLOUS DERMATOSIS)

Linear IgA disease is a recently recognized form of bullous dermatosis that is closely related to dermatitis herpetiformis, bullous pemphigoid, and chronic bullous disease of childhood.[69,70] Linear

GENERAL SEVERITY	BULLAE	SCARRING	CONJUNCTIVAL INVOLVEMENT
Mildest form (except herpetiform type)	Clear, tense	−	Rare
Severe (survive <2 years)	Large sheets	− (Atrophy)	Extensive
Moderate	Bullae	+	20%
Moderate-severe	Large, flaccid, ±hemorrhagic	+	Majority
Variable	Tense ±hemorrhagic	+	Occasionally

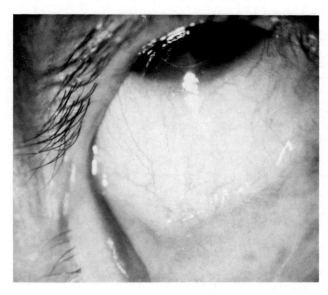

Fig. 25-21. Conjunctival scarring in linear IgA disease. (Courtesy of Eric Donnenfeld, Rockville Center, NY.)

deposition of IgA is seen along the epithelial basement membrane.[71] It occurs in adults and is characterized by tense blisters of varying size. The majority of cases have mucosal involvement.

Conjunctival inflammation occurs in many patients and can lead to scarring and symblepharon (Fig. 25-21).[69,72-74] In one recent review of 25 cases, conjunctival inflammation occurred in 72% and scarring in 40% of patients.[69]

CHRONIC BULLOUS DISEASE OF CHILDHOOD

Chronic bullous disease of childhood is an uncommon blistering disease that affects preschool-aged children. Large tense bullae occur mainly in flexural areas, such as the neck, axillae, and the groin. Annular lesions, such as those seen in erythema multiforme, also can be present. Chronic bullous disease of childhood runs a course of exacerbations and remissions, with gradually decreasing severity and resolution before the teens or adulthood. Linear IgA deposits are seen in the epithelial basement membrane.[75] In one recent study, ocular symptoms of pain, redness, grittiness, or discharge were present in 40% of children, and conjunctival scarring was seen in two of seven patients examined by an ophthalmologist.[69]

PEMPHIGUS VULGARIS

Pemphigus is another group of blistering skin diseases characterized by intraepithelial bulla formation. Autoantibodies are directed against an antigen located within the intercellular space of squamous epithelium, both epidermal and mucosal[76,77] (Fig. 25-22). IgG and complement components can be demonstrated in the intercellular spaces of early acantholytic lesions in nearly all cases.[78,79]

The most common type of pemphigus encountered in the United States is pemphigus vulgaris. A chronic disease, it most commonly occurs in the fourth and fifth decades of life, but can develop at any age. The skin lesions are flaccid, weeping bullae that erode, leaving large denuded areas. The mucous membranes are commonly involved, particularly the oral mucosa, and can be the site of onset.[80] Because the bullae form within the epithelium, and the substantia propria and dermis are not involved, scarring does not occur.

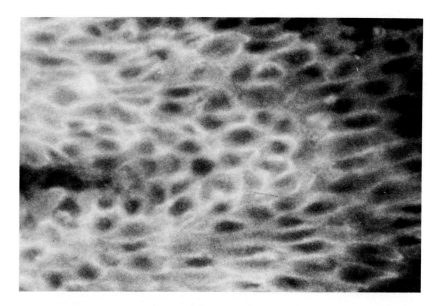

Fig. 25-22. Deposition of immunoglobulin in intercellular spaces in pemphigus vulgaris. (Courtesy of SF Bean, Houston.)

Ocular lesions occur in approximately 16% of patients[81] (Fig. 25-23). Intraepithelial conjunctival bullae are seen, mainly on the palpebral conjunctiva, and commonly near the inner canthus. The bullae rupture and nearly always heal without scarring. The cornea is not affected.

HYDROA VACCINIFORME

Patients with hydroa vacciniforme exhibit a congenitally abnormal sensitivity to sunlight. *Hydroa* refers to the vesicular nature of the eruption, and *vacciniforme* refers to the tendency for the lesions to heal without scarring. The sun-exposed areas, particularly the face and eyelids, are primarily involved (Fig. 25-24).

A hypertrophic conjunctivitis can occur. Conjunctival epithelial thickening and cyst formation are seen. The conjunctiva can be hyperemic, and vesicles, ulceration, and scarring can be present. Scarring and vascularization of the cornea also can occur.[82]

EXFOLIATIVE ERYTHRODERMA (EXFOLIATIVE DERMATITIS)

Exfoliative erythroderma refers to a group of papulosquamous eruptions that produce a diffuse erythroderma with desquamation (exfoliation) (Fig. 25-25). There are multiple causes; it often represents a generalized extension of a preexisting dermatosis, such as psoriasis, atopic dermatitis, pityriasis rubra pilaris, or ichthyosis. It can be associated with leukemia, lymphoma, tinea, or drug reaction, or it can be idiopathic. The prognosis is variable, depending on the underlying etiology; overall approximately 60% of patients recover within 8 to 10 months; 30% of patients die. Multiple recurrences can be seen in idiopathic cases.

OCULAR MANIFESTATIONS

Nonspecific conjunctival irritation can be caused by desquamation of scales from adjacent skin into the conjunctival sac. Chronic inflammation of the lid skin can produce cicatricial ectropion (Fig. 25-26). Some shrinkage of the lower conjunctival fornix can be seen. The cornea is not affected, except secondarily from ectropion or scaling.

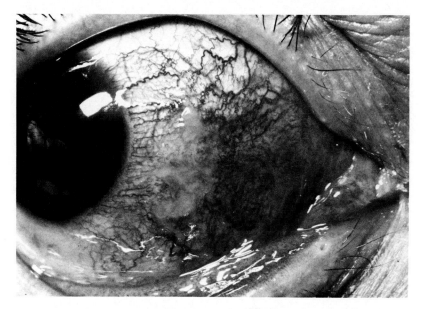

Fig. 25-23. Conjunctival lesion in pemphigus vulgaris. (From Roat MI and Thoft RA: Pemphigus. In Gold DH and Weingeist TA: The eye in systemic disease, Philadelphia, 1990, JB Lippincott.)

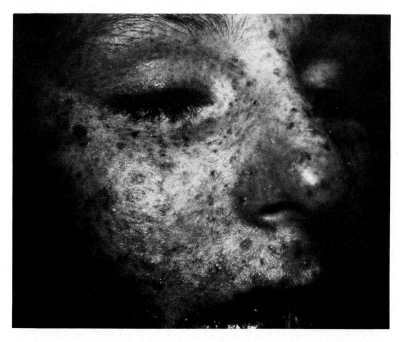

Fig. 25-24. Hydroa vacciniforme with papulovesicular lesions on exposed skin.

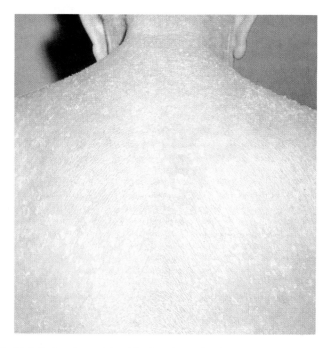

Fig. 25-25. Exfoliative dermatitis with chronic erythroderma and extensive skin scaling.

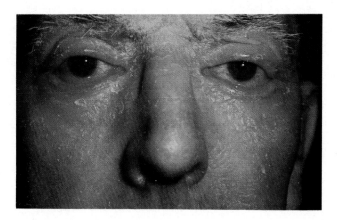

Fig. 25-26. Exfoliative dermatitis resulting in cicatricial ectropion.

ROSACEA

Rosacea is a dermatosis in which significant ocular morbidity can occur with relatively mild skin disease. It occurs primarily in the area of the forehead, nose, cheeks, and chin. Rosacea is a chronic disorder that affects women more than men, and its onset is usually between 25 and 50 years of age. It has a vascular component (erythema and telangiectasia) with or without an acneform component (papules, pustules, and nodules) (Fig. 25-27). No comedones are seen. Rhinophyma is an advanced form of the nasal disease in which there is hypertrophy of the nose with hyperplasia of sebaceous glands, fibrosis, and increased vascularity (Fig. 25-28). The skin condition is often overlooked, and certainly this disease is more common than realized.

The cause of rosacea and the relationship between the skin disease and the eye disease are not known. The associated blepharitis and meibomitis do not appear to be solely responsible for the eye complications. Attempts at relating the disease to staphylococcal infection have not been very successful: Cutaneous disease does not correlate well with the presence of mannitol-positive staphylococcal organisms, and organisms are still present on the eyelids and conjunctiva in most cases that respond to tetracycline treatment.

OCULAR MANIFESTATIONS

The most commonly associated eye findings are meibomitis and blepharitis. The lid margins are red and slightly thickened, and telangiectasia can be present. Inspissation of meibomian gland secretions, inflammation around the gland orifices, and foaming of the lid margins also may be present. Chalazia are frequently observed, as are staphylococcal infections of the lids.

The blood vessels of the conjunctiva can be dilated in a manner similar to the vessels of the skin of the eyelids, nose, and face. The dilated vessels most often are seen in the interpalpebral areas of the bulbar conjunctiva. They can be large and tortuous and can cause the misdiagnosis of infectious conjunctivitis. A nodular conjunctivitis, similar to a phlyctenule, also can be seen. These are small,

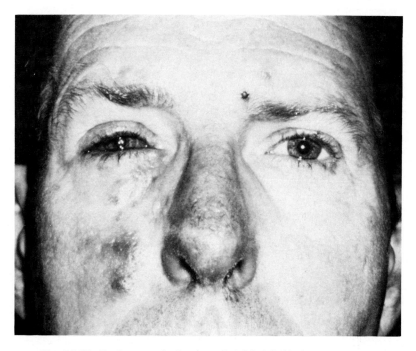

Fig. 25-27. Erythema and telangiectasia of facial skin in acne rosacea.

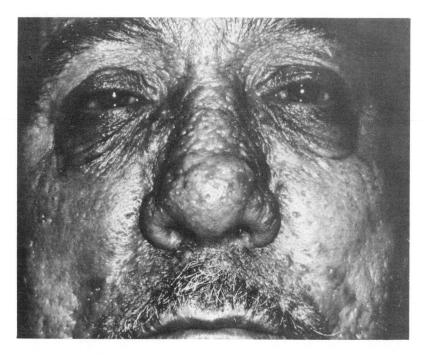

Fig. 25-28. Rhinophyma caused by acne rosacea.

gray, highly vascularized elevations of the bulbar conjunctiva, most often located near the limbus in the interpalpebral area. They can be sufficiently elevated to cause dellen formation.

The cornea can become extensively involved with scarring and vascularization. Rosacea keratitis is accompanied by pain, photophobia, and foreign body sensation. Superficial punctate keratopathy, involving the lower two thirds of the cornea, often accompanies the blepharitis or meibomitis.[83] Frequently, a leash of superficial vessels grows onto the cornea, most commonly in the inferior interpalpebral area, and can be associated with fluorescein staining and sometimes superficial infiltrates at the central edge (Fig. 25-29).

Progression usually occurs with a series of intermittent attacks. Ophthalmic remissions and exacerbations can occur independently of the course of the skin disease. Broad areas of pannus can form, and even the entire circumference of the limbus can be affected; but the disease usually remains worse inferiorly. Dense white scars can form, with heavy vascularization. Marginal or, less commonly, central corneal melting can develop (Fig. 25-30). Progressive thinning can occur during a single episode or with repeated bouts of inflammation. Perforation can occur, especially if topical corticosteroids have been used injudiciously.

Nodular episcleritis and scleritis occur rarely.[84]

TREATMENT

The patient with severe rosacea should be under the joint care of a dermatologist and ophthalmologist. The most effective treatment is systemic tetracycline 250 mg four times a day.[85,86] The reason that rosacea responds to tetracycline is not really known. If tetracycline cannot be tolerated, doxycycline (100 mg a day) can be tried instead.[87] Ampicillin and erythromycin (both 250 mg four times a day) also can be used, but they seem to be less effective. Lid hygiene should also be instituted, and any staphylococcal infection of the lid margins should be eliminated.

The tetracycline is continued four times a day for 1 month, and then decreased by 250 mg/day each month. Many patients require 250 to 500 mg/day to prevent recurrence of disease.

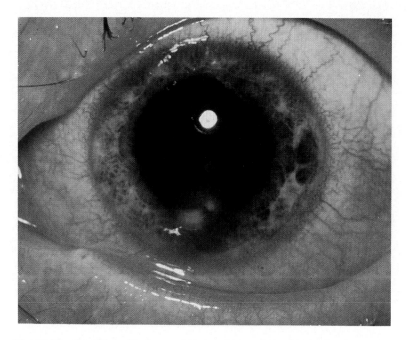

Fig. 25-29. Keratitis, with dense white opacities and vascularization in rosacea.

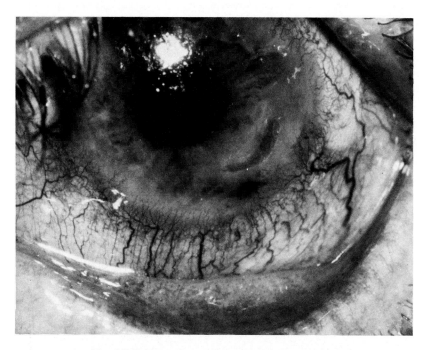

Fig. 25-30. Marginal corneal ulceration in rosacea.

Topical corticosteroid therapy can reduce ocular inflammation, vascular invasion, and infiltration. However, it is essential to ensure that infiltrates are not infectious before initiating treatment. In addition, attention must be paid to the length of treatment and the dose given, since this is a chronic disease, prone to superinfection, thinning, and perforation.

It may be necessary to perform a corneal graft if the cornea becomes extensively scarred, but the long-term results are not satisfactory.

SEBORRHEIC DERMATITIS

Seborrheic dermatitis is an oily skin eruption, seen as greasy scales on an erythematous patch of skin. The scalp, eyebrows, eyelids, nasolabial folds, retroauricular skin, chest, and back can be involved. Sebaceous gland dysfunction, with excess sebum production, is thought to be responsible for the skin findings. Nearly all patients with seborrheic blepharitis, and approximately one third of patients with meibomian gland dysfunction, have evidence of seborrheic dermatitis, but it is usually mild and easily overlooked.[88,89]

PSORIASIS

Psoriasis is a chronic skin disorder characterized by excessive proliferation of the epidermis. This is most often seen as geographic, demarcated, erythematous patches of skin covered with silvery white scales (Fig. 25-31). Auspitz sign is present; when hyperkeratotic scales are removed by scratching, small blood droplets appear within a few seconds.

It is a common disease that can be seen in any age group, but typically arises in the third decade. It usually lasts for life, but many patients experience remissions, which can last for years. It is more common in whites and women.

The primary defect in psoriasis is not known. Many patients have relatives with psoriasis, so heredity may be a factor. The psoriatic patient exhibits a tendency to accelerated epidermopoiesis in

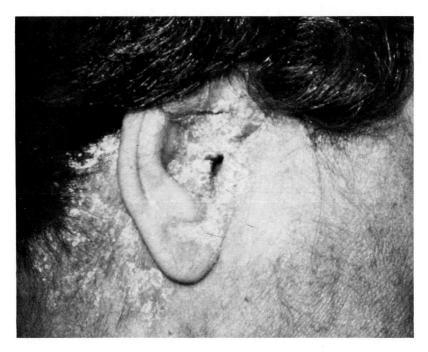

Fig. 25-31. Involvement of ear in psoriasis. Skin typically exhibits erythematous patches covered with silvery white scales.

response to external and internal stimuli. The nature of the stimuli is controversial, although it has been shown that the condition improves when the patient is in a warmer climate. Trauma, infection, and stress also may be trigger factors.

OCULAR MANIFESTATIONS

Ocular signs of psoriasis occur in approximately 10% of cases. The eyelids are frequently involved (Fig. 25-32) and can become swollen, red, and scaly. Scaling also may be seen at the base of the lashes. Trichiasis and madarosis occur in severe cases. A nonspecific conjunctivitis is common, and yellow plaquelike lesions can occur. Phlyctenule-like lesions can be seen at the limbus.

The cornea can be affected by superficial and deep opacities, vascularization, peripheral infiltration, and melting[90-93] (Fig. 25-33). Corneal involvement usually occurs when there is active disease in the skin of the lids.

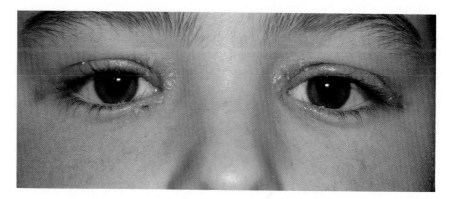

Fig. 25-32. Involvement of the lids in psoriasis.

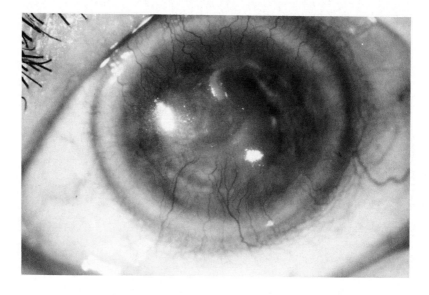

Fig. 25-33. Corneal ulceration and vascularization in psoriasis.

Treatment of psoriasis with psoralens and long ultraviolet light (PUVA) can cause superficial punctate keratitis.[94] Uveitis can occur, usually in patients with psoriatic arthritis.

TREATMENT

Treatment of the systemic and dermatologic problems should be undertaken by an internist and dermatologist, respectively. Topical therapy includes anthralin, tar, and corticosteroids. Systemic therapy with methotrexate, oral vitamin A (etretinate), and PUVA can be used in more severe cases.

Corneal melting is treated with lubrication, bandage contact lenses, tarsorrhaphy, and treatment of the systemic disease.

ICHTHYOSIS

Ichthyosis is a large group of disorders characterized by thickening (hyperkeratosis), fissuring, and scaling of the skin (Fig. 25-34). It can be hereditary or acquired. Acquired disease is usually associated with lymphoma. All involve retardation of desquamation or hyperproliferation of the epidermal cells. Four main hereditary groups exist (Table 25-3): (1) ichthyosis vulgaris (autosomal dominant); (2) recessive X-linked ichthyosis (steroid sulfatase deficiency); (3) lamellar ichthyosis, which includes both classic lamellar ichthyosis and congenital ichthyosiform erythroderma (autosomal recessive); and (4) epidermolytic hyperkeratosis (autosomal dominant). The heterozygous females in the X-linked form (carriers) do not develop the full-blown dermatosis but manifest some of the clinical features. Ichthyosis also is seen as part of the keratitis, ichthyosis, and deafness syndrome, which is discussed later.

OCULAR MANIFESTATIONS

Lid ectropion can be seen in lamellar ichthyosis.[95] In the X-linked form, diffuse dotlike or striate opacities can be seen on Descemet's membrane or immediately anterior to it (Fig. 25-35).[96-101] These

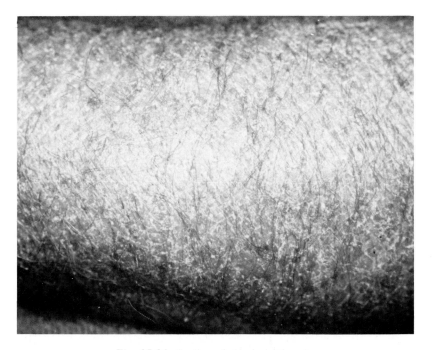

Fig. 25-34. Scaling of skin in ichthyosis.

TABLE 25-3. Major Forms of Ichthyosis

FEATURES	ICHTHYOSIS VULGARIS	X-LINKED ICHTHYOSIS	LAMELLAR ICHTHYOSIS*	EPIDERMOLYTIC HYPERKERATOSIS
Onset	<1 year	<1 year	Birth	Birth
Inheritance	AD†	X-R§	AR‡ (AD)	AD
Scales on skin	Fine, extensor surfaces	Brownish, extensor surfaces of extremities	White→brown, fine→large, over most of body	Often dark, warty, generalized
Palmoplantar hyperkeratosis	Mild	—	Moderate	Mild-severe
Associated disease	Atopy	Cryptorchidism, steroid sulfatase deficiency	Prematurity, sepsis, heat intolerance	Sepsis
Eye findings	None	Pre-Descemet opacities, band keratopathy, superficial nodular lesions, increased corneal nerve visibility	Ectropion, conjunctivitis (CIE), keratitis (CIE)	None

*At least two different forms; classic lamellar ichthyosis and congenital ichthyosiform erythroderma (CIE).
†Autosomal dominant.
‡Autosomal recessive.
§X-linked recessive.

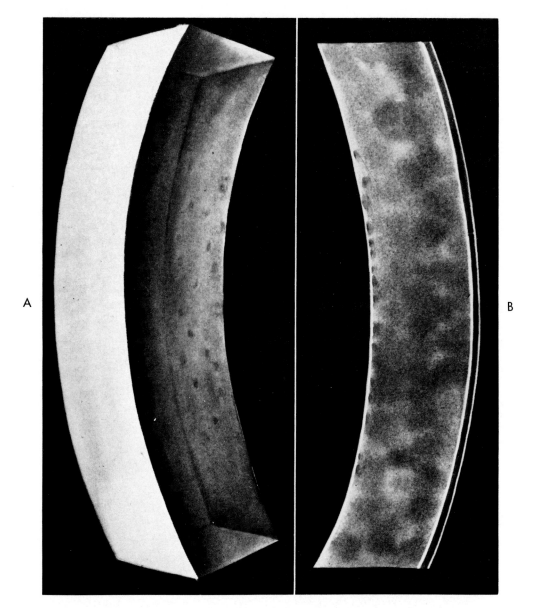

Fig. 25-35. Punctate or striate opacities on or anterior to Descemet's membrane in x-linked ichthyosis. **A,** Parallelepiped section. **B,** Optical section.

opacities usually are not present until adulthood in affected males. Larger white or gray deep stromal opacities also have been noted.[102] Small refractile bodies in the epithelium, superficial stroma and endothelium, prominent corneal nerves, and band keratopathy also have been reported.[103,104] Superficial nodular corneal degeneration and ulceration are rarely part of the picture (Fig. 25-36).

Conjunctivitis and keratitis can be present in the congenital ichthyosiform erythroderma form of lamellar ichthyosis (Fig. 25-37),[105] and superficial punctate keratopathy can be present in all forms.

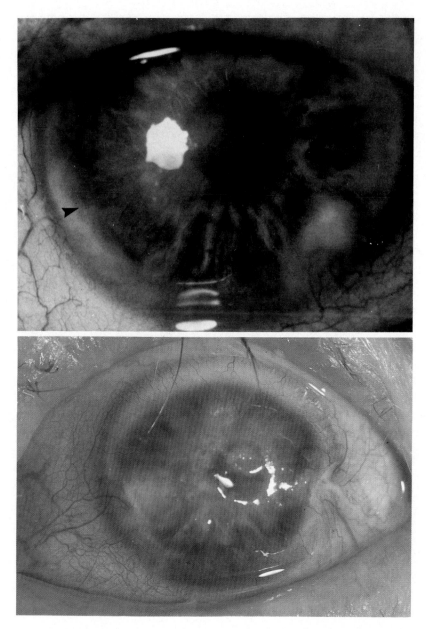

Fig. 25-36. Superficial nodular corneal degeneration and ulceration in ichthyosis.

KERATITIS, ICHTHYOSIS, AND DEAFNESS SYNDROME

Keratitis, ichthyosis, and deafness (KID) syndrome is a rare congenital syndrome.[106,107] Some cases exhibit autosomal dominant transmission,[108,109] whereas others are sporadic. The ichthyosis usually is present at an early age. Hyperkeratosis of the palms and soles with a characteristic dotted and waxy pattern in bas-relief is noted (Fig. 25-38). A reticulated pattern of hyperkeratosis on the face, perioral furrowing, heavy grain–leatherlike keratoderma, leukoplakia of the buccal mucosa, deep lingual fissuring along the dorsal midline of the tongue, and rugae of the buccal mucosa can be seen. Follicular plugging and scant or absent hair, eyebrows, and eyelashes are noted (Figs. 25-39

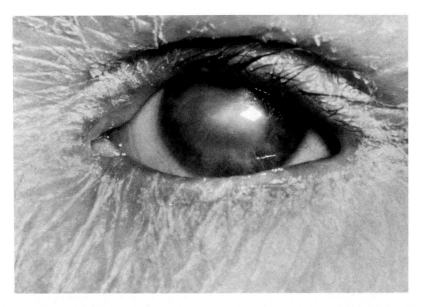

Fig. 25-37. Congenital ichthyosiform erythroderma with scaling of skin and corneal opacification.

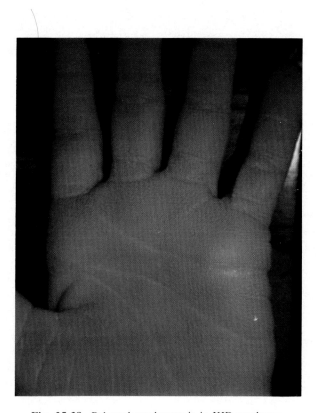

Fig. 25-38. Palmar hyperkeratosis in KID syndrome.

and 25-40). The nails can be thick and dystrophic (Fig. 25-41). Many patients have decreased sweating caused by hyperkeratosis and plugging of the eccrine glands.

Deafness is severe and is of the neurosensory type; it is present at birth or develops in the first 2 years of life. These patients also appear to be prone to fungal infections of the skin and squamous cell carcinoma. Hypoplasia of the cerebellum has been noted in some patients.[110-112]

Punctate epithelial keratopathy and vascularizing keratitis (Fig. 25-42) are prominent features. The pannus is superficial and can extend 360 degrees. It can be accompanied by numerous intraepithelial cysts. Corneal thinning and stromal opacification also occur.

Oral vitamin A (etretinate) can improve the skin condition.[109]

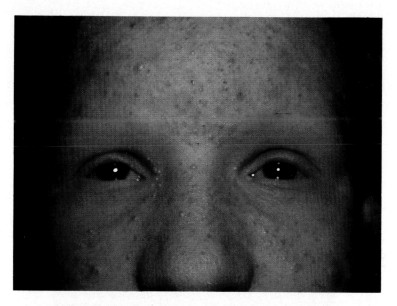

Fig. 25-39. Facial sebaceous dysfunction in KID syndrome.

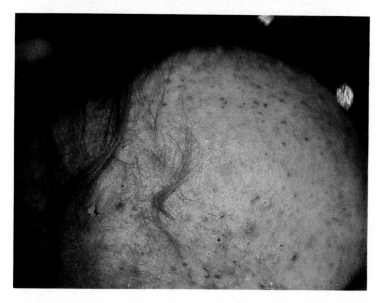

Fig. 25-40. Skin lesions as noted on scalp in KID syndrome. Note loss of hair.

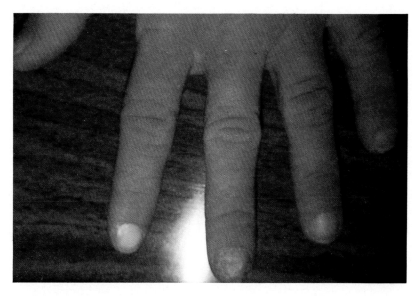

Fig. 25-41. Fingernail malformation in KID syndrome.

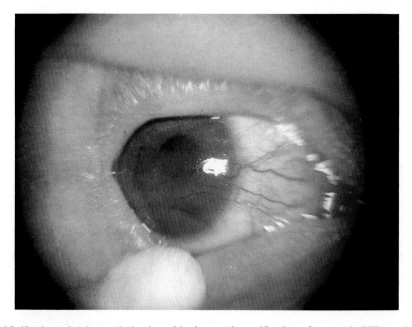

Fig. 25-42. Superficial vascularization, thinning, and opacification of cornea in KID syndrome.

JUVENILE XANTHOGRANULOMA

Juvenile xanthogranulomas are firm skin nodules that are reddish at first and then turn yellow-orange (Fig. 25-43). They usually appear before the end of the first year of life and resolve within 3 to 6 years. Histologically, a granulomatous infiltrate is present, containing lipid-laden macrophages, lymphocytes, foreign body giant cells, and Touton giant cells.

Xanthogranulomas can involve the iris and ciliary body (Fig. 25-44). The iris lesions can cause spontaneous anterior chamber hemorrhages and secondary glaucoma can ensue.[113,114] Multiple

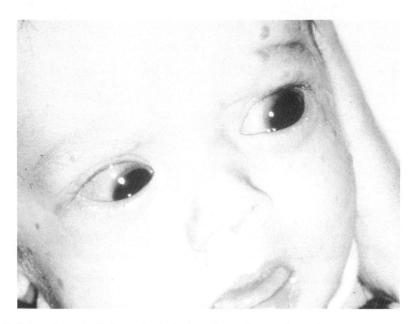

Fig. 25-43. Yellow-red papular lesions of skin in juvenile xanthogranuloma. These can occur as epibulbar lesions that can extend onto the cornea.

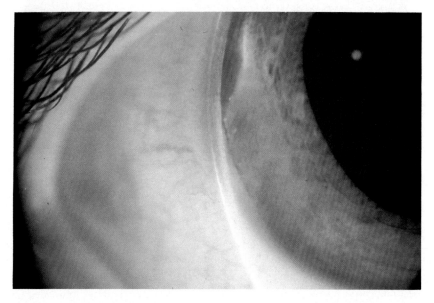

Fig. 25-44. Iris lesion in juvenile xanthogranuloma. (Courtesy of David A. Hiles, Pittsburgh.)

phlyctenule-like epibulbar lesions occasionally occur and can extend onto the cornea.[115] They are yellow-white to pink and can resemble the salmon-pink nodules seen in lymphoma. Corneal blood staining can result from hyphema, and corneal edema and enlargement can result from glaucoma.

KERATOSIS FOLLICULARIS SPINULOSA DECALVANS

The hallmarks of keratosis follicularis spinulosa decalvans (keratosis pilaris decalvans, follicular ichthyosis, Sieman's disease) are hyperkeratotic, conical, horny plugs at the hair follicle openings that give the skin a coarse texture. Sites of predilection are the face, scalp, eyebrows, neck, arms, and fingers. In addition, some loss of hair occurs at the lateral portion of the eyebrow and occiput. Skeletal hypoplasia, failure to thrive, deafness, and recurrent infections have been reported.[96,116]

Ocular Manifestations

Keratosis follicularis spinulosa decalvans affects the cornea only rarely. It may show circumferential pannus with diffuse, superficial, farinaceous opacities[117] (Fig. 25-45, *A*). Female carrier's may show recurrent erosions, epithelial or subepithelial opacities, and prominent corneal nerves. The epithelium can be thick and irregular and contain irregularly shaped nuclei, vacuoles, and keratotic spines (Fig. 25-45, *B,C*).

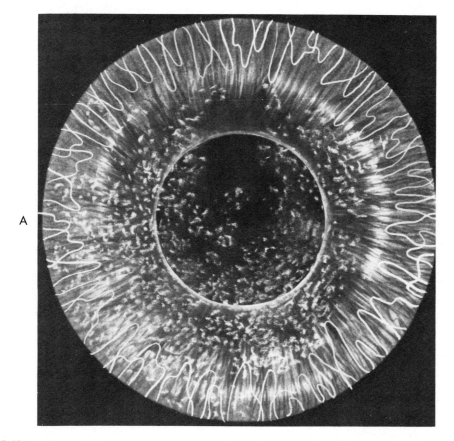

Fig. 25-45. In Sieman's disease, one may see circumferential pannus with diffuse superficial farinaceous opacities. **A,** Diagrammatic representation of corneal findings.   *Continued.*

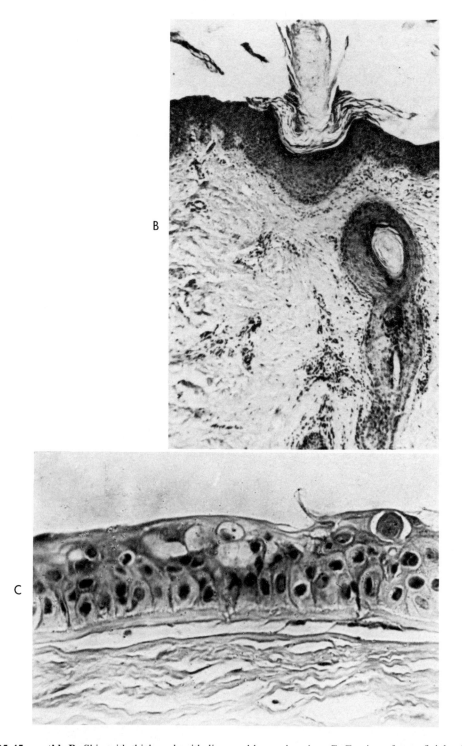

Fig. 25-45, cont'd. B, Skin with thickened epithelium and keratotic spine. **C,** Erosion of superficial epithelium. (Courtesy A. Franceschetti, Geneva, Switzerland.)

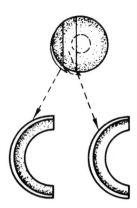

Fig. 25-46. In Kyrle's disease minute, yellow-brown opacities can be seen subepithelially and in anterior stroma. (From Tessler HH, Apple DJ, and Goldberg M: Arch Ophthalmol 90:278, 1973.)

KYRLE'S DISEASE

Kyrle's disease is characterized by multiple hyperpigmented keratotic papules that have a central plug. They can be located on any part of the body, with relative sparing of the palms, soles, and face. The cause is unknown; it can be associated with chronic renal failure or diabetes mellitus.[118]

OCULAR MANIFESTATIONS

The corneal lesions of Kyrle's disease have a unique appearance. They consist of minute, yellow-brown, subepithelial opacities (Fig. 25-46). Their greatest density and deepest penetration occur at the limbus, the least at the corneal center.[119] Posterior subcapsular cataracts also can be found.

KERATOSIS FOLLICULARIS (DARIER'S DISEASE)

In Darier's disease small, brown scaly papules affect mainly the scalp, face, and upper trunk (Fig. 25-47). The nails and oral mucosa are frequently affected. Histologic findings are diagnostic: focal acantholysis and abnormal cornification with dyskeratotic cells. Darier's disease is autosomally inherited.

OCULAR MANIFESTATIONS

Corneal involvement in Darier's disease is varied, but peripheral opacities and central epithelial irregularity in a radiating cobweb pattern are most often seen[120,121] (Fig. 25-48). In addition, a dense yellow peripheral pannus and a central stromal opacity can be noted. The eyelids may exhibit keratotic plaques, and sometimes staphylococcal blepharitis and trichiasis are seen.

DIFFERENTIAL DIAGNOSIS

Hyperkeratosis of the palms and soles can be associated with corneal disorders in the following diseases:
1. Richner-Hanhart syndrome
2. Pityriasis rubra pilaris
3. Hypohidrotic ectodermal dysplasia
4. Ichthyosis
5. Pachyonychia congenita
6. Papillon-Lefèvre syndrome
7. Keratosis follicularis (Darier's disease)

The skin lesions improve with oral retinoid therapy, but the corneal lesions do not.

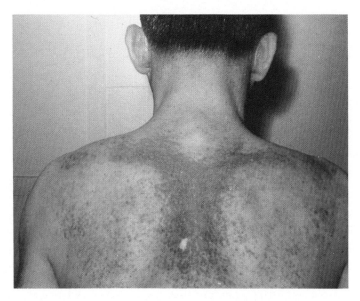

Fig. 25-47. Darier's disease, showing thick vegetative plaques and papulomatous growths covered with greasy crusts. (From Grayson M and Keates RH: Manual of diseases of the cornea, Boston, 1969, Little, Brown & Co.)

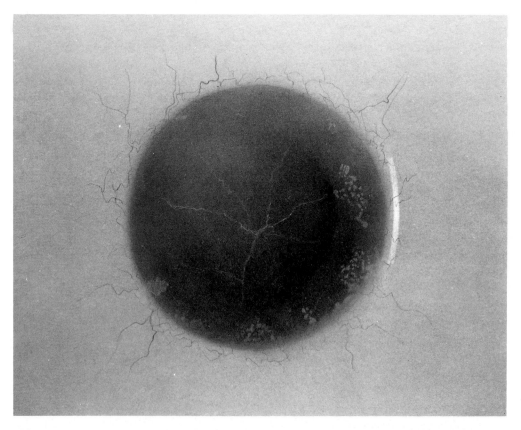

Fig. 25-48. Schematic illustration of peripheral opacities and central radiating lines in corneal epithelium of 43-year-old woman with Darier's disease. (From Blackman HJ, Rodrigues MM, and Peck GL: Ophthalmology 87:931, 1980.)

WERNER'S SYNDROME

Werner's syndrome is a rare autosomal recessive disorder marked by progeroid features. A cessation of growth occurs during the second decade, and graying of the hair, balding, atrophy of skin and muscles, high-pitched voice, trophic ulcers of the legs, painful hyperkeratotic skin lesions, metastatic calcification, osteoporosis, and hypogonadism are among the other features.

Bilateral posterior stellate cataracts appear usually between the ages of 20 and 35. Bullous keratopathy has followed cataract extraction in many cases.[122,123] Metastatic corneal calcification has been observed after both cataract extraction and penetrating keratoplasty.[124] Blue sclera,[119] iris telangiectasia, and retinitis pigmentosa have been reported.[125,126]

ACRODERMATITIS ENTEROPATHICA

This rare familial disease usually appears in early infancy and follows a characteristic clinical course. One sees a rash symmetrically distributed over the face and bony prominences (Fig. 25-49). The rash first goes through a vesiculobullous stage, then assumes a more erythematous, squamous, psoriasiform appearance. Dystrophy of the nails and alopecia, with loss of eyelashes and eyebrows, are also seen. The infant is withdrawn and irritable and has diarrhea.

This disease appears to result from faulty absorption of zinc. The synthesis of keratins is affected by the zinc deficiency. Systemic administration of zinc sulfate often results in rapid improvement.[127,128] Zinc treatment must be maintained for life.

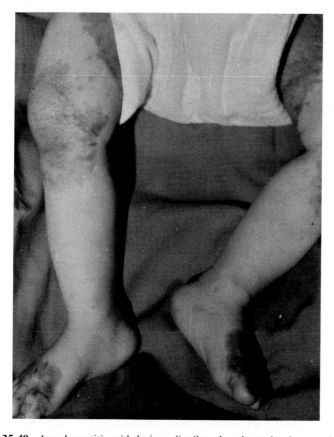

Fig. 25-49. Acrodermatitis with lesions distributed on buttocks, legs, and feet.

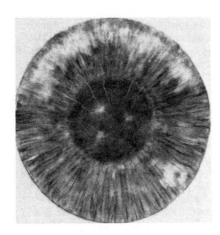

Fig. 25-50. Corneal lesions seen in some cases of acrodermatitis enteropathica are radiating, linear, white-brown, slightly whorl-like opacities passing from limbus about two thirds of the distance to the corneal center. (From Matta CS, Felker GV, and Ide CH: Arch Ophthalmol 93:140, 1975.)

OCULAR MANIFESTATIONS

Blepharitis, photophobia, and conjunctivitis can be seen. Bilateral superficial punctate lesions and nebulous subepithelial opacities of the cornea, mainly located in the upper paralimbal region, also are seen.[129,130] These are radiating, linear, white to light brown, slightly whorl-like opacities passing from the limbus about two thirds of the distance to the corneal center (Fig. 25-50). In some cases a corneal opacity occurs at the tips of these radiating lines, and in one case anterior corneal vascularization occurred.[131] Histologic examination of this case indicated thinning and loss of polarity of the epithelium and absence of Bowman's layer.[131]

MALIGNANT ATROPHIC PAPULOSIS (DEGO'S DISEASE)

Malignant atrophic papulosis is a rare systemic disease with skin, gastrointestinal, and central nervous system manifestations. The underlying process is a lymphocyte-mediated vasculitis, the etiology of which is unknown; it has been hypothesized that a transmissible agent (for example, a slow virus) is responsible.[132] The skin lesions may be the first sign of the disease and are pathognomonic. The lesions are firm, pink or pale red, smooth, dome-shaped papules, 2 to 5 mm in diameter, which can develop central necrosis, resulting in a porcelain white color (Fig. 25-51). Thin white scales can overlie the lesion, which can demonstrate pink, telangiectatic borders.[133]

Gastrointestinal involvement occurs in the majority of patients, usually manifested as cramps, pain, vomiting, or bleeding. Infarcts and vascular thromboses can affect the central nervous system and other organs. Approximately 50% of patients die within 3 years.

Conjunctival lesions can occur and are seen as avascular patches, sometimes accompanied by telangiectasias and microaneurysms.[134-136] They can be mistaken for a Bitot's spot. Ptosis, neuritis, diplopia, papilledema, and visual field abnormalities can result from neurologic involvement.

MELKERSSON-ROSENTHAL SYNDROME

Melkersson-Rosenthal syndrome consists of recurrent swelling of the lip or the face, intermittent facial nerve paralysis, and furrowed tongue. The corneal lesions consist of thickening and opacification of Bowman's layer. On retroillumination the lesions appear as a dense central horizontal core with graceful swirling rods in the nature of horse hair[137] (Fig. 25-52). There may be a diffuse punc-

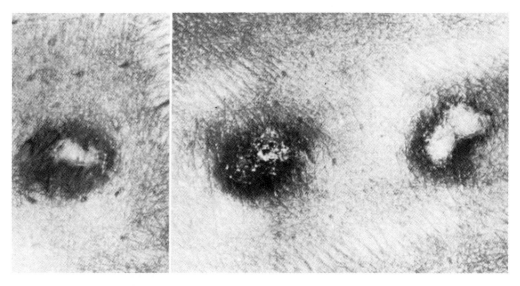

Fig. 25-51. Skin lesions with atrophic porcelain white centers are characteristic of malignant atrophic papulosis. (From Howsden SM et al: Arch Dermatol 112:1582, 1976.)

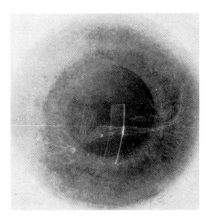

Fig. 25-52. Corneal lesions in Melkersson-Rosenthal syndrome are composed of graceful swirling lines. (From Mulvihill JJ et al: Arch Intern Med 132:116, 1973.)

tate keratopathy of the interpalpebral cornea, with focal epithelial thickening and opacification adjacent to the areas of opaque Bowman's layer. In addition, keratoconjunctivitis sicca occurs.

XERODERMA PIGMENTOSUM

Xeroderma pigmentosum is an autosomal recessive disorder characterized by intolerance to sunlight. It is caused by a defect in the repair of ultraviolet light–induced DNA damage. Prolonged erythema and edema occur with even minimal sun exposure. With time, the sun-exposed skin develops macules and atrophies, with hypopigmented plaques, telangiectasias, dryness, and scaling (Fig. 25-53). Beginning as early as the first decade, these children develop numerous malignant cutaneous tumors, particularly basal cell carcinomas and squamous cell carcinomas. There is a predilection for the circumoral and circumorbital areas.

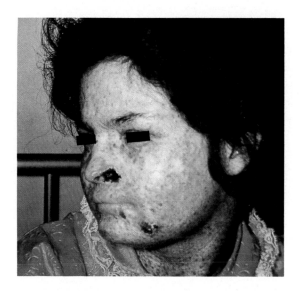

Fig. 25-53. Skin changes in xeroderma pigmentosum, including squamous and basal cell carcinomas of the skin.

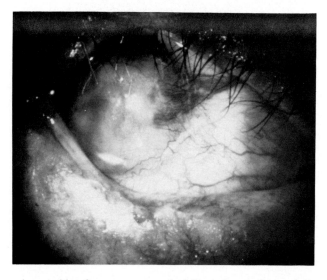

Fig. 25-54. Corneal scarring resulting from exposure and trichiasis in xeroderma pigmentosum. (From Sugar J: Metabolic disorders of the cornea. In Kaufman HE et al: The cornea, New York, 1989, Churchill-Livingstone.)

OCULAR MANIFESTATIONS

Most patients with xeroderma pigmentosum have photophobia, and many have conjunctivitis. The conjunctivae are dry and hyperemic. Telangiectasias and pigmented lesions occur on the bulbar conjunctiva. There can be recurrent inflammation, sometimes with membrane formation, and symblepharon can result.[138] Loss of cilia, ectropion, and entropion are common and can result in conjunctival or corneal exposure.[139] The cornea can become vascularized and scarred (Fig. 25-54), and limbal tumors, particularly squamous cell carcinoma, are frequently encountered.[140] Endothelial cell density is less than normal for cell age, and the coefficient of variation of cell size is increased, suggesting an increased rate of endothelial injury and loss due to ultraviolet exposure.[141]

The major treatment is avoidance of ultraviolet radiation. Close monitoring, for development of tumors, and early excision are essential. Lid deformities should be surgically corrected to prevent corneal complications.

ACANTHOSIS NIGRICANS

Acanthosis nigricans refers to a complex of skin findings observed in a number of internal diseases. A pigmented, velvety, rugated hypertrophy of the skin affects the face, neck, groin, axillae, and periumbilical area. Soft papillomas also can be seen in affected areas. Histologically the primary abnormality is papillomatosis of the epidermis with hyperkeratosis.

The lid skin can be involved, resulting in thickening and pigmentation.[142] Palpebral conjunctival epithelial hypertrophy, with hyperkeratosis, has been observed in some cases.[143] The cornea can be affected by infiltration and vascularization.

PAPILLON-LEFÈVRE SYNDROME

Papillon-Lefèvre syndrome is an extremely rare autosomal recessive syndrome manifested by periodontitis, causing premature shedding of teeth, hyperkeratosis of the palms and soles, and calcifications of the falx and tentorium. Occasionally the cornea can be involved, with peripheral vascularization and epithelial hypertrophy.

CUTIS VERTICIS GYRATA (ROSENTHAL-KLOEPFER SYNDROME)

In Rosenthal-Kloepfer syndrome the skin is thrown into convoluted folds and furrows, especially on the scalp. It may be accompanied by an acromegaloid habitus, cranial deformities, mental retardation, and epilepsy. These findings plus corneal leukomas were reported in the initial pedigree described by Rosenthal and Kloepfer.[123]

DERMOCHONDROCORNEAL DYSTROPHY OF FRANCOIS

This condition is transmitted as an autosomal recessive trait. Deformities of the hands and feet occur in the first 5 years of life. Xanthomalike nodules appear in the skin of the nose, ears, and extensor aspects of the elbows and joints of the fingers.

By the end of the first decade, white or brownish, irregular subepithelial opacities appear.[144] The corneal periphery is clear, and the stroma and endothelium are normal. Vision is somewhat decreased, but the corneal changes do not advance.

OTHER SKIN DISEASES

A number of other skin diseases that can affect the cornea or conjunctiva are described in Table 25-4.[145-150]

TABLE 25-4. Other Skin Diseases with Corneal or Conjunctival Findings

DISORDER	INHERITANCE	MAJOR FINDINGS	ANTERIOR SEGMENT FINDINGS
Hereditary benign intraepithelial dyskeratosis	AD*	Oral dyskeratoses	Conjunctival hyperemia; foamy gelatinous perilimbal plaques; corneal vascularization
Hereditary mucoepithelial dysplasia	AD	Mucosal dyskeratoses; follicular keratoses; alopecia; lung disease	Photophobia; tearing; conjunctival dyskeratoses; corneal vascularization; keratitis; cataracts
Dyskeratosis congenita	(?)X-R[†]	Reticulated hyperpigmentation; nail dystrophy; mucosal leukoplakia	Punctal stenosis; blepharitis; ectropion; madarosis; bullous conjunctivitis[145]
Epidermal nevus syndrome	?	Linear epidermal or sebaceous nevi; CNS and skeletal abnormalities	Nevus involving ocular surface; lid coloboma; limbal lipodermoids; corneal opacities[146]
Pili torti	AD	Twisted hairs	Corneal opacities[147]
Progressive facial hemiatrophy (Romberg-Parry syndrome)	—	Atrophy of the soft tissues of half the face (Fig. 25-55); seizures; trigeminal neuralgia	Ectropion, iritis; corneal exposure; band keratopathy (Fig. 25-56); bullous keratopathy; pupil and extraocular muscle abnormalities
Sjögren-Larsson syndrome	AR[‡]	Ichthyosis; mental retardation; spasticity	"Corneal dystrophy"[148]
Incontinentia pigmenti	X-D[§]	Vesicular lesions leave linear, whorled hyperpigmentation (Fig. 25-57)	Conjunctival pigmentation; corneal opacity; interstitial keratitis[149]
Papillon-LeFèvre syndrome	AR	Hyperkeratosis of palms and soles; periodontitis; calcification of falx cerebri	Peripheral corneal vascularization; corneal epithelial hypertrophy

Pachyonychia congenita (Jackson-Lawler type)	AD	Nail thickening (pachyonychia); palmoplantar hyperkeratoses; follicular keratosis	Corneal dyskeratoses
Pityriasis rubra pilaris	Sporadic or AD	Follicular squamous papules; palmar plantar keratoderma (Fig. 25-58)	Conjunctival and corneal keratinization; fibrovascular pannus; interstitial scarring; corneal epithelial erosions; corneal vascularization
Rothmund-Thomson syndrome	AR	Poikiloderma; atrophy, hypopigmentation, or hyperpigmentation; telangiectasia; hyperkeratosis; skeletal anomalies; hypogonadism	Cataracts; band keratopathy; keratoconus
Anhidrotic ectodermal dysplasia	X-R; AR	Hypohidrosis; hypotrichosis; defective dentition; absence of sebaceous glands	Keratitis sicca; peripheral pannus; tiny intraepithelial cysts; punctal atresia
Ectrodactyly-ectodermal dysplasia-cleft lip/palate (EEC) syndrome	AD	Lobster-claw deformity of hands; anomalies of the central face; sparse hair; hypohidrosis; deafness	Abnormal or absent meibomian glands; lacrimal drainage system abnormalities; conjunctival scarring; entropion; secondary corneal disease
Cutis verticis gyrata (Rosenthal-Kloepfer syndrome)	—	Convoluted folds and furrows in skin, especially the scalp; acromegaloid habitus; mental retardation; epilepsy	Corneal leukomas[150]

*Autosomal dominant.
†X-linked recessive.
‡Autosomal recessive.
§X-linked dominant.

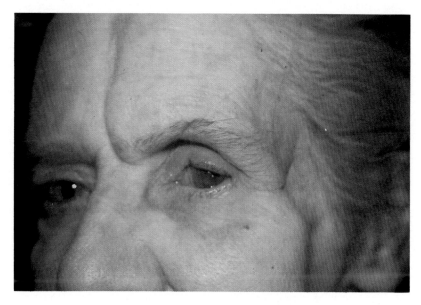

Fig. 25-55. Parry-Romberg syndrome of progressive hemifacial atrophy showing severe depression of zygomatic and temporal areas. (From Grayson M and Pieroni D: Am J Ophthalmol 70:42, 1970.)

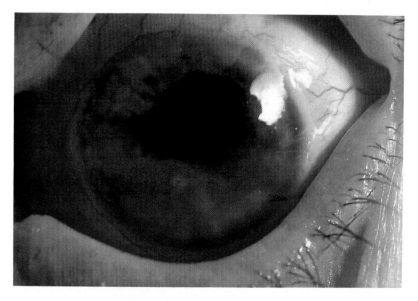

Fig. 25-56. Early corneal edema and band keratopathy in Parry-Romberg syndrome. (From Grayson M and Pieroni D: Am J Ophthalmol 70:42, 1970.)

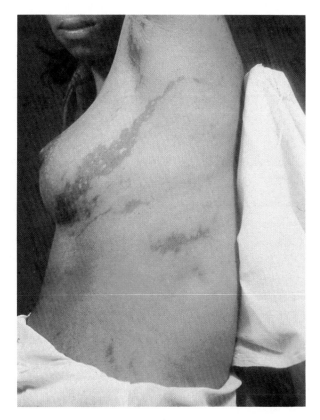

Fig. 25-57. Pigmented, whorl-like striae and hypertrophic skin changes are typical of incontinentia pigmenti.

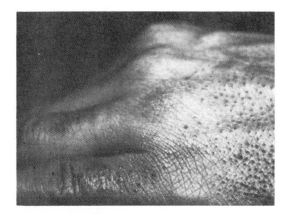

Fig. 25-58. Pityriasis rubra pilaris lesions exhibit spiny, keratotic, scaly, acuminate follicular papules on an erythematous base. (From Grayson M and Keates RH: Manual of diseases of the cornea, Boston, 1969, Little, Brown & Co.)

REFERENCES

1. Lever WF: Pemphigus and pemphigoid, J Am Acad Dermatol 1:2, 1979.
2. Wright PG: Cicatrizing conjunctivitis, Trans Ophthalmol Soc UK 105:1, 1986.
3. Mondino BJ and Brown SI: Ocular cicatricial pemphigoid, Ophthalmology 88:95, 1981.
4. Foster CS, Wilson LA, and Ekins MB: Immunosuppressive therapy for progressive ocular cicatricial pemphigoid, Ophthalmology 89:340, 1982.
5. Tauber J, Melamed S, and Foster CS: Glaucoma in patients with ocular cicatricial pemphigoid, Ophthalmology 96:33, 1989.
6. Norn MS and Kristensen EB: Benign mucous membrane pemphigoid. II. Cytology, Acta Ophthalmol (Copenh) 52:282, 1974.
7. Person JR and Rogers RS: Bullous and cicatricial pemphigoid: clinical, histopathologic, and immunopathologic correlations, Mayo Clin Proc 52:54, 1977.
8. Ralph RA: Conjunctival goblet cell density in normal subjects and in dry eye syndromes, Invest Ophthalmol 14:299, 1975.
9. Nelson JD and Wright JC: Conjunctival goblet cell densities in ocular surface disease, Arch Ophthalmol 102:1049, 1984.
10. Anderson SR et al: Benign mucous membrane pemphigoid. III. Biopsy, Acta Ophthalmol (Copenh) 52:455, 1974.
11. Carroll JM and Kuwabara T: Ocular pemphigus: an electron microscopic study of conjunctival and corneal epithelium, Arch Ophthalmol 80:683, 1968.
12. Galbavy EJ and Foster CS: Ultrastructural characteristics of conjunctiva in cicatricial pemphigoid, Cornea 4:127, 1985.
13. Furney N et al: Immunofluorescent studies of ocular cicatricial pemphigoid, Am J Ophthalmol 80:825, 1975.
14. Griffith MR et al: Immunofluorescent studies in mucous membrane pemphigoid, Arch Dermatol 109:195, 1974.
15. Rogers RS et al: Immunopathology of cicatricial pemphigoid: studies of complement deposition, J Invest Dermatol 68:39, 1977.
16. Proia AD, Foulks GN, and Sanfilippo FP: Ocular cicatricial pemphigoid with granular IgA and complement deposition, Arch Ophthalmol 103:1669, 1985.
17. Waltman SR and Yarran D: Circulating autoantibodies in ocular pemphigoid, Am J Ophthalmol 77:891, 1974.
18. Dantzig PI: Circulating antibodies in cicatricial pemphigoid, Arch Dermatol 108:264, 1973.
19. Leonard J et al: Immunofluorescent studies in ocular cicatricial pemphigoid, Br J Dermatol 118:209, 1988.
20. Meyer JR, Migliorati CA, Daniels RE, and Greenspan JS: Localization of basement membrane components in mucous membrane pemphigoid, J Invest Dermatol 84:105, 1985.
21. Thoft RA et al: Ocular cicatricial pemphigoid associated with hyperproliferation of the conjunctival epithelium, Am J Ophthalmol 98:37, 1984.
22. Mondino BJ, Brown SI, and Rabin BS: HLA antigens in ocular cicatricial pemphigoid, Br J Ophthalmol 62:265, 1978.
23. Bean SF et al: Ocular cicatricial pemphigoid, Trans Am Acad Ophthalmol Otolaryngol 81:806, 1976.
24. Waltman SR and Yarian D: Circulating autoantibodies in ocular pemphigoid, Am J Ophthalmol 77:891, 1974.
25. Patten JT, Cavanagh HD, and Allansmith MR: Induced ocular pseudopemphigoid, Am J Ophthalmol 82:272, 1976.
26. Fiore PM, Jacobs IH, and Goldberg DB: Drug-induced pemphigoid: a spectrum of diseases, Arch Ophthalmol 105:1660, 1987.
27. Pouliquen Y et al: Drug-induced cicatricial pemphigoid affecting the conjunctiva: light and electron microscopic features, Ophthalmology 93:775, 1986.
28. Lass JH, Thoft RA, and Dohlman CH: Idoxuridine-induced conjunctival cicatrization, Arch Ophthalmol 101:747, 1983.
29. Flach A: Symblepharon in sarcoidosis, Am J Ophthalmol 85:210, 1978.
30. Mondino BJ and Brown SI: Immunosuppressive therapy in ocular cicatricial pemphigoid, Arch Ophthalmol 96:453, 1983.
31. Hardy KM et al: Benign mucous membrane pemphigoid, Arch Dermatol 104:467, 1971.
32. Rogers RS, Seehaer JR, and Perry HO: Treatment of cicatricial (benign mucous membrane) pemphigoid with dapsone, J Am Acad Dermatol 6:215, 1982.
33. Fujikawa LS and Nussenblatt RB: The cornea and dermatologic disorders. In Smolin G and Thoft RA, editors: The cornea: scientific foundations and clinical practice, Boston, 1983, Little, Brown & Co.
34. Sainz de la Maza M, Tauber J, and Foster CS: Cataract surgery in ocular cicatricial pemphigoid, Ophthalmology 95:481, 1988.
35. Venning B et al: Mucosal involvement in bullous and cicatricial pemphigoid, Br J Dermatol 118:7, 1988.
36. Jordan RE, Triftshauser CT, and Schroeter AL: Direct immunofluorescent studies of pemphigus and bullous pemphigoid, Arch Dermatol 103:486, 1971.
37. Ahmed AR, Maize J, and Provost TT: Bullous pemphigoid: clinical and immunologic follow-up after successful therapy, Arch Dermatol 113:1043, 1977.
38. Soter NA and Wuepper KD: Erythema multiforme and Stevens-Johnson syndrome. In Samter M, editor: Immunological diseases, ed 4, Boston, 1988, Little, Brown & Co.
39. Howard GM: The Stevens-Johnson syndrome: ocular prognosis and treatment, Am J Ophthalmol 55:893, 1963.
40. Foster CS et al: Episodic conjunctival inflammation after Stevens-Johnson syndrome, Ophthalmology 95:453, 1988.
41. Arstikoitis MJ: Ocular aftermath of Stevens-Johnson syndrome, Arch Ophthalmol 90:376, 1973.
42. Dohlman CH and Doughman DJ: The Stevens-Johnson syndrome, Trans New Orleans Acad Ophthalmol 24:236, 1972.
43. Assaad D et al: Toxic epidermal necrolysis in Stevens-Johnson syndrome, Can Med Assoc J 118:154, 1978.
44. Lyell A: Toxic epidermal necrolysis: an eruption resembling scalding of the skin, Br J Dermatol 68:355, 1956.

45. Lyell A, Dick HM, and Alexander JOD: Outbreak of toxic epidermal necrolysis associated with staphylococci, Lancet 1:787, 1969.

46. Lyell A: A review of toxic epidermal necrolysis in Britain, Br J Dermatol 79:662, 1967.

47. Revuz J et al: Treatment of toxic epidermal necrolysis: Créteil's experience, Arch Dermatol 123:1156, 1987.

48. Amon RB and Dimond RL: Toxic epidermal necrolysis, Arch Dermatol 111:1433, 1978.

49. Revuz J et al: Toxic epidermal necrolysis. Clinical findings and prognosis factors in 87 patients, Arch Dermatol 123:1160, 1987.

50. Melish ME and Glasgow LA: The staphylococcal scalded-skin syndrome: development of an experimental model, N Engl J Med 282:1114, 1970.

51. McKay ALC, Arbuthnott JP, and Lyell A: Action of staphylococcal epidermolytic toxin in mouse skin: an electron microscopic study, J Invest Dermatol 65:423, 1975.

52. Stein KM et al: Demonstration of basal cell immunofluorescence in drug-induced toxic epidermal necrolysis, Br J Dermatol 86:246, 1972.

53. Roujeau J-C et al: Sjögren-like syndrome after toxic epidermal necrolysis, Lancet 1:609, 1985.

54. Binaghi M et al: Ocular complications of Lyell's syndrome, J Fr Ophthalmol 8:239, 1985.

55. Hintner H et al: Immunofluorescence mapping of antigenic determinants within the dermal-epidermal junction in mechanobullous diseases, J Invest Dermatol 76:113, 1981.

56. Yaoita H et al: Epidermolysis bullosa acquisita: ultrastructural and immunologic studies, J Invest Dermatol 76:288, 1981.

57. Woodley D et al: Identification of the skin basement autoantigen in epidermolysis acquisita, N Engl J Med 310:1007, 1984.

58. Woodley D: Epidermolysis bullosa acquisita, Prog Dermatol 22:1, 1988.

59. Schachner LA and Press S: Vesicular bullous and pustular disorders. In Schachner LA, and Hansen RC, editors: Pediatric dermatology, New York, 1988, Churchill Livingstone.

60. Gans LA: Eye lesions of epidermolysis bullosa: clinical features, management, and prognosis, Arch Dermatol 124:762, 1988.

61. Aurora A, Madhaven M, and Rao S: Ocular changes in epidermolysis bullosis letalis, Am J Ophthalmol 79:464, 1975.

62. Sorsby A, Frazer-Roberts JA, and Bran RT: Essential shrinking of the conjunctiva in a hereditary affection allied to epidermolysis bullosa, Doc Ophthalmol 5:118, 1951.

63. Zierhut M et al: Ocular involvement in epidermolysis bullosa acquisita, Arch Ophthalmol 107:398, 1989.

64. McDonnell PJ and Spalton DJ: The ocular signs and complications of epidermolysis bullosa, J R Soc Med 81:576, 1988.

65. Lang PG and Tapert MJ: Severe ocular involvement in a patient with epidermolysis bullosa acquisita, J Am Acad Dermatol 16:439, 1987.

66. McDonnell PJ et al: Eye involvement in junctional epidermolysis bullosa, Arch Ophthalmol 107:1635, 1989.

67. Huff JC: The immunopathogenesis of dermatitis herpetiformis, J Invest Dermatol 84:237, 1985.

68. Duke-Elder S and Leigh AG: System of ophthalmology, vol VIII: Diseases of the outer eye, St Louis, 1965, Mosby–Year Book, Inc.

69. Wojnarowska F et al: Chronic bullous disease of childhood, childhood cicatricial pemphigoid, and linear IgA disease of adults: a comparative study demonstrating clinical and immunopathologic overlap, J Am Acad Dermatol 19:792, 1988.

70. Wilson BD et al: Linear IgA bullous dermatosis. An immunologically defined disease, Int J Dermatol 24:569, 1985.

71. Leonard JN et al: Linear IgA disease in adults, Br J Dermatol 107:301, 1982.

72. Kelly SE et al: A clinicopathological study of mucosal involvement in linear IgA disease, Br J Dermatol 119:161, 1988.

73. Aultbrinker EA, Starr MB, and Donnenfeld ED: Linear IgA disease. The ocular manifestations, Ophthalmology 95:340, 1988.

74. Leonard J et al: The relationship between linear IgA disease and benign mucous membrane pemphigoid, Br J Dermatol 110:307, 1984.

75. Drabonski J, Chorzelski TP, and Jablonska S: The ultrastructural localization of IgA deposits in chronic bullous disease of childhood (CBDC), J Invest Dermatol 72:291, 1979.

76. Ahmed AR et al: Pemphigus: current concepts, Ann Intern Med 92:396, 1980.

77. Woo TT et al: Specificity and inhibition of the epidermal cell detachment induced by pemphigus IgG in vitro, J Invest Dermatol 81:115, 1983.

78. Jordan RE, Triftshauser CT, and Schroeter AL: Direct immunofluorescent studies of pemphigus and bullous pemphigoid, Arch Dermatol 103:486, 1971.

79. Jordan RE et al: Classical and alternate pathway activation of complement in pemphigus vulgaris lesions, J Invest Dermatol 63:256, 1974.

80. Meurer M et al: Oral pemphigus vulgaris: a report of ten cases, Arch Dermatol 113:1520, 1977.

81. Bean SF, Holubar K, and Gillet RB: Pemphigus involving the eyes, Arch Dermatol 111:1484, 1975.

82. Bennion SD, Johnson C, and Weston WL: Hydroa vacciniforme with inflammatory keratitis and secondary anterior uveitis, Pediatr Dermatol 4:320, 1987.

83. Jenkins MS et al: Ocular rosacea, Am J Ophthalmol 88:618, 1979.

84. Watson PG and Hayreh SS: Scleritis and episcleritis, Br J Ophthalmol 60:163, 1976.

85. Brown SI and Shahinian L: Diagnosis and treatment of ocular rosacea, Trans Am Acad Ophthalmol 85:779, 1978.

86. Knight AG and Vickers CFH: A follow-up of tetracycline-treated rosacea, Br J Dermatol 93:577, 1975.

87. Frucht-Pery J et al: The effect of doxycycline on ocular rosacea, Am J Ophthalmol 107:434, 1989.

88. McCulley JP and Sciallis GF: Meibomian keratoconjunctivitis: oculo-dermal correlates, CLAO J 9:130, 1983.

89. McCulley JP and Dougherty JM: Blepharitis associated with acne rosacea and seborrheic dermatitis, Int Ophthalmol Clin 25:159, 1985.

90. Kaldeck R: Ocular psoriasis, Arch Dermatol 68(suppl):44, 1953.

91. Boss JM et al: Peripheral corneal melting syndrome in association with psoriasis, Br Med J 282:609, 1981.

92. Cram DL: Corneal melting in psoriasis, J Am Acad Dermatol 5:617, 1981.

93. Catsarou-Catsari A et al: Ophthalmological manifestations in patients with psoriasis, Acta Derm Venereol (Stock) 64:557, 1984.

94. Backman HA: The effects of PUVA on the eye, Am J Optom Physiol Opt 59:86, 1982.

95. Shindle R and Leone C: Cicatricial entropion associated with lamellar ichthyosis, Arch Ophthalmol 89:62, 1973.

96. Franceschetti A: Hereditary skin disease (genodermatosis) and corneal affections. In Beard C et al, editors: Symposium on surgical and medical management of congenital anomalies of the eye, St Louis, 1968, Mosby–Year Book, Inc.

97. Franceschetti A and Maeder G: Dystrophie profonde de la cornée dans un casd'ichtyose congénitale, Bull Mem Soc Fr Ophtalmol 67:146:1954.

98. Savin LH: Corneal dystrophy associated with congenital ichthyosis and allergic manifestations in male members of a family, Br J Ophthalmol 40:82, 1956.

99. Sever RJ, Frost P, and Weinstein G: Eye changes in ichthyosis, JAMA 206:2283, 1968.

100. Vail D: Corneal involvement in congenital ichthyosis, Arch Ophthalmol 24:215, 1940.

101. Piccirillo A et al: Ocular findings and skin histology in a group of patients with X-linked ichthyosis, Br J Dermatol 119:185, 1988.

102. Friedman B: Corneal findings in ichthyosis, Am J Ophthalmol 39:575, 1955.

103. Francheschetti A and Schlaeppe V: Dégénérescence en bandelette et dystrophie, prédescemétique de la cornée dans un d'ichtyose congénitale, Dermatologica 115:217, 1957.

104. Jay B, Black RK, and Wells RS: Ocular manifestations of ichthyosis, Br J Ophthalmol 52:217, 1968.

105. Van Everdingen JJ, Rampen FH, and Van der Schaar WW: Normal tearing and tear production in congenital ichthyosiform erythroderma with deafness and keratitis, Acta Dermatol Venereol 62:76, 1982.

106. Skinner BA, Greist MC, and Norins AL: The keratitis, ichthyosis, and deafness (KID) syndrome, Arch Dermatol 117:285, 1981.

107. Baden HP and Alper JC: Ichthyosiform dermatosis, keratitis, deafness, Arch Dermatol 113:1701, 1977.

108. Tuppurainen K et al: The KID-syndrome in Finland: a report of four cases, Acta Ophthalmol (Copenh) 66:692, 1988.

109. Grob JJ et al: Keratitis, ichthyosis, and deafness (KID) syndrome: vertical transmission and death from multiple squamous cell carcinomas, Arch Dermatol 123:777, 1987.

110. Hsu HC, Lin GS, and Li WM: Keratitis, ichthyosis, and deafness (KID) syndrome with cerebellar hypoplasia, Int J Dermatol 27:695, 1988.

111. Hazen PG, Carney P, and Lynch WS: Keratitis, ichthyosis, and deafness syndrome with development of multiple cutaneous neoplasms, Int J Dermatol 28:190, 1989.

112. Madriaga J et al: Squamous cell carcinoma in congenital ichthyosis with deafness and keratitis, Cancer 57:2026, 1986.

113. Zimmerman LE: Ocular lesions of juvenile xanthogranuloma, Am J Ophthalmol 60:1011, 1965.

114. Cadera W, Silver MM, and Burt L: Juvenile xanthogranuloma, Can J Ophthalmol 18:169, 1983.

115. Cogan DG, Kuwabara T, and Parke D: Epibulbar nevo-xantho-endothelioma, Arch Ophthalmol 59:717, 1958.

116. Britton H et al: Keratosis follicularis spinulosa decalvans: an infant with failure to thrive, deafness and recurrent infections, Arch Dermatol 114:761, 1978.

117. Forgács J and Franceschetti A: Histologic aspect of corneal changes due to hereditary metabolic and cutaneous affections, Am J Ophthalmol 47:191, 1959.

118. Cunningham SR et al: Kyrle's disease, J Am Acad Dermatol 16:117, 1987.

119. Tessler HH, Apple DJ, and Goldberg MF: Ocular findings in a kindred with Kyrle disease: hyperkeratosis follicularis et parafollicularis in cutem penetrans, Arch Ophthalmol 90:278, 1973.

120. Blackman HJ, Rodrigues MM, and Peck GL: Corneal epithelial lesions in keratosis follicularis (Darier's disease), Ophthalmology 87:941, 1980.

121. Wright JC: Darier's disease, Am J Ophthalmol 55:134, 1963.

122. Rud E: Werner's syndrome in 3 siblings, Acta Ophthalmol 34:255, 1956.

123. Petrohelos MA: Werner's syndrome: a survey of 3 cases with review of the literature, Am J Ophthalmol 56:941, 1956.

124. Kremer I, Ingber A, and Ben-Sira I: Corneal metastatic calcification in Werner's syndrome, Am J Ophthalmol 106:221, 1988.

125. Kleeberg J: Werner's syndrome, Acta Med Orient 8:145, 1949.

126. Valero A and Gellei B: Retinitis pigmentosa, hypertension and uremia in Werner's syndrome, Br J Med 2:351, 1960.

127. Campo AG and McDonald CJ: Treatment of acrodermatitis enterpathica with zinc sulfate, Arch Dermatol 112:687, 1976.

128. Hirsch FS, Michel B, and Strain WH: Gluconate zinc in acrodermatitis enteropathica, Arch Dermatol 112:475, 1976.

129. Matta CS, Felker GV, and Ide CH: Eye manifestations in acrodermatitis enteropathica, Arch Ophthalmol 93:140, 1975.

130. Warshawsky RS et al: Acrodermatitis enteropathica. Corneal involvement with histochemical and electron micrographic studies, Arch Ophthalmol 93:194, 1975.

131. Cameron JD and McClain CJ: Ocular histopathology of acrodermatitis enteropathica, Br J Ophthalmol 70:662, 1986.

132. Soter NA, Livingston DL, and Mihm MC: Malignant atrophic papulosis. In Fitzpatrick TB et al, editors: Dermatology in general medicine, ed 3, New York, 1987, McGraw-Hill.

133. Lemmengson W: Epidermolysis bullosa, Klin Monatsbl Augenheilkd 122:350, 1953.

134. Howard RO and Nishida S: A case of Degos' disease with electron microscope findings, Trans Am Acad Ophthalmol Otolaryngol 73:1097, 1969.

135. Winkelman RK et al: Malignant papulosis of skin and cerebrum: a syndrome of vascular thrombosis, Arch Dermatol 87:54, 1963.

136. Feuerman I, Dollberg L, and Salvador O: Malignant atrophic papulosis with mucin in the dermis: a clinical and pathological study including autopsy, Arch Pathol 90:310, 1970.

137. Mulvihill JJ et al: Melkersson-Rosenthal syndrome, Hodgkin disease, and corneal keratopathy, Arch Intern Med 132:116, 1973.

138. Stenson S: Ocular findings in xeroderma pigmentosum: report of two cases, Ann Ophthalmol 14:580, 1982.

139. Reese A and Wilber J: The eye manifestations of xeroderma pigmentousum, Am J Ophthalmol 26:901, 1943.

140. Gaasterland D, Rodrigues M, and Mashell A: Ocular involvement in xeroderma pigmentosum, Ophthalmology 89:980, 1982.

141. Okubo K et al: The corneal endothelium in xeroderma pigmentosum, Ophthalmologica 195:178, 1987.

142. Lamba P and Lal S: Ocular changes in benign acanthosis nigricans, Dermatologica 1140:356, 1970.

143. Newman G and Carsten M: Acanthosis nigricans: conjunctival and lid lesions, Arch Ophthalmol 90:259, 1973.

144. François J: Heredo-familial corneal dystrophies, Trans Ophthalmol Soc UK 86:367, 1966.

145. Steir W, Van Voolen A, and Selmanowitz V: Dyskeratosis congenita: relationship to Fanconi's anemia, Blood 39:510, 1972.

146. Storer JS and Hawk RJ: Neonatal skin and skin disorders. In Schachner LA and Hansen RC, editors: Pediatric dermatology, New York, 1988, Churchill Livingstone.

147. Hurwitz S: Hair disorders. In Schachner LA and Hansen RC, editors: Pediatric dermatology, New York, 1988, Churchill Livingstone.

148. Williams ML: Ichthyosis and disorders of cornification. In Schachner LA and Hansen RC, editors: Pediatric dermatology, New York, 1988, Churchill Livingstone.

149. McCrary J and Smith JL: Conjunctival and retinal incontinentia pigmenti, Arch Ophthalmol 79:417, 1968.

OTHER SYSTEMIC DISORDERS

NUTRITIONAL DISORDERS

VITAMIN A DEFICIENCY

Vitamin A deficiency is relatively rare in the United States, but it is common in some developing countries. It is the leading cause of childhood blindness in the world.[1] It primarily occurs in preschool-aged children and is usually seen in association with other nutritional deficits, such as multiple vitamin deficiency and protein-calorie malnutrition (marasmus). In the well-fed populations of developed countries, vitamin A deficiency is rarely seen, but can result from systemic disease (for example, malabsorption, cystic fibrosis, liver disease) or dietary indiscretion.[2-8]

Clinical manifestations. A classification scheme of ocular findings in xerophthalmia that has been developed by the World Health Organization is illustrated in the box on p. 607. The earliest symptom of vitamin A deficiency is usually night blindness. This symptom is followed by conjunctival xerosis and keratinization, blepharitis, and meibomitis. Nonocular findings can include hyperkeratosis of the skin, lengthening of the eyelashes, enhanced keratinization and xerosis of other mucosal surfaces, increased intracranial pressure, and mental retardation.

In conjuctival xerosis the conjunctiva can be lusterless, wrinkled, red, and opaque.[9-11] The signs are first noted in the temporal quadrant, appearing as an unwettable portion of the conjunctiva. Later all portions of the conjunctiva can be involved, but the bulbar conjunctiva tends to be more affected

WHO CLASSIFICATION OF FINDINGS IN VITAMIN A DEFICIENCY

XN	Night blindness
X1A	Conjunctival xerosis
X1B	Bitot's spots
X2	Corneal xerosis
X3A	Corneal ulceration or keratomalacia involving < one third of corneal surface
X3B	Corneal ulceration or keratomalacia involving ≥ one third of corneal surface
XS	Corneal scar
XF	Xerophthalmic fundus

than the palpebral. A Bitot's spot (Fig. 26-1) is a small white-gray irregular plaque with a foamy surface. It is seen on the bulbar conjunctiva, usually temporal to the limbus, and is often bilateral.

Histologically the main feature is squamous metaplasia of the conjunctival and corneal epithelium[12-15] (Fig. 26-2). There is acanthotic thickening of the epithelium, with keratinization of the surface. Goblet cells are greatly reduced in number, resulting in a lack of mucin. A chronic inflammatory infiltrate is often present in the substantia propria. Bitot's spots are areas of marked keratinization.[15] The foamy appearance is caused by mucus and xerosis bacilli *(Corynebacterium xerosis)*.[16]

Non–vitamin A responsive Bitot's spots also can occur as a result of previous vitamin A deficiency.[1,11] In addition, not all cases of vitamin A deficiency manifest a Bitot's spot.

Corneal xerosis usually is seen in individuals with conjunctival xerosis (Fig. 26-3). The earliest sign is a superficial punctate keratopathy, which usually begins inferiorly. When the punctate keratopathy becomes confluent, the cornea develops a peau d'orange or ground-glass appearance. Keratinization, stromal edema, and rapid tear break-up also can be noted. Aqueous tear production may be normal.

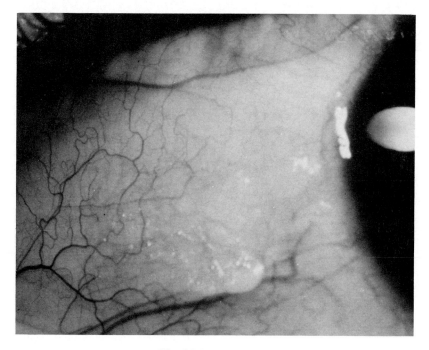

Fig. 26-1. Bitot's spot.

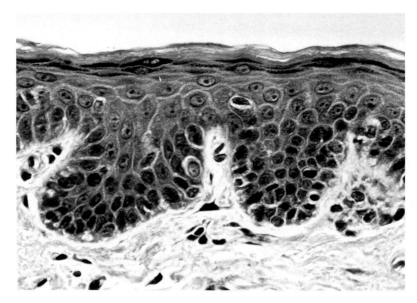

Fig. 26-2. Bitot's spot. Epidermalization of conjunctival epithelium with stratified squamous configuration, rete peg formation, absence of goblet cells, and keratinization of surface. (Hematoxylin-eosin stain; X800.) (Courtesy of Bruce L. Johnson, Pittsburgh.)

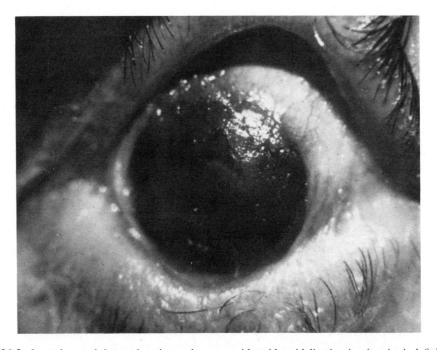

Fig. 26-3. Lusterless and dry conjunctiva and cornea with epidermidalization in vitamin A deficiency.

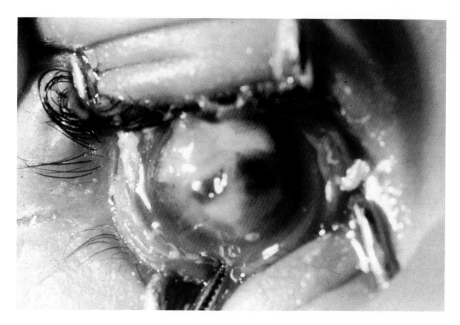

Fig. 26-4. Keratomalacia in vitamin A deficiency. (Courtesy of D. Paton, Houston.)

The preceding changes are readily reversible with vitamin A treatment.[17,18] However, these eyes are prone to corneal ulceration, often with severe visual consequences[10,19,20] (Fig. 26-4). The reason for the ulceration is not known, but minor trauma or conjunctival infection (for example, measles) often lead to marked stromal loss and scarring.[21-23]

The earliest and most common form of corneal ulceration are small, sharply punched-out lesions, most often affecting the peripheral nasal cornea.[17] These may begin as localized, sharply demarcated, areas of swollen, opaque, grayish-yellow stroma, which sloughs, leaving a descemetocele. Larger and more irregularly shaped ulcers also can occur.

Keratomalacia is an extreme form of corneal ulceration in vitamin A deficiency. It is particularly common in children with advanced starvation and those with systemic disease, such as diarrhea, parasitic infection, or measles, in addition to malnutrition. Keratomalacia can develop suddenly. There is generalized softening of the stroma, which turns yellow-white and sloughs, leaving a descemetocele or perforation. The cause is not known: Both clinically and histologically it appears that an inflammatory response does not play a significant role.

Treatment. Vitamin A can be administered orally, or parentally, if necessary. The recommended dose for children over 1 year of age is 200,000 IU on each of 2 consecutive days, followed by another dose 1 to 2 weeks later. Adjunctive topical vitamin A administration also appears to be beneficial.[24-26] Improvement is seen in 1 to 4 days, with complete resolution usually within 1 week.

RIBOFLAVIN DEFICIENCY

Riboflavin deficiency causes *cheilosis,* which is fissuring and ulceration of the oral mucous membranes, particularly at the corners of the mouth. Facial seborrhea and glossitis also occur. A fine desquamation occurs in the nasolabial folds and along the sides of the nose. The tongue has a purplish hue, and the filiform papillae are flattened out.

The patient complains of photophobia, irritation, and twitching and burning of the eyes. The lid margins and conjunctivae are injected. Increased prominence of the limbal vessels occurs early, and

TABLE 26-1. Neurologic Disorders with Corneal Manifestations

DISORDER	INHERITANCE	PATHOGENESIS	MAJOR SYSTEMIC FINDINGS	OCULAR FINDINGS
Familial dysautonomia (Riley-Day syndrome)	AR*	Dopamine-beta-hydroxylase deficiency	Autonomic instability; emotional lability; dysphagia	Tear deficiency; corneal anesthesia; retinal vascular tortuosity
Shy-Drager syndrome	—	Degeneration of central autonomic nervous system	Progressive autonomic instability in elderly; orthostatic hypotension; urinary incontinence; impotence; hypohidrosis	Dry eye; iris atrophy; convergence insufficiency; anisocoria; Horner's syndrome
Neurofibromatosis (von Recklinghausen's disease)	AD†	Unknown	Neurofibromas; other neural tumors; pigmented skin lesions	Corneal hypesthesia; plexiform neuroma of the upper lid; iris nodules; glaucoma
Myotonic dystrophy	AD	Unknown	Progressive muscle weakness; myotonia	Corneal exposure; cataracts; hypotony; ophthalmoplegia; ptosis; enophthalmos
Wilson's disease (Chapter 24)	AR	Impaired liver excretion of copper	Progressive neurologic impairment; liver dysfunction	Kayser-Fleischer ring; sunflower cataract
Ataxia-telangiectasia	AR	Unknown	Cerebellar ataxia; cutaneous telangiectasia; immunodeficiency	Conjunctival telangiectasias

*Autosomal recessive.
†Autosomal dominant.

these vessels can later extend onto the cornea. A superficial epithelial keratitis, corneal opacification, mydriasis, and increased iris pigmentation can be seen.[27]

NEUROLOGIC DISORDERS

FAMILIAL DYSAUTONOMIA (RILEY-DAY SYNDROME)

Familial dysautonomia is an autosomal recessively inherited disease that seems to be confined to Ashkenazi Jews (Table 26-1). There is a deficiency of plasma dopamine-beta-hydroxylase (DBH), the enzyme that catalyzes the conversion of dopamine to norepinephrine, this results in a deficiency of norepinephrine and epinephrine and elevation of serum and urine homovanillic acid, the breakdown product of dopamine.

Clinical manifestations. Patients with familial dysautonomia usually have a history of feeding difficulty from birth and show an extreme emotional lability. Autonomic instability is demonstrated by abnormal sweating, labile hypertension, and postural hypotension. Other findings include decreased lacrimation, corneal hypesthesia, absence of the fungiform papillae of the tongue (Fig. 26-5), diminished pain and temperature sensation, hyporeflexia, motor incoordination, episodic fever, and episodic vomiting. Few patients reach adulthood because of recurrent pulmonary infections and renal failure secondary to hypertension.

Ocular manifestations. Corneal complications result from tear deficiency and corneal anesthesia. There is a wide variation in the severity of corneal disease; some cases may be free of corneal disease, whereas others experience ulceration (Fig. 26-6), scarring, vascularization, or perforation.[28-31]

Although anisocoria and myopia have been seen in some patients, there seems to be little significance attached to these findings. Retinal vascular tortuosity, ptosis, and exotropia also have been observed.[32] Prompt pupillary constriction occurs after instillation of a dilute miotic (for example, 2.5% methacholine).[33]

Treatment. Early diagnosis of Riley-Day syndrome will permit routine protective care of the patient's cornea so that complications are minimized. Therapy includes artificial tear solutions, punctal

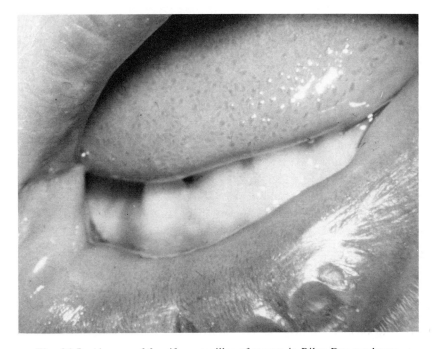

Fig. 26-5. Absence of fungiform papillae of tongue in Riley-Day syndrome.

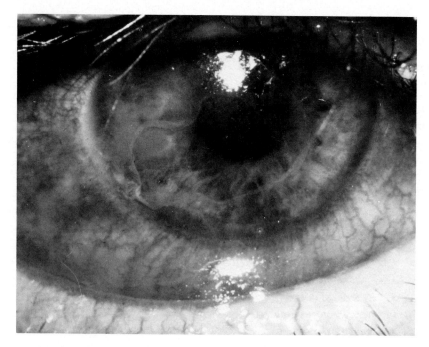

Fig. 26-6. Corneal ulcer in Riley-Day syndrome with severe hypolacrima.

occlusion, and tarsorrhaphy. (Treatment of dry eyes is discussed in Chapter 14; neurotrophic keratitis in Chapter 15.) Parenteral administration of pilocarpine or neostigmine will increase tear production[33-35]; however, the side effects prevent the therapeutic use of these drugs.

SHY-DRAGER SYNDROME

Shy-Drager syndrome is a progressive degenerative disorder of the autonomic nervous system, with onset usually in the sixth or seventh decade. Findings include orthostatic hypotension, urinary incontinence, impotence, and decreased sweating. The cornea and conjunctiva may become affected by keratoconjunctivitis sicca. Other eye findings are iris atrophy, convergence insufficiency, anisocoria, and Horner's syndrome.

OTHER NEUROLOGIC DISORDERS

Neurofibromatosis (von Recklinghausen's disease) is an autosomal dominant disease characterized by multiple neurofibromas, hyperpigmented lesions of the skin (Fig. 26-7), and other tumors of the central and peripheral nervous system. Plexiform neuromas can occur in the upper lid, simulating a "bag of worms" (Figs. 26-8 and 26-9). Increased visibility of the corneal nerves and decreased corneal sensation, sometimes leading to neurotrophic keratitis, also can be seen.

Myotonic muscular dystrophy is another autosomal dominant disease in which there is slowly progressive muscle weakness. Exposure keratitis can be noted in the inferior cornea. Orbicularis muscle weakness and a poor Bell's phenomenon contribute to the corneal exposure. Multicolored granular cortical opacities can be seen in the lens. Other ocular findings include hypotony, ophthalmoplegia, ptosis, and enophthalmos.

HEREDITARY DISORDERS AFFECTING MULTIPLE ORGAN SYSTEMS
EHLERS-DANLOS SYNDROME

This syndrome is produced by a group of hereditary disorders and is characterized by hypermobile joints and hyperextensibility of the skin. Some forms also exhibit skin fragility, easy bruising,

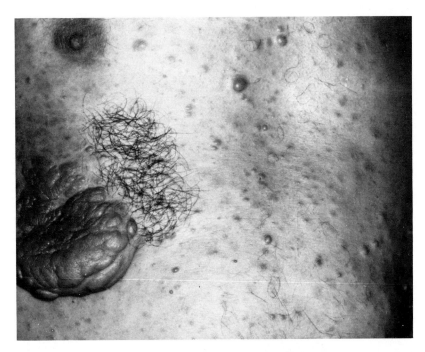

Fig. 26-7. Subcutaneous tumors are firm, nodular, and attached to nerve in neurofibromatosis.

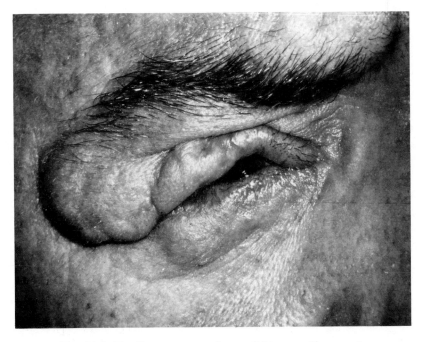

Fig. 26-8. Plexiform neuroma of upper lid in neurofibromatosis.

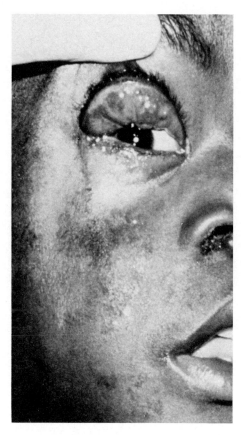

Fig. 26-9. Lid involvement in neurofibromatosis.

organ ruptures, hernias, or joint dislocation. Ehlers-Danlos type VI, known as the ocular form, is inherited as an autosomal recessive trait and appears to be caused by a deficiency of lysyl hydroxylase, the enzyme responsible for hydroxylation of lysine residues in collagen types I and III. In its absence, cross-linkage of the collagen molecules does not occur. Patients exhibit joint hypermobility, skin hyperextensibility, scoliosis, marfanoid habitus, and aortic rupture. Ocular signs include microcornea, recurrent intraocular bleeding, and susceptibility to rupture of the globe. A variant of this condition has been described, characterized by keratoglobus, blue sclera, ocular fragility, mild joint hypermobility, and normal lysyl hydroxylase (see Chapter 17).[36-40]

ALPORT'S SYNDROME

Alport's syndrome is a hereditary disorder consisting of nephritis and sensorineural deafness. It can be inherited as an autosomal dominant or X-linked trait. Progressive anterior and posterior lenticonus and spherophakia are seen. Subcapsular cataract, macular changes, albipunctate fundus, and optic nerve drusen also can occur.

The cornea may exhibit an arcus juvenilis[41] or keratoconus. Pigment dispersion is noted in some cases, with deposition of pigment on the cornea (Krukenberg spindle) and the lens capsule.[42] Some cases of severe corneal ulcers resistant to treatment have been observed.

LOWE'S OCULOCEREBRORENAL SYNDROME

Lowe's syndrome includes congenital bilateral cataracts, nystagmus, glaucoma, Fanconi's syndrome (aminoaciduria, renal tubular acidosis, hypercalciuria, glucosuria, hypouricemia), mental and psychomotor retardation, oculodigital sign of Franceschetti (ocular manipulation with the hands), hypotonia, and areflexia. The disease is often, but not always, transmitted as a sex-linked recessive trait. Most patients with Lowe's syndrome have been fair-haired boys; however, the disease also has been described in females and in a black individual.[43]

Ocular manifestations. Cataracts are found in all patients. The female carrier can have white, punctate, anterior and posterior lens opacities. Congenital glaucoma is present in approximately 60% of patients. A mild haze can occur in the cornea, involving the peripheral stroma.[44] Buphthalmos, stromal vascularization, and scarring also can occur, and exuberant corneal scarring (corneal keloid formation) has been described.[45,46] The cause of the corneal scarring is unclear, but it may be related to oculodigital manipulation or surgical procedures for glaucoma and cataract. Iris and retinal abnormalities also can be found.[47]

Rubella can cause both cataract and glaucoma, but usually not together in the same patient. It would be wise to check the mother of a boy with cataracts and glaucoma.

REFERENCES

1. Tielsch JM and Sommer A: The epidemiology of vitamin A deficiency and xerophthalmia, Annu Rev Nutr 4:183, 1984.
2. Fells P and Bors F: Ocular complications of self-induced vitamin A deficiency, Trans Ophthalmol Soc UK 89:221, 1969.
3. Olver J: Keratomalacia on a "healthy" diet, Br J Ophthalmol 70:357, 1986.
4. Matsuo T et al: Keratomalacia in a child with familial hypo-retinol-binding proteinemia, Jpn J Ophthalmol 32:249, 1988.
5. Sullivan WR, McCulley JP, and Dohlman CH: Return of goblet cells after vitamin A therapy in xerosis of the conjunctiva, Am J Ophthalmol 75:720, 1973.
6. Petersen RA, Petersen VS, and Robb RM: Vitamin A deficiency with xerophthalmia and night blindness in cystic fibrosis, Am J Dis Child 116:662, 1968.
7. Suan EP et al: Corneal perforation in patients with vitamin A deficiency in the United States, Arch Ophthalmol 108:350, 1990.
8. Brooks HL, Driebe WT, and Schemmer GG: Xerophthalmia and cystic fibrosis, Arch Ophthalmol 108:354, 1990.
9. Sommer A et al: Vitamin A responsive panocular xerophthalmia in a healthy adult, Arch Ophthalmol 96:1630, 1978.
10. Paton D: Keratomalacia: a review of its relationship to xerophthalmia and its response to treatment, Eye Ear Nose Throat Mon 46:186, 1967.
11. Paton D and McLaren, DS: Bitot spots, Am J Ophthalmol 50:568, 1960.
12. Dohlman CH and Kalevar V: Cornea in hypovitaminosis A and protein deficiency, Isr J Med Sci 8:1179, 1972.
13. Pirie A: Xerophthalmia, Invest Ophthalmol 15:417, 1976.
14. Sullivan WR, McCulley JP, and Dohlman CH: Return of goblet cells after vitamin A therapy in xerosis of the conjunctiva, Am J Ophthalmol 75:720, 1973.
15. Sommer A, Green R, and Kenyon KR: Clinical histopathologic correlations of vitamin A responsive and nonresponsive Bitot's spots, Arch Ophthalmol 99:2014, 1981.
16. Ganley JP and Payne CM: Clinical and electron microscopic observations of the conjunctiva of adult patients with Bitot's spots, Invest Ophthalmol Vis Sci 20:632, 1981.
17. Sommer A and Sugana T: Corneal xerophthalmia and keratomalacia, Arch Ophthalmol 100:404, 1982.
18. Sommer A: Nutritional blindness: xerophthalmia and keratomalacia, New York, 1982, Oxford University Press.
19. Smith RS, Farrell T, and Bailey T: Kerotomalacia, Surv Ophthalmol 20:213, 1975.
20. Venkataswamy G: Ocular manifestations of vitamin A deficiency, Br J Ophthalmol 51:854, 1967.
21. Seng WL et al: The effect of thermal burns on the release of collagenase from corneas of vitamin A-deficient rats, Invest Ophthalmol Vis Sci 19:1461, 1980.
22. Sandford-Smith JH and Whittle H: Corneal ulceration following measles in Nigerian children, Br J Ophthalmol 63:720, 1983.
23. Foster A and Sommer A: Childhood blindness from corneal ulceration in Africa: causes, presentation and treatment, Bull WHO 64:619, 1986.
24. Sommer A and Emran N: Topical retinoic acid in the treatment of corneal xerophthalmia, Am J Ophthalmol 86:615, 1978.
25. Van Horn DL et al: Topical retinoic acid in the treatment of experimental xerophthalmia in the rabbit, Arch Ophthalmol 99:317, 1981.
26. Ubels JL et al: The efficacy of retinoic acid ointment for treatment of xerophthalmia and corneal epithelial wounds, Curr Eye Res 4:1049, 1985.
27. Syndenstricker VP et al: The ocular manifestations of ariboflavinosis, JAMA 114:2437, 1940.
28. Liebman SD: Ocular manifestations of Riley-Day syndrome, Arch Ophthalmol 56:719, 1956.
29. Boruchoff SA and Dohlman CH: The Riley-Day syndrome: ocular manifestations in a 35-year-old patient, Am J Ophthalmol 63:523, 1967.
30. Dunnington JH: Congenital alacrima in familial autonomic dysfunction, Arch Ophthalmol 52:925, 1954.
31. Liebman SD: Riley-Day syndrome, Arch Ophthalmol 58:188, 1957.
32. Goldberg MF, Payne JW, and Brunt PW: Ophthalmologic studies of familial dysautonomia, Arch Ophthalmol 80:732, 1968.

33. Smith AA, Dancis J, and Breinin G: Ocular responses to autonomic drugs in familial dysautonomia, Invest Ophthalmol 4:358, 1965.

34. Kroop IG: The production of tears in familial dysautonomia: preliminary report, J Pediatr 48:328, 1956.

35. Pilger IS: Familial dysautonomia: report of case with stimulation of tear production by prostigmine, Am J Ophthalmol 43:285, 1957.

36. Biglan AW, Brown SI, and Johnson BC: Keratoglobus and blue sclera, Am J Ophthalmol 83:225, 1977.

37. Gregoratos N, Bartoscocas C, and Papas K: Blue sclera with keratoglobus and brittle cornea, Br J Ophthalmol 55:424, 1971.

38. Hymas SW, Dar H, and Newman E: Blue sclera keratoglobus, Br J Ophthalmol 53:53, 1969.

39. Stein R, Lazar M, and Adam A: Brittle cornea. A familial trait associated with blue sclera, Am J Ophthalmol 66:67, 1968.

40. Judisch F, Wariri M, and Krachmer J: Ocular Ehlers-Danlos syndrome with normal lysyl hydrolase activity, Arch Ophthalmol 94:1489, 1976.

41. Chavis RM and Groshong T: Corneal arcus in Alport's syndrome, Am J Ophthalmol 75:793, 1973.

42. Davies PD: Pigment dispersion in a case of Alport's syndrome, Br J Ophthalmol 54:557, 1970.

43. Johnson BL and Hiles DA: Ocular pathology of Lowe's syndrome in a female infant, J Pediatr Ophthalmol 13:204, 1976.

44. Wilson WA, Richards W, and Donnell GR: Oculo-cerebral-renal syndrome of Lowe, Arch Ophthalmol 70:5, 1963.

45. Cibis GW et al: Corneal keloid in Lowe's syndrome, Arch Ophthalmol 100:1795, 1982.

46. Sugar J: Metabolic disorders of the cornea. In Kaufman HE et al, editors: The cornea, New York, 1988, Churchill Livingstone.

47. Ginsberg J, Bore KE, and Fogelson MH: Pathological features of the eye in the oculocerbrorenal (Lowe) syndrome, J Pediatr Ophthalmol Strabismus 18:16, 1981.

CHAPTER 27

DRUGS AND METALS

Metals
- Gold
- Mercury
- Copper
- Silver
- Iron

Systemic drugs
- Phenothiazines
- Aminoquinolones
- Cytarabine
- Fluorouracil
- Retinoids

This chapter deals first with the deposition of metals in the conjunctiva and the cornea. The lesions caused by metal-containing therapeutic agents must be recognized because in many instances their effect can aggravate the initial disease. The effect of systemic drugs on the conjunctiva and cornea also is discussed. The adverse effects of topical drugs is reviewed in the next chapter.

METALS

GOLD

Gold can accumulate in the cornea after systemic administration of gold compounds, typically for rheumatoid arthritis.[1-5]* Both oral (for example, auranofin) and intramuscular (for example, gold sodium thiomalate or thiosulfate) preparations are used; their mechanism of action is not known.

The condition of gold deposition in the cornea is known as *corneal chrysiasis*. The presence of corneal deposits is related to the total dose of gold, the duration of treatment, and the intensity of gold therapy (total dose/duration of therapy).[3] The density of the deposits is correlated with the duration of treatment, but not the total dose.[3,4] In general, corneal changes are not seen until the total dose exceeds 1 g; the majority of patients receiving more than 1 g will exhibit corneal deposits.[3,4,6] The deposits in the cornea usually clear within 3 to 5 months after gold therapy is discontinued.

Stromal involvement appears to be most common. Slit-lamp microscopy reveals fine, dustlike, yellow-brown to purple-violet granules that affect mainly the posterior stroma and are denser inferiorly. On transillumination, the cornea can appear purple. Deposition also can occur in the corneal

---

*Roberts and Wolter's[5] article contains an excellent drawing of stromal deposits.

617

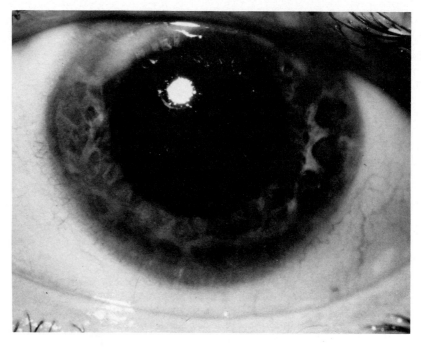

Fig. 27-1. Ulcerative and infiltrative corneal lesion seen in gold therapy for rheumatoid arthritis.

epithelium. In one large study[4] of patients relatively early in the course of therapy, deposits were seen only in the epithelium. The deposits are usually diffuse and can have a vortex pattern, as in Fabry's disease. In other cases they can be peripheral, or only central, like a Hudson-Stähli line.

Some fine gold granules in the conjunctiva also may be seen.[2] Histologically the conjunctival gold deposits are both intracellular and extracellular, found in the epithelium and superficial substantia propria.

A second type of corneal reaction is severe, consisting of marginal ulcerative keratitis (Fig. 27-1) and iritis. The keratitis is seen as a white, crescent-shaped ulcer bordering the limbus and associated with conjunctival hyperemia and pain. The keratitis is thought to be caused by a hypersensitivity reaction to the gold.[7] Infiltration without ulceration also can be seen. The infiltration may start as a flat, distinct, superficial white opacity at one side of the cornea, with no line of normal cornea between the opacity and the sclera. The ulceration and infiltration tend to remain in the anterior layers of the cornea, but spread from the periphery centrally and along the limbus.

Lens deposition (lenticular chrysiasis) occurs later than corneal deposition, usually after more than 3 years of therapy.[3,8,9] Several patterns of deposition can be seen: fine, diffuse, granular deposits, without a purplish hue, on or within the central anterior lens capsule; fine deposits within the anterior embryonic suture lines; flakelike deposits within the central cortex; and diffuse, anterior subcapsular deposits, with or without posterior subcapsular deposits.

The gold deposits in the cornea, conjunctiva, and lens do not interfere with vision and are not an indication to stop gold therapy. If keratitis occurs, however, therapy should be discontinued. The keratitis heals, but a vascularized scar can remain. Penicillamine therapy also appears to be effective.

Mercury

Chronic exposure to mercury can result in changes in the lens and cornea.[10,11] Exposure can occur through occupational exposure to mercury vapor and mercurial compounds or from chronic topi-

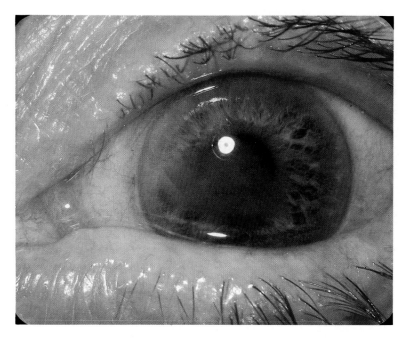

Fig. 27-2. Band keratopathy caused by mercurial toxicity (topical use of medication containing phenylmercuric nitrate as a preservative).

cal application of ophthalmic medications containing organomercurial compounds. These compounds serve as antiseptics or preservatives; examples are thimerosal, mercuric oxide, and phenylmercuric nitrate.

Bluish gray mercurial deposits can be seen around conjunctival blood vessels and in peripheral Descemet's membrane. In rare cases fine, glistening, particulate opacities have been seen in the central corneal stroma. Follicular conjunctivitis, punctate keratitis, subepithelial infiltrates, edema, and vascularization have been reported.[12] Calcific band keratopathy also can develop[13] (Fig. 27-2) (see Chapter 28). Chelation with ethylene diaminetetraacetic acid (EDTA) is effective in removing the mercury deposits.

Mercurialentis consists of a rose-brown or pinkish homogeneous opacity that can involve the whole anterior surface of the lens, but sometimes is limited to an anterior subcapsular disc.[14] Phenylmercuric nitrate and acetate penetrate the eye readily and can bind persistently to sulfhydryl groups in the lens. This reaction occurs more readily than with other mercurial antimicrobial preservatives, such as thimerosal. Mercurialentis has not been seen with thimerosal at the normal concentration used in ophthalmic solutions (0.005%).

Thimerosal in contact lens solutions can elicit a delayed hypersensitivity reaction in some patients.[15] Sterile corneal infiltrates (see Chapter 9), papillary conjunctivitis, and contact lens–induced keratoconjunctivitis may be related to thimerosal hypersensitivity.

COPPER

Chalcosis is the term used to describe deposition of copper in tissues. Deposition in the eye most commonly results from copper-containing intraocular foreign bodies. Pure copper tends to cause a violent purulent reaction that usually leads to panophthalmitis and loss of the eye. Alloy metals less than 85% copper tend to cause chalcosis.[16]

Copper has an affinity for basement membranes, such as Descemet's membrane and the lens cap-

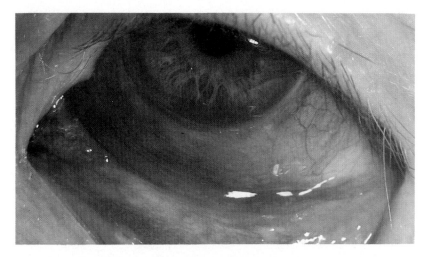

Fig. 27-3. Silver pigmentation of conjunctiva in argyrosis.

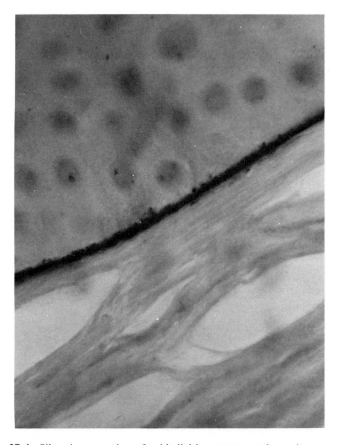

Fig. 27-4. Silver impregnation of epithelial basement membrane in argyrosis.

sule, but deposition can occur in any tissue.[17] Corneal deposition is seen as yellow-brown, red, blue, or green coloration of peripheral Descemet's membrane. The iris can be slightly greenish, the vitreous yellowish green-blue. Iridescent, multicolored particles are seen beneath the anterior lens capsule and can take on the form of a sunflower.[18]

The deposition of copper in the cornea and lens in systemic diseases, such as Wilson's disease, is described in Chapter 24.

SILVER

Argyrosis is the deposition of silver in mucous membranes and skin, usually after long-term use of silver-containing medications. Colloidal silver, silver protein, and silver nitrate are topical antibacterial agents that are used rarely in the United States today but are relatively common in other countries. A silver nitrate compound, Argyrol, was used extensively early in this century. If ocular argyrosis occurs at all today it is usually a result of industrial exposure to organic salts of silver.[19]

After both topical and systemic administration, the manifestations are similar. Silver deposition can result in a slate gray discoloration of the conjunctiva (Fig. 27-3), lids, and nasolacrimal apparatus.[20-22] The nasal conjunctiva tends to be most affected because of pooling of tears. The cornea also can be affected: Fine blue, gray, green, or gold opacities are found in the deep stroma and Descemet's membrane.[23-25] Iridescent anterior subcapsular lens opacities also can occur.[21]

Histologically the silver is deposited intracellularly in the substantia propria of the conjunctiva, in the basement membrane of the conjunctival epithelium (Fig. 27-4), in conjunctival vascular endothelium, and in Descemet's membrane[24,26,27] (Fig. 27-5).

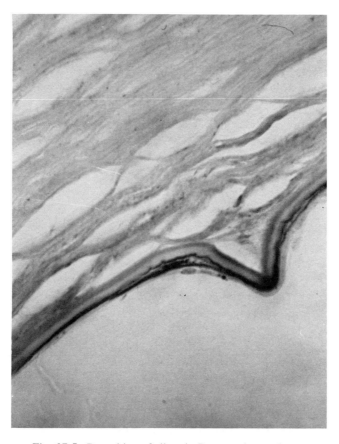

Fig. 27-5. Deposition of silver in Descemet's membrane.

The silver deposition rarely interferes with vision and gradually fades after cessation of exposure. If the appearance is unacceptable, the following treatment can reduce the discoloration: A sterile solution containing 6% sodium thiosulfate and 0.25% potassium ferricyanide, prepared within 30 minutes of use, is injected into the skin or subconjunctival tissue.

IRON

Iron deposition, or *siderosis,* can occur as a result of the presence of an iron-containing foreign body, systemic hemochromatosis, or systemic iron administration, or as a degenerative change in the epithelium (Table 27-1). When iron is released from particles inside the eye, the surrounding tissues develop a rust-brown discoloration, and their function can be impaired. In general, iron-containing particles in the anterior chamber or cornea are better tolerated than those in the posterior segment. In the anterior chamber, iron compounds are slowly released and carried away by the flow of aqueous, so the deposits affect only the tissues adjacent to the foreign body.

The cornea is seldom discolored by intraocular iron, but it can display a rust-brown color due to fine deposits in the deepest layers. These impart a gray and dirty appearance, but on oblique illumination it can appear greenish blue or golden. Histopathologic examination of one case demonstrated iron deposits only within keratocytes, and there was no relationship between siderosome accumulation and cell degeneration.

An iron-containing foreign body buried in the conjunctiva or cornea can lead to localized brownish red pigmentation of the adjacent tissues (Fig. 27-6). If it is allowed to remain long enough and is large enough, it can cause more diffuse pigmentation of the cornea by spreading through the epithelium, stroma, and endothelium.[28]

Coats' white ring is a small ring of iron deposition remaining after removal of a superficial corneal metallic foreign body (see Chapter 16).[29,30] It is made up of discrete white dots and is most common in the interpalpebral area.

After persistent hemorrhage in the anterior chamber, iron deposition can be seen in the posterior stroma (Fig. 27-7). The development of such "corneal blood staining" appears to be related to both the elevation of intraocular pressure and the duration of the hyphema. In a rabbit model the corneal blood staining was uniformly accompanied by endothelial cell injury.[31] After resolution of the hemorrhage, the corneal deposits gradually fade; however, penetrating keratoplasty may be necessary.

Systemic hemochromatosis usually does not involve the cornea.[32,33] Scleral iron deposition can occur and is usually only evident histologically. However, rusty discolorization anterior to the horizontal recti has been noted. Such deposition can rarely occur after numerous blood transfusions or

TABLE 27-1. Corneal Iron Deposition

CONDITION	COLOR	LOCATION	PATTERN
Hereditary spherocytosis (Dalgleisch line)	Brown	Epithelium	Horizontally oval
Coats' white ring	White	Epithelium, anterior stroma	Small interpalpebral circle
Hudson-Stähli line	Brown	Epithelium	Linear, junction of inferior and middle thirds
Fleischer ring	Brown	Epithelium	Base of cone in keratoconus
Stocker line	Brown	Epithelium	Linear, central to pterygium
Ferry line	Brown	Epithelium	Linear, central to filtering bleb
Blood staining	Yellow-brown-red	Deep stroma	Diffuse, central
Intraocular foreign body	Yellow-brown-red	Deep stroma	Diffuse central

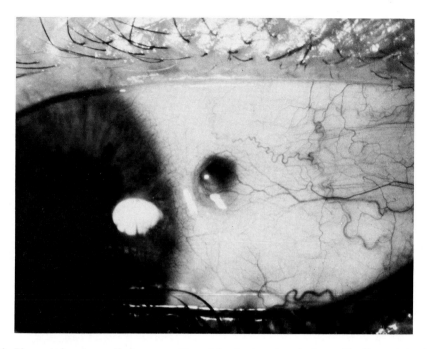

Fig. 27-6. Pigmented spot near limbus caused by retained subconjunctival metallic (ferrous) foreign body.

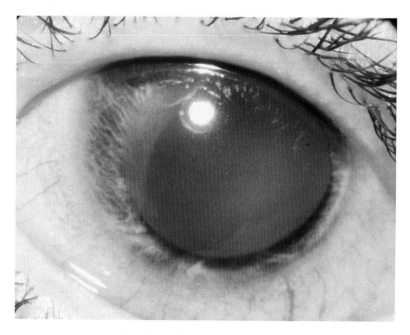

Fig. 27-7. Blood staining of cornea.

TABLE 27-2. Systemic Medications That Affect the Cornea and Conjunctiva

DRUG	USES	EFFECTS
Adriamycin (doxorubicin)	Malignancy	Nonspecific conjunctivitis, lacrimation
Alkylating agents (busulfan, chlorambucil, cyclophosphamide, melphalan)	Malignancy, systemic inflammatory diseases	Blepharoconjunctivitis, dry eye, hyperpigmentation, corneal opacities and edema (nitrosourea)[44]
Aminoquinolones (amodiaquine, chloroquine, hydroxychloroquine)	Malaria, rheumatoid arthritis	Vortex keratopathy, yellow discoloration of the conjunctiva
Amiodarone	Cardiac arrhythmias	Vertex keratopathy, halos, blurred vision
Antacids		Band keratopathy (hypercalcemia), bluish discoloration of conjunctiva, corneal deposits[45]
Clofazimine	Leprosy	Reddish pigmentation of the skin and conjunctiva, vortex keratopathy
Cytarabine (Ara-C, cytosine arabinoside)	Malignancy, herpes simplex	Corneal epithelial microcysts, conjunctivitis
Diethylcarbamazine	Filariasis	Punctate keratitis, corneal opacities (related to dead organisms), nonspecific conjunctivitis
Fluorouracil	Malignancy	Blepharitis, lacrimation, punctal stenosis, cicatricial ectropion, conjunctivitis
Gold-containing compounds	Rheumatoid arthritis	Corneal and lens deposits, keratitis, ulceration
Indomethacin	Antiinflammatory	Nonspecific conjunctivitis, photosensitivity, edema, vortex keratopathy, superficial punctate keratitis, crystalline deposits
Iron dextran	Iron deficiency	Conjunctival erythema, edema, scleral pigmentation
Methotrexate	Malignancy, systemic inflammatory diseases, psoriasis	Blepharoconjunctivitis, hypopigmentation, hyperpigmentation, lacrimation, dry eye
Naproxen	Antiinflammatory	Vortex keratopathy, ?corneal ulcers
Perhexilene	Arrhythmias	Vortex keratopathy,[46] dry eye
Phenothiazines	Psychosis	Deposits, first on anterior lens surface, then near Descemet's membrane, and only in extreme cases in the epithelium
Phenylbutazone	Antiinflammatory	Peripheral vascularization, corneal opacities, keratitis, scarring, ulceration, (?) due to lupoid reaction to drug[12]
Practolol	Angina, hypertension	Conjunctival inflammation,[47] scarring, keratinization, dry eye,[48] dense yellow or white stromal opacities, ulceration
Quinacrine (Atabrine)	Antimalarial, anthelmintic	Yellow, white, brown, blue, or gray deposits in conjunctiva and cornea

TABLE 27-2. Systemic Medications That Affect the Cornea and Conjunctiva—cont'd

DRUG	USES	EFFECTS
Retinoids (etretinate, isotretinoin)	Psoriasis, acne	Blepharoconjunctivitis, dry eyes, fine subepithelial opacities[49]
Suramin	Onchocerciasis, trypanosomiasis	Vortex keratopathy, keratitis
Tamoxifen	Breast carcinoma	Vortex keratopathy
Thioxanthene derivatives (chlorprothixene, thiothixene)	Antipsychotics	Fine particulate corneal deposits, keratitis[12]
Tilorone	Immunoadjuvant, malignancy, graft vs host	Vortex keratopathy[50]
Vitamin D		Calcium deposits in cornea and conjunctiva

markedly prolonged iron therapy.[34] A bilateral circular pigmented line of the corneal epithelium can be seen in hereditary spherocytosis (Dalgleisch lines).[35]

Iron deposition in the corneal epithelium occurs with aging and with conditions that disturb the normal pattern of epithelial migration over the cornea. The typical form of iron deposition is the *Hudson-Stähli line,* which occurs in the majority of patients over 50 years of age.[36] It is seen as a brown, green, yellow, or white irregular horizontal line in the central deep epithelium, at the juncture of the lower and middle thirds of the cornea. Histologically, iron is present in the basal corneal epithelial cells.[37] Such iron deposits can be found in nearly all corneas of any age,[36,37] suggesting that this is a normal, progressive process related to epithelial turnover.

Epithelial iron lines also occur adjacent to acute elevations of the corneal surface: central to filtering blebs (Ferry),[38] or pterygia (Stocker)[39] at the base of the cone in keratoconus (Fleischer),[40] around Salzmann's nodules,[41] inside the rim of corneal grafts,[42] and around radial keratotomy incisions and other refractive procedures.[43]

SYSTEMIC DRUGS

A wide variety of medications can affect the conjunctiva or cornea when administered systemically. Some of the more common ones are discussed below, others are listed in Table 27-2.

PHENOTHIAZINES

Phenothiazines are a group of medications used primarily in the treatment of psychoses. Their action is believed to be related to blockage of dopamine receptors in the central nervous system. The incidence of ocular side effects is low, but is dose and drug dependent. Chlorpromazine is the drug most commonly associated with pigmentary deposits in the eye. The deposits are first seen in the lens, as anterior, subcapsular yellow-brown-white dots in the pupillary aperture[51] (Fig. 27-8). In more advanced cases similar deposits can be seen near Descemet's membrane (Fig. 27-9). They tend to involve the interpalpebral cornea and are accompanied by similar granules in the interpalpebral conjunctiva. In extreme cases pigmented streaks or lines can be seen in the interpalpebral corneal epithelium.[52] The distribution of the deposits suggests that exposure to light contributes to their formation.

The deposits in the lens, cornea, and conjunctiva have no adverse effects. They tend to subside slowly with cessation of drug administration.

AMINOQUINOLONES

Chloroquine (Aralen) and hydroxychloroquine (Plaquenil) are aminoquinolones used as antimalarial agents and in treating rheumatoid arthritis, systemic lupus erythematosus, and other systemic in-

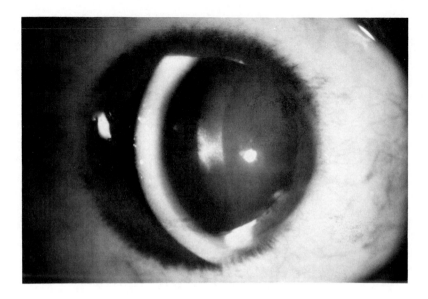

Fig. 27-8. Lens deposits resulting from thorazine administration.

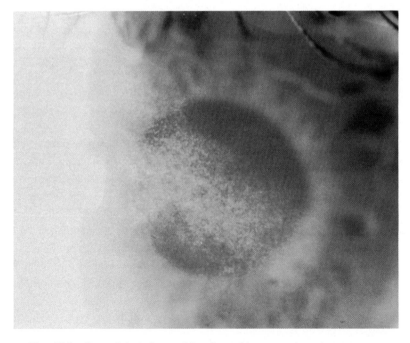

Fig. 27-9. Corneal deposits resulting from chlorpromazine administration.

flammatory diseases. Their major ocular side effect is retinopathy, which can result in permanent visual loss. Ocular toxicity is most common with chloroquine, but it also can occur with hydroxychloroquine. Chronic administration of chloroquine can also produce deposits in the cornea that are visible with the biomicroscope. They are seen as many fine yellowish or white dots in the epithelium.[53-55] At first they may appear as a Hudson-Stähli line or as an increase in an existing iron line, but the most common appearance is as an epithelial vortex (Fig. 27-10). These deposits usually do not disturb the surface of the epithelium. They also can be seen in individuals who work in the manufacturing of chloroquine.

The corneal deposits do no harm and disappear after the medication is discontinued or if the dose

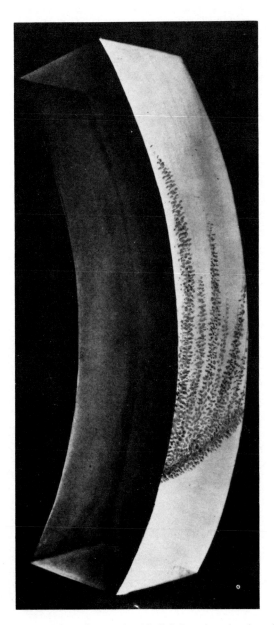

Fig. 27-10. Diagrammatic representation of corneal epithelial deposits related to chloroquine administration.

is reduced. They are not a contraindication to continued use of the drug, and there appears to be no correlation between corneal deposition and retinopathy.

Similar deposits can be seen with administration of quinacrine, indomethacin,[56] amiodarone (Fig. 27-11),[57,58] naproxen,[59] suramin,[60] tamoxifen, clofazimine,[61] and other medications. Many of the drugs associated with this picture exhibit cationic amphiphilia, and it has been hypothesized that these drugs form complexes with polar intracellular lipids, which cannot be metabolized by lysosomal phospholipases.[62,63] The complexes accumulate in the epithelial cells, resulting in a condition similar to Fabry's disease.

CYTARABINE

Cytarabine (Ara-C, cytosine arabinoside) is an antimetabolite used in the treatment of leukemias and other malignancies, as well as systemic herpes simplex infection. Ocular complications are common in patients receiving high dose (> 3 g/m^2) chemotherapy. Conjunctivitis and ocular irritation are most common, but corneal epithelial cysts can also occur[64] (Fig. 27-12). These cysts can produce marked photophobia, tearing, and reduced vision. Symptoms usually develop 5 to 7 days after initiation of therapy and reverse 1 to 2 weeks after cessation. The incidence and severity appear to be reduced by prophylactic use of corticosteroids.[65] In one study 2-deoxycytidine was found to be equally effective, with a theoretically lower risk of complications.[66]

FLUOROURACIL

Fluorouracil (5-FU) is another antimetabolite used systemically in the treatment of malignancies, particularly carcinoma of the colon, rectum, breast, stomach, and pancreas. It also has been injected subconjunctivally to reduce scar formation after filtering surgery.[67] Systemic administration is associated with excess tearing, conjunctival irritation, occlusion of the lacrimal puncta (Fig. 27-13), and blepharitis.[68,69] In addition, limbal conjunctivitis can occur (Fig. 27-14). Cicatricial ectropion can result from topical administration to the facial skin.[70]

Subconjunctival 5-FU for filtering surgery can lead to persistent epithelial defects, subepithelial scarring, and corneal ulceration.[71-73]

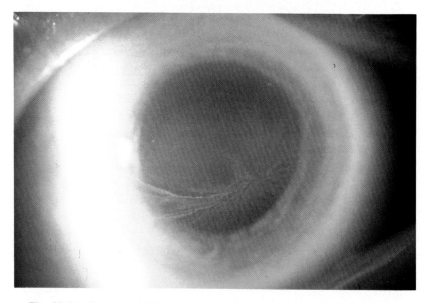

Fig. 27-11. Corneal epithelial pigmentation due to amiodarone administration.

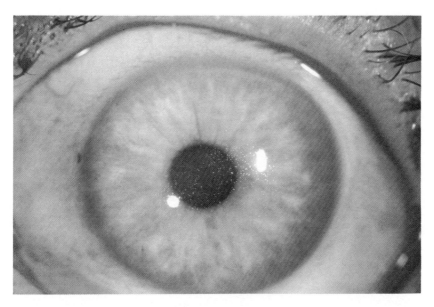

Fig. 27-12. Corneal epithelial cysts related to cytarabine therapy.

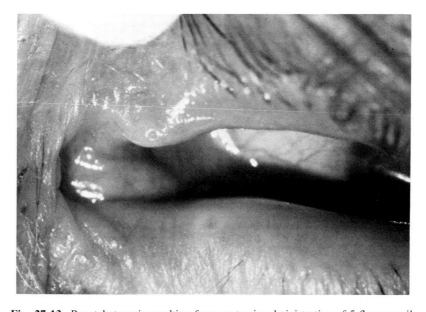

Fig. 27-13. Punctal stenosis resulting from systemic administration of 5-fluorouracil.

RETINOIDS

Etretinate and isotretinoin (Accutane) are vitamin A–related compounds that are used in the treatment of psoriasis, cystic acne, and other skin disorders. They are commonly associated with blepharoconjunctivitis, dry eyes, and transient blurred vision. Fine, round subepithelial opacities also have been observed in the central and peripheral corneas of patients on these medications.[49] The opacities usually do not interfere with vision.

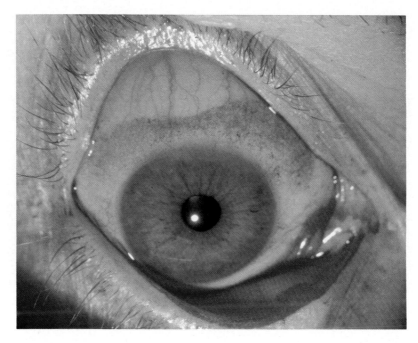

Fig. 27-14. Superior limbal staining with rose bengal related to systemic administration of 5-fluorouracil.

REFERENCES

1. Hashimoto A et al: Corneal chrysiasis: a clinical study in rheumatoid arthritis receiving gold therapy, Arthritis Rheum 15:309, 1972.
2. Kincaid MC et al: Ocular chrysiasis, Arch Ophthalmol 100:1791, 1982.
3. McCormick SA et al: Ocular chrysiasis, Ophthalmology 92:1432, 1985.
4. Bron AJ, McLendon BF, and Camp AV: Epithelial deposition of gold in the cornea in patients receiving systemic therapy, Am J Ophthalmol 88:354, 1979.
5. Roberts WH and Wolter JR: Ocular chrysiasis, Arch Ophthalmol 56:48, 1956.
6. Hashimoto A et al: Corneal chrysiasis: a clinical study in rheumatoid arthritis patients receiving gold therapy, Arthritis Rheum 15:309, 1972.
7. Rodenhäuser JH and von Behrend T: Type 2 incidence of eye involvement after parenteral gold therapy, Dtsch Med Wochenschr 94:2389, 1969.
8. Gottlieb NL and Major JC: Ocular chrysiasis correlated with gold concentrations in the crystalline lens during chrysotherapy, Arthritis Rheum 21:704, 1978.
9. Weidle EG: Lenticular chrysiasis in oral chrysotherapy, Am J Ophthalmol 103:240, 1987.
10. Gourlay JS: Mercurialentis, Trans Ophthalmol Soc 74:441, 1954.
11. Locket Z and Nazroo IA: Eye changes following exposure to metallic mercury, Lancet 1:528, 1952.
12. Fraunfelder FT: Drug-induced ocular side effects and drug interactions, ed 3, Philadelphia, 1989, Lea & Febiger.
13. Kennedy RE, Roca PD, and Platt DS: Further observations on atypical band keratopathy in glaucomatous patients, Trans Am Ophthalmol Soc 72:107, 1974.
14. Burn RA: Mercurialentis, Proc R Soc Med 55:322, 1962.
15. Wilson LA, McNatt J, and Reitschel R: Delayed hypersensitivity to thimerosal in soft contact lens wearers, Ophthalmology 88:804, 1981.
16. Oae NA, Tso MOM, and Rosenthal AR: Chalcosis in the human eye, Arch Ophthalmol 94:1379, 1976.
17. Rosenthal AR, Appleton B, and Hopkins JL: Intraocular copper foreign bodies, Am J Ophthalmol 78:671, 1974.
18. Rao NA, Tso MOM, and Rosenthal R: Chalcosis in the human eye, Arch Ophthalmol 94:1379, 1976.
19. Moss AP et al: The ocular manifestations and functional effect of occupational argyrosis, Arch Ophthalmol 97:906, 1979.
20. Yanoff M and Scheie HG: Argyrosis of the conjunctiva and lacrimal sac, Arch Ophthalmol 72:57, 1964.
21. Bartlett RE: Generalized argyrosis with lens involvement, Am J Ophthalmol 38:402, 1954.
22. Spencer WH et al: Endogenous and exogenous ocular and systemic silver deposition, Trans Ophthalmol Soc UK 100:171, 1980.
23. Weiler HH et al: Argyria of the cornea due to self-administration of eyelash dye, Ann Ophthalmol 14:822, 1982.
24. Hanna C, Fraunfelder FT, and Sanchez J: Ultrastructural study of argyrosis of the cornea and conjunctiva, Arch Ophthalmol 92:18, 1974.
25. Gutman FA and Crosswell HH: Argyrosis of the cornea without clinical conjunctival involvement, Am J Ophthalmol 65:183, 1968.

26. Spencer WH et al: Endogenous and exogenous ocular and systemic silver deposition, Trans Ophthalmol Soc UK 100:171, 1980.

27. Karcioglu ZA and Caldwell DR: Corneal argyrosis: histologic, ultrastructural and microanalytic study, Can J Ophthalmol 20:257, 1985.

28. Zuckerman BD and Lieberman TW: Corneal rust ring, Arch Ophthalmol 63:254, 1960.

29. Coats G: Small superficial opaque white rings in the cornea, Trans Ophthalmol Soc UK 32:53, 1912.

30. Nevins RC, Davis WH, and Elliott JH: Coats' white ring of the cornea—unsettled metal fettle, Arch Ophthalmol 80:145, 1968.

31. Gottsch FD et al: Corneal blood staining. An animal model, Ophthalmology 93:797, 1986.

32. Cibis PA, Brown EB, and Hong SM: Ocular aspects of systemic siderosis, Am J Ophthalmol 44:158, 1957.

33. Davies G et al: Deposition of melanin and iron in ocular structures in haemochromatosis, Br J Ophthalmol 56:338, 1972.

34. Salminen L, Paasio P, and Ekfors T: Epibulbar siderosis induced by iron tablets, Am J Ophthalmol 93:660, 1982.

35. Dalgleisch R: Ring-like corneal deposits in a case of congenital spherocytosis, Br J Ophthalmol 49:40, 1965.

36. Gass JD: The iron lines of the superficial cornea, Arch Ophthalmol 71:348, 1964.

37. Barraquer-Somers E, Chan CC, and Green WR: Corneal epithelial iron deposition, Ophthalmology 90:729, 1983.

38. Ferry AP: A new iron line of the superficial cornea, Arch Ophthalmol 79:142, 1968.

39. Stocker FW: Eine pigmentierte hornhautline bei ptergium, Schweiz Med Wochenschr 20:19, 1939.

40. Fleischer B: Über keratoconus und eigenartige figuren bildung in der cornea, Munchen Med Wochenschr 53:625, 1906.

41. Reinach NW and Baum J: A corneal pigmented line associated with Salzmann's nodular degeneration, Am J Ophthalmol 91:677, 1981.

42. Mannis MJ: Iron deposition in the corneal graft, Arch Ophthalmol 101:1858, 1983.

43. Koenig SB et al: Corneal lines after refractive keratoplasty, Arch Ophthalmol 101:1862, 1983.

44. Kapp JP et al: Limitations of high dose intra-arterial 1,3-bis(2-chloroethyl)-1-nitrosoures (BCNU) chemotherapy for malignant gliomas, Neurosurgery 10:715, 1982.

45. Fischer FP: Bismuthiase secondaire de la cornee, Ann Oculist (Paris)183:615, 1950.

46. Gibson JM et al: Severe ocular side effects of perhexilene maleate: case report, Br J Ophthalmol 68:553, 1984.

47. Garner A and Rahi AHS: Practolol and ocular toxicity: antibodies in serum and tears, Br J Ophthalmol 60:684, 1976.

48. Wright P: Untoward effects associated with practolol administration: oculomucocutaneous syndrome, Br Med J 1:595, 1975.

49. Fraunfelder FT, LaBraico JM, and Meyer SM: Adverse ocular reactions possibly associated with isotretinoin, Am J Ophthalmol 100:534, 1985.

50. Weiss JN, Weinberg RS, and Regelson W: Keratopathy after oral administration of tilorone hydrochloride, Am J Ophthalmol 89:46, 1980.

51. McClanahan WS et al: Ocular manifestations of chronic phenothiazine derivative administration, Arch Ophthalmol 75:319, 1966.

52. Johnson AW and Buffaloe WJ: Chlorpromazine epithelial keratopathy, Arch Ophthalmol 76:664, 1966.

53. Bernstein HN: Chloroquine ocular toxicity, Surv Ophthalmol 12:415, 1967.

54. Carr RE et al: Ocular toxicity of antimalarial drugs, Am J Ophthalmol 66:738, 1968.

55. Lawwill T, Appleton B, and Alstatt L: Chloroquine accumulation in human eyes, Am J Ophthalmol 65:530, 1968.

56. Burns DA: Indomethacin, reduced retinal sensitivity, and corneal deposits, Am J Ophthalmol 66:825, 1968

57. Kaplan LJ and Cappaert WE: Amiodarone keratopathy, Arch Ophthalmol 100:601, 1982.

58. Wilson FM, Schmitt TE, and Grayson M: Amiodarone-induced cornea verticillata, Ann Ophthalmol 12:657, 1980.

59. Szmyd L and Perry HD: Keratopathy associated with the use of naproxen, Am J Ophthalmol 99:598, 1985.

60. Teich SA et al: Toxic keratopathy associated with suramin therapy, N Engl J Med 314:1455, 1986.

61. Walinder PE, Gip L, and Stempa M: Corneal changes in patients treated with clofazimine, Br J Ophthalmol 60:526, 1976.

62. Lullman H, Lullmann-Rauch R, and Wassermann O: Lipidosis induced by amphiphilic cationic drugs, Biochem Pharmacol 27:1103, 1978.

63. D'Amico DJ and Kenyon KR: Drug-induced lipidoses of the cornea and conjunctiva, Int Ophthalmol 4:67, 1981.

64. Hopen G et al: Corneal toxicity with systemic cytarabine, Am J Ophthalmol 91:500, 1981.

65. Lass J et al: Topical corticosteroid therapy for corneal toxicity from systemically administered cytarabine, Am J Ophthalmol 94:617, 1982.

66. Lazarus HM et al: Comparison of the prophylactic effects of 2-deoxycytidine and prednisolone for high-dose intravenous cytarabine-induced keratitis, Am J Ophthalmol 104:476, 1987

67. Heuer DK et al: 5-Fluorouracil and glaucoma filtering surgery. III. Intermediate follow-up of a pilot study, Ophthalmology 93:1537, 1986.

68. Caravella LP, Burns JA, and Zangmeister M: Punctal-canalicular stenosis related to systemic fluorouracil therapy, Arch Ophthalmol 99:284, 1981.

69. Imperia PS, Lazarus HM, and Lass JH: Ocular complications of systemic cancer chemotherapy, Surv Ophthalmol 34:209, 1989.

70. Galentine P et al: Bilateral cicatricial ectropion following topical administration of 5-fluorouracil, Ann Ophthalmol 13:575, 1981.

71. Knapp A et al: Serious corneal complications of glaucoma filtering surgery with postoperative 5-fluorouracil, Am J Ophthalmol 103:183, 1987.

72. Shapiro MS et al: 5-Fluorouracil toxicity to the ocular surface epithelium, Invest Ophthalmol Vis Sci 26:580, 1985.

73. Capone A et al: In vivo effects of 5-FU on ocular surface epithelium following corneal wounding, Invest Ophthalmol Vis Sci 28:1661, 1987.

TOXIC AND ALLERGIC REACTIONS TO TOPICAL OPHTHALMIC MEDICATIONS

FRED M. WILSON II, MD*

Toxic reactions
- Toxic papillary keratoconjunctivitis
- Toxic papillary keratoconjunctivitis with scarring (pseudopemphigoid)
- Toxic follicular conjunctivitis
- Toxic follicular conjunctivitis with scarring (pseudotrachoma)
- Anesthetic toxicity
- Toxic calcific band-shaped keratopathy

Allergic reactions
- Allergic contact dermatoconjunctivitis
- Anaphylactoid blepharoconjunctivitis
Miscellaneous reactions
Recovery from drug reactions
Prevention of drug reactions

Toxic and allergic reactions to topical ophthalmic medications are common and troublesome. They are second in frequency only to keratoconjunctivitis sicca among all external ocular diseases.[1]

Toxicity is the result of direct chemical irritation of tissues by drugs or preservatives. Allergy requires sensitization of and the induction of ocular inflammation by the patient's immune system. Contrary to widespread belief, toxic reactions are much more common than allergic ones, the former accounting for about 90% of all reactions (Table 28-1).

TOXIC REACTIONS

TOXIC PAPILLARY KERATOCONJUNCTIVITIS

Toxic papillary keratoconjunctivitis is the most common of all adverse reactions to topical medications (Table 28-1). It results from the ability of certain medications to be irritating simply by being applied repeatedly to the ocular surface. The toxic effects usually take at least 2 weeks to develop.

Punctate staining, more prominent with rose bengal red than with fluorescein, is the most common finding. The staining is usually most pronounced on the inferonasal conjunctiva and cornea (Fig. 28-1), where medications gravitate on their way to the lacrimal outflow system. Worsening of preexisting corneal staining can occur, even before the typical inferonasal staining, if corneal surface dis-

*Professor of Ophthalmology, Co-Director, Cornea and External Ocular Disease Service, Indiana University School of Medicine, Department of Ophthalmology, 702 Rotary Circle, Indianapolis, IN 46202.

TABLE 28-1. Relative Frequencies of Various Types of Adverse Reactions to Topical Ophthalmic Medications[1]

TYPE OF REACTION	RELATIVE FREQUENCY (%)
TOXIC REACTIONS	**90**
Toxic papillary reactions	76
Toxic follicular reactions	9
Toxic calcific band keratopathy	2
Pseudopemphigoid	2
Pseudotrachoma	1
ALLERGIC REACTIONS	**10**
Allergic contact reactions	10
Anaphylactoid reactions	Very rare

ease precedes development of the drug reaction (Fig. 28-2). Rarely, ointments are trapped beneath the upper eyelid, producing staining along the upper limbus. Medications toxic to the epithelium also can cause, or inhibit the healing of, chronic epithelial defects of the cornea, sometimes producing pseudodendrites or pseudogeographic ulcers, which can be mistaken for herpes simplex keratitis[1,2] (Fig. 28-3).

Other signs include hyperemia, nonspecific papillary conjunctivitis, and scant mucoid or mucopurulent discharge. Itching is absent and eosinophils are not seen in conjunctival scrapings.

The main causes of toxic papillary reactions (see box on p. 635) are aminoglycoside antibiotics, antiviral agents, and the preservative benzalkonium chloride (Zephiran). Benzalkonium is an especially common offender because it is one of the most frequently used preservatives (in concentrations

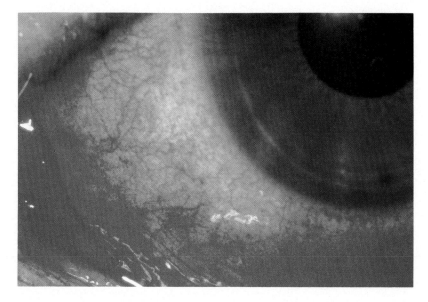

Fig. 28-1. Characteristic punctate staining, with rose bengal red, of inferonasal bulbar conjunctiva in toxic papillary keratoconjunctivitis secondary to neomycin. Such staining occurs in association with toxic reactions to many other drugs and preservatives and several other types of medication-induced toxicities and allergies. Similar, but usually less impressive, staining can be seen with fluorescein.

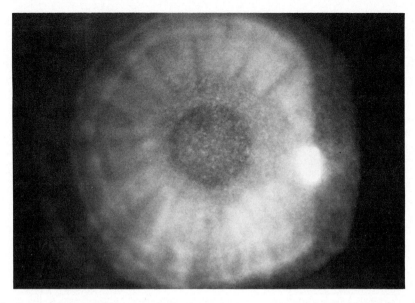

Fig. 28-2. Toxic keratitis secondary to neomycin. Extensive punctate staining of the cornea, in this case with fluorescein, can precede or develop in conjunction with the typical inferonasal staining of toxic papillary kerato-conjunctivitis (and other medication-induced reactions) when preexisting ocular surface disease, such as kerato-conjunctivitis sicca, is present. Such corneal staining develops eventually, even in the absence of predisposing surface disease.

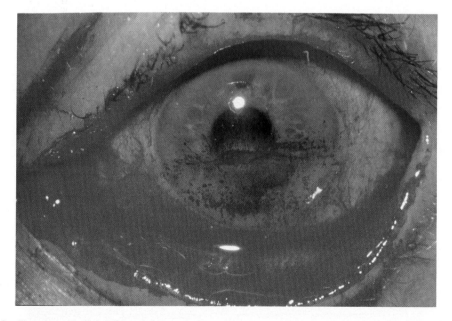

Fig. 28-3. Chronic epithelial defect of the cornea secondary to neomycin toxicity (rose bengal red stain). Such toxic epithelial defects are often mistaken for herpes simplex dendrites or geographic ulcers. The toxic lesions have relatively smooth and rolled-under edges and change very little with time, whereas herpetic defects have finely irregular edges and change their shapes fairly rapidly. Note also the drug-induced staining of the inferonasal bulbar conjunctiva.

MAIN CAUSES OF TOXIC PAPILLARY REACTIONS

AMINOGLYCOSIDE ANTIBIOTICS
Neomycin
Gentamicin
Tobramycin

NEARLY ALL "CONCENTRATED" OR "FORTIFIED" ANTIBIOTICS AND ANTIFUNGAL AGENTS

ANTIVIRAL AGENTS
Idoxuridine
Vidarabine
Trifluorothymidine*

TOPICAL ANESTHETIC AGENTS
Proparacaine
Tetracaine

PRESERVATIVES†
Benzalkonium

---

*Trifluorothymidine is the least toxic of the three antiviral agents.
†Chlorobutanol is occasionally toxic to the dry eye.

from 0.004% to 0.02%) and because it is a surfactant with detergent-like properties. Damage to corneal epithelium occurs even at the lower concentrations.[1-3]

The factors that predispose to toxic papillary reactions include (1) keratoconjunctivitis sicca, (2) other ocular surface problems, (3) prolonged use of medications, and (4) use of multiple preparations. The dry eye is especially susceptible, so even relatively nontoxic preservatives, such as chlorobutanol, can cause toxicity. The major problem is that benzalkonium is still present in several artificial-tear preparations, and patients with dry eye who use such tears often are made worse by them sooner or later. These difficulties have led to the advent of an artificial tear (Tears Naturale II) with a preservative (polyquaternium-1, Polyquad) that is presumably nontoxic to epithelial cells; artificial tears and contact lens solutions that are preserved with sorbic acid or sorbate (also thought to be nontoxic); preservative-free tears such as Refresh, Celluvisc, and Hypotears PF that are dispensed in small, sterile, "unit-dose" containers; and preservative-free lubricating ointments (Aqua-Tears, Duolube, Duratears Naturale, Hypotears, Lacri-Lube NP, and Refresh PM).

The mainstay of treatment of toxic papillary reactions, and virtually all other reactions, is the withdrawal of offending medications and preservatives. Preservative-free artificial tears or lubricants may be prescribed if necessary. Topical corticosteroids are of no value (and are usually preserved with benzalkonium). Patching or therapeutic soft contact lenses are sometimes helpful for treating chronic epithelial defects or keratopathy.

Toxic Papillary Keratoconjunctivitis with Scarring (Pseudopemphigoid)

Prolonged and severe toxic papillary reactions can lead to conjunctiva scarring or keratinization, worse below, producing a clinical picture that mimics cicatricial pemphigoid (Fig. 28-4). Corneal pannus also can develop. This kind of reaction is probably most often the result of long-standing and severe toxic papillary keratoconjunctivitis, although evidence exists that type-III (antigen-antibody-mediated) hypersensitivity might play a role in some cases.[4,5] Progression ceases when the causative medications are stopped.

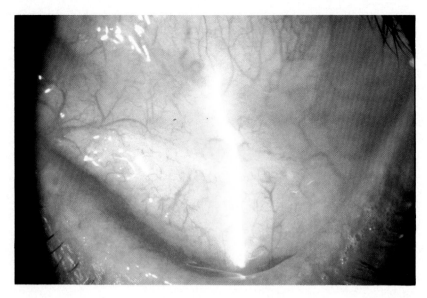

Fig. 28-4. Pseudopemphigoid from the chronic use of dipivalyl epinephrine. Conjunctival scarring and cicatricial foreshortening of the inferior conjunctival fornix.

Pseudopemphigoid is usually caused by the long-term use of glaucoma medications, perhaps because of the chronicity of their use (see box below).

Toxic Follicular Conjunctivitis

The exact mechanism by which toxic follicular conjunctivitis develops is uncertain, although it is presumed to be toxic rather than allergic.[1] Itching, eczematoid dermatitis, eosinophils in conjunctival scrapings, and positive cutaneous patch tests are all absent unless the patient also happens to react allergically to the causative drug. Even ocular hyperemia and punctate staining are often, but not invariably, lacking or unimpressive; these findings, too, if present, can indicate superimposed toxic papillary or allergic reactions. The toxic follicular response itself probably results from the ability of certain drugs to act as nonantigenic mitogens (as do, for example, phytohemagglutinin and pokeweed mitogen) to induce mitoses and lymphoblastic transformations of lymphocytes by nonimmunologic means.

Toxic follicular reactions come about slowly, usually requiring at least several weeks, and sometimes years, to develop. Follicular conjunctivitis is the main finding (Fig. 28-5). This represents a proliferation of subepithelial conjunctival lymphocytes. True lymphoid follicles, with germinal centers containing lymphoblasts, are present[1] (Fig. 28-6). The follicles are most prominent in the lower

---

ANTIGLAUCOMA AGENTS: MAIN CAUSES OF DRUG-INDUCED PSEUDOPEMPHIGOID*

Echothiophate
Epinephrine
Dipivalyl epinephrine
Pilocarpine

---

*Some of these reactions, especially those caused by epinephrine or dipivalyl epinephrine, may have associated type-III hypersensitivity and so may not be purely toxic.

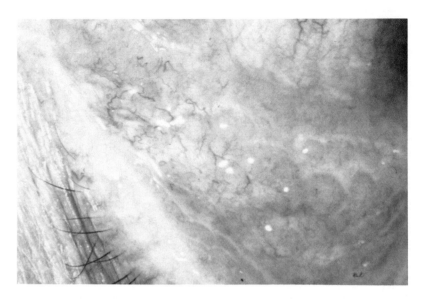

Fig. 28-5. Toxic follicular conjunctivitis caused by topical dipivalyl epinephrine. Similar reactions can be produced by epinephrine itself, antiviral agents, miotic drugs, and certain cycloplegic agents (atropine and homatropine).

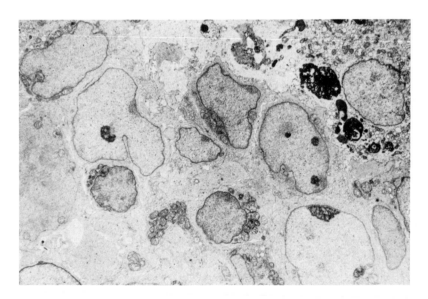

Fig. 28-6. Electron microscopy of germinal center of dipivalyl epinephrine-induced follicle from patient shown in Fig. 28-5. That this is a true lymphoid follicle is indicated by the presence of the large, pale lymphoblasts with prominent nuclei (and often nucleoli) and the dark, irregular "tingible bodies" *(upper right)*. Tingible bodies are macrophages that have engulfed nuclear material and are evidence of follicular maturity. As is also characteristic of lymphoid follicles, masses of lymphocytes (produced by the metabolically active lymphoblasts) were found more peripherally (not shown here). (Original magnification, ×3000.) (From Wilson FM II: Trans Am Ophthalmol Soc 81:854, 1983.)

CAUSES OF DRUG-INDUCED TOXIC FOLLICULAR CONJUNCTIVITIS*

ANTIVIRAL AGENTS

Idoxuridine
Vidarabine
Trifluorothymidine

ANTIGLAUCOMA AGENTS

Pilocarpine
Echothiophate
Epinephrine
Dipivalyl epinephrine
Carbachol

CYCLOPLEGIC AGENTS

Atropine
Homatropine

*With prolonged use, these drugs can cause conjunctival scarring, producing a pseudotrachoma syndrome.

fornix and the inferior palpebral conjunctiva but can occur at the limbus, in the superior palpebral conjunctiva, and the semilunar fold. As mentioned previously, hyperemia and punctate staining are usually mild, if present at all. The same is true of mucoid or mucopurulent discharge. The exudate seldom shows any purulence clinically, although a few neutrophils sometimes can be found in conjunctival scrapings.

The causes of toxic follicular conjunctivitis are shown in the box above. No preservatives are known to produce follicular reactions, and only a few specific drugs do so. Although various drugs and preservatives cause toxic papillary reactions in susceptible individuals, only the drugs listed in the box above are known to induce follicles.

The factors that predispose to toxic follicular conjunctivitis are prolonged use of one of the causative drugs and individual susceptibility. Some evidence suggests that the use of old or outdated medications that have undergone deterioration might also predispose to the problem.[6]

The best treatment is withdrawal of the drug that is causing the reaction. Occasionally, substitution of a new and fresh preparation of the same drug can be helpful. Topical corticosteroid slows but does not prevent the development of the follicular hypertrophy and would hardly ever be useful as treatment except, perhaps, as a temporizing measure. Of course, simple observation, with continuation of the offending drug, is permissible if the drug is needed and the symptoms are not severe.

Toxic Follicular Conjunctivitis with Scarring (Pseudotrachoma)

Long-standing toxic follicular conjunctivitis can lead to conjunctival scarring and corneal pannus, producing (with the follicles) a *pseudotrachoma* syndrome (Fig. 28-7). Even preauricular lymphadenopathy can be present, representing lymphocytic hypertrophy in the regional lymph node. Punctal occlusion can occur in the absence of other evidence of conjunctival scarring. Molluscum contagiosum of the eyelid margin is another cause of pseudotrachoma.

Anesthetic Toxicity

Toxic keratoconjunctivitis secondary to the abuse of topical anesthetic agents is an uncommon but potentially severe problem. It is primarily a particularly severe form of toxic papillary keratoconjunctivitis, although it has some features of its own that warrant consideration as a separate entity.

The chronic use of topical anesthetic is extremely toxic to epithelial microvilli, organelles, and

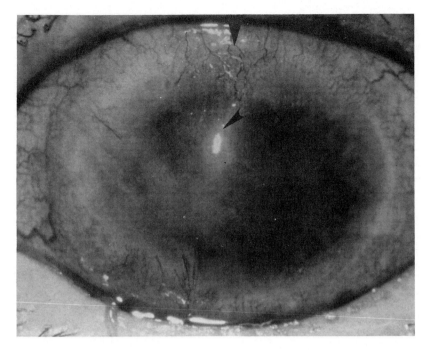

Fig. 28-7. Pseudotrachoma secondary to idoxuridine. Corneal pannus *(large arrow)* and corneal infiltrate *(small arrow)*. Although the infiltrate is probably of herpetic origin, it is often uncertain whether corneal vascularization is secondary to drug toxicity or to underlying disease. Associated conjunctival follicles and scarring, which were clearly drug induced, combined to create a trachoma-like picture.

desmosomes (intercellular bridges), and to cellular metabolism, mitosis, and migration.[2] The loss of microvilli causes instability of the tear film, adding to the drying and neurotrophic keratopathy that result from the loss of corneal sensation. Some of the inflammation might be secondary to a superimposed antibody-mediated reaction.

Anesthetic toxicity develops within a few days to weeks. The ability of the drug to relieve pain is short-lived, so the patient soon begins to use it more frequently (often every few minutes), with progressively less relief or response and more rebound pain as the effect of the drop wears off. Patients who abuse topical anesthetics sometimes have psychologic or psychiatric problems and continually gain access to the drug on their own, although physicians are occasionally at fault for providing the medication.

Clinical manifestations can include severe ocular pain, lid swelling, hyperemia, mucopurulent discharge, extensive punctate staining, chronic epithelial defects of the cornea, Wessely–immune ringlike or disciform stromal infiltrates, corneal edema, superficial or deep corneal vascularization, and iridocyclitis with keratic precipitates (Fig. 28-8). The corneal stroma does not show ulceration or necrosis as often occurs with bacterial, fungal, or acanthamoebic corneal ulcers, and corneal cultures are negative or noncontributory. Hypopyon and hyphema also have developed secondary to anesthetic toxicity.

Treatment of anesthetic abuse requires stopping the drug and substituting other means for relieving pain and encouraging healing, for example, cycloplegia, patching, therapeutic soft contact lenses, or systemic analgesic agents. Topical corticosteroid can reduce pain and inflammation to some extent. Hospitalization and psychiatric consultation are occasionally advisable.

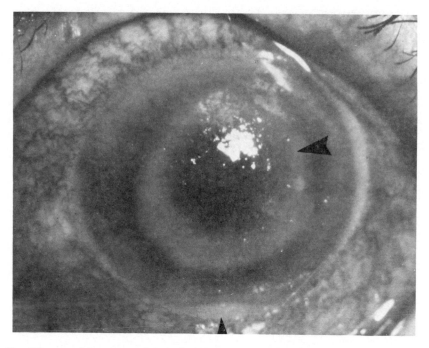

Fig. 28-8. Keratitis caused by abuse of topical proparacaine. Hyperemia, chronic epithelial defect, stromal edema surrounded by a Wessely–immune ringlike infiltrate *(large arrow),* and small hypopyon *(small arrow)* without stromal ulceration or necrosis. (Courtesy of Merrill Grayson, Indianapolis.)

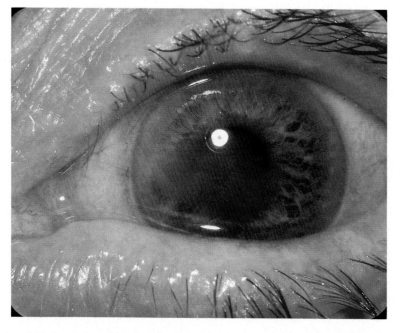

Fig. 28-9. Toxic calcific band-shaped keratopathy induced by phenylmercuric nitrate preservative in pilocarpine eye drops.

Toxic Calcific Band-Shaped Keratopathy

Medications preserved with phenylmercuric nitrate can cause deposition of calcium in the cornea (Fig. 28-9) and mercury in the lens.[2,7,8] The preservative is believed to damage protein in the superficial corneal stroma, so the calcium is then deposited as a degenerative change.[9] The mercury itself accumulates in the anterior lens capsule (mercurialentis).[10] A closely related preservative, phenylmercuric acetate, also can cause mercurialentis but not band keratopathy.[10] These deposits appear only after months or years of exposure to the mercurial preservatives.[2]

Unlike other forms of calcific band keratopathy, the preservative-induced form sometimes begins centrally, rather than peripherally. Eventually, the calcium extends as a horizontal band across the interpalpebral zone of the cornea. The deposits lie superficially in Bowman's layer. Mercurialentis appears as a circular, pink to rose-brown dusting of the central anterior lens capsule.

The band keratopathy can be removed by debridement and chelation therapy as is used for other forms of calcific band keratopathy. Obviously the medication containing the phenylmercuric preservative should be stopped.

ALLERGIC REACTIONS

Allergic Contact Dermatoconjunctivitis

Allergic contact dermatoconjunctivitis is the second most common type of drug reaction (see Table 28-1).[1] Allergic contact reactions occur after sensitization of thymus-derived lymphocytes (T cells) in the regional lymph nodes and represent type-IV (delayed) hypersensitivity. Topical medications act as haptens (partial antigens) and must combine with tissue proteins to form complete antigens that can sensitize lymphocytes in nearby lymph nodes. The lymphocytes then return to the site of application and accumulation of the medication, combine with the drug-protein antigen, and produce inflammation by releasing various lymphokines.

These reactions usually take weeks to years to develop, depending on the amount of hapten applied, the degree of its penetrability, and the extent to which it is a sensitizer.[2] However, allergic contact reactions can appear in as little time as 48 hours if the patient has been sensitized previously to the drug involved.

The only important predisposing factor, other than individual susceptibility and the prolonged use of medication, is the presence of preexisting cutaneous disease of the eyelids, which permits enhanced penetration of the hapten. It should be remembered that cross sensitization to similar haptens is to be expected. For example, a patient who is allergic to one aminoglycoside antibiotic will probably react to any of the other ones.

The hallmark of this kind of reaction is eczematoid blepharitis and periocular dermatitis (Fig. 28-10). If the cause is an eye drop, the eczema begins at the nasal aspect of the lower eyelid (where drugs first spill onto the skin (Fig. 28-11). The dermatitis is preceded by generalized hyperemia of the conjunctiva and the same findings as occur with toxic papillary reactions and can finally spread extensively to affect the upper eyelid, the temporal and malar regions, and the cheek. If the cause is an ointment or a nonophthalmic substance, such as a cosmetic, the eczema appears first wherever the hapten has been applied, for example, the upper eyelid, and the eye itself can be uninflamed. Itching is prominent, and eosinophils are present in conjunctival scrapings in about 25% of cases because the sensitized lymphocytes can produce an eosinophil chemotactic factor.[1,2] Rarely, contact allergy can be associated with marginal corneal infiltration and ulceration.[2,11,12]

The most common causes of allergic contact dermatoconjunctivitis are shown in the box on p. 643. Thimerosal use (in contact lens care solutions) is often associated with and may be at least partially responsible for a specific clinical syndrome (*contact lens–induced keratoconjunctivitis*, see Chapter 7) seen in people who wear contact lenses. Severe inflammation of the conjunctiva and cornea can occur, but there is seldom any dermatitis, probably because insufficient amounts of the pre-

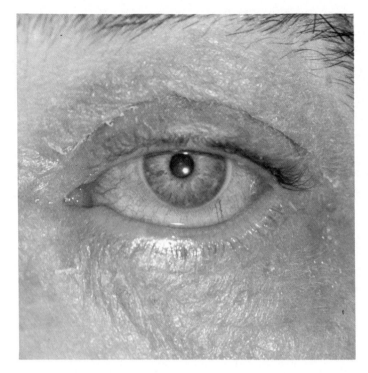

Fig. 28-10. Periocular cutaneous eczema of allergic contact dermatoconjunctivitis secondary to idoxuridine.

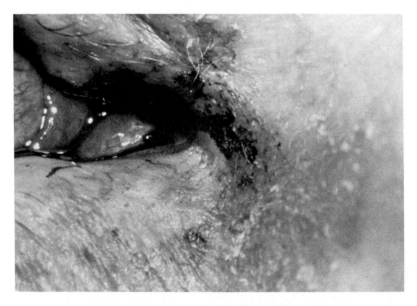

Fig. 28-11. Early allergic contact dermatoconjunctivitis affects the skin of the medial canthal area and inferonasal eyelid. This example was caused by dipivalyl epinephrine. Rose bengal red stain has been instilled (appears black).

MAIN CAUSES OF DRUG-INDUCED ALLERGIC CONTACT REACTIONS

AMINOGLYCOSIDE ANTIBIOTICS
Neomycin
Gentamicin
Tobramycin

ANTIVIRAL AGENTS
Idoxuridine
Vidarabine
Trifluorothymidine (rarely)

CYCLOPLEGIC AGENTS
Atropine
Homatropine

PRESERVATIVES OR OTHER ADDITIVES
Thimerosal*
Chlorhexidine*
Edetate (EDTA)

*Thimerosal and (very rarely) chlorhexidine cause contact allergy almost exclusively in people who wear contact lenses.

servative are present in and on the contact lens to result in any significant spillover to the skin. Nevertheless, a type-IV allergic contact reaction may be responsible.

Secondary infection of eczematoid dermatitis is not uncommon, usually by *Staphylococcus* or *Streptococcus,* less often by *Candida.*[2,13] Any of these organisms alone can cause spreading eczema, with or without a preexisting drug allergy. Such *infectious eczematoid dermatitis* should be suspected whenever cutaneous ulcerations are present in the affected skin; relatively remote areas such as the nose, forehead, lower face, or neck are involved; or the eczema fails to clear after the supposedly causative drug is withdrawn. Patients with atopic eczema are highly susceptible both to drug-induced and infectious eczematoid reactions.

Once the skin is broken down, even poorly sensitizing drugs can induce contact allergy; this type of reaction should be treated by stopping all topical medications whenever possible. Cool compresses may be used for relief of discomfort. Contact allergy does respond well to topical corticosteroid, but I prefer not to prescribe it because secondary infection may develop, and some of the ingredients (or even the steroid itself[14-16]) could possibly lead to further contact reactions. If infection is unlikely, I sometimes apply a topical steroid ointment once to the affected skin, in the office only; this approach can achieve considerable and rapid relief while avoiding the risks of ongoing treatment. Any suspicion of infection is reason for taking cultures (or at least scrapings) and perhaps for prescribing appropriate oral antibiotic therapy.

ANAPHYLACTOID BLEPHAROCONJUNCTIVITIS

Anaphylactoid reactions to topical ophthalmic medications are rare. I have seen only six cases in the past 23 years.

These reactions are mediated by previously formed immunoglobulin-E (IgE) humoral antibodies (type-I, immediate hypersensitivity). Patients who have had prior sensitization to a drug and already have circulating IgE antibodies to it can upon reexposure react within seconds or minutes by manifesting urticaria (in the epidermis) or angioedema (in the dermis) of the eyelids, as well as chemosis and itching (Fig. 28-12). The eye is mildly to moderately hyperemic and has only a watery or slight mucoid discharge. Itching is intense. Although eosinophils are present in the conjunctival stroma, few if any are detected in scrapings because they do not quickly reach the conjunctiva surface. Systemic anaphylactoid symptoms, and even true anaphylaxis, are possible but fortunately are extremely rare.[17,18]

The causes of anaphylactoid reactions are few and include some medications (bacitracin and sulfacetamide) that otherwise seldom cause either allergic or toxic reactions (see box on p. 644).

Therapy of anaphylactoid blepharoconjunctivitis should include immediate instillation of a vaso-

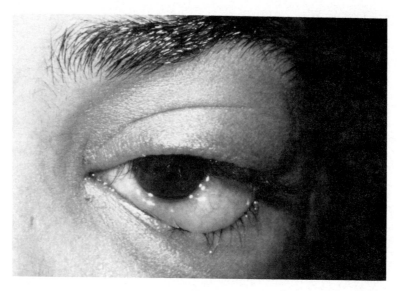

Fig. 28-12. Anaphylactoid blepharoconjunctivitis. Erythema and angioedema of the eyelids, conjunctival edema (chemosis).

constricting agent and topical corticosteroid and the application of a cold compress. An oral antihistamine should be given if the problem persists for more than a few minutes, and one should be prepared to treat systemic anaphylaxis if necessary. The offending drug should never be used again.

MISCELLANEOUS REACTIONS

Several other kinds of adverse effects of topical ophthalmic medications are possible,[2] many of which are seldom encountered, including *phototoxic* and *photoallergic reactions* (requiring interaction between drugs and light and, in the case of photoallergy, participation of the patient's immune system), *cutaneous changes secondary to the application of fluorinated corticosteroids, drug-induced alterations of melanin* (producing hyperpigmentation or hypopigmentation), and *cumulative depositions of drugs* (for example, pigmentation secondary to mercury or silver, the deposition of silver being referred to as argyria in the skin and argyrosis in the conjunctiva).

A more common cumulative deposition is the so-called *adrenochrome deposit*, which is an accumulation of oxidized and polymerized epinephrine in preexisting conjunctiva cysts. These deposits appear as discrete, dark brown to black, round spots, one to several millimeters in diameter, in the subepithelial conjunctiva of patients who have been treated chronically with epinephrine or dipivalyl epinephrine eyedrops for glaucoma (Fig. 28-13). The deposits are harmless and should not be mistaken for melanomas.

MAIN CAUSES OF ANAPHYLACTOID REACTIONS TO TOPICAL OPHTHALMIC MEDICATIONS

ANTIMICROBIAL AGENTS
 Penicillin
 Bacitracin
 Sulfacetamide

ANESTHETIC AGENTS
 Proparacaine
 Benoxinate
 Tetracaine

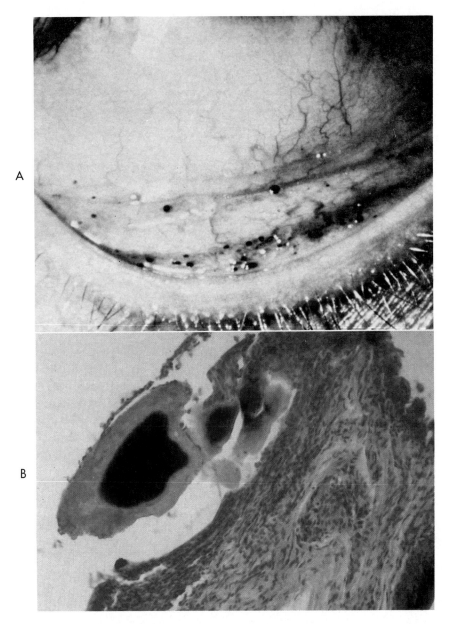

Fig. 28-13. A, Adrenochrome deposits of oxidized and polymerized epinephrine in lower palpebral conjunctiva. **B,** Histopathologic appearance of conjunctival adrenochrome deposit. Deposit lies within a conjunctival cyst and consists of a dark central area of fully oxidized and polymerized drug, surrounded by a lighter peripheral zone of incomplete polymerization. (Hematoxylin-eosin stain; ×100.) (From Wilson FM II: Surv Ophthalmol 24:57, 1979.)

Antibiotics and steroids can alter the normal microbial flora of the eyelids and conjunctiva, sometimes predisposing to the development of opportunistic infections. Steroids also can inhibit wound healing, exert biotropism (drug-induced reactivations of latent infections by dermatophytes, *Candida* and possibly, herpes simplex), and enhance the activity of the enzyme collagenase (leading to corneal "melting" and perforation).

RECOVERY FROM DRUG REACTIONS

Except for anaphylactoid reactions, drug reactions often resolve slowly after the causative medications are stopped. Some reactions improve or clear within a few days to a week or two, but many require at least 2 or 3 weeks to clear completely. If a topical steroid is stopped abruptly along with other medications, the patient actually can appear worse for several days as a result of "rebound inflammation," which can occur when a steroid is suddenly withdrawn.

PREVENTION OF DRUG REACTIONS

An effort to make an accurate diagnosis is probably the single most important measure that can be taken to prevent drug-induced diseases.[19] Lack of diagnosis tends to lead to excessive and prolonged treatment—excessive treatment because the practitioner hopes to cover all possibilities ("shotgun therapy") and prolonged treatment because it is impossible to know the prognosis and natural history of the disease without first knowing the diagnosis. This approach can cause the *overtreatment syndrome* in which harmful therapy is continued past the time when the underlying disease has improved or resolved because the adverse effects of treatment are misinterpreted as a failure or insufficiency of therapy; more medications are then prescribed, producing a relentless cycle interrupted only when treatment is much reduced or stopped.

The second most important factor in prevention is knowledge of and respect for the potential toxicities and allergenicities of specific drugs and preservatives (Table 28-2).[1,2]

The third most common problem is the mistaken belief on the part of both patients and practitioners that adverse drug reactions should clear quickly after medications are stopped. As discussed earlier, many reactions resolve slowly. Even when a drug reaction is correctly suspected, reducing treatment will be of little benefit if more drugs are prescribed a week or two later because the patient has not improved.

Finally, prevention requires dispelling the idea that most drug reactions are allergies and not toxicities. This misconception leads one to expect that almost any change in therapy should solve the

TABLE 28-2. Potential Toxicities and Allergenicities of Preservatives and Other Additives in Topical Ophthalmic Medications

PRESERVATIVE OR ADDITIVE	TOXICITY	ALLERGENICITY
Benzalkonium	++++	0
Boric acid	+	0
Chlorhexidine	+	+*
Chlorobutanol	+	0
Edetate (EDTA)	0	+
Parabens	0	+
Phenol	+	0
Phenylethyl alcohol	+	0
Phenylmercuric acetate	++†	0
Phenylmercuric nitrate	++†	0
Polyquaternium-1	0	+
Sodium bisulfate or thiosulfate	+	0
Sorbic acid or sorbate	0	+
Thimerosal	0	+++*

*Thimerosal and (very rarely) chlorhexidine cause contact allergy almost only in people who wear contact lenses (contact lens–induced keratoconjunctivitis); these patients nearly always have contact allergy only on the eye itself and do not manifest cutaneous eczema.

†Phenylmercuric nitrate causes toxic calcific band-shaped keratopathy and mercurialentis, whereas phenylmercuric acetate causes only mercurialentis.

BENIGN (RELATIVELY NONTOXIC AND NONALLERGIC) TOPICAL OPHTHALMIC MEDICATIONS

ANTIMICROBIAL AGENTS
Sulfacetamide
Erythromycin
Bacitracin
Polymyxin B

OCULAR LUBRICANTS
Preservative-free artificial tears and ointments
Preserved artificial tears and ointments without benzalkonium

---

problem (because the patient is thought simply to be "allergic" to a particular medication); but no improvement can occur if the patient is actually suffering from toxicity and the new medications are as toxic as the previous ones.

Adverse reactions to topical ophthalmic medications usually result from diagnostic uncertainty, leading to the prescribing of inappropriately numerous or potent medications for unnecessarily prolonged periods. Problems can occur, but they are much less frequent when medications are prescribed prudently and wisely. When possible, and especially when the diagnosis is in doubt, it is usually best to prescribe relatively "bland" medications that are unlikely to cause irritation or allergy, as discussed in the box above, for example, erythromycin, bacitracin, sulfacetamide, polymyxin B, or artificial tears and lubricating ointments without benzalkonium (especially for patients who have dry eyes).

Although generally benign, such medications can be very useful. Potency, "newness," and popularity are not necessarily indicative of efficacy, although these features too often influence the selection of drugs. Medications should be prescribed for specific purposes and with specific goals in mind. If the goals are not attained within 2 or 3 weeks, the treatment probably should be changed or stopped and reevaluated. It is usually pointless to treat for several months with an antibiotic-steroid preparation, an antiviral agent, or an aminoglycoside antibiotic. Any conditions that may respond to such a regimen (and there are very few) should do so within a few days; continuing the treatment too long almost always makes the patient worse.

Admittedly, rapid and accurate diagnosis of the red or irritated eye is not always easy or possible. When the diagnosis is in doubt, it is generally better to prescribe relatively harmless drugs, or even placebo therapy, unless the eye is imminently and seriously threatened. Intensive therapy and polypharmacy are neither necessary nor efficacious for most external ocular diseases. Such treatment is apt to obscure spontaneous or therapy-induced improvement and to make diagnosis more difficult.

ACKNOWLEDGMENTS

This work was supported in part by grants from the Indiana Lions Eye Bank, Inc., Indianapolis, and Research to Prevent Blindness, Inc., New York.

This material was presented in part in a thesis (1983) written for partial fulfillment of membership requirements of the American Ophthalmological Society.[1]

DISCLAIMER

The author has no proprietary interest in any of the medications discussed.

REFERENCES

1. Wilson FM II: Adverse external ocular effects of topical ophthalmic therapy: an epidemiologic, laboratory, and clinical study, Trans Am Ophthalmol Soc 81:854, 1983.
2. Wilson FM II: Adverse external ocular effects of topical ophthalmic medications, Surv Ophthalmol 24:57, 1979.
3. Gardner SK: Ocular drug pentration and pharmacokinetic principles. In Lamberts W and Potter DE, editors: Clinical ophthalmic pharmacology, Boston, 1987, Little, Brown & Co.
4. Pattern JT, Cavanagh HD, and Allansmith MR: Induced ocular pseudopemphigoid, Am J Ophthalmol 82:272, 1976.
5. Ostler HB et al: Drug-induced cicitrization of the conjunctiva. In O'Connor GR, editor: Immunologic diseases of the mucous membranes: pathology, diagnosis, and treatment, New York, 1980, Masson Publishing.
6. Theodore FH and Schlossman A: Ocular allergy, Baltimore, 1958, Williams & Wilkins.
7. Kennedy RE, Roca PD, and Landers PH: Atypical band keratopathy in glaucomatous patients, Am J Ophthalmol 72:917, 1971.
8. Kennedy RE, Roca PD, and Platt DS: Further observations on atypical band keratopathy in glaucoma patients, Trans Am Ophthalmol Soc 72:107, 1974.
9. Galin MA and Ostbaum SA: Band keratopathy in mercury exposure, Ann Ophthalmol 6:1257, 1974.
10. Garron LK et al: A clinical pathologic study of mercurialentis medicamentosus, Trans Am Ophthalmol Soc 74:295, 1966.
11. Theodore FH and Schlossman A: Ocular allergy, Baltimore, 1958, Williams & Wilkins.
12. Thygeson P: Marginal corneal infiltrates and ulcers, Trans Am Acad Ophthalmol Otolaryngol 51:198, 1947.
13. Thygeson P: Etiology and treatment of blepharitis, Arch Ophthalmol 36:445, 1946.
14. Fisher AA: Contact Dermatitis, ed 2, Philadelphia, 1973, Lea & Febiger.
15. Smolin G: Medrysone hypersensitivity. Report of a case, Arch Ophthalmol 85:478, 1971.
16. Theodore FH and Schlossman A: Ocular allergy, Baltimore, 1958, Williams & Wilkins.
17. Carter ES Jr and Cope CB: Anaphylaxis due to topical penicillin, J Allergy 25:270, 1954.
18. McCuiston CF: Penicillin-sensitivity test, N Engl J Med 25:1114, 1957.
19. Wilson FM II: Prevention of iatrogenic drug-induced external ocular disease. In Frielaender MH, editor: Prevention of eye disease, New York, 1988, Mary Ann Liebert, Inc.

CHEMICAL INJURIES

A wide variety of chemicals can cause ocular surface injury. In most cases the injury is relatively mild and recovery is rapid; however, some chemicals cause severe ocular damage and even permanent blindness. Burns of the external eye from strong acids or alkalies are the most common serious chemical injuries. The severe effects of these agents result mainly from an alteration of the local concentration of hydrogen and hydroxide ions. If ionization in solution is weak, the agent will be relatively harmless, as demonstrated by the potentially acidic substance carbon dioxide, which is lipid soluble and penetrates the epithelial layer of the cornea well. The carbolic acid is not harmful because ionization is weak. The amount of damage also depends on the amount and concentration of the chemical, the time that the eye is exposed to the chemical, and the ability of the chemical to penetrate the eye. Many chemicals also have specific toxic effects, such as acting as organic solvents, binding to proteins, inactivating enzymes, or impairing other metabolic processes.

Any chemical injury should be treated as an acute ophthalmic emergency. This is the only situation, outside of the operating room, where literally seconds can affect the outcome. Regardless of the nature of the specific chemical, prompt irrigation with any benign fluid, such as water, can lessen or prevent blinding sequelae. This must be performed wherever the injury occurs; by the time the patient arrives at the emergency room or the ophthalmologist's office, most of the damage already has been done. Nevertheless, irrigation is repeated to ensure elimination of the chemical from the ocular surface. Of course, any solid material should be located and removed. The chemical(s), their concentrations, and the duration of exposure also should be determined. The patient should be asked to bring the chemical container or its label, particularly if the agent is uncommon, or has a mixture of ingredients. Toxicology books, such as *Grant's Toxicology of the Eye*,[1] poison control centers, package inserts, and manufacturers also can provide valuable information.

ALKALI BURNS
ALKALINE CHEMICALS

The most caustic alkalies are ammonium hydroxide, sodium hydroxide, calcium hydroxide, potassium hydroxide, and magnesium hydroxide. As evident from their names, each is a combination of a cation and hydroxide (OH$-$) and readily dissociates in solution, releasing large amounts of the toxic hydroxide.

Ammonia. Ammonia (NH_3), a common cleaning agent, is found in fertilizers and refrigerants and is used in the manufacturing of other chemicals. Ammonia can become dissolved in water, including tears, and form ammonium hydroxide (NH_4OH), which is very caustic. The ammonia penetrates ocular tissues readily, since it is both lipid and water soluble; it can reach the anterior chamber in less than a minute.[2] Thus it can cause extensive internal ocular injury and is not readily removed by topical irrigation.

Sodium hydroxide. Sodium hydroxide (NaOH) is commonly referred to as lye or caustic soda and is used as a cleanser and in manufacturing. Injuries probably most commonly occur during its use in the unclogging of household drains. In these cases a combination of crystals and solution explode out of the drain into the eyes. Lye also appears to be a common choice in deliberate attempts at blinding. Sodium hydroxide penetrates the eye quickly, but not as quickly as ammonia; peak anterior chamber alkalinity occurs 3 to 5 minutes after exposure.[2] Severe injuries are common.

Calcium hydroxide. Lime, plaster, cement, mortar, and whitewash contain calcium hydroxide [$Ca(OH)_2$] and are common sources of ocular injury. The solids usually fall or are splashed into the eye and can become trapped in the fornices, resulting in prolonged ocular exposure. Calcium hydroxide penetrates relatively poorly; it reacts with the epithelial cell membrane to form calcium soaps, which precipitate and hinder further penetration. Therefore it tends to cause more superficial injury but early opacification. This often suggests a worse outcome than is actually observed.

Others. Potassium hydroxide (KOH), also known as caustic potash, is commonly used as a cleanser and in manufacturing. Its penetration and severity are similar to those of sodium hydroxide. Magnesium hydroxide [$Mg(OH)_2$] is a component of flares and fireworks and therefore is seen in the context of thermal and sometimes concussive injuries. By itself, magnesium hydroxide causes minor epithelial injury.

PATHOGENESIS

Strongly alkaline chemicals result in disruption of cells because the high pH causes saponification and dissociation of fatty acids in the cell membranes. A local pH of 11.5 or greater appears to be associated with permanent injury. In the stroma, the hydroxyl ions cause swelling of collagen fibers, which results in their thickening and shortening. They also lead to hydrolyzation of interfibrillar glycosaminoglycans.[3] The severity of stromal injury also is related to the nature of the cation, which influences penetration, and itself can bind collagen and glycosaminoglycans.[4]

Injury to conjunctiva, corneal nerves, keratocytes, endothelium, and limbal blood vessels also can occur by the same mechanisms. Stimulation of the free nerve endings in the corneal and conjunctival epithelium is responsible for the intense pain associated with alkali injury.[5] The effect of alkali injury on the goblet cell population is unclear; some have found decreased goblet cell density, as in cicatricial pemphigoid and other scarring diseases.[6] Others, surprisingly, found goblet cell density to be increased significantly.[7]

Intraocular structures, including the iris, lens, trabecular meshwork, and ciliary body also can be affected depending on aqueous pH. Aqueous pH can remain alkaline for up to 3 hours after injury, regardless of external irrigation.[2,8] Aqueous glucose and ascorbate levels are decreased and can remain so for prolonged periods.[9-11]

Stromal ulceration commonly occurs in alkali-burned corneas. Several factors contribute to stromal ulceration, including persistent epithelial defects, tear deficiency, inflammation, release of proteolytic enzymes, antioxidant deficiency,[12,13] anesthesia, and impairment of collagen synthesis. One type of proteolytic enzyme, collagenase, appears to play a significant role and has been the subject of a great deal of investigation. Epithelium, fibroblasts, and polymorphonuclear leukocytes (PMNs) are capable of releasing collagenase, and collagenase activity has been detected in ulcerating corneas after alkali burns.[2,14] Collagenase appears within 9 hours after the burn and reaches a peak at 14 to 21 days.

Production of plasmin by epithelial cells, PMNs, and keratocytes also may play a role in stromal ulceration (see Chapter 15). It also has been proposed that the host's immunologic response contributes to ulceration,[15,16] as suggested by the following findings: In rabbits, if a second eye is burned 2 to 4 weeks after the first, the rate of ulceration in the second eye is much higher than in the first. In addition, administration of convalescent serum from burned rabbits increases the rate of ulceration.

Localized corneal ascorbate deficiency has been observed after alkali burns and may play a role in corneal ulceration.[11,17,18] Aqueous levels of ascorbate are normally 20 times higher than in plasma, presumably because of active transport by the ciliary body. Damage to the ciliary body can impair or eliminate this function and lead to a relative ascorbate deficiency. Ascorbate is required for collagen synthesis, the conversion of monocytes to fibroblasts, and in the formation of normal rough endoplasmic reticulum and plays a role in the synthesis of glycosaminoglycans.

CLINICAL MANIFESTATIONS

Acute. Within minutes after a severe alkali injury, extensive injury can incur to all cell types in the cornea, including epithelium, keratocytes, nerves, vessels, and endothelium. Damage to cellular and

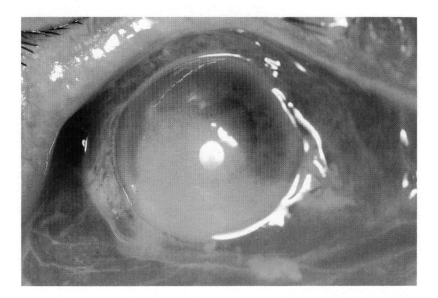

Fig. 29-1. Alkali burn with injection and chemosis of conjunctiva and increased relucency of cornea.

vascular components of the conjunctiva, iris, and ciliary body and to the lens epithelium also can occur in the first few hours. The conjunctiva is injected and can exhibit areas of necrosis, which appear white and devoid of blood vessels (Figs. 29-1 to 29-3). Large epithelial defects can be present, involving the entire cornea and extending into the fornices. The corneal stroma is often cloudy and edematous; in severe injuries it can be opaque. The anterior chamber may be shallow and exhibit fibrin formation.

The intraocular pressure can rise rapidly.[19-21] This early increase appears to be caused by the

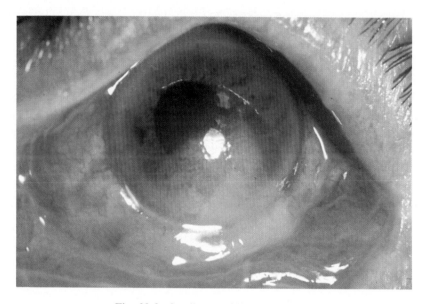

Fig. 29-2. Small area of limbal ischemia.

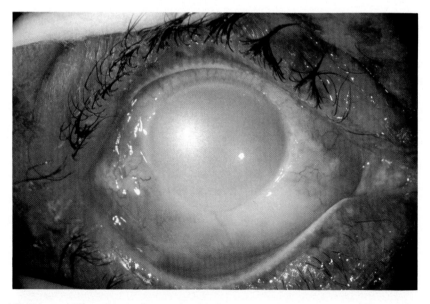

Fig. 29-3. Alkali burn with total loss of corneal epithelium, stromal haze, and ischemia of approximately one third of the limbus.

TABLE **29-1.** Hughes-Roper-Hall Classification of Chemical Burns

GRADE	CLINICAL FINDINGS	PROGNOSIS
Grade I	Corneal epithelial damage; no limbal ischemia (Fig. 29-1)	Good
Grade II	Cornea hazy but iris detail seen; ischemia at less than one third of limbus (Fig. 29-2)	Good
Grade III	Total loss of corneal epithelium; stromal haze blurring iris details; ischemia at one third to one half of limbus (Fig. 29-3)	Guarded
Grade IV	Cornea opaque, obscuring view of iris or pupil; ischemia at more than one half of limbus (Fig. 29-4)	Poor

shrinkage of collagen in the cornea and trabecular meshwork, with compression of the anterior chamber and trabecular outflow channels. Within a few hours other mechanisms can come into play: increased episcleral venous pressure, blockage of the trabecular meshwork with inflammatory debris, and possibly prostaglandin release from damaged intraocular structures. Although these mechanisms can contribute to a pressure rise, ciliary body injury also can occur, leading to decreased aqueous outflow. Over the first few days the balance between these factors is precarious, and the eye can fluctuate between hypotony and marked pressure elevation.

The severity of injury and the prognosis for healing of the eye can be estimated based on initial examination. A useful classification scheme developed by Hughes[22,23] and modified by Roper-Hall[24] divides the injuries into four groups (Table 29-1). A more detailed classification scheme has been devised by Ralph,[25] as shown in the box on p. 654. These schemes are helpful, particularly for those unaccustomed to caring for patients with chemical injuries. They can be used as an indication of the likelihood of complications and the long-term prognosis. Clearly the most important prognostic signs are the degree of limbal necrosis (ischemia) and the cloudiness of the corneal stroma. Signs of anterior chamber injury, such as a fixed, dilated pupil, iridocyclitis, and a sustained increase in intraocular pressure, also indicate more severe injury. These signs are considered only in Ralph's scheme.

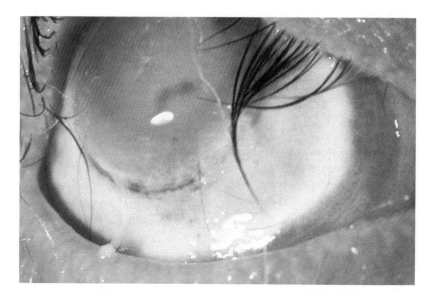

Fig. 29-4. Marbleization of cornea and severe limbal ischemia.

CLASSIFICATION OF CHEMICAL BURNS

CONJUNCTIVA	SCORE
Perilimbal hyperemia	0
Chemosis	1

LIMBUS	
No ischemia	0
Spotty limbal ischemia	1
Ischemia < one third of circumference	2
Ischemia one third to one half of circumference	3
Ischemia > one half of circumference	4

CORNEAL EPITHELIUM	
Clouded epithelium	1
Epithelial loss ≤50%	2
Epithelial loss >50%	3

CORNEAL STROMA	
Mild stromal haze; iris details visible	2
Moderate stromal haze; iris details barely visible	3
Severe stromal haze; no iris details visible	4

INTRAOCULAR STRUCTURES	
Oval, fixed pupil or aqueous cells	2
Sustained increase of intraocular pressure during first 24 hours	3

TOTAL SCORE	PROGNOSIS
0-3	Insignificant injury; rapid recovery without sequelae
4-6	Mild injury with rapid replacement of damaged epithelium and clearing of any stromal haze; return of visual acuity to baseline usually occurs within 1 to 2 weeks
7-9	Moderately severe injury, usually with a delay of 1 to 3 weeks in complete reepithelialization; some reduction in visual acuity may result from persistent stromal haze; peripheral pannus is common
10-12	Severe burn, with sluggish regrowth of epithelium and frequent development of pannus; stromal loss is common and perforation can occur; visual acuity usually permanently reduced by pannus and stromal haze
13-17	Most severe burns with worst prognosis; prolonged epithelial recovery, with dense pannus formation and stromal loss; perforation is common; cataract is expected; end result, after many months or years, is dense corneal scarring and vascularization, phthisis, or loss of the globe

Adapted from Ralph RA: Chemical burns of the eye. In T Duane, editor: Clinical ophthalmology, vol 4, Hagerstown, Md, 1988, Harper & Row.

Early reparative phase. Typically the epithelium begins to grow in from the periphery of the defect within a few days. Depending on the extent of injury, however, it can take 1 to 2 weeks to reach the cornea. In the meantime symblepharon can develop as a result of fusion of the denuded palpebral and bulbar conjunctival surfaces. Its progression across the cornea can be agonizingly slow, taking many weeks, especially in cases with marked stromal injury. The epithelial healing rate depends on the extent of limbal involvement, the amount of tissue necrosis, adequacy of lid function, tear production, and patient age. Peripheral vascularization and inflammatory cell infiltration often accompanies the epithelium.

With time the stroma gradually clears, and anterior chamber inflammation subsides. However, fibrotic membranes can form on the iris, endothelium, or lens, and the lens can become swollen and

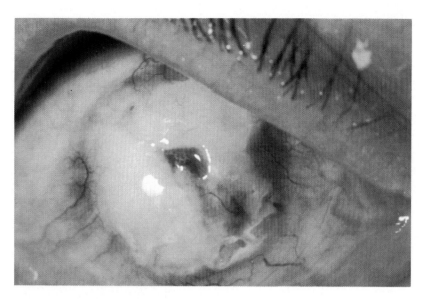

Fig. 29-5. Perforation of cornea after alkali burn.

cloudy. The intraocular pressure can range from hypotony to a glaucoma difficult to control, but usually is not as labile as in the acute phase.

Stromal ulceration can occur anytime after the first 7 to 10 days, but most typically begins 2 to 3 weeks after injury. It occurs only in areas in which epithelium and superficial vessels are not present. In most cases the epithelium covers the cornea before there is significant thinning, and vessels are seen peripherally or not at all; however, the longer the epithelium is not intact the greater the likelihood of ulceration. In severe cases epithelial healing can take months, and progressive stromal ulceration can occur before the epithelium reaches the central cornea (Fig. 29-5). If perforation can be avoided, healing will eventually be realized, albeit often with severe vascularization and scarring.

Late reparative phase. If initial epithelial healing is achieved without marked vascularization and scarring, the eye can look fairly good at this stage, even after severe burns. A closer inspection, however, can often indicate obstacles yet to be dealt with. Conjunctival scarring can progress for weeks after injury and can lead to closure of the lacrimal gland ductules, entropion, trichiasis, and impaired lid closure (Fig. 29-6). In addition to aqueous tear deficiency, the lipid component of tears can be reduced by scarring of the meibomian gland orifices, and sometimes tear surfacing also is impaired. Corneal sensation often is reduced because of nerve injury. Although it is not readily evident, there also may be extensive endothelial and keratocyte injury.

All of these problems can take their toll with time. In the more severe cases corneal scarring and vascularization progress for 6 to 12 months after injury. Damage to the endothelium can lead to retrocorneal fibrous membrane formation. The trabecular meshwork, iris, and ciliary body also can be affected by fibrous proliferation. Pupillary membranes and cataracts are often present and must be removed before visual rehabilitation. Intraocular pressure can remain elevated, or the eye can become hypotonous and subsequently phthisical.

TREATMENT

Immediate. The chemically injured eye must be copiously irrigated as soon as possible (see box on p. 656).[26,27] In most cases the fate of the eye is determined in the first few minutes after injury; therefore, irrigation is best performed at the site of injury with any nontoxic liquid. After the patient

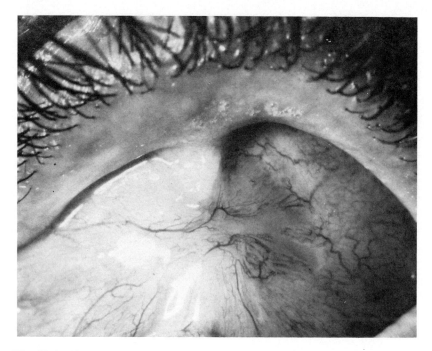

Fig. 29-6. Cicatrization of conjunctiva and symblepharon formation after alkali burn.

arrives at the emergency room or doctor's office, irrigation should be repeated. It is useful to determine the pH in the inferior cul-de-sac before irrigation, using litmus paper, but not if it delays irrigation. Theoretically an isotonic, neutral pH, buffered solution would be the ideal irrigation fluid, but these do not appear to be superior to water, Ringer's lactate, normal saline, or similar solutions.

Irrigation usually is accomplished by running the solution through intravenous tubing, retracting the lids, and manually holding the tubing so that the fluid drips into the eye. Irrigation tubes attached to polymethylmethacrylate scleral contact lenses (Medi-Flow therapeutic lens, Mor-Tan, Inc., Torrington, WY 82240) and a perforated silicone tube shaped to lie in the conjunctival fornix (Oklahoma eye irrigating tube, Edward Weck and Co., Inc., Long Island City, NY 11101) are commercial products designed to facilitate this process. Irrigation is continued for a minimum of 30 minutes or until

---

INITIAL TREATMENT OF ALKALI INJURY

1. Irrigate at the site of injury with water or other nontoxic liquid.
2. Irrigate on presentation with water or intravenous solution for at least 30 minutes, or until pH is neutral.
3. Remove any solid material. This may be facilitated by 0.01% EDTA solution on swab or irrigation.
4. Use cycloplegia to decrease pain: atropine 1% twice a day, or scopolamine 0.25% two to four times a day.
5. Use prophylactic antibiotics (for example, sulfacetamide, gentamicin, or erythromycin, four times a day) to reduce the incidence of infection.
6. Control intraocular pressure, primarily with drugs that reduce aqueous inflow (for example, timolol and acetazolamide).
7. Use topical corticosteroids (for example, prednisolone acetate 1% four times a day) for 7 to 10 days to decrease pain and inflammation.
8. If opposing conjunctival surfaces are denuded of epithelium, consider physical separation with scleral shell or plastic wrap (combined with bandage contact lens).

---

the pH becomes neutral. Topical anesthetic agents or lid block may be required for this initial treatment.

Removal of solid material is essential and may require double eversion of the lid to properly ensure that this area is free of chemical. The sticky paste or powder of calcium hydroxide can be particularly difficult to remove. Irrigation with a 0.01 to 0.05 M solution of ethylenediaminetetraacetic acid (EDTA) and cotton swabs soaked in the same solution can help loosen it.[4]

Paracentesis with removal of aqueous or irrigation has been recommended,[5,27-29] but its benefit has not been established,[30] and there are significant risks. Therefore I do not recommend this procedure.

A cycloplegic drop is usually instilled for comfort, and a prophylactic antibiotic administered. If the injury is relatively mild (for example, grade I), the eye can be patched and the patient reexamined the next day. With more severe burns, particularly with bilateral injury, the patient should be admitted to the hospital.

Early (1 to 2 weeks). The role of the ophthalmologist in the early period of treatment is to ease discomfort, control intraocular pressure, and promote epithelial healing. A cycloplegic, such as scopolamine or atropine, is used to increase comfort, and a relatively nontoxic antibiotic is applied 2 to 4 times a day to lessen the risk of infection. Intraocular pressure elevation is treated primarily with drugs that decrease inflow, such as timolol and carbonic anhydrase inhibitors.

If conjunctival epithelial injury is extensive, affecting both the palpebral and bulbar conjunctiva, or synechiae begin to form, measures can be taken to physically separate the two conjunctival surfaces. Whether these affect the final result is unclear. They certainly do not prevent subepithelial scarring, but they may reduce forniceal shortening. In most cases, I prefer to use a symblepharon ring, in combination with a bandage contact lens (Fig. 29-7). Alternatively, the palpebral surface can be lined with a thin plastic material, such as plastic food wrap, or adhesions can be lysed daily with a glass rod.

Epithelial healing can be promoted by lubrication, patching, bandage contact lenses, or tarsorrhaphy. Bandage contact lenses are helpful when epithelial healing is prolonged or there is recurrent epithelial loss. The lens is left in place until adequate adhesion is achieved, which may require as

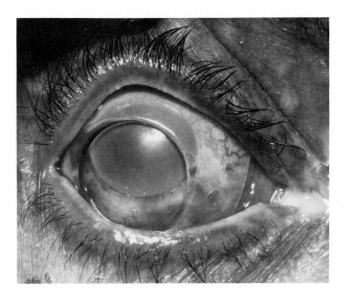

Fig. 29-7. Symblepharon ring and bandage contact lens.

long as 3 months. Incomplete lid closure, entropion, ectropion, or trichiasis may develop and should be corrected as much as possible. Bandage contact lenses are also helpful in ameliorating the effects of these conditions.

Both fibronectin[31,32] and epidermal growth factor (EGF)[33-38] promote epithelial healing after alkali injury in rabbits (see also Chapter 15). In these models, however, epithelial defects recur, even with continued fibronectin or EGF treatment. The incidence of secondary epithelial breakdown was reduced by combined use of EGF and fibronectin,[39] or by the addition of topical steroid treatment to EGF or fibronectin treatment.[40] Clinical trials of these medications are currently underway.

The use of topical corticosteroids is controversial. The steroids reduce inflammation and provide some comfort, but they have the potential to promote stromal ulceration.[41,42] Because the risk of stromal ulceration is low in the first 10 days after injury,[42] I use 1% prednisolone acetate four times a day during the first 7 to 10 days. After this point topical corticosteroids are applied only if the epithelium is intact. In cases with marked inflammation and progressive scarring and vascularization, I gradually taper the steroid dose until the eye is stable, but, whether this regimen affects the final outcome is debatable.

As mentioned earlier, aqueous and stromal levels of ascorbate are decreased after alkali burns. In experimental animals administration of ascorbate prevented alkali-related corneal ulceration, if treatment was begun before the onset of ulceration.[11,17,43] When ascorbate was compared with a control group receiving citrate, however, the incidence of ulceration and perforation was much less in the citrate group.[44] Unlike ascorbate, citrate also was effective if begun after the onset of stromal ulceration.[45] Citrate has been found to decrease PMN activity, including mediator release, and phagocytosis.[46,47] A clinical trial of ascorbate and citrate therapy is being conducted, in which patients receive both topical (10%) and systemic ascorbate or citrate. The topical therapy is given hourly, 14 times a day.

Intermediate (2 weeks to 6 months). The major complication in the intermediate period is stromal ulceration. The main goal is to promote epithelial healing, as described earlier, because this will prevent further ulceration. Cultures should be obtained regularly because of the possible role of microbial infection. A variety of substances have been suggested to reduce the progression of ulceration, including collagenase inhibitors, heparin,[48] citrate, and medroxyprogesterone[49]; however, no agent has been clearly demonstrated to be of benefit clinically.

If medical treatment is not successful, a conjunctival flap can often halt ulceration. Ipsilateral conjunctiva is preferred, but if it is necrotic or scarred, contralateral conjunctiva or oral mucosa can be used.[50] Tissue adhesive also can be used to impede ulceration or to seal a small perforation. Larger perforations can be repaired by lamellar or penetrating keratoplasty, but the grafts usually succumb to ulceration as well. Covering the grafts with conjunctiva or mucosa may increase their resistance.

Long-term (longer than 6 months). If there is severe scarring of the cornea or conjunctival sac, one may resort to keratoplasty or reconstructive plastic surgery. Although results of penetrating keratoplasty have been encouraging in some instances, the overall prognosis for the marbleized corneas from alkali burns is still guarded. The odds of success are primarily determined by the severity of the injury; however, results can be improved by paying special attention to the ocular environment in which the graft is placed. Lid scarring and distortion, trichiasis, symblepharon, inflammation, and tear and mucus deficiency can threaten the graft.

Penetrating keratoplasty should be delayed until the eye is healed completely and inflammation has resolved, a process that usually requires at least 1 year and often 1½ to 2 years.[51] Lid position abnormalities and trichiasis should be corrected first, and glaucoma should be controlled. Fresh donor tissue with healthy epithelium is important to lessen the risk of early epithelial defects. The graft epithelium should be protected during and after surgery; bandage contact lens wear, continuous patching, or suture tarsorrhaphy are used for at least 4 to 6 weeks after surgery. While the eye is open it must be kept well lubricated with artificial tears and ointments. Ocular inflammation should be minimized with topical or systemic corticosteroids.

The risk of rejection is relatively high because of the presence of corneal vessels.[52] The ability of HLA matching and immunosuppressives, such as cyclosporin and FK506, to increase the rate of graft survival is currently being investigated.

In addition, the grafts often opacify because of poor epithelial healing. If epithelial defects occur they are slow to heal, and stromal ulceration or wound separation can develop. If there has been extensive limbal injury, the host epithelium is abnormal with less capacity for healing and maintenance of corneal clarity. Eventually the abnormal epithelium grows over the graft and can become affected by recurrent defects, superficial opacification, and vascularization.

Conjunctival transplantation was designed to provide healthy epithelium for resurfacing of corneas damaged by chemical and thermal burns[53-55] to prevent recurrent epithelial breakdown and reduce central corneal scarring and vascularization. A superficial lamellar keratectomy is performed first. In the traditional form, four circular areas of perilimbal conjunctiva is taken from the fellow eye and sutured at the limbus (Fig. 29-8). Alternatively a crescentic lamellar graft containing several clock hours of limbus can be transplanted,[56] but it clearly cannot remove deep corneal scarring or replace damaged endothelium. If the injury is unilateral, conjunctiva can be obtained from the fellow eye. If this is not possible, donor limbal epithelium can be used, and the procedure is called *keratoepithelioplasty*.[57]

Conjunctival transplantation is indicated in cases with recurrent epithelial breakdown or persistent epithelial defects. This procedure appears to be useful only late in the reparative period after a burn, after primary healing of the epithelium and subsidence of inflammation, or after penetrating keratoplasty. It also can be an alternative to penetrating keratoplasty when corneal scarring and vasculariza-

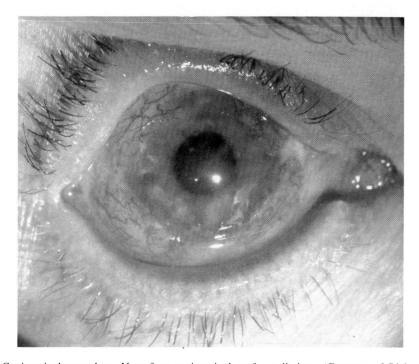

Fig. 29-8. Conjunctival transplant. Note four conjunctival grafts at limbus. (Courtesy of Richard A. Thoft, Pittsburgh.)

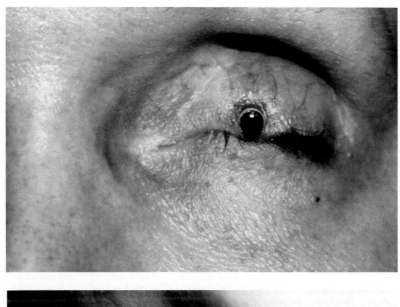

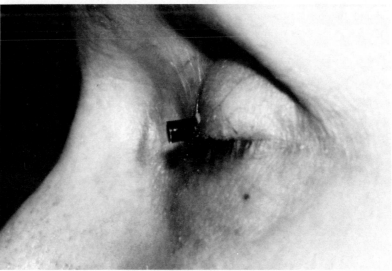

Fig. 29-9. Keratoprosthesis, front and side views. (Courtesy of Massimo Busin, Bonn, Germany.)

tion are relatively superficial. In such cases the pannus and opacified anterior stroma are removed before placement of the conjunctival grafts. The surface environment should be optimized, as with keratoplasty.

Keratoprosthesis. In cases with severe bilateral injury and multiple failed keratoplasties, keratoprostheses can be used as a last resort to obtain useful vision[58-60] (Fig. 29-9). These devices are fraught with complications and are successful for only a few years at best, but they can provide good visual acuity, albeit with a very narrow field.

ACID BURNS

Exposure of the eye to weak acids tends to result in less severe injury than exposure to weak alkalies, but strong acids can cause devastating injury (Fig. 29-10). In general the clinical manifesta-

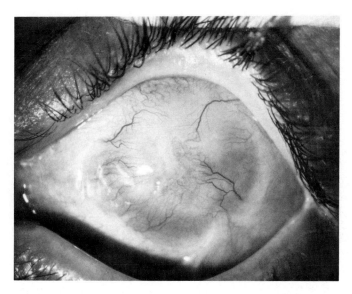

Fig. 29-10. Corneal scarring resulting from severe acid burn.

tions and treatment of acid burns are similar to those of alkali burns, so emphasis will be placed on those features that are unique.

ACIDIC CHEMICALS

Sulfuric acid (H_2SO_4) is probably the most commonly encountered acid in ocular burns. It is widely used in industry, but most burns result from battery explosions. Lead-acid batteries contain a 20% to 25% solution of sulfuric acid. When it is exposed to an electric current, hydrogen and oxygen gases are released, producing an explosive mixture.[61] This mixture is ignited when a match or lighter is used to illuminate the engine compartment, or jumper cables are connected improperly, resulting in sparks. The ocular injury is a combination of acid burn and contusion or laceration resulting from the explosion.

Sulfurous acid (H_2SO_3) is formed when sulfur dioxide gas combines with the water in tears or cornea. Sulfurous acid is highly soluble in both lipid and water and therefore penetrates rapidly. It also damages the corneal nerves, resulting in anesthesia.

Hydrofluoric (HF) acid is widely used in industry and tends to cause severe injury. Although it is a weak acid, the fluoride ion is a strong solvent and can dissolve cellular membranes.[62] This characteristic, plus its low molecular weight and small size, enables HF to penetrate tissues easily.

Hydrochloric (HCl) acid solutions release hydrogen chloride gas, which is irritating to the eye, but usually not damaging; however, concentrated solutions can cause severe damage. Exposure to small amounts of chromic acid (Cr_2O_3), used in the chrome-plating industry and in washing laboratory glassware, can cause chronic conjunctivitis and a brownish discoloration of the conjunctival epithelium.

Nitric (HNO_3) acid burns are unusual in that the epithelial opacities are yellowish rather than white. High concentrations of silver nitrate ($AgNo_3$) can result in opacification of the cornea that may be permanent[63] (Fig. 29-11). Some injuries have occurred as a result of inadvertent neonatal prophylaxis, with a solution much more concentrated than the usual 1%. The use of solid silver nitrate sticks to cauterize lesions on the lids or conjunctiva has resulted in severe corneal injury, as well as cataract formation. Thermal injury, acid burn, and silver deposition occur.

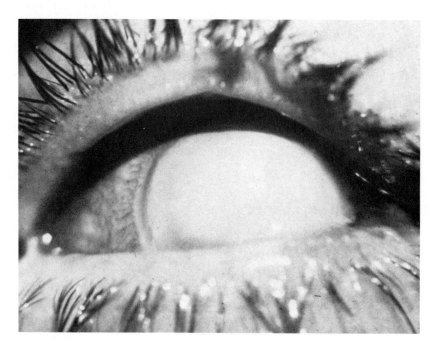

Fig. 29-11. Diffuse opacity of cornea resulting from concentrated silver nitrate solution.

PATHOGENESIS

When exposed to an acidic environment, proteins coagulate and precipitate. In the cornea acids coagulate the epithelial cells, shrink stromal collagen, and precipitate glycosaminoglycans.[64] Fortunately, this process occurs on the surface and tends to inhibit further penetration of the chemical. Deeper injury can occur, however, especially where the anion penetrates well, or the anion itself is toxic, as exemplified by hydrofluoric acid, in which the fluoride both penetrates well and dissolves membranes.

Collagen shrinkage can lead to increased intraocular pressure, as occurs in alkali injury.[19,65] Intraocular damage can occur; lowering of aqueous pH, and increased aqueous protein and prostaglandin levels have been observed after experimental hydrochloric acid injury.[65] Ciliary body damage can result in decreased aqueous and stromal levels of ascorbate, as occurs in severe alkali burns.[17,18]

CLINICAL MANIFESTATIONS

Although no classification scheme has been designed specifically for acid burns, both the Hughes-Roper-Hall (Table 29-1) and Ralph (see box on p. 654) schemes for alkali burns are applicable. The most important prognostic indicators are limbal ischemia and evidence of intraocular injury. Corneal opacification is an indication of severity but is less significant in acid injuries because epithelial and anterior stromal coagulation can occur without extensive deep stromal or anterior chamber injury. The epithelium of the cornea and conjunctiva can turn white and opaque or, with nitric or chromic acid burns, yellow-brown. This necrotic epithelium sloughs within a few days, sometimes revealing a clear stroma.

As in alkali burns, corneal anesthesia, conjunctival scarring, stromal ulceration, iritis, glaucoma, and lens opacification can occur. Any acid can cause these complications if it is sufficiently concentrated and the exposure is long enough. Certain acids, however, such as sulfurous acid and hydrofluoric acid, are more likely to produce severe burns because they penetrate the corneal stroma more readily or the anions are more toxic.

TREATMENT

The treatment of acid burns is the same as for alkali burns of the same severity. The primary emergency treatment is irrigation. Although less time is generally required for neutralization of the tears, a minimum of 20 to 30 minutes of irrigation is still recommended. Specific neutralizing chemicals have been suggested for hydrofluoric acid burns, including benzalkonium chloride, calcium chloride, and calcium gluconate, but these are toxic themselves and should be avoided.[62,66]

OTHER CHEMICALS

TEAR GAS

Tear gasses disarm their targets by causing ocular stinging, smarting, and tearing through selective stimulation of sensory nerve endings in the cornea. A variety of active ingredients, or lacrimators, may be used, the most common of which is chloroacetophenone. The mechanism of effect is not understood, but the active agents in tear gasses are toxic to sulfhydryl- or thiol-containing enzymes.[1] At the concentrations encountered in normal use, no ocular injury occurs; however, at high concentrations severe damage can result.

Tear gas weapons come in explosive and solvent spray types. The explosive type includes cartridges for pistols, grenades, and canisters, all of which contain concentrated lacrimator and explosives or combustibles. Direct blasts from these weapons at close range expose the eye to mechanical damage, flying debris, and sometimes thermal injury, as well as concentrated lacrimator. The solvent spray type, such as mace, also can cause damage if the chemical is sprayed directly into the eye at close range.

Corneal epithelial loss, stromal edema, and stromal scarring can occur (Fig. 29-12). The lacrimator appears to be able to penetrate the cornea and appears to be toxic to the endothelium.[67,68]

OTHERS

Most organic solvents are not acidic or alkaline and do not exhibit much chemical reactivity with tissues. Epithelial injury can occur, but deeper involvement is unusual. The chemicals are readily eliminated by a few minutes of irrigation.

A few chemicals cause an epithelial injury in which the symptoms are delayed until several hours

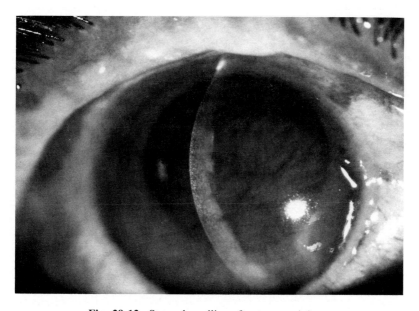

Fig. 29-12. Stromal swelling after tear gas injury.

after exposure, similar to what is seen in ultraviolet keratitis. Superficial punctate keratopathy is the most common finding, but diffuse epithelial loss, stromal edema, and, rarely, stromal scarring and vascularization can occur. Such chemicals include Diving Mask Defogger, formaldehyde, hydrogen sulfide, mustard gas, osmic acid, and poison ivy.[1]

REFERENCES

1. Grant WM: Toxicology of the eye, ed 3, Springfield, Ill, Charles C Thomas.
2. Pfister RR et al: Collagenase activity of intact corneal epithelium in peripheral alkaline burns, Arch Ophthalmol 86:308, 1971.
3. Cejkova J et al: Alkali burns of the rabbit cornea. II. A histochemical study of glycosaminoglycans, Histochemistry 45:71, 1975.
4. Grant WM and Kern HLL: Action of alkalies on the corneal stroma, Arch Ophthalmol 54:931, 1955.
5. Pfister RR: Chemical injuries of the eye, Ophthalmology 90:12146, 1983.
6. Nelson JD and Wright JC: Conjunctival goblet cell densities in ocular surface disease, Arch Ophthalmol 102:1049, 1984.
7. Ohji M et al: Goblet cell density in thermal and chemical injuries, Arch Ophthalmol 105:1686, 1987.
8. Paterson CA, Pfister RR, and Levinson RA: Aqueous humor pH changes after experimental alkali burns, Am J Ophthalmol 79:414, 1975.
9. Pfister RR, Friend J, and Dohlman CH: The anterior segments of rabbits after alkali burns, Arch Ophthalmol 86:189, 1971.
10. Levinson RA, Paterson CA, and Pfister RR: Ascorbic acid prevents corneal ulceration and perforation following experimental alkali burns, Invest Ophthalmol 15:986, 1976.
11. Pfister RR and Paterson CA: Ascorbic acid in the treatment of alkali burns of the eye, Ophthalmology 87:1050, 1980.
12. Nirankari VS et al: Superoxide radical scavenging agents in treatment of alkali burns, Arch Ophthalmol 99:886, 1981.
13. Wright P: The chemically injured eye, Trans Ophthalmol Soc UK 102:85, 1982.
14. Berman MB et al: Characterization of collagenolytic activity in the ulcerating cornea, Exp Eye Res 11:255, 1971.
15. Ben-Hanan I et al: Further evidence for the involvement of immunoregulatory processes in corneal alkali burns: effects of immunosuppression and convalescent serum, Ophthalmic Res 18:288, 1986.
16. Ben-Hanan Y et al: Indications for the role of the immune system in the pathogenesis of corneal alkali burns, Br J Ophthalmol 67:635, 1983.
17. Levinson RA, Paterson CA, and Pfister RR: Ascorbic acid prevents corneal ulceration and perforation following experimental alkali burns, Invest Ophthalmol 15:986, 1976.
18. Pfister RR and Paterson CA: Additional clinical and morphological observations on the favorable effect of ascorbate in experimental ocular alkali burns, Invest Ophthalmol Vis Sci 16:478, 1977.
19. Chiang TS, Moorman LR, and Thomas RP: Ocular hypertensive response following acid and alkali burns in rabbits, Invest Ophthalmol 10:270, 1971.
20. Paterson CA and Pfister RR: Intraocular pressure changes after alkali burns, Arch Ophthalmol 91:211, 1974.
21. Stein MR, Naidoff MA, and Dawson CR: Intraocular pressure response to experimental alkali burns, Am J Ophthalmol 75:99, 1973.
22. Hughes WF: Alkali burns of the eye. I. Review of the literature and summary of present knowledge, Arch Ophthalmol 35:423, 1946.
23. Hughes WF: Alkali burns of the eye. II. Clinical and pathologic course, Arch Ophthalmol 36:189, 1946.
24. Roper-Hall MJ: Thermal and chemical burns, Trans Ophthalmol Soc UK 85:631, 1965.
25. Ralph RA: Chemical burns of the eye. In Duane T, editor: Clinical ophthalmology, vol 4, Hagerstown, Md, 1988, Harper & Row.
26. Brown SI, Tregakis MP, and Pearce DB: Treatment of the alkali burned cornea, Am J Ophthalmol 74:361, 1972.
27. Hughes WF: Alkali burns of the eye: review of the literature and summary of present knowledge, Arch Ophthalmol 35:423, 1946.
28. Bennett TO, Payman GA, and Rutgard J: Intracameral phosphate buffer in alkali burns, Can J Ophthalmol 13:93, 1978.
29. Paterson CA, Pfister RR, and Levinson RA: Aqueous humor pH changes after experimental alkali burns, Am J Ophthalmol 79:414, 1975.
30. Grant WM: Experimental investigation of paracentesis in the treatment of ocular ammonia burns, Arch Ophthalmol 44:399, 1950.
31. Caron LA et al: Topical fibronectin in a rabbit alkali burn model of corneal ulceration, Invest Ophthalmol Vis Sci 26 (suppl):176, 1985.
32. Tenn PF et al: Fibronectin in alkali-burned rabbit cornea: enhancement of epithelial wound healing, Invest Ophthalmol Vis Sci 26 (suppl):92, 1985.
33. Frati L et al: Selective binding of the epidermal growth factor and its specific effects on the epithelial cells of the cornea, Exp Eye Res 14:135, 1972.
34. Savage CR and Cohen S: Proliferation of corneal epithelium induced by epidermal growth factor, Exp Eye Res 15:361, 1973.
35. Watanabe K, Nakagawa S, and Nishida T: Stimulatory effects of fibronectin and EGF on migration of corneal epithelial cells, Invest Ophthalmol Vis Sci 28:205, 1987.
36. Singh G and Foster CS: Epidermal growth factor in alkali-burned corneal epithelial wound healing, Am J Ophthalmol 103:802, 1987.
37. Chung JH and Fagerholm P: Treatment of rabbit corneal alkali wounds with human epidermal growth factor, Cornea 8:122, 1989.

38. Reim M et al: Effect of epidermal growth factor in severe experimental alkali burns, Ophthalmic Res 20:327, 1988.

39. Singh G and Foster CS: Treatment of nonhealing corneal ulcers and recurrent corneal erosions. In Cavanagh HD, editor: The cornea: transactions of the World Congress on the Cornea III, New York, 1988, Raven Press.

40. Singh G and Foster CS: Growth factors in treatment of nonhealing corneal ulcers and recurrent erosions, Cornea 8:45, 1989.

41. Brown SI, Weller CA, and Vidrich AM: Effect of corticosteroids on corneal collagenase of rabbits, Am J Ophthalmol 70:744, 1970.

42. Donshik PC et al: Effect of topical corticosteroids on ulceration in alkali-burned corneas, Arch Ophthalmol 96:2117, 1978.

43. Pfister RR, Paterson CA, and Hayes SA: Effect of topical 10% ascorbate solution on established corneal ulcers after severe alkali burns, Invest Ophthalmol Vis Sci 16:22:382, 1982.

44. Pfister RR, Nicolaro ML, and Paterson CA: Sodium citrate reduces the incidence of corneal ulcerations and perforations in extreme alkali-burned eyes: acetylcysteine and ascorbate have no favorable effect, Invest Ophthalmol Vis Sci 21:486, 1981.

45. Pfister RR, Haddox JL, and Lank KM: Citrate or ascorbate/citrate treatment of established corneal ulcers in the alkali-injured rabbit eye, Invest Ophthalmol Vis Sci 29:1110, 1988.

46. Pfister RR: The effects of chemical injury on the ocular surface, Ophthalmology 90:601, 1983.

47. Paterson CA, Williams RN, and Parker RV: Characteristics of polymorphonuclear leukocyte infiltration into the alkali burned eye and the influence of sodium citrate, Exp Eye Res 39:701, 1984.

48. Aronson SB et al: Pathogenetic approach to therapy of peripheral corneal inflammatory disease, Am J Ophthalmol 70:65, 1970.

49. Newsome DA and Gross J: Prevention by medroxyprogesterone of perforation in the alkali-burned rabbit cornea: inhibition of collagenolytic activity, Invest Ophthalmol Vis Sci 16:21, 1977.

50. Ballen PH: Mucous membrane grafts in chemical (lye) burns, Am J Ophthalmol 55:302, 1963.

51. Kramer SG: Late numerical grading of alkali burns to determine keratoplasty prognosis, Trans Am Ophthalmol Soc 81:97, 1983.

52. Abel R et al: The results of penetrating keratoplasty after chemical burns, Trans Am Acad Ophthalmol Otolaryngol 79:584, 1975.

53. Thoft RA: Conjunctival transplantation, Arch Ophthalmol 95:1425, 1977.

54. Thoft RA: Conjunctival transplantation as an alternative to keratoplasty, Ophthalmology 86:1084, 1979.

55. Thoft RA: Indications for conjunctival transplantation, Ophthalmology 89:335, 1982.

56. Kenyon KR and Tseng SCG: Limbal autograft transplantation for ocular surface disorders, Ophthalmology 96:709, 1989.

57. Thoft RA: Keratoepithelioplasty, Am J Ophthalmol 97:1, 1983.

58. Aquavella JV, et al: Keratoprosthesis: results, complications, and management, Ophthalmology 89:655, 1982.

59. Cardonna H: Prosthokeratoplasty, Cornea 2:179, 1983.

60. Barron BA: Prosthokeratoplasty. In Kaufman HE et al, editors: The cornea, New York, 1988, Churchill Livingstone.

61. Holekamp TLR and Becker B: Ocular injuries from automobile batteries, Trans Am Acad Ophthalmol Otolaryngol 83:805, 1977.

62. McCulley JP et al: Ocular hydrofluoric acid burns. In Henkind P et al, editors: Acta XXIV International Congress Ophthalmology, New York, 1982, JB Lippincott.

63. Grayson M and Peroni D: Severe silver nitrate injury to the eye, Am J Ophthalmol 70:227, 1970.

64. Friedenwald JS, Hughes WF, and Herrmann H: Acid burns of the eye, Arch Ophthalmol 35:98, 1946.

65. Paterson CA et al: The ocular hypertensive response following experimental acid burns in the rabbit eye, Invest Ophthalmol Vis Sci 18:67, 1979.

66. McCulley JP: Chemical injuries. In Smolin G and Thoft RA, editors: The cornea: scientific foundations and clinical practice, Boston, 1983, Little, Brown & Co.

67. Oaks LW, Dorman JE, and Petty RW: Tear gas burns of the eye, Arch Ophthalmol 63:689, 1960.

68. Laibson PR, and Oconor J: Explosive tear gas burns of the eye, Trans Am Acad Ophthalmol Otolaryngol 74:811, 1970.

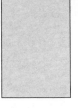

LIMBAL TUMORS

The limbus is a unique portion of the ocular surface that is often involved in disease processes. Many types of limbal lesions can occur: inflammatory, traumatic, congenital, degenerative, metabolic, and neoplastic (see boxes on pp. 667 and 670). This chapter is concerned primarily with neoplastic tumors, but some other conditions that simulate neoplasms, such as traumatic and inflammatory tumors, are also discussed. Some neoplasms that primarily involve nonlimbal conjunctiva, but can also affect the limbus and cornea, are discussed. Strictly corneal tumors are rare; most tumors involving the cornea arise near the limbus. The most common true neoplasms arise from the squamous epithelial cells, or the melanocytes within the epithelium. Congenital lesions are discussed in Chapter 5.

OBTAINING SPECIMENS

It is often not possible to distinguish tumors clinically; histopathologic examination is required. Cytology is a simple procedure that can aid in the diagnosis of external lesions. It is used mainly to identify diffuse neoplastic processes causing conjunctivitis; a cytology specimen containing neoplastic cells points to the correct diagnosis and the need for biopsy. After topical anesthesia the surface of

LIMBAL LESIONS

NEOPLASTIC
EPITHELIAL TUMORS

Papillomata
Benign hereditary dyskeratosis
Actinic keratosis
Squamous dysplasia and carcinoma in situ (CIN)
Invasive squamous cell carcinoma
Mucoepidermoid carcinoma
Spindle cell carcinoma

LYMPHOID TUMORS

Lymphoid hyperplasia
Lymphoma

SEBACEOUS CELL CARCINOMA
MELANOCYTIC LESIONS

Nevi
Primary acquired melanosis
Malignant melanoma

FIBROUS HISTIOCYTOMA
KAPOSI'S SARCOMA

SYSTEMIC DISEASE

Juvenile xanthogranuloma
Gaucher's disease (pigmented pseudopingueculae)
Multiple endocrine neoplasia (type IIB)
Neurofibromatosis (neurofibroma, schwannoma)
Ochronosis (alkaptonuria)

INFLAMMATORY

Follicles
Leprosy
Sarcoid
Phlyctenule
?Nodular fasciitis

CONGENITAL
CHORISTOMAS

Dermoids and lipodermoids
Ectopic lacrimal gland
Osseous choristomas
Vascular hamartomas

DEGENERATIVE

Pterygium
Pingueculae
Amyloid

POSTTRAUMATIC

Pyogenic granuloma
Corneal or conjunctival inclusion cyst (Fig. 30-1)
Filtering bleb (Fig. 30-2)
Uveal prolapse (Fig. 30-3)
Intrastromal air (Fig. 30-4)
Foreign body granuloma
Keloid (Fig. 30-5)

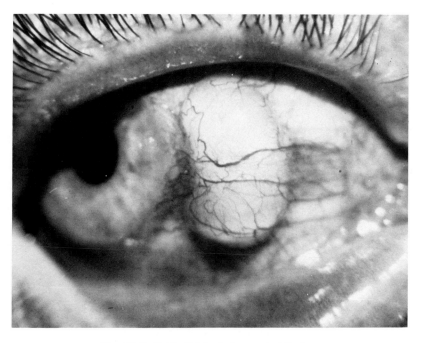

Fig. 30-1. Epithelial inclusion cyst at limbus.

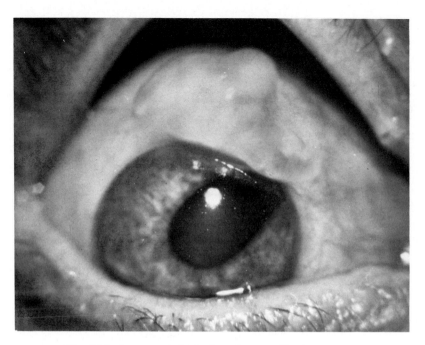

Fig. 30-2. Large cystic bleb after glaucoma filtering surgery.

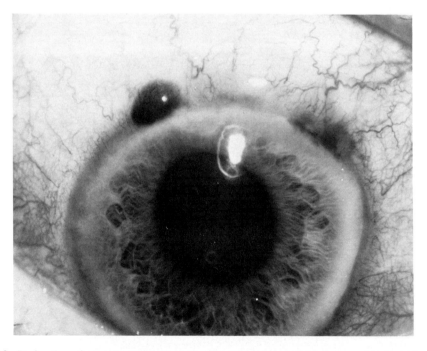

Fig. 30-3. Perforation of cornea with uveal prolapse in Terrien's marginal degeneration (see Chapter 16).

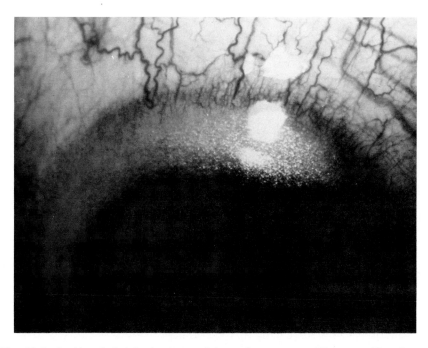

Fig. 30-4. Accidental air injection into periphery of cornea resembling crystalline change.

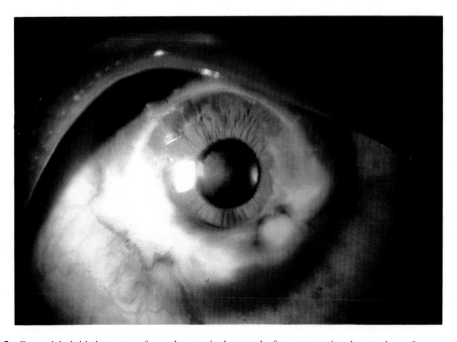

Fig. 30-5. Corneal keloid that arose from the surgical wound after penetrating keratoplasty for a corneal leukoma. (Courtesy of Massimo Busin, Bonn, Germany.)

CHARACTERISTICS OF LIMBAL LESIONS

RAPIDLY GROWING

Pseudoepitheliomatous hyperplasia
Nodular fasciitis
Pyogenic granuloma
Mucoepidermoid carcinoma

NO GROWTH

Dermoid
Ectopic lacrimal gland
(?)Juvenile xanthogranuloma

PAPILLARY

Benign noninfectious papilloma
Infectious ([?]papillomavirus) papilloma
Intraepithelial neoplasia

HYPERKERATOTIC

Benign hereditary dyskeratosis
Intraepithelial neoplasia (rare)
Invasive squamous cell carcinoma
Actinic keratosis
Pseudoepitheliomatous hyperplasia

CHILDREN (FIRST DECADE)

Benign hereditary dyskeratosis
Dermoid
Ectopic lacrimal gland
Juvenile xanthogranuloma
Nevi

BILATERAL

Benign hereditary dyskeratosis
Dermoid
Infectious papilloma

EXTEND OVER CORNEA (> 1 MM)

Intraepithelial neoplasia
Invasive squamous cell carcinoma
Mucoepidermoid carcinoma
Dermoid
Ectopic lacrimal gland
Juvenile xanthogranuloma
Malignant melanoma
Primary corneal epithelial dysplasia

PIGMENTED

Nevi
Malignant melanoma
Primary acquired melanosis
Congenital melanosis
Kaposi's sarcoma (reddish)

METASTASIZE

Mucoepidermoid carcinoma
Malignant melanoma
Invasive squamous cell carcinoma (rare)

CORNEAL STROMA EXTENSION

Dermoid
Ectopic lacrimal gland
Juvenile xanthogranuloma
Invasive squamous cell carcinoma (rare)
(?)Mucoepidermoid carcinoma

ASSOCIATED WITH INFLAMMATION

Pyogenic granuloma
Benign hereditary dyskeratosis
Primary acquired melanosis
Nevi

HEREDITARY

Benign hereditary dyskeratosis

the mass is scraped with a stainless steel blade. The material is spread on a slide and immediately fixed with a spray cytologic fixative, or with alcohol.

In nearly all cases a biopsy is preferable; more cells are obtained, the architecture is preserved, and the diagnosis is more likely to be accurate. Often the lesion can be completely removed without an extensive procedure. In other cases, such as primary acquired melanosis or suspected pagetoid spread of sebaceous cell carcinoma, multiple small biopsies are taken. Topical or infiltrative local anesthesia is sufficient, and no suturing is necessary. Handling of the specimen with forceps should be minimized to prevent crushing.

It is important to make a drawing of the lesion and the site(s) of biopsy. Each specimen should be marked and preserved separately. It is best to place them flat on a carrier, such as a tongue blade, and indicate their orientation.

INFLAMMATORY AND POSTTRAUMATIC LESIONS

PYOGENIC GRANULOMA

Pyogenic granulomas are exuberant growths of granulation tissue after injury, usually by trauma or infection. They most commonly occur after conjunctival surgery (for example, for strabismus or pterygia) (Fig. 30-6). Rarely, they can arise on the cornea, usually in an area with fibrovascular pannus.[1-3] They grow acutely, are intense red due to the high vascular content, and can have a narrower base, giving a pedunculated appearance (Fig. 30-7). Simple excision is usually sufficient; however, they can recur. Because Kaposi's sarcoma can have a similar appearance, it should be considered in the differential diagnosis.

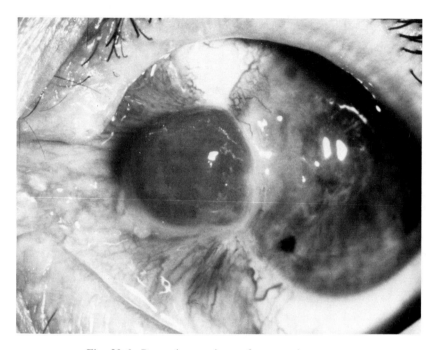

Fig. 30-6. Pyogenic granuloma after pterygium surgery.

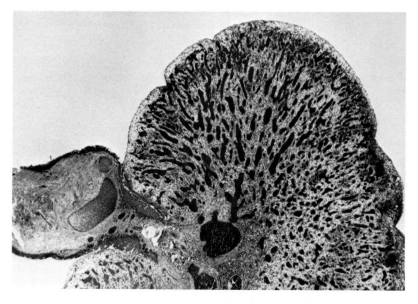

Fig. 30-7. Pyogenic granuloma of conjunctiva. Smooth-surfaced mass composed of vascularized granulation tissue with acute and chronic inflammatory cells. Pedunculated base is seen on left. (Hematoxylin-eosin stain, ×50.) (Courtesy of Bruce L. Johnson, Pittsburgh.)

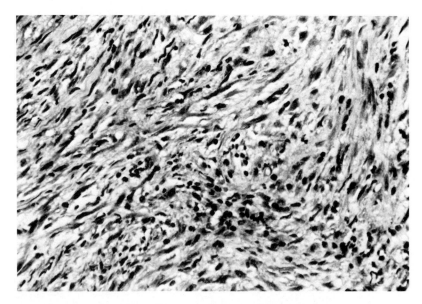

Fig. 30-8. Nodular fasciitis. Loosely coherent spindle-shaped fibroblasts, intercellular myxoid material, and chronic inflammatory cells. (Hematoxylin-eosin stain, ×500.) (Courtesy of Bruce L. Johnson, Pittsburgh.)

NODULAR FASCIITIS

Nodular fasciitis is a rare acute reactive (nonneoplastic) proliferation of immature connective tissue. Histologically, these tumors are composed of highly cellular, generally nonencapsulated proliferations of immature fibroblasts, vascular endothelial cells, pools of mucinous material, and chronic inflammatory cells and can be mistaken for sarcomas (Fig. 30-8). The lesions usually can be removed by simple excision.

INTRASTROMAL CYSTS

After trauma epithelial cysts can form within the corneal stroma. Epithelial cells are implanted in the stroma during penetrating or perforating injury, and proliferate, forming an interlamellar cyst. This cyst can be clear or become translucent as it fills with desquamated epithelium.[4]

Intraepithelial or intrastromal hemorrhage also can occur in vascularized corneas. Rarely these can lead to ulceration of the overlying stroma, presumably because of impairment of the passage of nutrients from the aqueous.[5]

FIBROUS HISTIOCYTOMA

Fibrous histiocytomas are solitary confined lesions composed of a mixture of fibroblasts and lipid-filled macrophages (histiocytes) that are most often found in the dermis or subcutaneous fibrous tissue. They are the most common mesenchymal orbital tumors in adults, but rarely arise from the conjunctiva, episclera, or sclera. They can grow at the limbus and extend over the peripheral cornea.[6-9] They are yellow-white and can appear as nodules at the limbus (Fig. 30-9) or infiltrative lesions extending into the corneal stroma from the limbus. It is not clear whether the pathologic process in these external lesions is reactive or neoplastic. Simple excision is usually curative.

LYMPHOID TUMORS

The conjunctiva is part of the mucosal immune system and normally contains abundant lymphoid tissue. This tissue can be affected by localized or systemic lymphoid proliferations, both benign and

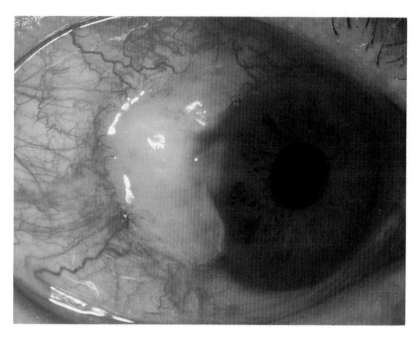

Fig. 30-9. Fibrous histiocytoma.

malignant. The tumors appear as single or multiple elevated masses that generally assume the contour of the globe. They are invariably salmon colored, exhibit sharply demarcated borders, lack gross blood vessels, are not tender or ulcerated, and have smooth overlying conjunctiva (Fig. 30-10). Approximately 15% to 20% of cases are bilateral. In the great majority of cases there is no history or evidence of systemic disease.

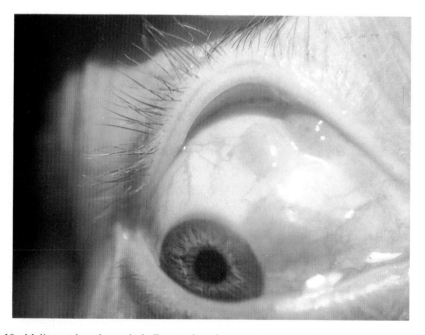

Fig. 30-10. Malignant lymphoma in bulbar conjunctiva, appears as smooth, raised, salmon pink tumor.

Histologically conjunctival lymphoid tumors can be divided into polyclonal T–cell rich pseudolymphomas and monoclonal B-cell lymphomas.[10-14] The monoclonal B-cell tumors can then be subdivided into well-differentiated, intermediate, and poorly differentiated lymphomas. Polyclonal tumors and well- and intermediately differentiated B-cell tumors have a very good prognosis; the risk of extraocular manifestations appears to be low.[15,16] However, the risk of systemic disease is much higher for poorly differentiated B-cell lymphomas. Further immunochemical differentiation, for example, T-cell and B-cell subsets, has not proved clinically useful.[14,15] The course of conjunctival lymphoid tumors seems to be better than that of orbital lymphoid tumors, possibly because the conjunctiva normally contains lymphoid tissue, but the orbit does not.[10] Even when spread occurs, the course is often slow, and survival prolonged.

The current treatment recommendations by Jakobiec and colleagues are as follows[7]:

1. All patients should be evaluated for evidence of systemic disease, including chest x-ray, whole-body CT, complete peripheral blood count, Coomb test, antinuclear antibodies, latex fixation, serum protein immunoelectrophoresis, bone marrow biopsy, bone scan, and liver-spleen scan.

2. If nonocular disease is not detected, patients receive 1500 to 2000 rads of radiotherapy to the involved area, with shielding of the eyeball. This treatment is necessary because of the possibility of dedifferentiation and spread.

3. Systemic noninvasive evaluations are repeated every 6 months for 5 years.

EPITHELIAL TUMORS

Tumors of the epithelium can be classified as benign, dysplastic or precancerous, and malignant. Benign tumors include cysts, papillomata, and keratoses. Dysplastic growths include squamous dysplasia and carcinoma in situ, which are referred to as conjunctival intraepithelial neoplasia and actinic keratoses. Invasive squamous cell carcinoma and mucoepidermoid carcinoma are malignant neoplasms.

The following terms are often used to describe epithelial growths and should be understood:

- *Squamous metaplasia*   Transformation of columnar or glandular epithelium into stratified squamous epithelium, sometimes with keratinization
- *Acanthosis*   Thickening of the prickle (malpighian) cell layer
- *Hyperkeratosis*   Increased keratin in the granular cell layer
- *Dyskeratosis*   Keratinization of individual cells at an abnormally deep level
- *Parakeratosis*   Nuclei present in the keratin layer
- *Dysplasia*   Cells show atypical size and shape, increased nuclear-cytoplasmic ratio, and mitotic figures; maturation and polarity are disturbed
- *Neoplasia*   New growth, tumor formation; a mass of abnormal cells
- *Pseudoepitheliomatous hyperplasia*   A benign reactive epithelial proliferation

PAPILLOMATA

A papilloma is a circumscribed, elevated epithelial tumor. It consists of villous or arborescent fibrovascular outgrowths covered by neoplastic epithelium. Clinically the epithelium is translucent, and through it one can see the capillaries in the connective tissue core. The tumor can arise from a thin central stalk (pedunculated type) or broad based (sessile type).

Conjunctival papillomatous lesions can be seen in young and old patients alike. They can be viral papillomas, other benign lesions, or malignant growths, and it can be difficult or impossible to clinically distinguish among them. Table 30-1 lists some differentiating features.

The lesions seen in the younger age group are most often caused by viral infection with human papilloma virus.[17-19] Different serotypes of this virus are thought to be responsible for verrucae of the

TABLE 30-1. Clinical Characteristics of Conjunctival Papillomata

INFECTIOUS (VIRAL)	NONINFECTIOUS (UNKNOWN CAUSE)
Usually in children or young adults	Usually in older adults
May be bilateral	Nearly always unilateral
May be multiple	Nearly always single
Usually on palpebral conjunctiva, fornix, or caruncle, especially below; less commonly at limbus	Usually on bulbar conjunctiva or at limbus
Pedunculated	Sessile or diffuse
Smooth surface	More surface irregularity and thickening
May occur with verrucae on eyelid or elsewhere	No such association
Multiple lesions may appear after excision of single lesion	Each recurrence usually single
Transmissible	Not transmissible
Usually little or no conjunctivitis; rarely moderate conjunctivitis	Occasionally marked conjunctivitis ("masquerade syndrome")
Occasionally fine ("toxic") epithelial keratitis	Cornea involved only by direct extension or mechanical factors
Rarely, if ever, malignant	Benign, dysplastic, or malignant
Spontaneous resolution common	Spontaneous resolution uncommon

From Wilson FM II and Oster HB: Am J Ophthalmol 77:103, 1974.

face, hands, and feet and genital and anal warts. In one case the virus isolated from a conjunctival papilloma was the same type as that commonly associated with condyloma accuminatum of the genitals.[17]

Papillomata in children can affect any portion of the conjunctiva, including the limbus. These transmissible lesions can be multiple and, if improperly removed, can become alarmingly widespread (Fig. 30-11). A fine epithelial keratitis can be seen. Viral papillomata are best left untreated; a 2-year waiting period is recommended, since many of the papillomata resolve spontaneously by that time. If treatment becomes necessary, however, simple excision should be combined with cryotherapy of the base and surrounding epithelium.

The papillomata in older persons are commonly dysplastic or malignant. The lesions in older individuals tend to be sessile and affect the limbus or bulbar conjunctiva (Fig. 30-12). The tumor can drape over the cornea or extend into the corneal epithelium or stroma. Growth into the cornea suggests dysplasia or malignancy. Papillary lesions in adults should be excised, particularly if they arise at the limbus, extend onto the cornea, or exhibit continued growth. Simple excision with cryotherapy of the base and surrounding epithelium is usually curative. The tumor usually can be scraped from the corneal surface, without dissection into the stroma, and cryotherapy is performed at the limbus.

BENIGN HEREDITARY DYSKERATOSIS

Benign hereditary dyskeratosis is a rare condition transmitted in a dominant fashion.[20,21] It affects descendants of a kindred of individuals from Halifax and Warren counties in North Carolina, with Halowar Indian, black and white heritage, and a high rate of consanguineous marriage. Cases have been seen in other parts of the country in individuals who have relocated from this area.[22,23]

Benign hyperkeratotic lesions of the bulbar conjunctiva are typically seen at the limbus. The conjunctival lesions are raised, granular, semitransparent, and horseshoe-shaped (Fig. 30-13). They are usually bilateral, can be both nasal and temporal, and are located in the interpalpebral fissure, extending superiorly and inferiorly. They commonly appear during the first year of life and gradually progress. The lesions do not extend over the cornea or threaten vision, but corneal opacities can rarely occur and are usually deep and associated with vascularization. These lesions can be associated

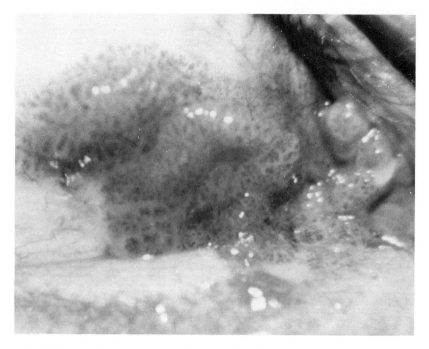

Fig. 30-11. Viral papilloma extending from limbal bulbar conjunctiva to caruncle.

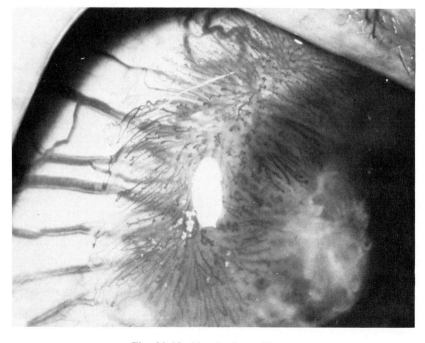

Fig. 30-12. Neoplastic papilloma.

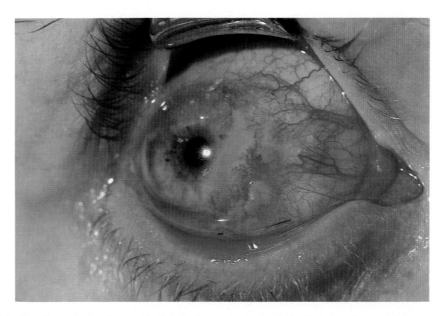

Fig. 30-13. Hereditary benign intraepithelial dyskeratosis: leukoplakic limbal lesions with large conjunctival feeder vessels and corneal pannus adjacent to lesions. (From McLean IW et al: Ophthalmology 88:164, 1981.)

with conjunctival injection, foreign body sensation, papillary hypertrophy of the tarsal conjunctiva, iritis, and rubeosis iridis. Oral lesions, such as white spongy lesions on the buccal and labial mucosa and the ventral aspect of the tongue, also can be seen.

Histologically the lesions are composed of hyperplastic epithelium, with acanthosis and dyskeratosis, but no other signs of atypia. Increased vascularization and a moderate inflammatory reaction in the conjunctival connective tissue may occur. These lesions do not evolve into truly dysplastic or carcinomatous tumors. There is no treatment, even after complete excision the lesions commonly recur.

SQUAMOUS DYSPLASIA AND CARCINOMA IN SITU (INTRAEPITHELIAL NEOPLASIA)

Dysplasia and intraepithelial neoplasia of the conjunctival epithelium are uncommon tumors that most often are seen in older, fair-skinned people. They grow slowly and are usually asymptomatic. They nearly always arise at the limbus and are more common in the interpalpebral area. The lesions appear as raised, somewhat gelatinous masses, which may be gray and slightly red, depending on the vascularity[24] (Fig. 30-14). Some dysplastic lesions have a papillary appearance, and rarely they can be hyperkeratotic and appear white (leukoplakic). In many cases the abnormal epithelium extends onto the peripheral cornea, where it can appear translucent, frosted, or white and can be associated with underlying vessels. If neglected for prolonged periods, extensive corneal involvement can develop (Fig. 30-15).

The main histopathologic feature of both dysplasia and carcinoma in situ is anaplasia of the epithelial cells. There is a high nuclear: cytoplasmic ratio, the normal polarity of the epithelium is lost, mitotic figures are more frequent, and there is dysmaturation, with dyskeratosis. The process is called "dysplastic" if only a partial thickness of the epithelium layer is replaced by atypical cells (Fig. 30-16) and carcinoma in situ if there is total replacement of the epithelial layer (Fig. 30-17); in both cases the basement membrane is intact. The usefulness of distinguishing between dysplasia and carcinoma in situ is controversial, and some prefer just to use the term "conjunctival intraepithelial neo-

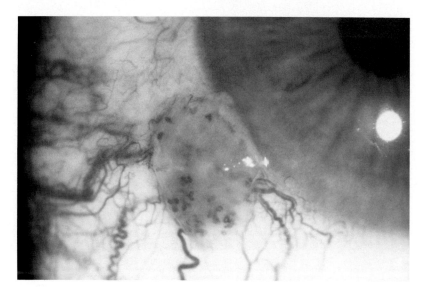

Fig. 30-14. Dysplastic lesion arising at limbus.

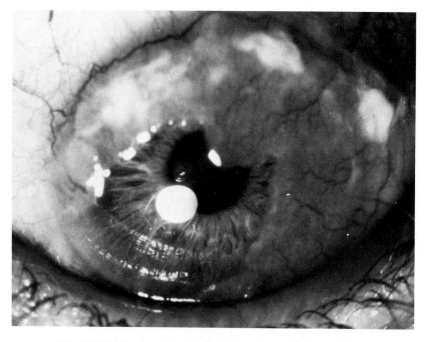

Fig. 30-15. Carcinoma in situ involving the corneal epithelium.

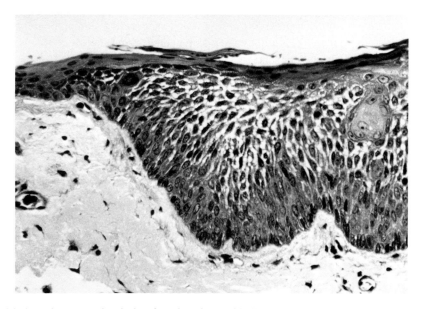

Fig. 30-16. Moderately severe dysplasia of conjunctival epithelium. Note thickening (acanthosis) of epithelial layer with moderate atypia and loss of cellular polarity, not involving the full thickness of the epithelium. (Hematoxylin-eosin stain, ×500.) (Courtesy of Bruce L. Johnson, Pittsburgh.)

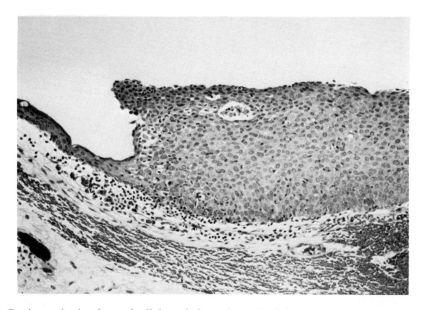

Fig. 30-17. Carcinoma in situ. Loss of cellular polarity and acanthosis involving the full thickness of the epithelial layer. (Hematoxylin-eosin stain, ×200.) (Courtesy of Bruce L. Johnson, Pittsburgh.)

plasia" (CIN) for both. If invasion into the subepithelial connective tissue occurs, the diagnosis of invasive squamous cell carcinoma is made.

Actinic keratoses are similar to solar keratoses, which arise on the skin and can be considered a type of dysplastic lesion. Histologically they are differentiated from other dysplastic lesions by their surface keratinization and elastotic degeneration of the collagen in the substantia propria.

The treatment is excision, down to bare sclera, incorporating a margin of apparently normal conjunctiva 2 to 3 mm wide. The extent of the tumor is best visualized by the application of rose bengal red (Fig. 30-18); areas with tumor exhibit punctate staining.[25] Portions extending over the cornea can be scraped off with a Kimura spatula or scalpel blade (for example, Bard-Parker #64). Occasionally an adherent fibrovascular pannus is present and must be removed with sharp dissection. The limbus is carefully cleaned and scraped and then scrubbed with absolute alcohol. The limbus, base, and conjunctival margin are then frozen with a retinal cryoprobe in a rapid double freeze-thaw manner.[26] One must be careful to avoid extensive deep freezing because in a few cases ciliary body damage has lead to phthisis.

A significant proportion of these lesions recur, even with the treatment described previously. Therefore these patients must be followed regularly, with rose bengal staining and reexcision of any suspicious areas.

PRIMARY CORNEAL EPITHELIAL DYSPLASIA

Primary corneal epithelial dysplasia is a rare condition that mainly affects the corneal epithelium, without a limbal mass. It probably arises at the limbus and, for unknown reasons, spreads in a relatively flat manner over the cornea rather than accumulating at the limbus or extending into the conjunctiva.[27-29] The abnormal epithelium appears frosted or opalescent, is usually not vascularized, and has smooth or fringelike (fimbriated) edges. They can be multiple, extend from the limbus or lie free

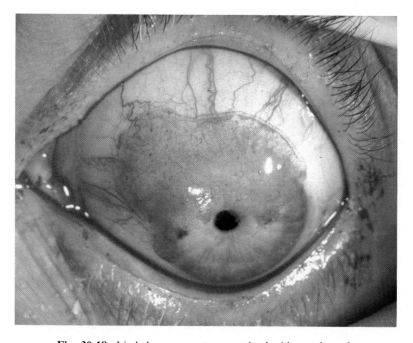

Fig. 30-18. Limbal squamous tumor stained with rose bengal.

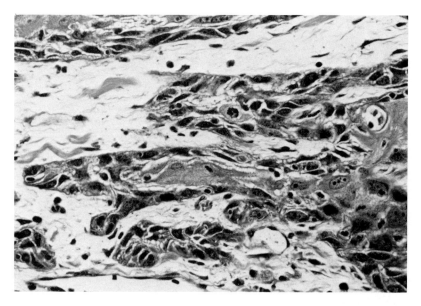

Fig. 30-19. Invasive squamous cell carcinoma. Atypical epithelial cells have invaded conjunctival stroma. (Hematoxylin-eosin stain, ×600.) (Courtesy of Bruce L. Johnson, Pittsburgh.)

in the cornea, and can be unilateral or bilateral. They progress slowly, waxing and waning in their extent. The treatment is simple removal (scraping), although the lesions can recur.

INVASIVE SQUAMOUS CELL CARCINOMA

Invasive squamous cell carcinoma can arise from preexisting epithelial dysplasia or carcinoma in situ. The anaplastic cells pass through the basement membrane and invade the subepithelial tissues of the conjunctiva or cornea (Fig. 30-19). If left undetected, the invasion can extend into the deeper layers of the cornea, the sclera, or even into the eye. Only very rarely will they metastasize.[30]

Excision is the recommended treatment. Wide local excision, including lamellar sclerectomy if necessary, is combined with cryotherapy of the base and margins.[26] If intraocular invasion has occurred, enucleation is indicated; exenteration is required for treatment of orbital extension.

MUCOEPIDERMOID CARCINOMA

Mucoepidermoid carcinoma is a more aggressive form of epithelial carcinoma in which there is proliferation of both squamous cells and mucin-producing goblet cells.[31-33] Mucoepidermoid carcinoma is usually seen in the elderly and most commonly arises at the limbus, although they can be found elsewhere in the conjunctiva. It is more likely than squamous cell carcinoma to invade the substantia propria, invade the globe, or metastasize to regional lymph nodes. For this reason it is important to make the distinction histologically (Fig. 30-20). Mucin production can be present in only a small portion of the tumor, and in some cases it was noted in only the intraocular portion.[32,34] Wide local excision with cryotherapy is the treatment.

SPINDLE CELL CARCINOMA

Spindle cell carcinoma is a variant of squamous cell carcinoma in which the cells are spindle-shaped, appearing similar to fibroblasts[35,36] (Fig. 30-21). Their epithelial origin, however, has been

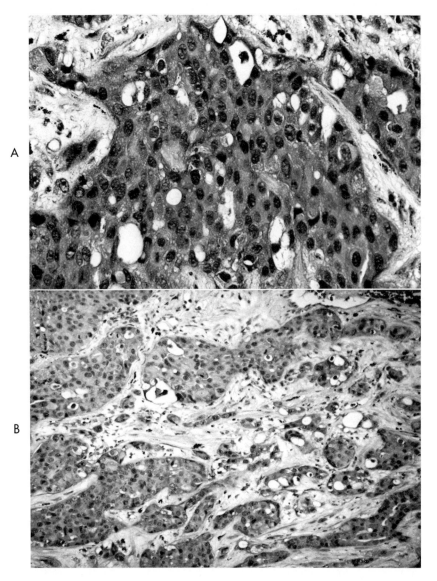

Fig. 30-20. Mucoepidermoid carcinoma. **A,** Nests of abnormal cells invading stroma. (Hematoxylin-eosin stain, ×200.) **B,** Multiple mucus-filled spaces are present within squamous cells. (Hematoxylin-eosin stain, ×500.) (Courtesy of Bruce L. Johnson, Pittsburgh.)

supported by electron microscopy and immunohistochemistry.[37] These tumors also are relatively aggressive and are capable of intraocular extension.

SEBACEOUS CELL CARCINOMA

Although it is not a primary tumor of the conjunctiva or cornea, sebaceous cell carcinoma is important to mention because of its tendency to spread in a pagetoid fashion into the conjunctiva and cornea. Tumors of the sebaceous glands in the lids (meibomian, Zeis) or caruncle can spread up the gland ducts onto the epithelial surface, sometimes without a noticeable primary nodule (Fig. 30-22). These patients can present with chronic unilateral conjunctivitis, blepharoconjunctivitis, or keratoconjunctivitis (masquerade syndrome)[38,39] (Fig. 30-23). Clues to the correct diagnosis are eyelid thickening and deformity, lash loss, marked mucoid discharge, unilaterality, and an abnormal, thick pap-

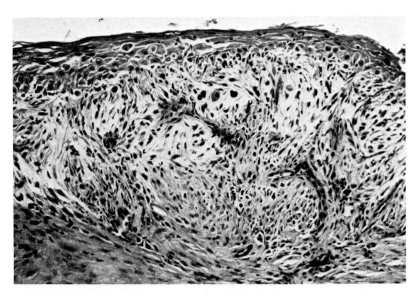

Fig. 30-21. Spindle-cell variant of squamous cell carcinoma. Pleomorphic and hyperchromatic spindle-shaped cells extend from the surface epithelium and infiltrate the stroma. (Hematoxylin-eosin stain, ×250.) (Courtesy of Bruce L. Johnson, Pittsburgh.)

illary conjunctival appearance (see Chapter 7). Whenever pagetoid spread of sebaceous cell carcinoma is suspected, multiple conjunctival biopsies should be taken. If the lid is thickened or a nodule is present, a wedge biopsy should be performed.

KAPOSI'S SARCOMA

This previously rare tumor has become more common because it frequently occurs in patients with acquired immune deficiency syndrome (AIDS).[40-43] The lesions are nodular or diffuse, blue-red or deep brown, and elevated and are usually found in the inferior forniceal conjunctiva[44] (Fig. 30-24). Kaposi's sarcoma usually develops in patients with an established history of the disease, but it can be a presenting manifestation. It also is more common in patients with lymphoma and leukemia. Most lesions are slowly progressive and rarely invasive.[43] Complications are usually related to the bulk of the tumor: entropion, discomfort, and obstruction of vision.

Histopathologically the tumor is composed of spindle-shaped cells with elongated oval nuclei, capillaries, and vascular slits without an apparent endothelial lining. It probably arises from vascular cells, endothelial cells, or pericytes.[44]

These tumors can be treated with simple excision, radiation, or chemotherapy. Usually, because of the general status of the AIDS patient, simple excision or local radiation is performed.

PIGMENTED LESIONS

The melanocytes in the conjunctiva are analogous to those of the epidermis.[45] They normally are located within the basal layer of the epithelium and have delicate branching dendritic processes that contain little or no pigment. When stimulated to produce excess amounts of melanin, the melanocytes typically secrete the pigment into the adjacent epithelial or underlying stromal cells. Blacks tend to develop pigmentation of nonmelanocytic lesions, such as papillomas, through this mechanism.

The conjunctival melanocyte is most likely derived from the neural crest cells. In histologic sections stained with hematoxylin and eosin, conjunctival melanocytes are solitary dendritic cells with clear cytoplasm. The cells vary in size, number, and melanin content.

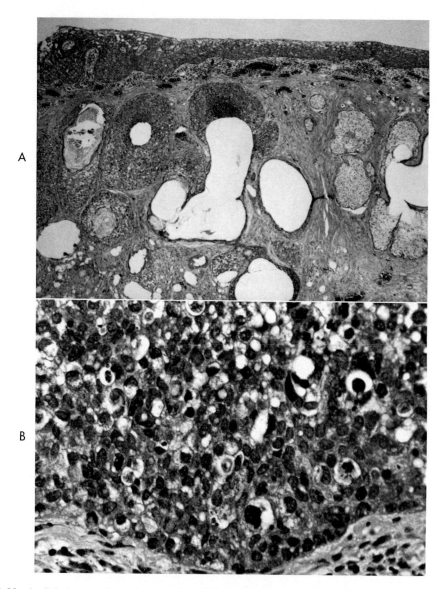

Fig. 30-22. A, Sebaceous cell carcinoma arising from the meibomian glands of the tarsus. Note normal gland tissue on the right, and spread of abnormal cells superficially (pagetoid growth) on the left. (Hematoxylin-eosin stain, ×4.) **B,** Higher magnification of anaplastic superficial cells, with vacuolated cytoplasm, large nuclear forms, and abnormal mitotic figures. (Hematoxylin-eosin stain, ×500.) (Courtesy of Bruce L. Johnson, Pittsburgh.)

The following conditions can cause pigmentation of the cornea, limbus, or neighboring conjunctiva[46,47]:

I. Benign epithelial melanosis
II. Congenital subepithelial melanosis
   A. Melanosis oculi
   B. Oculodermal melanocytosis (nevus of Ota)
III. Primary acquired melanosis
IV. Conjunctival nevi
   A. Intraepithelial (junctional)
   B. Subepithelial

   C. Compound
V. Blue nevi
VI. Secondary pigmentation
   A. Chronic conjunctival disorders
      1. Trachoma
      2. Vernal conjunctivitis
      3. Vitamin A deficiency
   B. Skin diseases

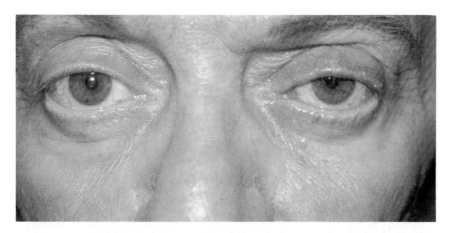

Fig. 30-23. Sebaceous cell carcinoma of left eye, producing conjunctivitis, thickening and erythema of upper lid, and loss of lashes. (Courtesy of Richard A. Thoft, Pittsburgh.)

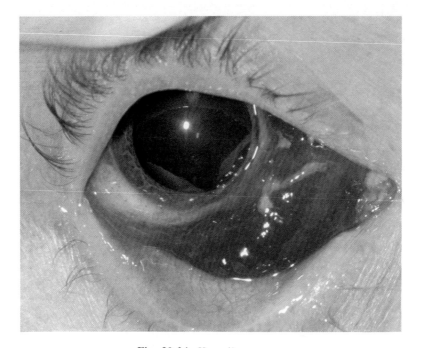

Fig. 30-24. Kaposi's sarcoma.

    1. Xeroderma pigmentosum
    2. Acanthosis nigricans
  C. Chemicals
    1. Arsenic
    2. Phenothiazines
    3. Epinephrine products
    4. Gold
    5. Quinacrine
  D. Systemic disorders
    1. Addison's disease

    2. Folic acid deficiency anemias[48]
    3. Pregnancy
    4. Thyroid disease
    5. Alkaptonuria
    6. Alport's syndrome
  E. Miscellaneous
    1. Striate melanokeratosis
    2. Mascara particle inclusions
    3. Uveal tissue
    4. Hematogenous pigmentation

Some of these conditions are discussed in the following sections.

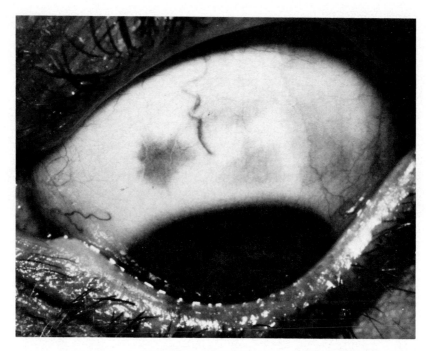

Fig. 30-26. Melanosis oculi.

Benign Epithelial Melanosis

Discrete pigmented lesions can appear at birth or early childhood, representing melanin in the basal layers of the conjunctival epithelium. These benign lesions are seen more frequently in more deeply pigmented races. They do not exhibit any malignant potential; they are always stationary. The pigmentation most often affects the perilimbal and interpalpebral areas and can extend into the peripheral corneal epithelium. It is bilateral, fairly symmetric, flat, and uninflamed.

Pigmentation also can be seen around an Axenfeld's loop, an intrascleral nerve loop approximately 4 mm from the limbus (Fig. 30-25), and around the anterior ciliary vessels. These spots occur regularly in blacks and less frequently in whites, especially those with lightly pigmented irides.

Congenital Subepithelial Melanosis

Abnormal melanin-containing cells are found in the episclera and sclera, creating a slate blue-gray coloration (Fig. 30-26). This condition is thought to result from incomplete migration of melanocytes destined for the surface epithelium. An increase in the number and size of melanocytes may be observed in the uvea, sclera, episclera, dermis of the eyelid, optic nerve meninges, and orbital soft tissues. These cases are more common in whites and are usually unilateral, congenital, and stationary. However, there is an increased risk of uveal malignant melanoma; therefore lifelong observation is required.

The condition is called *melanosis oculi* if it is restricted to the globe, and *congenital oculodermal melanocytosis (nevus of Ota)* if it involves both the globe and the periorbital skin. It is usually unilateral and occurs mainly in Asians and blacks (Fig. 30-27). Malignant melanoma can occur, but the incidence does not appear to be higher than normal.

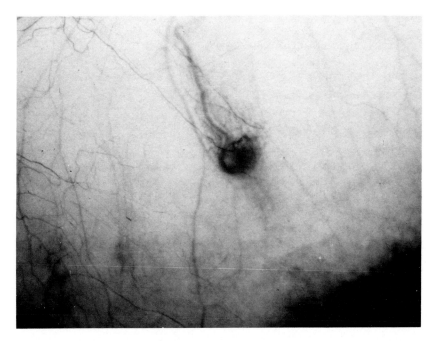

Fig. 30-25. Axenfeld's loop.

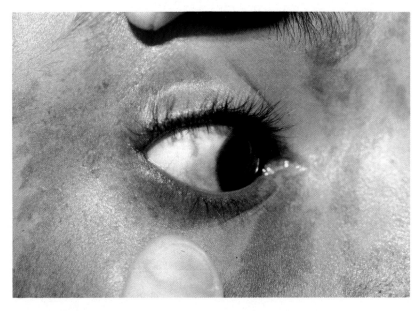

Fig. 30-27. Nevus of Ota. (Courtesy of Kenneth Cheng, Pittsburgh.)

MELANOCYTOMA

Melanocytoma is a congenital, jet-black, slowly progressive pigmented tumor, composed of large polyhedral cells that are loaded with melanin. They are found in the deep substantia propria and episclera; therefore the lesion often does not move with the conjunctiva. It rarely can occur in the limbal area and can be mistaken for a malignant melanoma.[49,50]

CONJUNCTIVAL NEVI

Nevi are common conjunctival lesions and are similar to those of the skin. They occasionally are noted at birth, but more commonly appear during the first two decades. They consist of clusters of rounded, benign-appearing melanocytes and are classified according to the following layer(s) in which they are found:

1. Intraepithelial (junctional)
2. Subepithelial
3. Compound (intraepithelial plus subepithelial)

The nevi are initially located between the basal epithelium and the epithelial basement membrane (junctional) and gradually extend into the substantia propria in the ensuing decades, becoming compound and then subepithelial. Therefore most conjunctival nevi are compound or subepithelial; junctional nevi are found only during the first two decades.

Conjunctival nevi occur mainly at the limbus, or in the bulbar conjunctiva (Fig. 30-28), plica, caruncle, or lid margin; palpebral conjunctival or forniceal nevi are relatively rare. They may be focal or diffuse, but usually not multifocal. Subepithelial and compound nevi typically elevate the conjunctival surface, a process that often increases with time. All nevi are freely movable over the globe. Approximately 20% to 30% of nevi are nonpigmented. Limbal nevi can slightly overlap the peripheral cornea (Fig. 30-29), but they do not extend into the corneal stroma. (The lesion can be lifted off the cornea, revealing that the base ends at the limbus.) They can grow, especially in childhood, be-

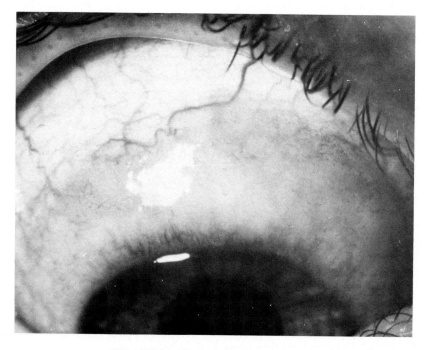

Fig. 30-28. Cystic nevus of limbal area.

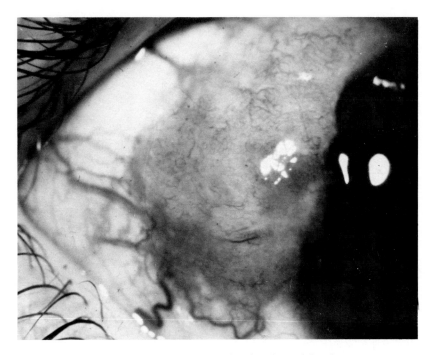

Fig. 30-29. Pigmented nevus overlapping the peripheral cornea.

come more pigmented, develop clear cysts, or be associated with inflammation. Rarely do they progress to melanoma, but approximately 25% of conjunctival melanomas arise from preexisting nevi.[51,52]

Pigmented lesions of the tarsal or forniceal conjunctiva should be excised because of the relatively greater likelihood that these lesions are malignant. Other lesions that are growing, increasing in vascularity, fixed to the underlying sclera, or associated with inflammation should be biopsied or excised, although most will be benign. Nevi can recur after excision.

Blue Nevi

Blue nevi and cellular blue nevi arise from congenital nests of melanocytes in the dermis of the skin or substantia propria of the conjunctiva. They are hamartomas, resulting from incomplete migration of neural crest cells destined for the surface epithelium. When they occur in the skin they are blue, but in the conjunctiva they appear brown or black. They lack cysts, are clearly subepithelial, and move freely with the conjunctiva.

Primary Acquired Melanosis

Bilateral acquired racial melanosis, seen commonly in blacks, is a brown lesion located at the limbus.[53,54] There is no malignant potential, and no treatment is necessary.

Primary acquired melanosis is a unilateral idiopathic pigmentation of the conjunctival epithelium that most often occurs in whites. The pigmentation is caused by proliferation of intraepithelial melanocytes. It is patchy or diffuse and can appear tan, black, or golden brown (Figs. 30-30 and 30-31). The onset is usually during the fourth decade or later. Any portion of the conjunctiva can be involved, and it can extend onto the lid margin or the cornea when there is adjacent melanosis. It begins as flat lesions that can wax and wane and change location, but it generally progress slowly. Increased activity can be associated with signs of inflammation, including hyperemia and subepithelial

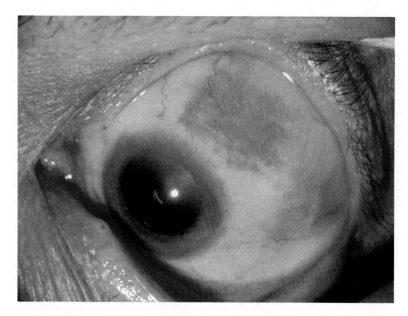

Fig. 30-30. Acquired melanosis.

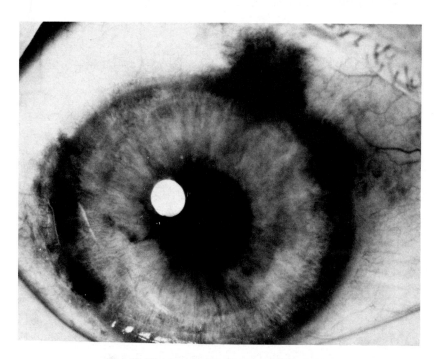

Fig. 30-31. Acquired melanosis of limbal area.

infiltrates. Ultraviolet light (Wood's lamp) is useful in detecting the full extent of the melanosis.[55]

Their most significant feature is their tendency for development of nodules of invasive malignant melanoma. The span between onset and malignant change is variable, but probably averages 5 to 10 years. The risk of development of malignancy can be estimated by determining the histology of the lesion in multiple locations.[53,54,56-58] Multiple biopsies are taken from the different areas of pigmentation and evaluated microscopically. The following classification scheme for primary acquired melanosis of the conjunctiva has been developed by Spencer and Zimmerman[57]:

I. Benign acquired melanosis
   A. With minimal melanocytic hyperplasia
   B. With atypical melanocytic hyperplasia
      1. Mild to moderately severe
      2. Severe (in situ malignant melanoma)
II. Malignant acquired melanosis
   A. With superficially invasive melanoma (tumor thickness < 1.5 mm)
   B. With deeply invasive melanoma (tumor thickness > 1.5 mm)

More recently it has become apparent that the pattern of epithelial involvement and the presence of epithelioid cells are most predictive of the risk of malignancy in stage I acquired melanosis.[54] When atypical melanocytes are arranged in nests or exhibit pagetoid epithelial spread the risk of melanoma approaches 90%. In addition, lesions with conspicuous epithelioid cell content are more likely to progress to melanoma.

Treatment. Multiple biopsies should be taken from the portions of pigmented conjunctiva in patients with primary acquired melanosis to estimate the risk of malignancy. All areas with atypia should be excised, if possible. If large areas of the conjunctiva are affected cryotherapy can be performed instead.[52,59,60] It is important to follow regularly all patients with acquired melanosis (three to four times a year), and those with biopsies indicating a high risk of melanoma should be followed especially closely. Photography is often helpful, and a Wood's lamp can assist in detecting the presence of early pigmentation. Any nodular lesion or otherwise suspicious lesion should be biopsied. The treatment of malignant melanoma is discussed later.

OTHER CAUSES OF MELANOSIS

Melanosis can occur after radiation, in metabolic disorders such as Addison's disease (Fig. 30-32), as a result of drug deposition (for example, epinephrine, arsenic, thorazine), and in chronic con-

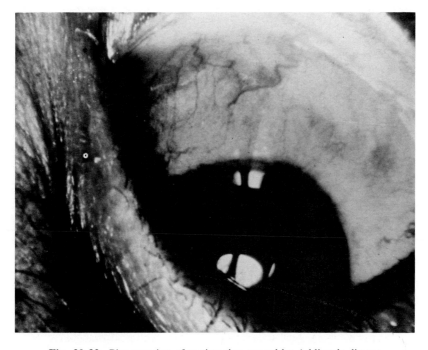

Fig. 30-32. Pigmentation of conjunctiva caused by Addison's disease.

junctival disorders such as trachoma, vernal conjunctivitis, and vitamin A deficiency. In xeroderma pigmentosum and acanthosis nigricans, pigmentation also can be seen. The pigmentation of alkaptonuria always must be considered in a differential diagnosis.

Striate melanokeratosis consists of lines of pigment extending out from the normal limbal pigmentation centrally across the cornea. This is seen mainly in blacks but can occur after severe inflammation and injury in other races.

MALIGNANT MELANOMA

Malignant melanoma can arise in clear conjunctiva (10%), from a preexisting nevus (20% to 30%), or from primary acquired melanosis (60% to 70%).[57] It can develop at any age but is rare before the third decade.[61] Clinically the lesions can be pigmented or nonpigmented, are elevated, and can affect any portion of the conjunctiva (Figs. 30-33 and 30-34). Because nevi rarely affect the tarsal or forniceal conjunctiva, when pigmented epithelial lesions are present in these areas, malignant melanoma should be suspected. Malignant melanomas can be fungating, plaquoid, or ulcerative. They can extend onto the peripheral cornea but only rarely are localized to the cornea.

The overall prognosis is 70% to 80% survival at 10 years.[54] Conjunctival melanomas are closer in behavior to melanomas of the skin than to melanomas of the uvea, in that they tend to invade the lymphatics and spread first to regional lymph nodes. In many cases further spread can be prevented by surgical excision or radiation of involved nodes. The total thickness of the tumor is important in prognosis: Lesions 1.5 mm or less in thickness are much less likely to metastasize than thicker tumors, but even lesions less than 0.8 mm thick can be lethal.[57,62] Metastases also are more likely if the tumor involves the fornix or caruncle, invades the sclera or orbit, infiltrates the epithelium in a pagetoid pattern, or recurs.

Melanomas should be treated by wide local excision, including lamellar sclerectomy or keratectomy if the tumor is fixed to the globe, followed by cryotherapy. If the melanoma arose from primary acquired melanosis, the remaining melanotic areas should also be treated.

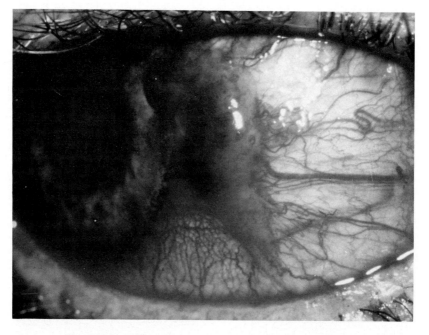

Fig. 30-33. Limbal melanoma with extensive vascularization.

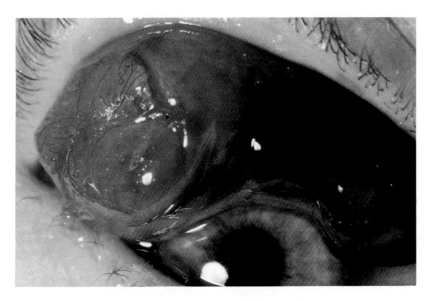

Fig. 30-34. Larger limbal malignant melanoma.

REFERENCES

1. Ferry AP and Zimmerman LE: Granuloma pyogenicum of limbus simulating recurrent squamous cell carcinoma, Arch Ophthalmol 74:229, 1965.
2. Boockvar W, Wessely Z, and Ballen P: Recurrent granuloma pyogenicum of limbus, Arch Ophthalmol 91:42, 1974.
3. Googe JM et al: Pyogenic granulomas of the cornea, Surv Ophthalmol 29:188, 1984.
4. Bloomfield SE, Jakobiec FA, and Iwamoto T: Traumatic intrastromal corneal cyst, Ophthalmology 87:951, 1980.
5. Searl SS et al: Corneal hematoma, Arch Ophthalmol 102:1647, 1984.
6. Grayson M and Pieroni D: Solitary xanthoma of the limbus, Br J Ophthalmol 54:562, 1970.
7. Jakobiec FA: Fibrous histiocytoma of the corneo-scleral limbus, Am J Ophthalmol 78:700, 1974.
8. Iwamoto R, Jakobiec FA, and Darrell RW: Fibrous histiocytoma of the corneoscleral limbus. The ultrastructure of a distinctive inclusion, Ophthalmology 88:1260, 1981.
9. Faludi JE, Kenyon KR, and Green WR: Fibrous histiocytoma of the corneoscleral limbus, Am J Ophthalmol 80:619, 1975.
10. Knowles DM and Jakobiec FA: Ocular adnexal lymphoid neoplasms: clinical histopathologic, electron microscopic, and immunologic characteristics, Hum Pathol 13:148, 1982.
11. Knowles DM and Jakobiec FA: Immunologic characterization of ocular adnexal lymphoid neoplasms, Am J Ophthalmol 87:603, 1979.
12. Jakobiec FA, Iwamoto T, and Knowles DM: Ocular adnexal lymphoid tumors: correlative ultrastructural and immunologic marker studies, Arch Ophthalmol 100:84, 1982.
13. Ellis JH et al: Lymphoid tumors of the ocular adnexa: clinical correlation with the working formulation classification and immunoperoxidase staining of paraffin sections, Ophthalmology 92:1311, 1985.
14. Sigelman J and Jakobiec FA: Lymphoid lesions of the conjunctiva: relation of histopathology to clinical outcome, Ophthalmology 85:818, 1978.
15. Jakobiec FA et al: Ocular adnexal monoclonal lymphoid tumors with a favorable prognosis, Ophthalmology 93:1547, 1986.
16. McNally L, Jakobiec FA, and Knowles DM: Clinical morphologic, immunophenotypic, and molecular genetic analysis of bilateral ocular adnexal lymphoid neoplasms in 17 patients, Am J Ophthalmol 103:555, 1987.
17. Lass JH et al: Detection of human papillomavirus DNA sequences in conjunctival papilloma, Am J Ophthalmol 96:670, 1983.
18. Volcker HE and Holbach L: Pedicled papilloma of the conjunctiva with papilloma virus. Immunohistochemical detection of species specific papilloma-virus antigens, Klin Monatsbl Augenheilkd 187:212, 1985.
19. McDonnell J et al: Demonstration of papillomavirus capsid antigen in human conjunctival neoplasia, Arch Ophthalmol 104:1801, 1986.
20. Yanoff M: Hereditary benign intraepithelial dyskeratosis, Arch Ophthalmol 79:291, 1968.
21. Yanoff M and Fine BS: Ocular pathology, New York, 1975, Harper & Row.
22. McLean IW et al: Hereditary benign intraepithelial dyskeratosis, Ophthalmology 88:164, 1981.
23. Reed JW, Cashwell LF, and Klintworth GK: Corneal manifestations of hereditary benign intraepithelial dyskeratosis, Arch Ophthalmol 97:297, 1979.
24. Blodi FC: Squamous cell carcinoma of the conjunctiva, Doc Ophthalmol 34:93, 1973.

25. Wilson FM II: Rose bengal staining of epibulbar squamous neoplasms, Ann Ophthalmol 7:21, 1976.

26. Fraunfelder FT and Wingfield D: Management of intraepithelial conjunctival tumors and squamous cell carcinomas, Am J Ophthalmol 95:359, 1983.

27. Waring GO, Ross Am, and Ekins MB: Clinical and pathologic description of 17 cases of corneal intraepithelial neoplasia, Am J Ophthalmol 97:547, 1984.

28. Campbell RJ and Bourne WM: Unilateral central corneal epithelial dysplasia, Ophthalmology 88:1231, 1981.

29. Brown HH et al: Keratinizing corneal intraepithelial neoplasia, Cornea 8:220, 1989.

30. Zimmerman LE: The cancerous, precancerous, and pseudocancerous lesions of the cornea and conjunctiva. Proceedings of the Second Annual International Corneoplastic Conference, London, 1969, Pergamon Press.

31. Rao NA and Font RL: Mucoepidermoid carcinoma of the conjunctiva: a clinicopathologic study of five cases, Cancer 38:1699, 1976.

32. Brownstein S: Mucoepidermoid carcinoma of the conjunctiva with intraocular invasion, Ophthalmology 88:1226, 1981.

33. Gamel JW, Eiferman RA, and Guibor P: Mucoepidermoid carcinoma of the conjunctiva, Arch Ophthalmol 102:730, 1984.

34. Searl SS et al: Invasive squamous cell carcinoma with intraocular mucoepidermoid features: conjunctival carcinoma with intraocular invasion and diphasic morphology, Arch Ophthalmol 100:109, 1982.

35. Cohen BH et al: Spindle cell carcinoma of the conjunctiva, Arch Ophthalmol 98:1809, 1980.

36. Wise AC: A limbal spindle cell carcinoma, Surv Ophthalmol 12:244, 1967.

37. Battifora H: Spindle cell carcinoma: ultrastructural evidence of squamous origin and collagen production by tumor cells, Cancer 37:2275, 1976.

38. Foster CS and Allansmith MR: Chronic unilateral blepharoconjunctivitis caused by sebaceous carcinoma, Am J Ophthalmol 86:218, 1978.

39. Wolfe JT et al: Sebaceous carcinoma of the eyelid: errors in clinical and pathologic diagnosis, Am J Surg Pathol 8:597, 1984.

40. Curran JW, and the Centers for Disease Control Task Force on Kaposi's Sarcoma and Opportunistic Infections: Epidemiologic aspects of the current outbreak of Kaposi's sarcoma and opportunistic infections, N Engl J Med 306:248, 1982.

41. Holland GN et al: Ocular disorders associated with a new severe acquired cellular immunodeficiency syndrome, Am J Ophthalmol 93:393, 1982.

42. Macher A et al: Multicentric Kaposi's sarcoma of the conjunctiva in a male homosexual with the AIDS, Ophthalmology 90:879, 1983.

43. Shuler JD et al: Kaposi sarcoma of the conjunctiva and eyelids associated with the acquired immunodeficiency syndrome, Arch Ophthalmol 107:858, 1989.

44. Weiter JJ, Jakobiec FA, and Iwamoto T: The clinical and morphologic characteristics of Kaposi's sarcoma of the conjunctiva, Am J Ophthalmol 89:546, 1980.

45. Zimmerman LE: Melanocytes, melanocytic nevi and melanocytomas, Invest Ophthalmol 4:11, 1965.

46. Folberg R et al: Benign conjunctival melanocytic lesions: clinicopathologic features, Ophthalmology 96:436, 1989.

47. Jakobiec FA, Folberg R, and Iwamoto T: Clinicopathologic characteristics of premalignant and malignant melanocytic lesions of the conjunctiva, Ophthalmology 96:147, 1989.

48. Gilliam JN and Cox AJ: Epidermal changes in vitamin B_{12} deficiency, Arch Dermatol 107:231, 1973.

49. Verdaguer J, Valenzuela H, and Strozzi L: Melanocytoma of the conjunctiva, Arch Ophthalmol 91:363, 1974.

50. Lee JS, Smith RE, and Minckler DS: Scleral melanocytoma, Ophthalmology 89:178, 1982.

51. Folberg R, McLean IW, and Zimmerman LE: Malignant melanoma of the conjunctiva, Hum Pathol 16:136, 1985.

52. Jakobiec FA et al: Cryotherapy for conjunctival primary acquired melanosis and malignant melanoma: experience with 62 cases, Ophthalmology 95:1058, 1988.

53. Folberg R, McLean IW, and Zimmerman LE: Primary acquired melanosis of the conjunctiva, Hum Pathol 16:129, 1985.

54. Folberg R, McLean IW, and Zimmerman LE: Conjunctival melanosis and melanoma, Ophthalmology 91:673, 1984.

55. Reese AB: Tumors of the eye, Hagerstown, MD, 1976, Harper & Row.

56. Jakobiec FA: The ultrastructure of conjunctival melanocytic tumors, Trans Am Ophthalmol Soc 82:599, 1984.

57. Spencer WH and Zimmerman LE: Conjunctiva. In Spencer WH, editor: Ophthalmic pathology: an atlas and textbook, ed 3, vol I, Philadelphia, 1985, WB Saunders.

58. Jakobiec FA, Folberg R, and Iwamoto T: Clinicopathologic characteristics of premalignant and malignant melanocytic lesions of the conjunctiva, Ophthalmology 96:147, 1989.

59. Jakobiec FA et al: The role of cryotherapy in the management of conjunctival melanoma, Ophthalmology 89:502, 1982.

60. Brownstein S et al: Cryotherapy for precancerous melanosis (atypical melanocytic hyperplasia) of the conjunctiva, Arch Ophthalmol 99:1224, 1981.

61. McDonnell JM et al: Conjunctival melanocytic lesions in children, Ophthalmology 96:986, 1989.

62. Silvers D et al: Melanoma of the conjunctiva: a clinicopathologic study. In Jakobiec FA, editor: Ocular and adnexal tumors, Birmingham, AL, 1978, Aesculapius Publishing Co.

INDEX